Foot and Ankle Instability

Beat Hintermann • Roxa Ruiz

Foot and Ankle Instability

A Clinical Guide to Diagnosis and Surgical Management

Springer

Beat Hintermann
Centre of Excellence for Foot and Ankle Surgery
Clinic of Orthopaedics and Traumatology
Kantonsspital Baselland
Liestal
Switzerland

Roxa Ruiz
Centre of Excellence for Foot and Ankle Surgery
Clinic of Orthopaedics and Traumatology
Kantonsspital Baselland
Liestal
Switzerland

ISBN 978-3-030-62925-0 ISBN 978-3-030-62926-7 (eBook)
https://doi.org/10.1007/978-3-030-62926-7

This Springer imprint is published by the registered company Springer Nature Switzerland AG
The registered company address is: Gewerbestrasse 11, 6330 Cham, Switzerland

To Esteban, Mathias, Sabrina, and Valeria

Foreword

It is my pleasure to write the foreword to this extraordinary textbook. I have personally written, edited, and authored numerous textbooks, and it was therefore no surprise that I became completely absorbed and engrossed in reading this book. I have heard these authors present their ideas on foot and ankle instabilities over the past decade, but seeing it in print validates their tremendous contributions to our field. The book is very well organized, easy to follow, and extraordinarily well illustrated. The topic of foot and ankle instabilities has never previously been covered comprehensively enough, and this clearly represents a lifelong interest and passion of the authors. Drs. Hintermann and Ruiz present a remarkably well researched and referenced summary of the existing literature, but, more importantly, have compiled their own ideas with their original research to provide the reader with new, compelling and clear approaches to instabilities of the foot and ankle. Coming from two leaders in the field of foot and ankle surgery, it is refreshing to read their own opinions in addition to a synopsis of the relevant literature.

Each chapter is systematically organized according to anatomy, biomechanics, clinical implications, injury mechanism, history and clinical findings, imaging, and various operative and nonoperative treatment alternatives, outcomes, complications, and conclusions. This makes the reading of the book very clear to follow, and along with the bullet points summarizing each section can be a quick resource for the reader to get an overview of each topic. The anatomy dissections have been caringly and meticulously done by the authors themselves and are beautifully presented. The clinical examples of each deformity are very well covered, and with the accompanying anatomic dissections make each section very readable, understandable, and exciting to learn from.

There are many statements and summaries in the book which are a consolidation of the findings in the literature with the authors' recommendations and opinions. I will highlight a few important aspects of the book which for me were innovative and thoroughly presented:

"Injuries of the Chopart joint are frequently missed or misdiagnosed, and often lead to a poor outcome." We are accustomed to diagnosing and treating these injuries associated with high-energy trauma and associated fractures, but midtarsal sprains resulting from low-energy inversion injuries have historically not received enough attention. I like the fact that this is presented as injuries of the Chopart joint "complex" to include all aspects of anatomy, pathomechanics, and treatment of the subtle inversion injury.

I have had a career-long interest in the adult flatfoot deformity, and it is not an exaggeration to say that after reading the chapters on the deltoid-spring ligament complex, my understanding of the pathological basis for diagnosis and treatment has been greatly enhanced if not clarified. I have always been fascinated by the etiopathogenesis of the adult flatfoot and have never subscribed to the belief that this is always the result of a rupture of the PTT. I have believed that there are too many instances of deltoid-spring failure as the primary pathology, and this is very well supported by the statement here: *"Loss of support of the deltoid-spring ligament complex is the main underlying cause of flatfoot deformity."* This concept is clearly and elaborately presented, with various treatment options for acute and chronic deltoid and spring ligament injury and peritalar instability. The deltoid does not only prevent medial ankle instability in the coronal plane, and integral to understanding of the flat foot deformity is their description:

"besides preventing foot pronation, the deltoid-spring ligament complex plays a crucial role in the maintenance of the plantar arch." The inclusion of their comprehensive classification to medial ankle instability is timely and elaborates and defines the pathologic anatomy very well, making it the new standard for descriptive work on these injuries. The reader will find this chapter on deltoid and spring ligament instability enticingly straightforward and very well thought out.

Here I highlight some of their statements (all are direct quotes) which I think are essential to our treatment of these foot and ankle instabilities:

- Conservative treatment *(of ankle sprains)* should not mean neglecting the injury.
- Despite conservative treatment *(of ankle sprains),* up to 40% of the patients complain about persistent pain and/or instability.
- No tilting is necessary at either the ankle or subtalar level to experience functional instability.
- There is need for better criteria to define lateral ankle ligament injuries that need primary surgical repair.
- Meticulous reconstruction of isometricity is mandatory for normal joint motion.
- Tenodesis procedures may change the biomechanics of the ankle joint complex, resulting in increased joint load, limited motion, subsequent pain, and progression of the degenerative disease.
- Specific studies are necessary to define the potential risks for developing secondary osteoarthritis, and how it can be prevented.
- Ligament injuries with bony avulsions and fractures *(of Chopart's joint)* need surgical treatment.
- As none of the syndesmotic stress tests are sensitive or specific, the diagnosis of syndesmotic injuries should not be made based on the medical history and physical examination alone.
- The first and most critical step of syndesmotic reduction is anatomic reduction of the fibula including restoration of length, alignment, and rotation.
- As the deltoid is the primary restraint against talar abduction and pronation, loss of its integrity may result in progressive destabilization of the foot with overpronation.
- In complete tears of the deep deltoid with a talar tilt >5°, surgical reconstruction might be critical.
- Inadequate primary treatment and/or reconstruction of the medial ankle ligaments result in persistent instability which may lead to chronic overload of the PT tendon.

I recommend this book to anyone with an interest in managing injury and deformity of the foot and ankle. From the beginner surgeon to the expert in the field, this book is a valuable compendium of research and brilliant new ideas in our field.

Mark Myerson, MD
Visiting Professor of Orthopedic Surgery, University of Colorado
Past President American Orthopedic Foot and Ankle Society
Editor Foot and Ankle Clinics N. America
Executive Director and Founder, Steps2Walk
Denver, CO, USA

Preface

"We can only diagnose what we know." This statement is still true today, as it was over a quarter of a century ago, when we started our orthopedic career. Even the rapid progress in imaging techniques has not changed this. As surgeons, we are obliged to understand the pathology, based on the morphologic changes and resulting pathomechanics. Moreover, the decision process for successful treatment is based on combining the latter and the knowledge of available treatment modalities and their possibilities as well as limitations.

This book is thus written as a monograph, characterized by its uniform approach through all six main chapters. It not only intends to be an update of the morphological and mechanical changes underlying various pathologies, however, also provides an up-to-date overview of the available treatment techniques in the form of an operative manual, based on the lifelong experience of both authors.

It is based on lifelong meticulous documentation of cases which is an additional workload for every surgeon, but mandatory to recognize, understand, and get an insight into many underlying processes that may affect patient outcome. To be able to assess the outcome many years after surgical treatment and to be able to compare the outcome with the initial situation has the unique potential to critically analyze the effectiveness of selected treatment and additionally, to understand failures.

For the opportunity to complete this book, we are grateful to a number of people, starting with the staff members, co-workers, and residents who have accompanied us over the years. We would like to especially thank and acknowledge Tamara Horn Lang, PhD, for her support in editing the text and the scientific team for building up the database. And finally, we thank all our patients; they are the ones who continuously inspire us to develop and evaluate new techniques to make things better.

Teaching and sharing the experience with others may be one of the highest privileges we have as surgeons. The effort invested in preparing this book has been immense; however the learning process has been very rewarding. It was a privilege to work together as a team on holidays, weekends, and nights. If *Foot and Ankle Instability* offers useful information to our colleagues and provides a new platform of knowledge from which others can advance and evolve further treatment of the unstable foot and ankle, we will have reached our goal.

Liestal, Switzerland

Beat Hintermann
Roxa Ruiz

Contents

About the Authors

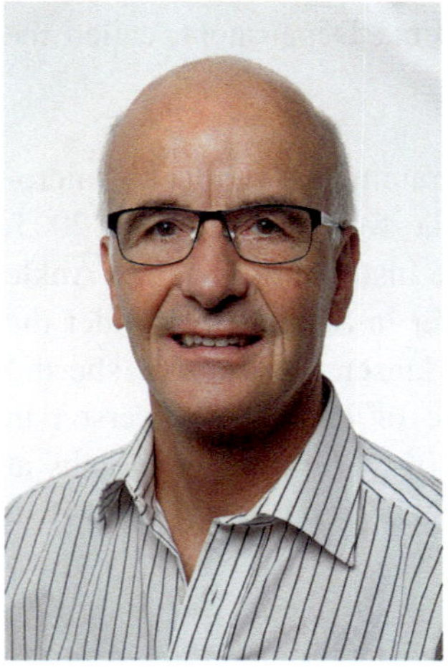

Beat Hintermann, born in 1956, was trained in orthopedic surgery and traumatology at the Hospitals of Neuchâtel, St. Gallen, Davos, and thereafter at the Orthopedic Department of the University of Basel. After finishing his residency program, he completed a research fellowship in Biomechanics at the University of Calgary/Canada (Benno Nigg, 1991–1992) and two clinical traveling fellowships to Asia and the USA/United Kingdom, respectively. As an associate Professor of the University of Basel, he was in charge of the Orthopaedic Trauma Unit at the University Hospital of Basel from 1994 to 2006. Since 2006, he is the Chair for the Orthopaedic Department at the teaching hospital in Liestal. For over 20 years, his main orthopedic interest is the ankle and hindfoot. In 2019, he founded the Center of Excellence for Foot and Ankle in Liestal that he chairs since. During his tenure, new and innovative techniques and procedures have been introduced such as ankle arthroscopy, stabilizing procedures, correcting osteotomies, arthrodeses of the hindfoot complex, and total ankle replacement.

Besides having published over 250 peer-reviewed articles in orthopedic surgery, in particular relating to ankle arthroscopy, ankle instability, ankle osteoarthritis, total ankle replacement, and foot and ankle trauma, he is the author of five medical textbooks related to reconstructive surgery of the ankle and hindfoot complex. He has received several awards for his clinical and biomechanical research.

Beat Hintermann was the main conceptor of the H3 ankle (Hintermann Series, former Hintegra) which is after 20 years of clinical use the best documented three-component prosthesis on the market. It was approved by the US FDA on June 4, 2019. He also developed the H2 ankle with Roxa Ruiz which was approved by the US FDA.

Over the last decade, he has put tremendous efforts into teaching orthopedic surgeons and those to-be, around the entire world as well as at his clinic, which was honored by several national Foot and Ankle societies and institutions. In 2017, he was appointed as Visiting Professor of the Ruijin University of Shanghai, China. He is regularly a faculty member of international Foot and Ankle meetings and organizer of Practical Instructional courses both in Switzerland and abroad.

Beat Hintermann is married, has two children, and lives in Liestal, Switzerland. Besides running, skiing, and mountaineering, he enjoys traveling and photography.

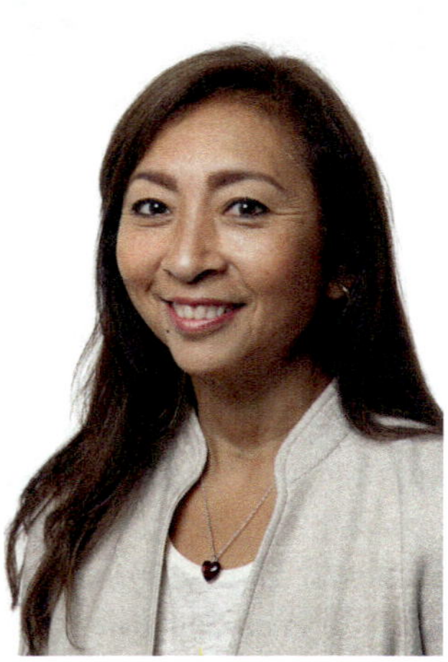

Roxa Ruiz, born in 1965, finished medical school in 1992 in Lima (Peru). Thereafter, she underwent the educational program in orthopedic trauma in Peru that also included services in the emergency departments of medical units in Lima. In 1998, she entered the Central Military Hospital of Lima as a senior resident. From 2010 onwards, she was working as a senior attending and afterwards also as the head of one of the two units of the Orthopedic Trauma Department, called the "War Service."

After having received specific training in hand and microsurgery, her main interest was the foot and ankle. In 2003, Roxa Ruiz did a fellowship at the Institute of Foot and Ankle of the Harborview Medical Center in Seattle/USA under the guidance of Prof. Sigvard Ted Hansen Jr. In 2008, she did a fellowship under the guidance of Dr. Mark Myerson in Baltimore/USA. Thereafter, in 2011, she spent 3 months at the Kantonsspital Liestal under the guidance of Prof. Beat Hintermann.

As a pioneer in her country, she opened a new chapter in the Peruvian Orthopaedic and Trauma Society for foot and ankle surgery, for which she also served as the first president. In 2014, she was honored by being incorporated as a guest Professor in the Post Grade Unit of the Mayor University of San Marcos in Lima, Peru. Additionally, she served as an International AO Faculty in many courses, including ones in Davos. Since 2016, she has been working as a senior attending surgeon at the Kantonsspital Baselland in Liestal, Switzerland.

Over the last years, she put tremendous efforts into teaching activities around the entire world, and she is regularly a faculty member at International Foot and Ankle meetings. She is the author of numerous scientific papers, book chapters, and coconceptor of the H2 ankle prosthesis (Hintermann Series).

Roxa Ruiz is married, has two children, and lives in Liestal, Switzerland. Besides skiing, swimming, and hiking, she enjoys cooking and gardening.

Abbreviations

2D	Two dimensional
3D	Three dimensional
AITFL	Anterior inferior tibiofibular ligament (part of syndesmotic ligaments)
Ant	Anterior
AP	Anteroposterior
AFT	Anterior fibular tubercle (Wagstaffe-Le Fort tubercle)
ATFL	Anterior tibiofibular ligament
ATT	Anterior tibial tubercle (Chaput's tubercle)
ATTL	Anterior tibiotalar ligament (part of deep deltoid ligament)
BL	Basset ligament
CFL	Calcaneofibular ligament
CL	Cervical ligament
cm	Centimeter
CT	Computed tomography
DDelt	Deep deltoid ligament
DLCCL	Dorsolateral calcaneocuboid ligament
DP	Dorsoplantar
DTNL	Dorsal talonavicular ligament
EDB	Extensor digitorum brevis
FDL	Flexor digitorum longus
FHL	Flexor hallucis longus
FTCL	Fibulotalocalcaneal ligament
HMA	Heel moment arm
ICNL	Inferior calcaneonavicular ligament (part of spring ligament)
IML	Intermalleolar ligament
ITCL	Interosseous talocalcaneal ligament
LCNL	Lateral calcaneonavicular ligament (part of bifurcate ligament)
LHT	Lateral hook test
LPL	Long plantar ligament (part of inferior calcaneocuboid ligament)
LTCL	Lateral talocalcaneal ligament
MCCL	Medial calcaneocuboid ligament (part of bifurcate ligament)
MCS	Medial clear space
Mid	Middle
mm	Millimeter
MPOCNL	Medioplantar oblique calcaneonavicular ligament (part of spring ligament)
MRI	Magnetic resonance imaging
OCL	Osteochondral lesion
PITFL	Posterior inferior tibiofibular ligament (part of syndesmotic ligament)
Post	Posterior
PTFL	Posterior talofibular ligament
PT(T)	Posterior tibial (tendon)
PTTL	Posterior tibiotalar ligament (part of deep deltoid ligament)

SDelt	Superficial deltoid ligament
SMCNL	Superomedial calcaneonavicular ligament (part of spring ligament)
SPL	Short plantar ligament (part of inferior calcaneocuboid ligament)
Spect CT	Single-photon emission computed tomography
ST	Sinus tarsi
STTL	Superficial tibiotalar ligament (part of superficial deltoid ligament)
TaH	Talar head
TaN	Talar neck
TAS	Tibial articular surface angle
TCL	Tibiocalcaneal ligament (part of superficial deltoid ligament)
TFCS	Tibiofibular clear space
TFIL	Tibiofibular interosseous ligament
TFO	Tibiofibular overlap
TNL	Tibionavicular ligament (part of superficial deltoid ligament)
TSL	Tibiospring ligament (part of superficial deltoid ligament)
TT	Tibiotalar tilt angle
TTFL	Transverse tibiofibular ligament
US	Ultrasonography
WB	Weight-bearing
X-rays	Roentgen radiation, composed of X-rays

1 Introduction

The ankle joint complex and its surrounding ligaments represent a complex mechanical structure with its mechanical properties highly dependent on the integrity of the ligaments. While an acute inversion/supination trauma may typically result in lateral ankle instability, a trauma that includes an acute adduction of the foot may cause an additional loss of stability of the lateral Chopart joint. An external/abduction trauma, while the foot is fixed in a neutral to dorsiflexed position, may cause injuries to the inferior tibiofibular (syndesmotic) ligaments. Injuries to the medial side, as is the case for an eversion/pronation trauma, in contrast, may lead to various types of instability patterns depending on different preexisting conditions such as deformities and function of the posterior tibial muscle. On the lateral side, inappropriate treatment may typically result in chronic instability, whereas on the medial side, it may result in progressive destabilization of the hindfoot as can be seen in an acquired flatfoot deformity. Therefore, proper diagnosis and appropriate treatment is mandatory to prevent the patient from experiencing chronic instability and progressive destabilization of the ankle and foot, respectively.

Proper medical history taking and physical examination remain the "single most" important tool in the diagnostic process of an unstable foot and ankle. Though tremendous progress has been made in the last two decades, current imaging modalities are not able to replace the clinical workup. While MRI may be helpful in assessing acute injuries, weight bearing CT scans offer better information in most chronic conditions. The introduction of arthroscopy brought new insights on articular pathologies, mainly of the ankle joint; but, with this, the surgeons learned to avoid the anatomy. Knowledge of the anatomy is mandatory for any surgical procedure, however. Therefore, in this book emphasis is given on describing the anatomy so the surgeon can understand the pathology to successfully plan the surgeries and estimate their effect.

The talus has a unique function coupled to its anatomical shape. It provides the functional coupling between the lower leg and foot. As this bone does not have direct muscle attachments, it is often called "bony meniscus." This unique construct may explain why the joints around the talus are highly exposed to injuries that, if not properly treated, may result in an unstable foot and ankle. The key for successful treatment is the full understanding of the resulting pathomechanics and involved morphologic structures. Therefore, emphasis is also given to work up the current knowledge on the biomechanics of the foot and ankle as well as the changes caused by instability. This, in turn, will help the surgeon to plan and to perform successful reconstructive surgeries.

Finally, the best treatment results from thoroughly understanding the pathology, knowing the expectations of the patient and being aware of the availability of various surgical and nonsurgical techniques. When considering surgical treatment, knowing their possibilities and limitations is mandatory for success. Main focus of this book is thus given to step-by-step instructions—in form of an operational manual, based on the authors' lifelong experience.

B. Hintermann, R. Ruiz, *Foot and Ankle Instability*, https://doi.org/10.1007/978-3-030-62926-7_1

2 Lateral Ankle Instability

Lateral ankle ligament injuries are the most common injuries in sports and recreational activities [1–4] and account for about 25% of the injuries that occur in running and jumping sports [5]. Seventy-five percent of all ankle injuries are ankle sprains [2–4, 6–9], and 85% of these sprains are caused by an inversion trauma [10]. Although most of these ligamentous ankle injuries can be treated successfully with physical rehabilitation and nonoperative treatment, 20–40% of the patients with these injuries will go on to experience chronic instability and subsequent disability [4, 11–18].

Some of these patients can be treated satisfactorily with late repair or reconstruction of the lateral ligaments [16, 19–29]. However, in spite of surgery, some patients will be left with persistent disability including subjective or objective instability, persistent talar tilt, stretching of the ligaments, pain, stiffness, or limitation of the range of motion [16, 30]. Some of the reasons for these displeasing results may be attributed to a lack of respecting the biomechanics of the unstable ankle joint complex when operative treatment is carried out. In case of nonanatomic ligament reconstructions, the altered joint anatomy changes the kinematics, which may lead to several unsatisfactory results [20, 31]. These may include having residual subtalar instability [32, 33] or having highly restricted subtalar motion with an increased development of arthrosis [30, 34, 35].

There is, apparently, need for a better understanding of the anatomy and function of the ligament structures, as well as their susceptibility to injury and resultant instability. This will give an overall understanding of the biomechanics of the ankle. Furthermore, it may then allow to establish a rational for the daily practice when dealing with patients suffering from an acute or chronic unstable condition of the ankle joint complex.

2.1 Anatomy of the Lateral Ligaments of the Ankle

- The lateral ankle ligaments form a complex construct that spans the ankle and subtalar joint.
- Each ligament has its isometric position to guide motion and to provide stability.
- The anterior talofibular and calcaneofibular ligaments are confluent and have a common insertion area on the anterior aspect of the distal fibula.

Anatomy textbooks and the orthopedic literature contain various descriptions of lateral ankle ligament anatomy [36–42]. The major lateral ligaments are the anterior talofibular ligament (ATFL), the calcaneofibular ligament (CFL), and the posterior talofibular ligament (PTFL).

2.1.1 Anterior Talofibular Ligament

The anterior talofibular ligament (ATFL) can be considered as being an intra-articular reinforcement of the anterolateral part of the rather weak ankle joint capsule. The ATFL is a broad flat ligament between 15 and 20 mm long, 6 and 10 mm wide, and 2 mm thick. It runs 45° medially from the fibula towards the talus in the coronal plane. The ATFL originates at the anterior edge of the fibula, just lateral to the articular cartilage of the lateral malleolus (Fig. 2.1). The center of its attachment is 10 mm proximal to the tip of the fibula as measured along the long axis of the fibula [36]. The insertion on the talus begins directly distal to the articular surface and the center is 18 mm proximal to the subtalar joint.

B. Hintermann, R. Ruiz, *Foot and Ankle Instability*, https://doi.org/10.1007/978-3-030-62926-7_2

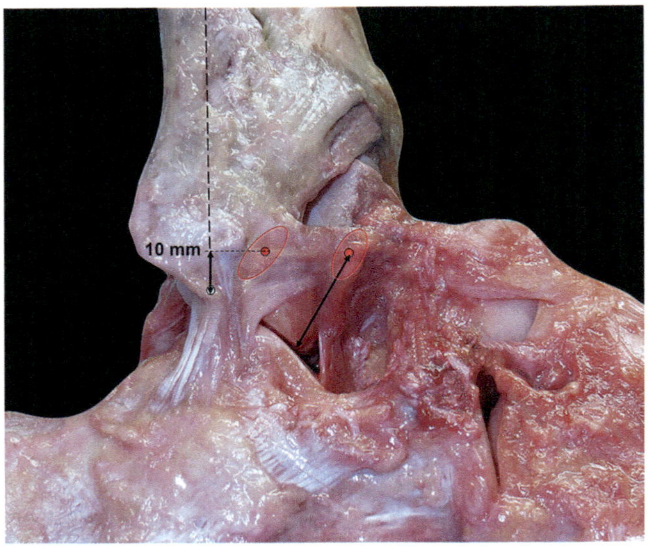

Fig. 2.1 The anterior talofibular ligament (ATFL) runs from the anterior border of fibula to the neck of talus with an angle of 105° to the ground. Its fibular insertion is 10 mm above the tip of the fibula and its talar insertion 18 mm above the subtalar joint

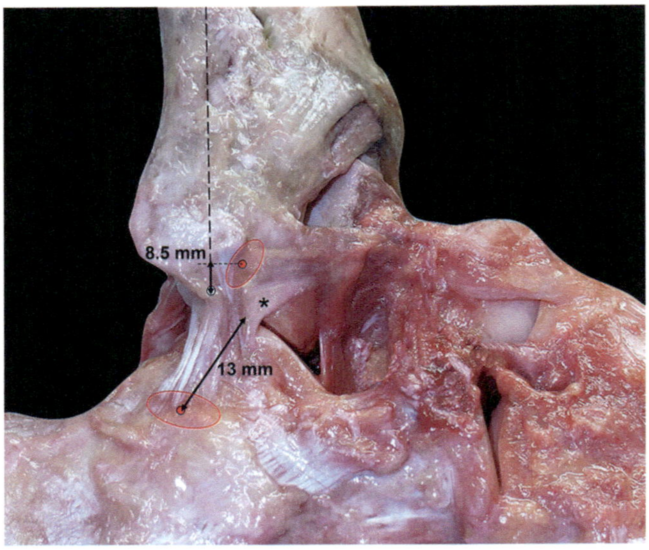

Fig. 2.2 The calcaneofibular ligament (CFL) crosses the subtalar joint perpendicularly, originating from the lateral calcaneus 13 mm below the subtalar joint. Its insertion on the anterior aspect of the fibula is 8.5 mm above its tip. The fan-shaped lateral talocalcaneal ligament (LTCL, asterisk) is contiguous with the CFL inferiorly, broadening to insert along the entire inferior portion of the ATFL

2.1.2 Calcaneofibular Ligament

The calcaneofibular ligament (CFL) is a cylindrical structure that lies deep to the peroneal tendons, underneath the tendon sheath, and superficial to the joint capsule. Structurally, the CFL is 2.5 times stronger than the ATFL and is 20–30 mm long, 4–8 mm wide, and 3–5 mm thick. In contrary to popular belief, the CFL does not originate from the apex of the tip of the lateral malleolus. Its attachment on the anterior edge of distal fibula is centered 8.5 mm from the distal tip just below the origin of the ATF ligament [36] (Fig. 2.2). As is the case for the ATFL, the CFL has most of its attachment fibers running on the lateral surface of the fibula. The calcaneal insertion begins 13 mm distal to the subtalar joint with its proximal edge on a line nearly perpendicular to the joint [36, 43].

The angle between the CFL and ATFL was measured on 50 cadavers. In the sagittal plane, the average angle was 105° ranging from 70° to 140° (Fig. 2.3). In the coronal plane, the average angle was 100° ranging from 60° to 140° [44].

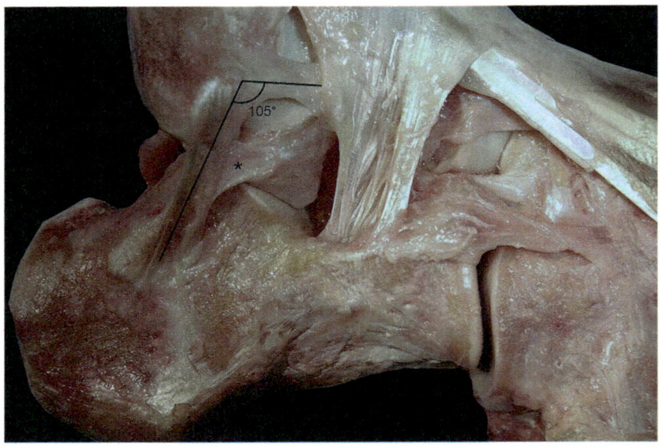

Fig. 2.3 The LTCL is a completely discrete ligament (asterisk). Notice the angulation between the CFL and the ATFL of 105° (varying from 70° to 140°)

2.1.3 Lateral Talocalcaneal Ligament

The lateral talocalcaneal ligament (LTCL) varies in configuration, from a distinct rectangular structure spanning the subtalar joint to a fan-shaped ligament contiguous with the CFL inferiorly and broadening to insert along the entire inferior portion of the ATFL. Burks et al. [36] found three basic ligament patterns: a ligament combined with the CFL (Fig. 2.1), a completely discrete ligament (Fig. 2.2), and a missing ligament.

2.1.4 Posterior Talofibular Ligament

The posterior talofibular ligament (PTFL) is a thick and rather long ligament. On average, it is 30 mm long, 5 mm wide, and 5–8 mm thick. The PTFL originates from the medial surface of the fibula and runs medially in a horizontal fashion to the posterior aspect of the talus (Fig. 2.4). The fibular attachment is centered 10 mm proximal to the tip in the digital fossa [36]. The attachment on the talus involves nearly the entire non-articular portion of the posterior talus up to the groove for the flexor hallucis longus tendon. The ligament is confluent with the joint capsule

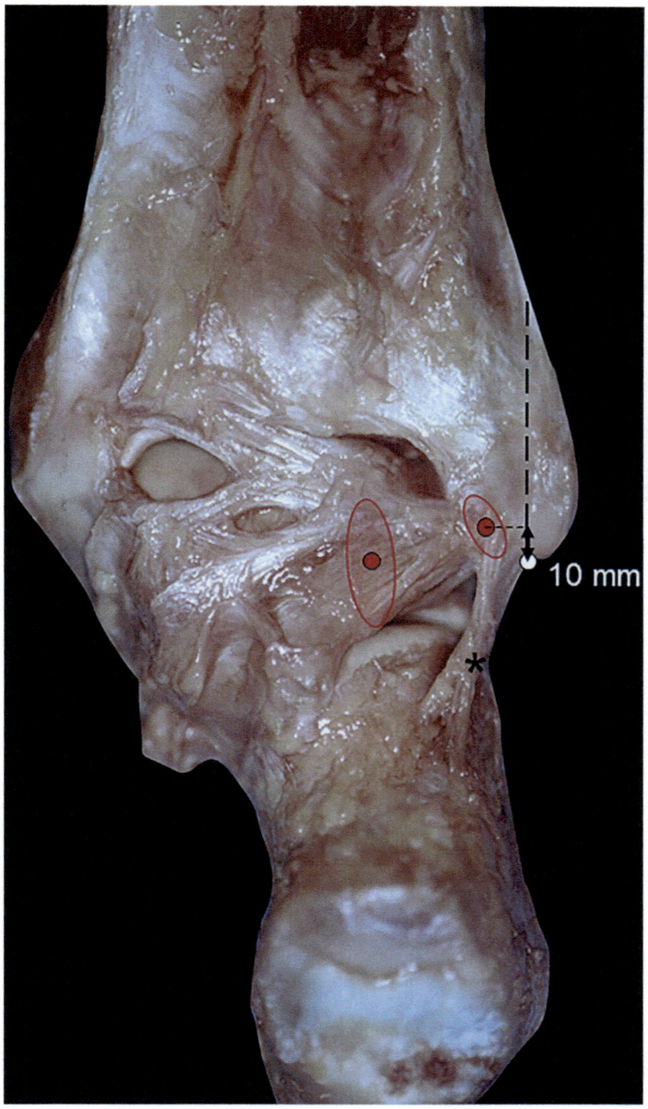

Fig. 2.4 The strong posterior talofibular ligament (PTFL) originates 10 mm above the tip of fibula and runs in a horizontal direction to the posterior aspect of the talus (CFL, asterisk)

and is well vascularized by vessels which supply the talus and the fibula via the digital fossa [42].

2.2 Biomechanics of Lateral Ankle Instability

- Loss of ligamentous support results in mechanical changes of the ankle joint complex.
- Lateral ankle instability is in most instances a rotational one, given by the freedom of the talus to move laterally, out of the ankle mortise.
- Ankle instability occurs in the absence of radiographically demonstrable talar tilt.

Besides providing stability, the ankle ligaments also have a significant role in preserving the mechanics of the ankle joint complex.

2.2.1 Stabilizing Function

Each of the lateral ligaments has a role in stabilizing the ankle and/or subtalar joint, depending on the position of the foot (Fig. 2.5). In dorsiflexion, the PTFL is maximally stressed and the CFL is taut, while the ATFL is loose. On the opposite, in plantarflexion the ATFL is taut, and the CFL and PTFL become loose [42, 45, 46].

Sequential sectioning of the lateral ligaments in cadavers has demonstrated the function of these ligaments in different positions and under various loading conditions. Johnson and Markolf [47] studied the laxity after sectioning the ATFL and found the most changes to occur in plantarflexion. They observed a smaller change in laxity in dorsiflexion, suggesting that the ATFL limits talar tilt throughout motion but has greatest influence on stability in plantarflexion. Others further confirmed the above findings, stating that talar tilt is limited in plantarflexion and in neutral position by the ATFL, and in dorsiflexion by the CFL plus the PTFL [46, 48]. In conclusion, the ATFL and CFL appear to synergistically work together to provide lateral stability to the ankle throughout the full range of motion, in such a way that when one is relaxed the other is strained and vice versa [20, 43, 49, 50].

2.2.2 Mechanical Changes with Loss of Ligamentous Support

In an attempt to elucidate how the ligaments contribute to this functional interplay with the bone structures of the ankle joint complex [13, 51–55], most reports have focused on the lateral ligaments and the role they play in maintaining lateral ankle stability [1, 46, 56, 57]. Although the magnitude of talar tilt has been shown to vary significantly [46, 58], there is a consensus that some tilt occurs with the loss of stabilization through these ligaments [1, 17, 56] (Fig. 2.6).

Recently it was reported in a study of ten matched pairs of specimens that stiffness and peak torque did not significantly decrease after sectioning the ATFL but decreased significantly after sectioning of the CFL [59]. Peak pressure in the tibiotalar joint decreased and mean contact area increased significantly after CFL release. Significantly more inversion of the talus and calcaneus as well as calcaneal medial displacement was seen with weight-bearing inversion after sectioning of the CFL.

2.2.3 Rotational Instability

Cass and Settles [58] studied the kinematics of ankle instability after lateral ligament sectioning in a model where axial

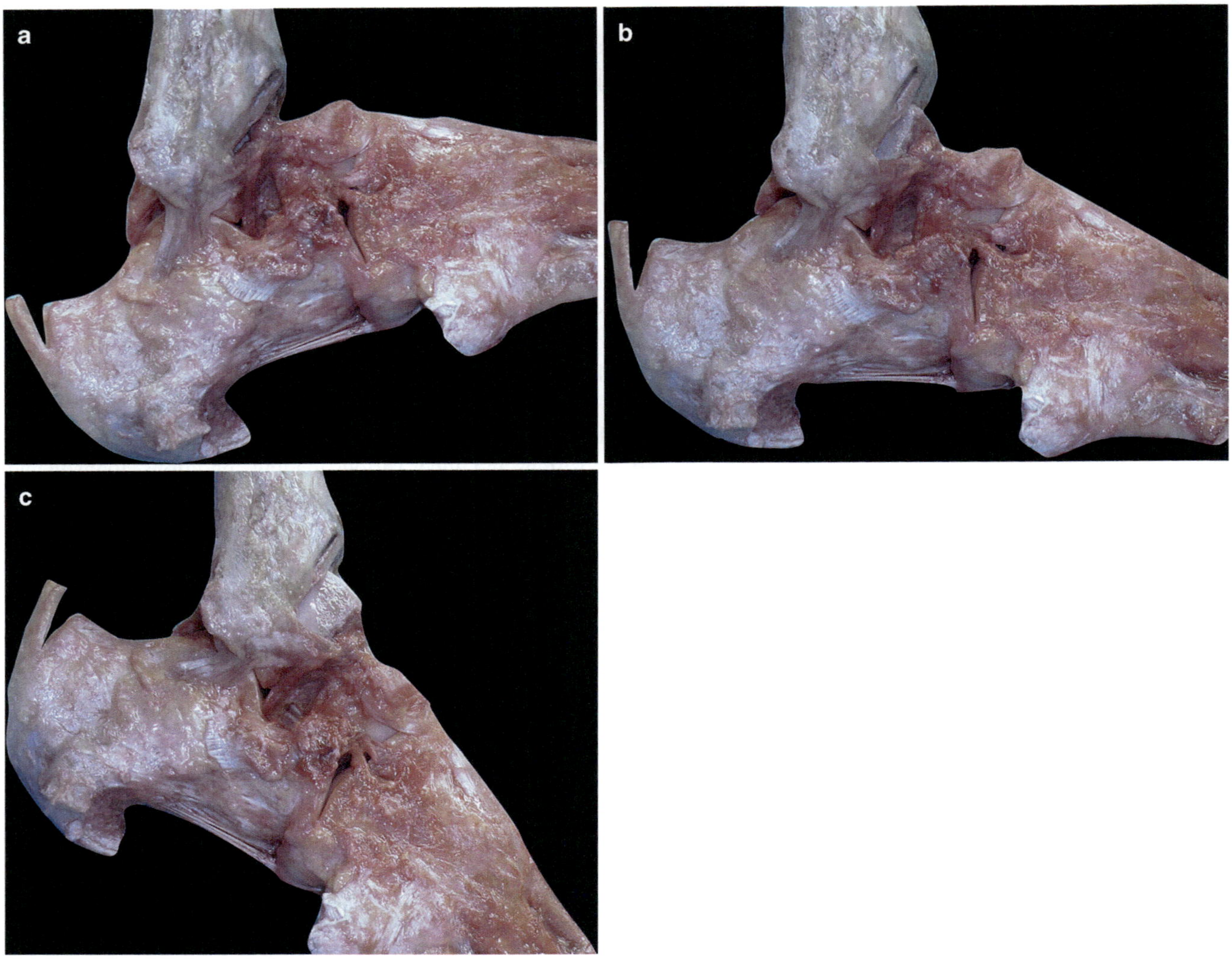

Fig. 2.5 Lateral view of the ankle joint complex while the foot is (**a**) in dorsiflexion, (**b**) in neutral position, and (**c**) in plantarflexion. While in dorsiflexion the PTFL and CFL are taut and the ATFL is loose, in plantarflexion the ATFL is taut, and the CFL and PTFL become loose

rotation was not constrained. They found no tilting of the talus to occur in the mortise with isolated release of the ATFL or CFL. However, after both ligaments were released, an average talar tilt of 20.6° occurred. External rotation of the leg occurred with inversion averaging 11.1° in the intact specimen. A further external rotation of 4.9° occurred after ATFL release when compared to the intact inverted specimen and 12.8° further after an additional CFL release. The authors concluded that the ATFL and CFL ligaments work in tandem to prevent tilting of the talus, and that the articular surfaces themselves do not seem to prevent tilting of the talus in the mortise.

Thus, inversion is accompanied by a mandatory external rotation of the leg [44, 60–62]. In the intact specimen, this external rotation occurs at the subtalar joint [58, 63]. After loss of ligamentous support, the external rotation increases, but not at the subtalar joint [58, 64]. Rather, this increase occurs between the tibia and the talus. One may thus speculate that ankle instability, at least in one form, is an axial rotational one (Fig. 2.7).

This rotational concept may explain why symptoms of ankle instability occur in the absence of radiographically demonstrable talar tilt. The role of the subtalar joint, therefore, also needs to be considered in ankle joint instability [65, 66].

2.3 Conclusions and Clinical Implications

- No tilting is necessary at either the ankle or subtalar level to experience functional instability.
- Repair of the anterior talofibular ligament alone can provide successful clinical results for treatment of ankle instability.

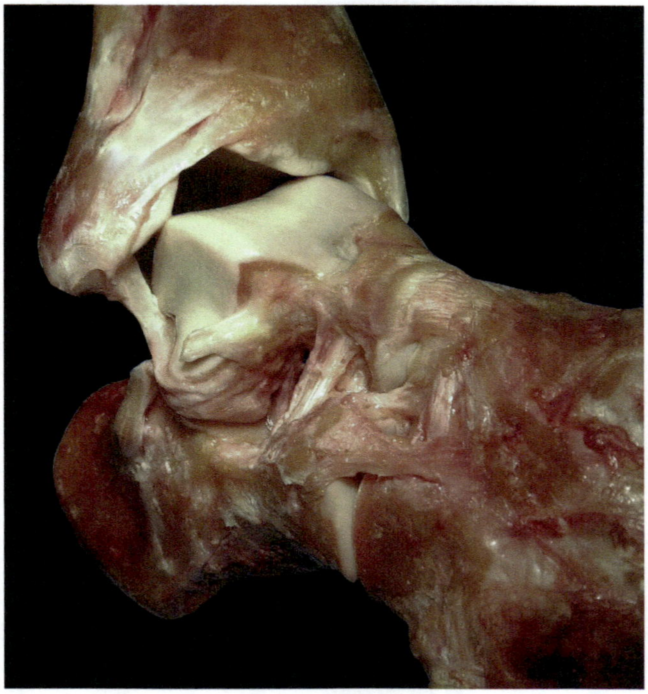

Fig. 2.6 After dissection of the ATFL and CFL, the talus will show some varus tilt and anterolateral extrusion out of ankle mortise when supination forces are applied to the foot

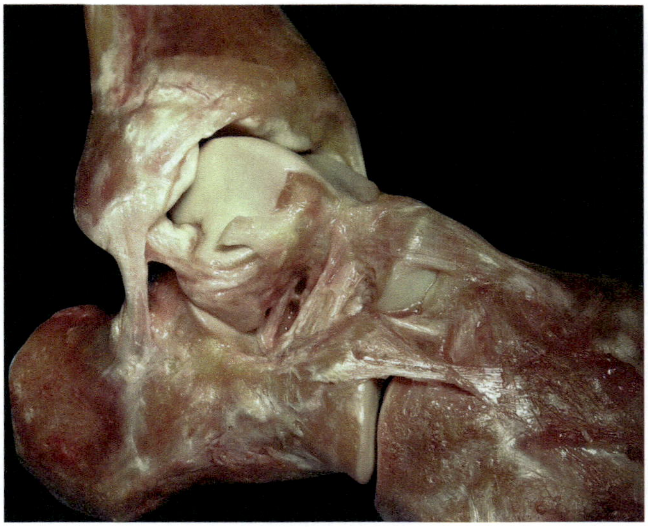

Fig. 2.7 Loss of the ATFL support results in anterolateral rotational instability of the ankle

There is general agreement that motion between the tibia and the foot is a complex combination of ankle and subtalar joint motion limited by osseous shape and soft tissue interaction. The complex pattern of ankle joint motion is guided by the close relationship between the geometry of the ligaments and the shape of the articular surfaces [60]. The slackening and tightening of the ankle ligaments may be explained in terms of their instantaneous position with respect to the moving axis of rotation. The pattern of rotation has been shown to be more isometric for the CFL and talocalcaneal ligament (TCL) with respect to all others.

Obviously, besides maintaining lateral ankle stability, the lateral ankle ligaments play a significant role in maintaining rotational ankle stability (Fig. 2.8). It has been shown that loss of the ATFL and/or CFL leads to a measurable increase in inversion without any additional tilting of the talus or subtalar gapping (Fig. 2.7). It has also been shown that the loss of the ATFL allows an increase in external rotation of the leg to occur. The loss of the ATFL restraint unlocks the subtalar joint, allowing for further inversion. It is this increase in inversion which may lead to symptomatic instability. Considering this, no tilting is necessary at either the ankle or subtalar level to nevertheless experience functional instability.

These rotational concepts may explain why repair of the ATFL alone can provide successful clinical results for treatment of ankle instability [12, 19]. It may also explain why reconstructions that simply tenodese the fifth metatarsal to the fibula, thereby preventing external rotation, cure ankle instability [67]. Most of the common tenodesis procedures [68–70], however, do significantly restrict subtalar motion and thus alter the physiological interplay of the ankle and subtalar joint motion. As they interfere with the hindfoot mechanics, these tenodesis procedures should be avoided [20, 71].

In conclusion, appreciating the anatomy and mechanics of the rearfoot complex aids in understanding the pathomechanics of lateral ankle sprains and chronic ankle instability. Mechanical instability of the ankle may be due to the specific insufficiencies of pathologic laxity, arthrokinematic restrictions, synovial irritation, or degenerative changes to the joints of the ankle complex. Functional instability is driven by insufficiencies in proprioception, neuromuscular control, postural control, and strength [72].

2.4 Injury Pattern of Lateral Ankle Ligaments

- Most frequently, the tear is located at the proximal insertion along the fibula, thus involving both the anterior talofibular and calcaneofibular ligaments.
- The posterior talofibular ligament is rarely affected by the injury.
- Associated injuries to the peroneal tendons are common.

The most common tear site of the ATFL and CFL are their proximal attachments, with the deep layers being more often affected than the superficial layers [36, 43] (Fig. 2.9). The

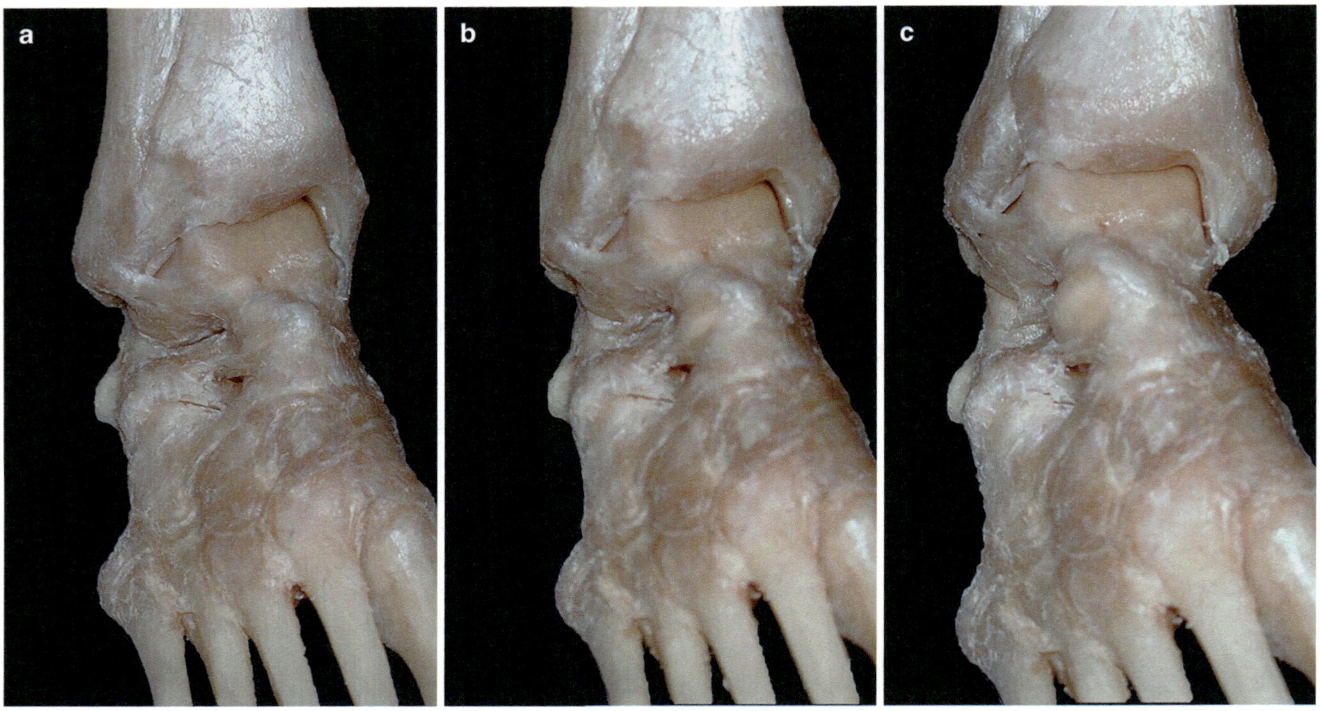

Fig. 2.8 The lateral ankle ligaments play an important role in maintaining rotational stability of the ankle. (**a**) pronation position, (**b**) neutral position, and (**c**) supination position of the foot

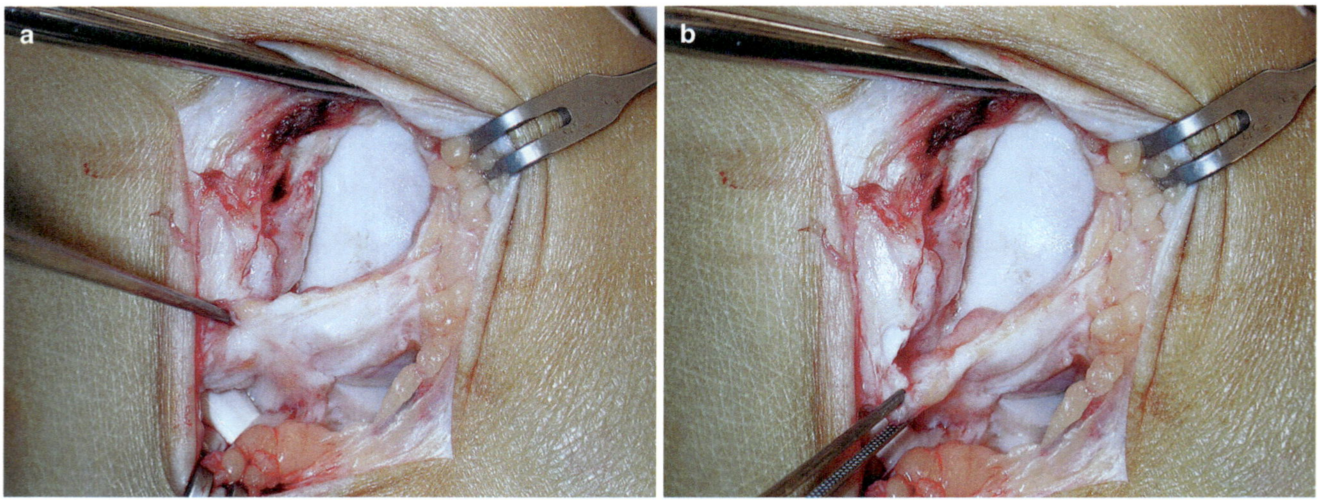

Fig. 2.9 (**a**) The most common injury site of the lateral ankle ligaments is at the proximal insertion of the ATFL/CFL complex. Very often the superficial layers remain intact, while the deep layers are detached. (**b**) After dissecting the superficial layers that remained connected to the periosteum, the extent of the tear with complete detachment from the fibula becomes visible

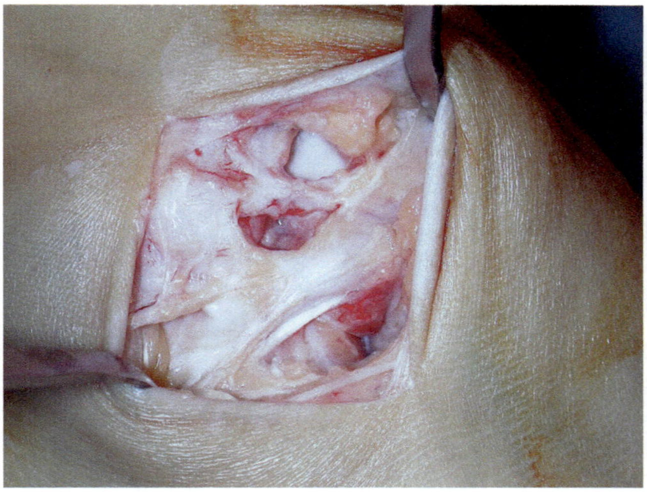

Fig. 2.10 Another case showing the complete detachment of the ATFL/CFL complex from the fibula with some superficial layers remaining intact while the deep layers are torn

rupture typically starts at the proximal site of the common insertion area and continues distally, leaving the ATLF/CFL complex intact, however detached from the fibula (Fig. 2.10). A special type of injury is an avulsion fracture of the lateral ankle ligaments at the fibula that is most commonly seen among children and patients over 40 years of age [73] (Fig. 2.11). The clinical characteristics are different from those of ligament rupture, and, unlike nonoperative treatment of lateral ligament rupture, nonoperative treatment of avulsion fractures does not yield satisfactory results [74]. Tears at the talar end of the ATFL (Fig. 2.12), in contrast, are less common since bone density is greater than at the fibular enthesis, and stress is dissipated away from the talar enthesis by the "wrap-around" fibrocartilaginous character of the ligament near the talar articular facet [75].

2.5 History and Clinical Presentation

- Patients most commonly report on having sustained a supination sprain.
- In the acute situation, pain and swelling can help the surgeon identify the location and extent of the lesion.
- Stress testing should be done with hanging feet.

Patients with an acute injury of the lateral ankle ligaments usually report on a sustained inversion-supination trauma and pain in the anteromedial part of the ankle joint. After a fracture has been ruled out, a careful physical examination is carried out starting with examining the swelling, deformity, and ecchymosis, as they are indicative of acute injury (Fig. 2.13). In cases where lateral ankle instability has become a chronic problem, making an accurate diagnosis may be more demanding, as pain is often missing and local symptoms may be subtle. To assess stability of the lateral ankle ligaments, two provocative maneuvers are essential, best done with the patient sitting upright with their feet hanging. The anterior drawer test assesses the integrity of the ATFL (Fig. 2.14) [49, 76–81] but its reliability was found to be poor, likely because the average amount of clinically meaningful talocrural laxity is small and varies considerably, making it difficult to perceive with a manual test [82]. If the ATFL is ruptured, in 50% of the cases a dimple sign can be seen in the anterior aspect of the joint (Fig. 2.15). The talar tilt test for the ATFL and CFL are shown in Fig. 2.16.

The foot's shape and overall alignment of the hindfoot are assessed with the patient standing (Fig. 2.17a–c). Any deformity is reassessed with the patient in the tiptoe position to determine if the deformity is affected by the eccentric pull of the Achilles tendon (Fig. 2.17d). To exclude that the hindfoot varus is not forefoot driven, the Coleman bloc test can be done [83] (Fig. 2.17e).

2.6 Imaging

- Radiographs serve to rule out a fracture.
- MRI may help to identify a ligament injury in the acute situation; however, it does not provide information about the resulting instability.
- MRI and CT scans may serve to identify associated lesions.

Standard non-weight-bearing X-rays (Fig. 2.18a, b), and, if necessary, CT scans are taken after an acute injury to exclude a fracture (Fig. 2.18c, d). A MRI can serve to further assess damage to the cartilage (Fig. 2.18e, f). In the case of chronic instability, standard weight-bearing X-rays are taken

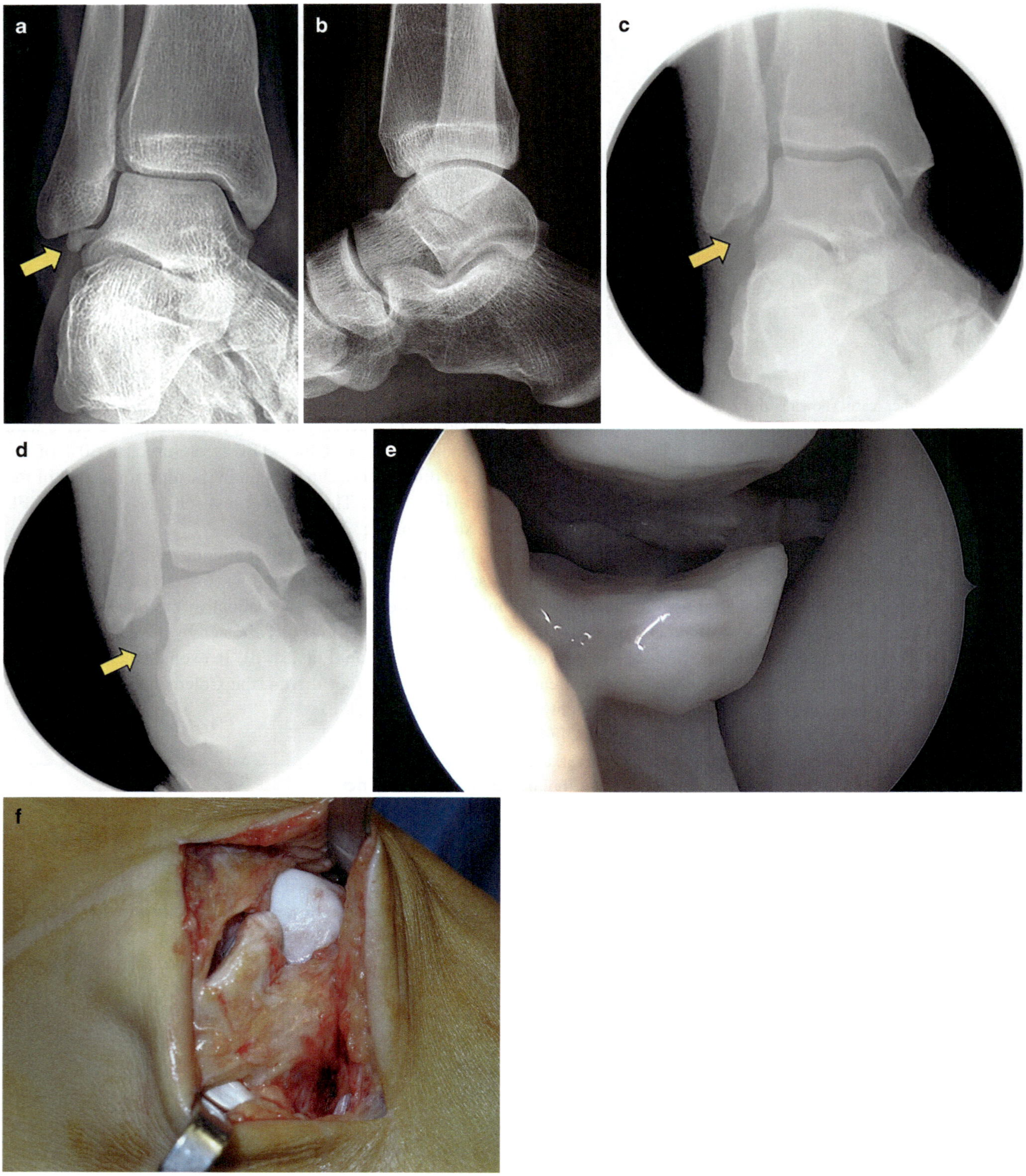

Fig. 2.11 Avulsion of the lateral ankle ligaments (arrow) in a chronically unstable ankle after experiencing a severe sprain. (**a**) AP radiograph showing the detached fragment (arrow). (**b**) In the lateral view, the fragment is seen at the anterior aspect of distal fibula. (**c**) Under fluoroscopy, the fragment is seen to be close to its origin when the foot is in neutral position (arrow); whereas (**d**) when varus stress is applied, the fragment is seen to move away from the fibula (arrow). (**e**) Arthroscopy shows a complete detachment of the fragment with the ATFL/CFL complex. (**f**) Surgical exploration evidences the detached fragment at the fibular site with an intact ATFL/CFL complex

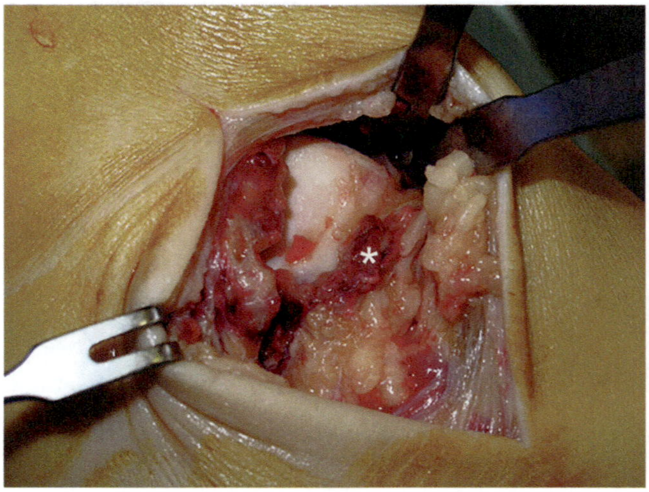

Fig. 2.12 An acute tear of the ATFL at its distal insertion on the talar neck (asterisk)

to assess any concomitant abnormalities such as hindfoot misalignment or cavovarus deformity (Fig. 2.19). A coalition can best be seen with a CT scan (Fig. 2.20a–c) or MRI (Fig. 2.20d). It may also evidence osteochondral lesions (Fig. 2.21) [84].

If the manual anterior drawer test suggests abnormal laxity, stress radiographs may be performed to demonstrate the degree of laxity of the ankle joint [85]. However, due to the tendency of examinees to protect their ankle joints through muscular contraction during the examination, thereby stiffening their ankle joint [86, 87], the sensitivity and accuracy of this procedure is low unless the examination is performed with the use of anesthetics or regional nerve block [88].

An alternative diagnostic tool may be stress ultrasound [76, 89–91]. It is easily available, economical, and portable.

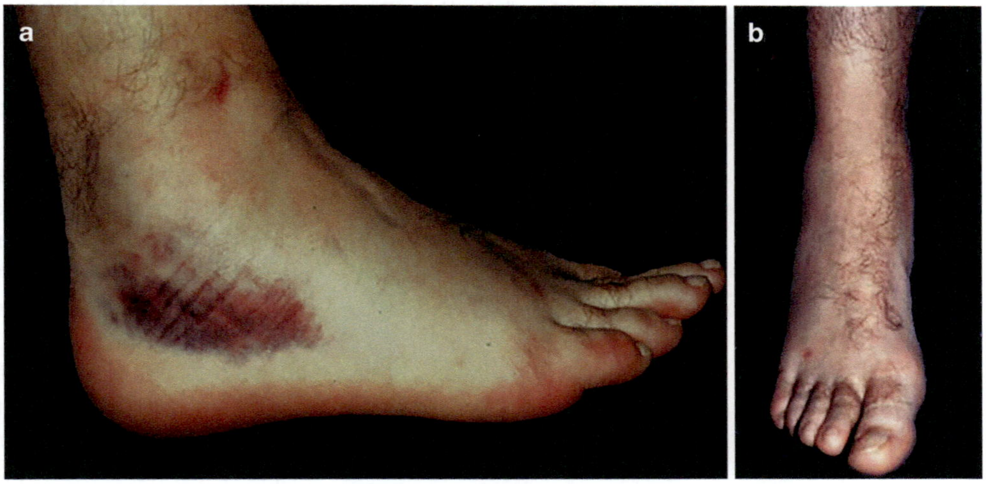

Fig. 2.13 Swelling and ecchymosis after an acute ankle sprain. (**a**) lateral view, (**b**) anterior view

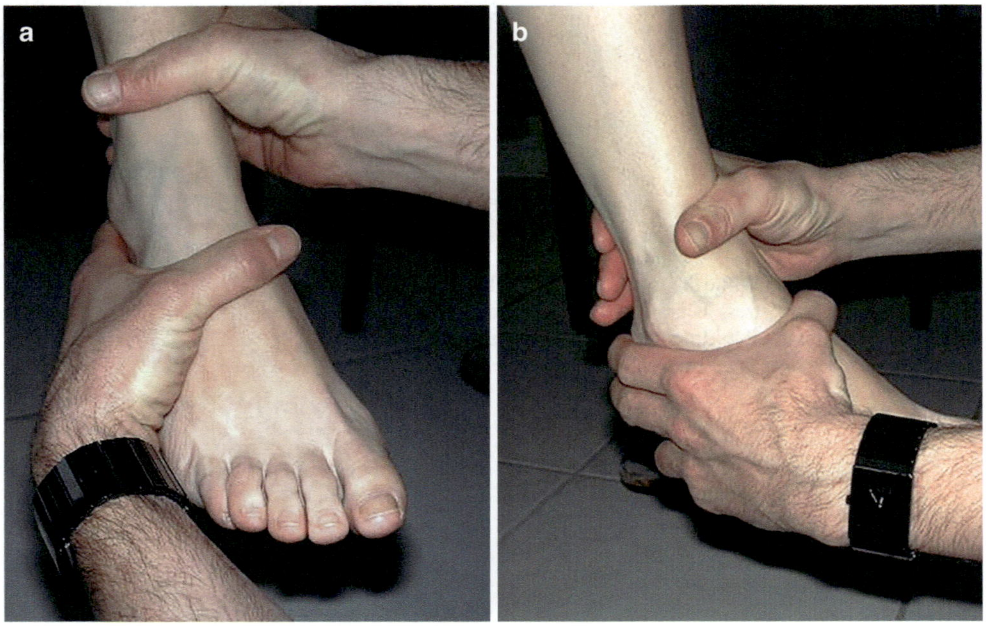

Fig. 2.14 Anterior drawer test. (**a**) With the foot hanging, the distal tibia is held with one hand while the other hand holds the foot at the heel. (**b**) While the foot is in slight plantar flexion, the heel is then pulled towards anterior

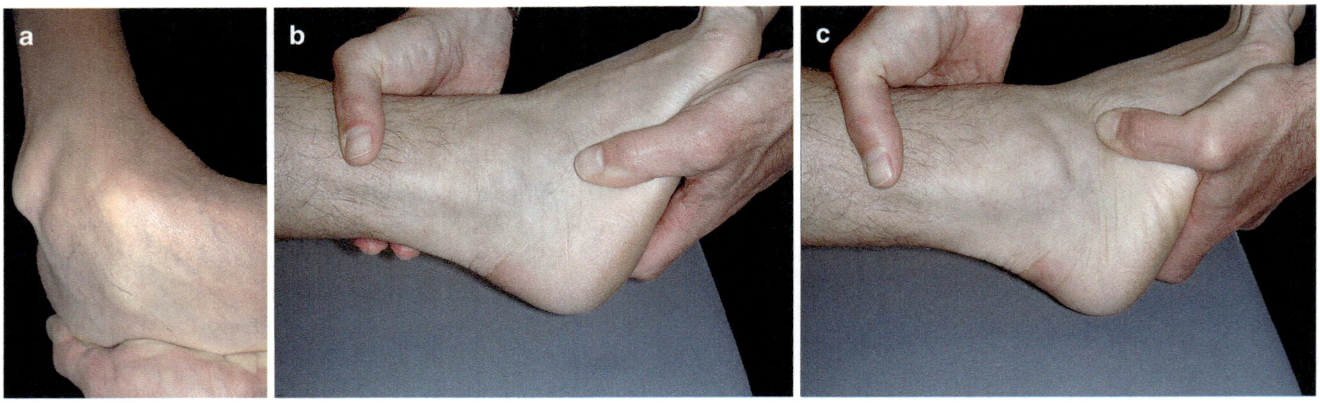

Fig. 2.15 Dimple sign. (**a**) While supination stress is applied, a dimple sign can often be seen at anterior ankle. (**b**) It can also be seen when the distal tibia and the heel are taken by the investigator, and (**c**) then the foot is pushed towards medial

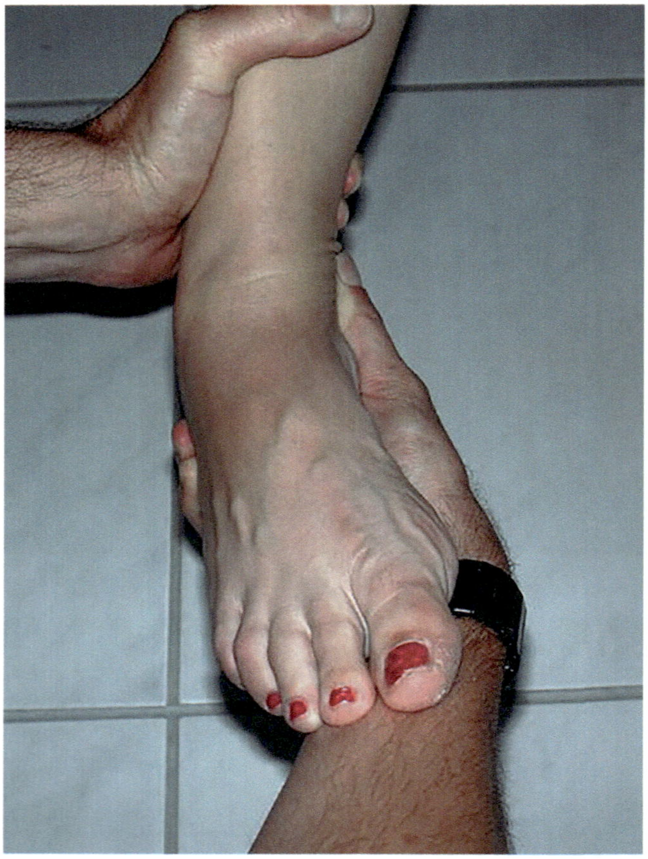

Fig. 2.16 Talar tilt test. While the foot is taken in slight plantar flexion by the heel and varus stress is applied, the investigator can feel the opening of the lateral ankle. Important for correct testing is that the patient is relaxed. This can be best achieved when the patient is sitting with hanging feet

MRI after suffering an acute ankle sprain revealed that isolated lateral ligament ankle injuries are not as common as believed (Fig. 2.22). The injury pattern seems complex and most patients appear to have more injuries than expected [92]. While more than half of the referred athletes evidenced lateral ligament injuries without syndesmotic involvement, about 20% evidenced a syndesmotic injury regardless of the involvement of the lateral ligaments [93]. Despite these findings in the assessment of ligament injuries [76, 94–96], the questions remain whether an MRI is justified immediately after an acute ankle sprain or whether it should be considered after a few days, when the normal course of symptoms is absent [97–99]. In the recent past, surgeons have often considered MRI findings for the morphological evaluation of the injured lateral ankle ligaments when deciding among the operative options for reconstruction and repair. This is done in particular for arthroscopic lateral ankle ligament repair procedures that require the presence of substantial ligament tissues to achieve firm postoperative ligament stability [100, 101]. Ligament intensity has a strong negative linear relationship with material biomechanical strength properties [102, 103]. A lower signal intensity in the ATFL ligament, based on preoperative MRI findings, is associated with a better clinical outcome, particularly a higher rate of return to sport [104]. Furthermore, MRI also demonstrates the healing process of the ligament as indicated by normalized ligament signal intensity [105].

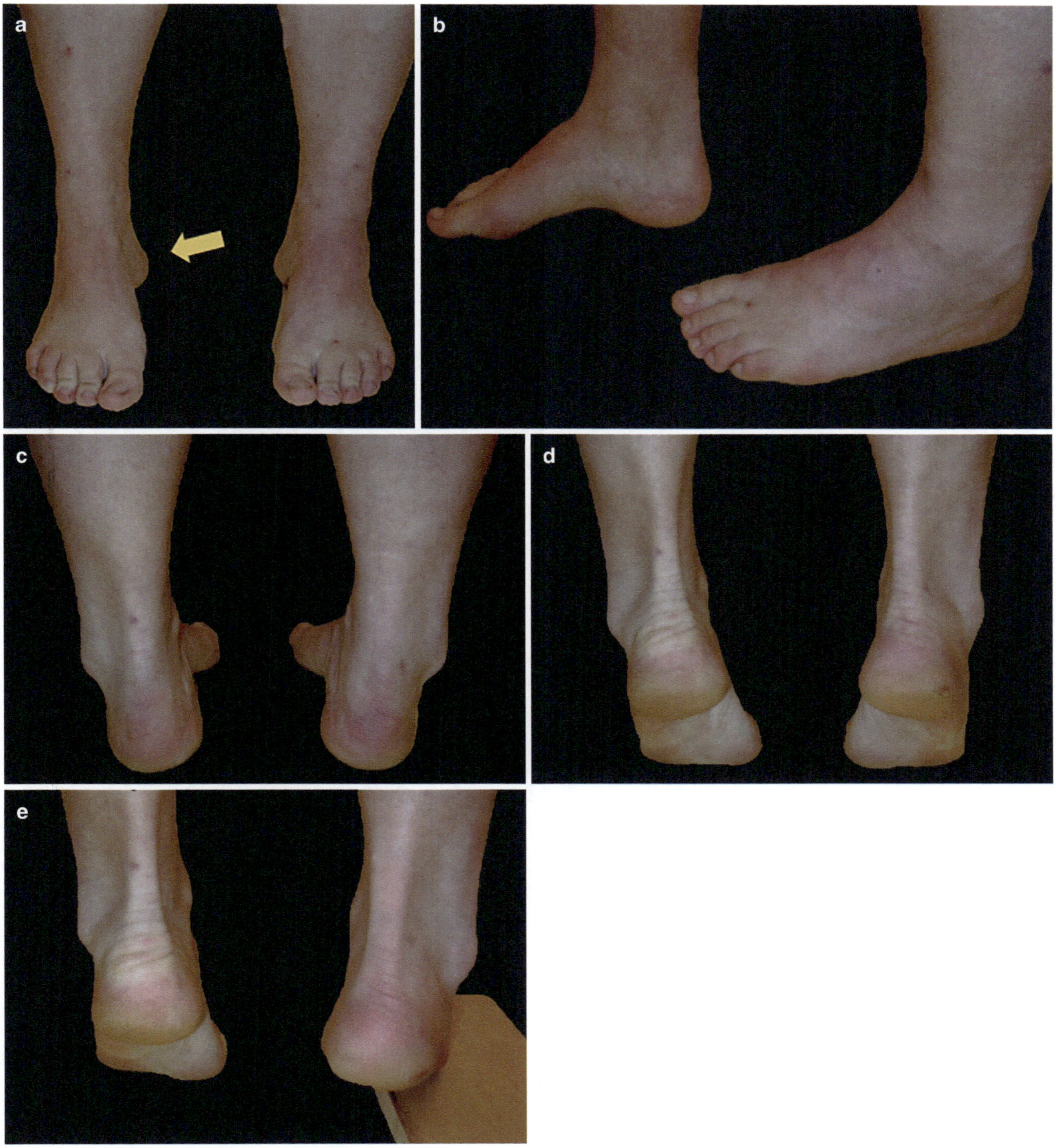

Fig. 2.17 Clinical assessment of the foot shape and hindfoot alignment is done with the patient weight-bearing. (**a**) Anterior view showing the peek-a-boo of the calcaneus due to the cavovarus deformity (arrow). (**b**) The high-arch configuration with shortening and some adduction of the forefoot. (**c**) Varus malalignment of the hindfoot that is associated with an external rotation of the foot is seen from posterior; typically, the lateral malleolus is very prominent, whereas the medial malleolus has disappeared. (**d**) In tiptoe position, while the heel cord is activated, no further varus malalignment is seen, meaning that it is a fixed deformity. (**e**) When performing the Coleman bloc test, no decrease of varus can be seen, which confirms that the hindfoot varus is not driven by a forefoot pronation

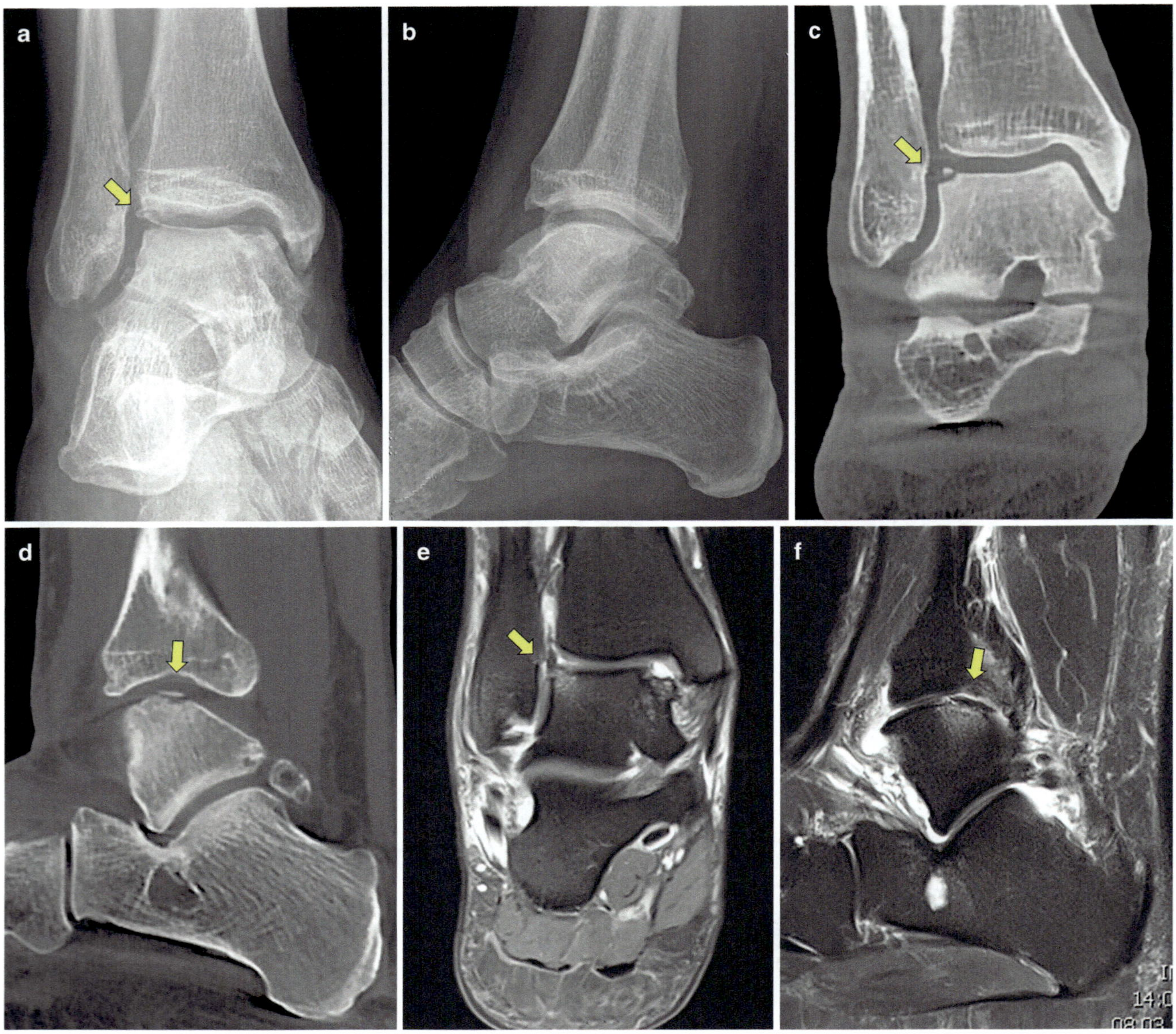

Fig. 2.18 Images taken from a 32-year-old female patient after a severe inversion sprain of her left ankle while jogging, with a history of an osteochondral lesion on the medial talus that was asymptomatic after arthroscopic microfracturing 3 years earlier. On plain non-weight-bearing radiography, (**a**) the AP view evidenced an osteochondral flake at the lateral talar dome (arrow), which cannot be seen on (**b**) the lateral view. Whereas, CT scan shows the detached fragment in both, the AP (**c**) and lateral view (**d**), with little displacement. MRI additionally shows a fracture of the cartilage in the coronal plane (**e**) and sagittal plane with perifocal edema indicating instability of the fragment (**f**)

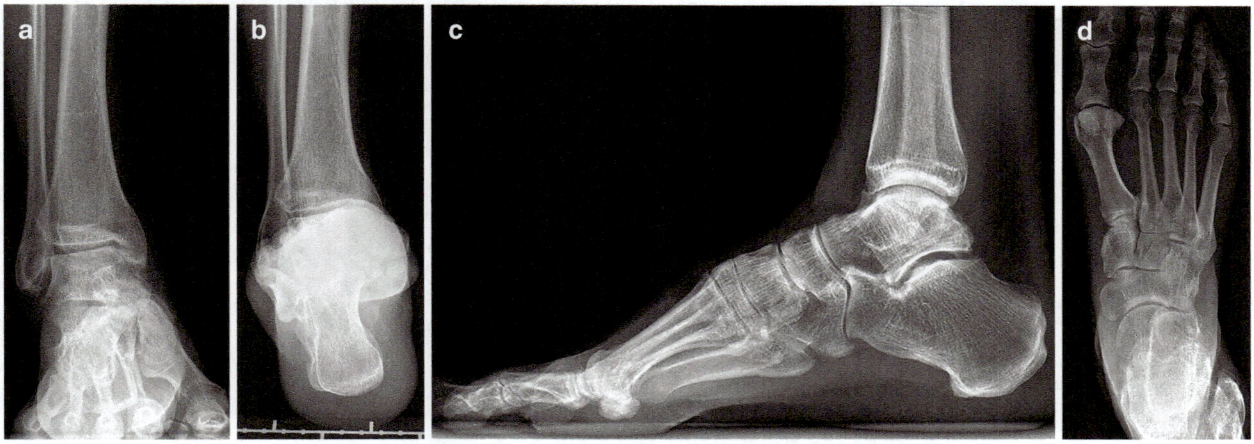

Fig. 2.19 Weight-bearing standard X-rays in a 46-year-old male patient with recurrent sprains after a severe sprain of his right ankle. (**a**) The AP view evidences a varus distal tibial articular surface angle, a varus tilt of the talus and some valgus of the calcaneus. There is obviously an incompetence of the lateral ankle ligaments. (**b**) The Saltzman hindfoot alignment view confirms the varus malalignment of the hindfoot. (**c**) On the lateral view, a high arch and a gapping of the subtalar joint can be seen. (**d**) On the DP view of the foot, some supination with a decreased talocalcaneal angle and some coverage of the cuboid by the navicular can be seen

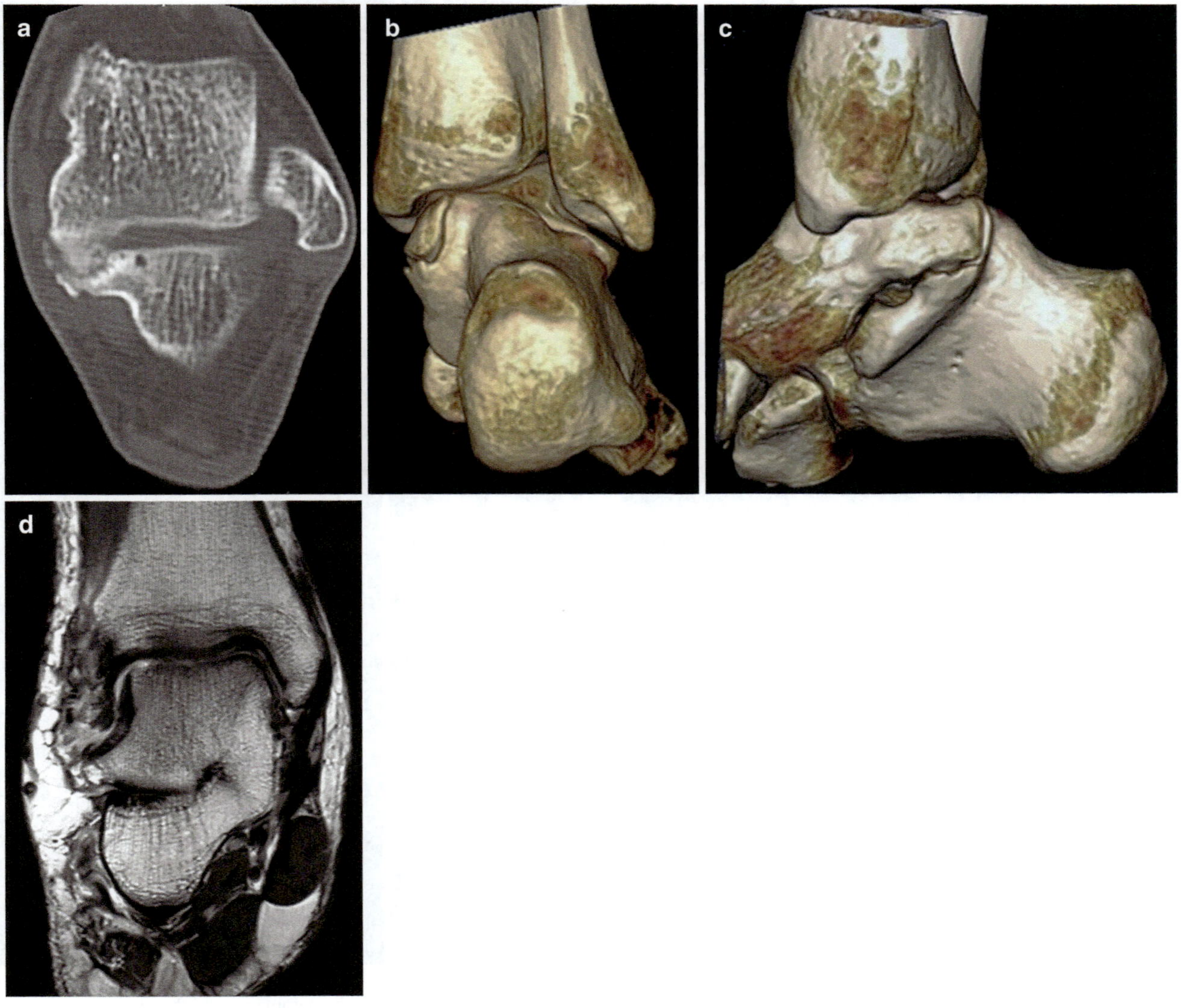

Fig. 2.20 Talocalcaneal (subtalar) coalition in a 32-year-old female patient suffering from chronic lateral ankle instability. (**a**) CT scan evidenced an incomplete coalition. (**b**) 3D CT scan showed the incomplete coalition with associated medialization of the talus. (**c**) The extent of the incomplete coalition is best seen on the medial view. (**d**) A coalition can also be seen with the aid of an MRI (not the same patient)

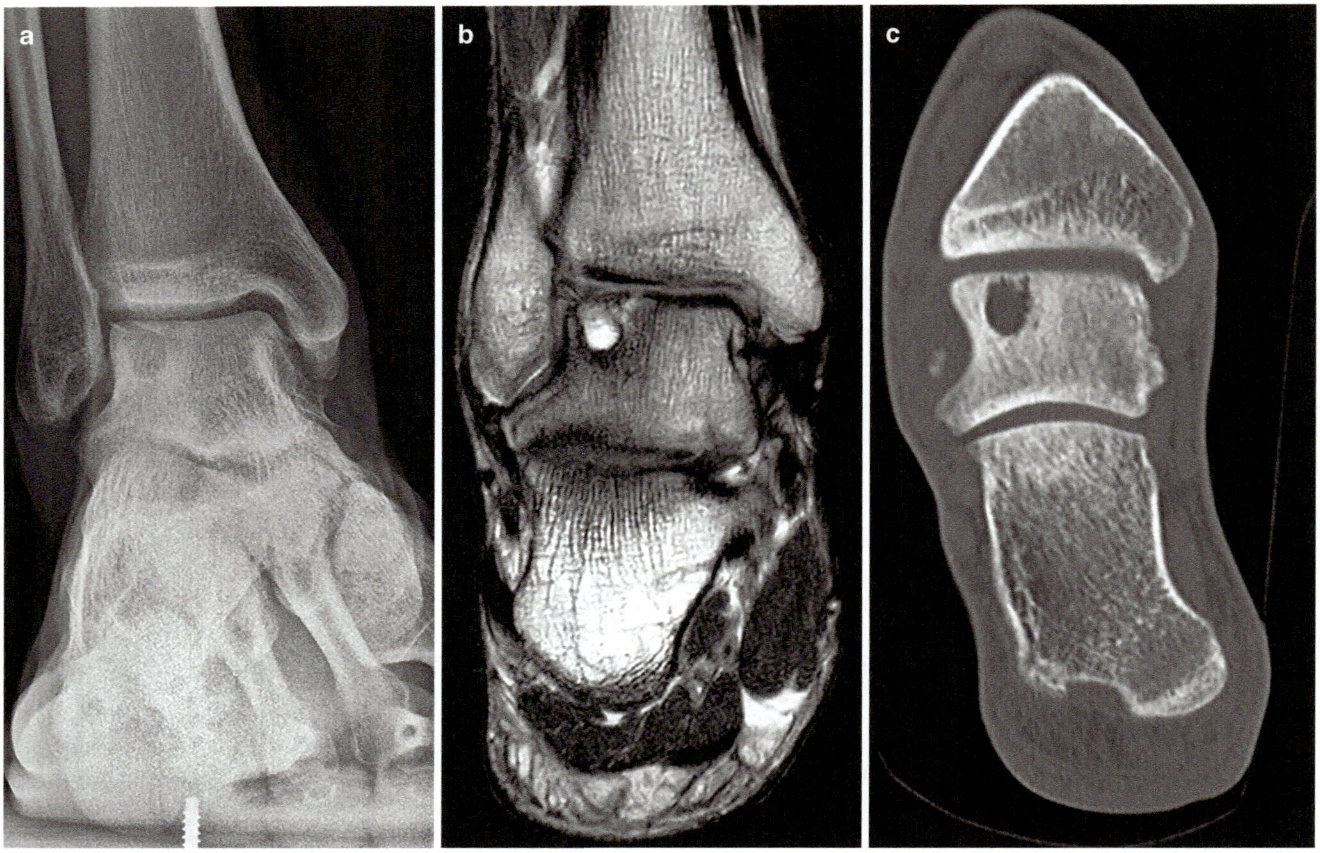

Fig. 2.21 Cystic osteochondral lesion in a 38-year-old male patient suffering from recurrent sprains of his left ankle. (**a**) AP radiograph of the ankle showing the cyst that involves the articular space. (**b**) The extent of chondral lesion can better be visualized with MRI. (**c**) CT scan may help to assess the state of the subchondral bone, especially rule out fractures

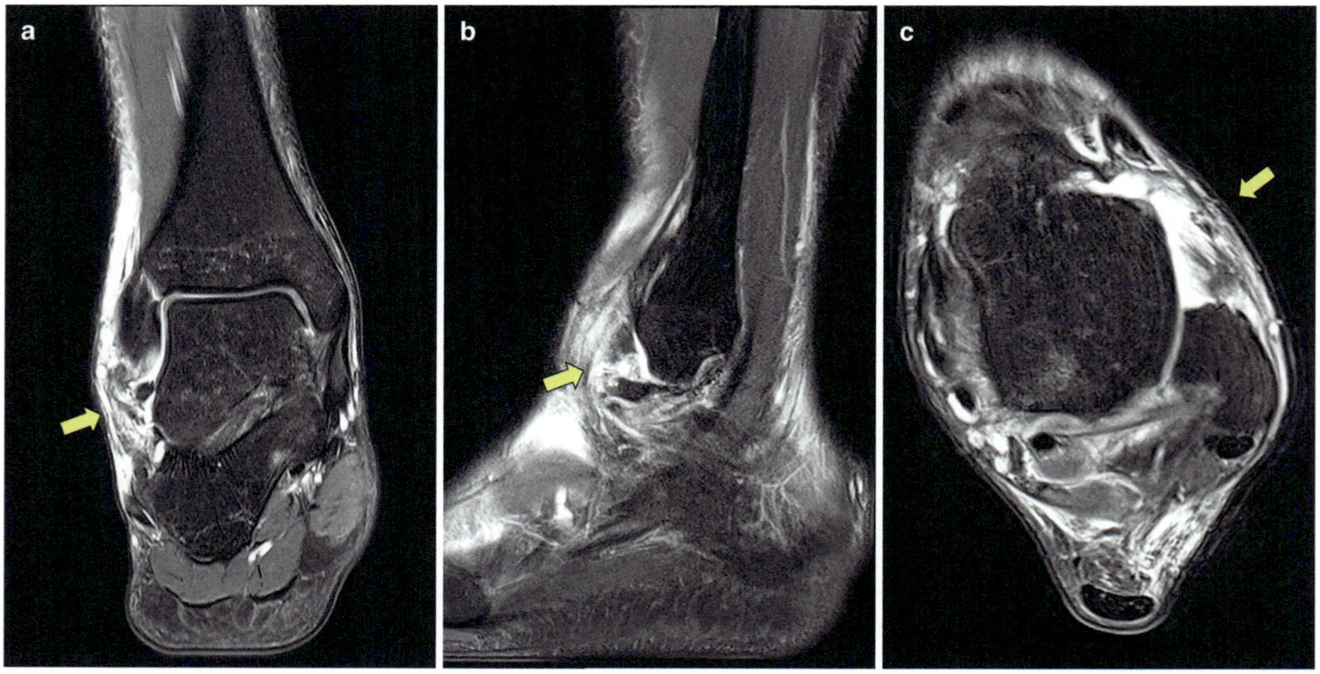

Fig. 2.22 MRI may be helpful to visualize morphologic changes of the soft tissue structures such as the ligaments after an acute sprain or in chronically unstable joints. Here, after an acute sprain, the ATFL is ruptured (arrow) and there is a hematoma around the fibula as well as fluid in the peroneal tendon sheet seen in (**a**) the coronal plane, (**b**) sagittal plane and (**c**) horizontal plane

2.7 Arthroscopy

- Arthroscopy is an excellent tool to identify accompanied intra-articular lesions.
- Arthroscopy also serves to identify the extent of ligament lesions and to understand the resulting instability pattern.

Arthroscopy has become a useful adjuvant tool to understand the severity and complexity of the unstable ankle prior to surgical reconstruction (Fig. 2.23) [106–109]. Direct arthroscopic visualization ensures not only to visualize and assess the lateral ankle ligaments after an acute sprain (Fig. 2.24) or in the chronically unstable condition (Fig. 2.25), but also to detect associated osteochondral lesions (Fig. 2.26). Besides this, it permits to understand the instability pattern (Fig. 2.27) [94, 110].

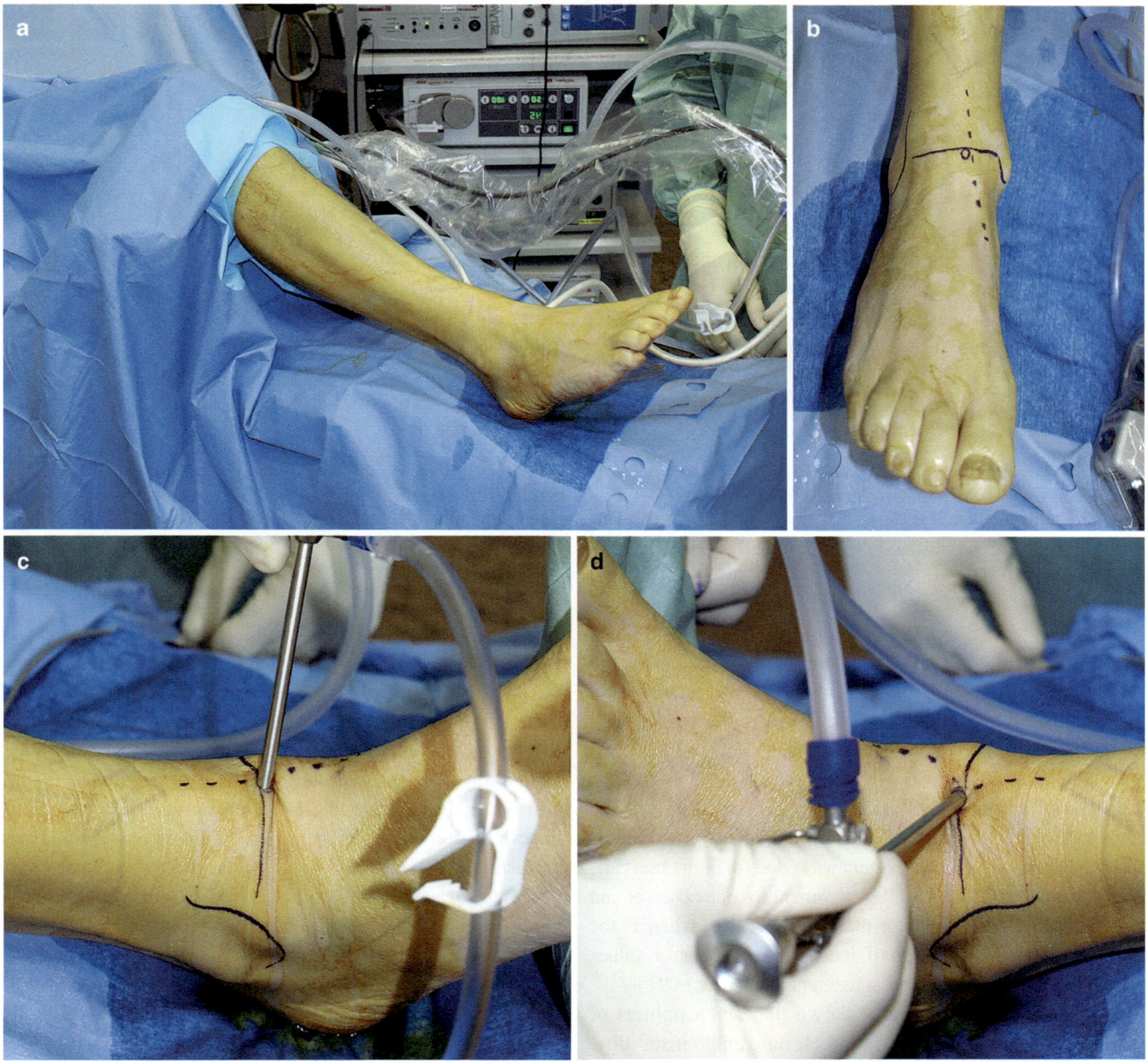

Fig. 2.23 *Surgical Technique: The author's preferred technique for ankle arthroscopy*. (**a**) The patient is in a supine position. A leg holder applied to the thigh is used to flex the knee 60–80°. This allows to investigate the foot in a "hanging" position. (**b**) A central portal is used at the lateral border of anterior tibial tendon (dotted line). (**c**) The 4.5-mm 30° standard arthroscope is introduced into the lateral gutter while the foot is maximally dorsiflexed to avoid damage to the cartilage. (**d**) The medial gutter can also be visualized with this central approach

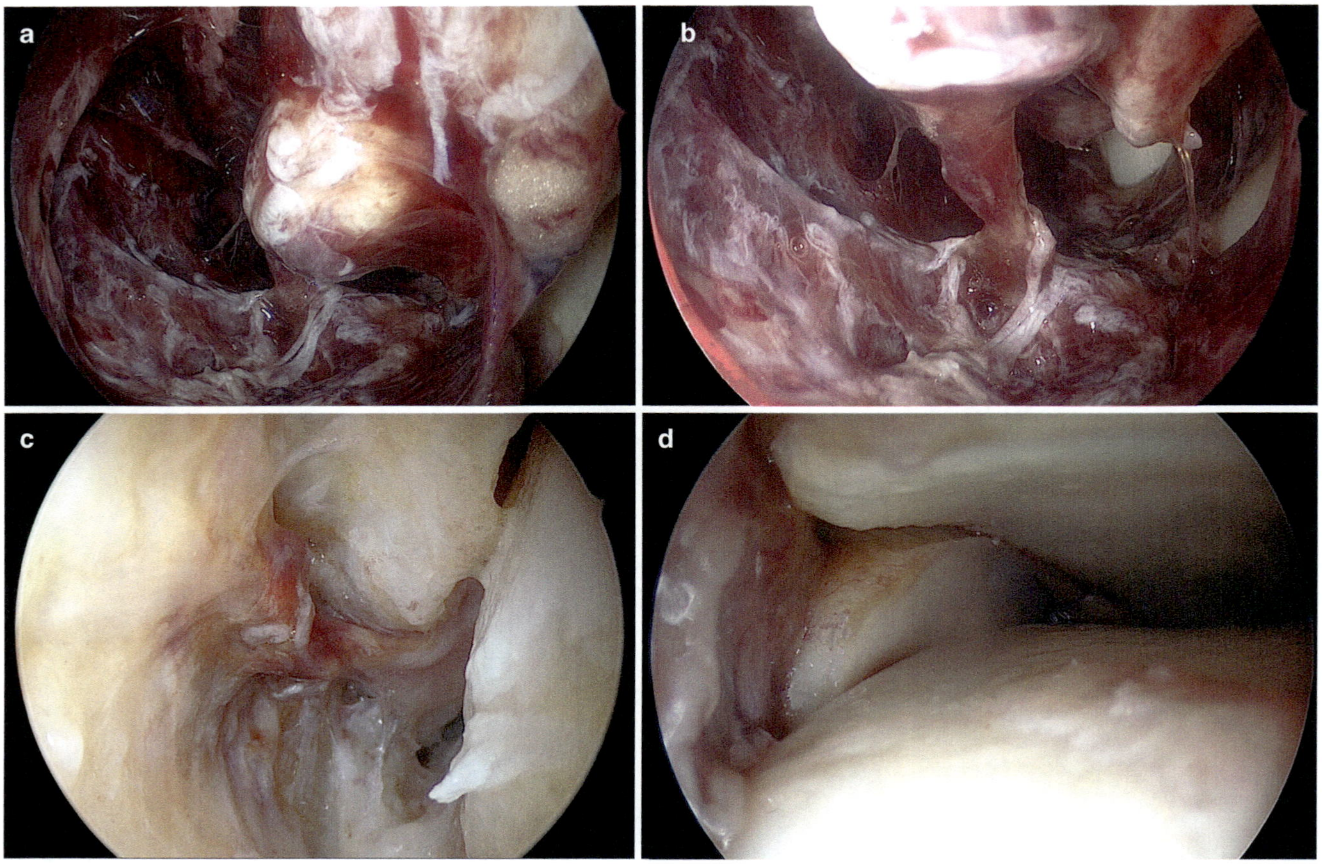

Fig. 2.24 *Surgical Technique: Arthroscopic findings in an acute injury*. (**a**) A complete rupture of the ATFL/CFL complex, with a remaining stump of the ATFL at its insertion site on the anterior fibula. (**b**) While moving the arthroscope more posteriorly, the peroneal tendons are visualized, which is a sign of complete detachment of the ATFL and CFL including disruption of the peroneal tendon sheet. (**c**) After a heavy sprain in this chronically unstable ankle, the scarred lateral ligaments are disrupted from the fibula. (**d**) In the same ankle, the anterior inferior tibiofibular (syndesmotic) ligament is also injured resulting in an instability of the fibula in its incisura. Notice also the gapping of the lateral joint space without any force applied to the foot

As evaluated for both the lateral and medial side, the ankle joint is graded as follows (Table 2.1) [107]:

Recently, the French arthroscopic society proposed a classification based on the condition of the ATFL [111] (Table 2.2). Sixty-nine arthroscopic videos of the anterior ankle in patients with chronic ankle instability were retrospectively analyzed. The intra- and interobserver reliability of the classification were evaluated: the intra-observer agreement was good for both observers, the κ value being 0.67 with 75% agreement for one observer and 0.68 with 76% agreement for the other observer, whereas the inter-observer agreement was fair to good, with the κ values ranging from 0.59 to 0.88 and agreement from 70% to 91%.

Arthroscopy has especially shown that abnormalities of different structures are involved in chronic ankle instability, and there is no single entity causing it, especially regarding the lateral and medial ligaments. For instance, the degree of lateral ligament lesions has no correlation with cartilage lesions of the talus, whereas medial ligament lesions have been shown to be associated with cartilage damage of the talus [106, 107, 112, 113]. The long-term outcome of these once-in-a-lifetime cartilage lesions remains unknown. This, in turn, emphasizes the need for accurate diagnosis and treatment of acute ligamentous injuries to the ankle to prevent secondary problems such as chronic instability and cartilage damage. Preoperative arthroscopy can therefore give essential information on the status of the chronic unstable ankle joint to facilitate the correct choice of surgical treatment [114].

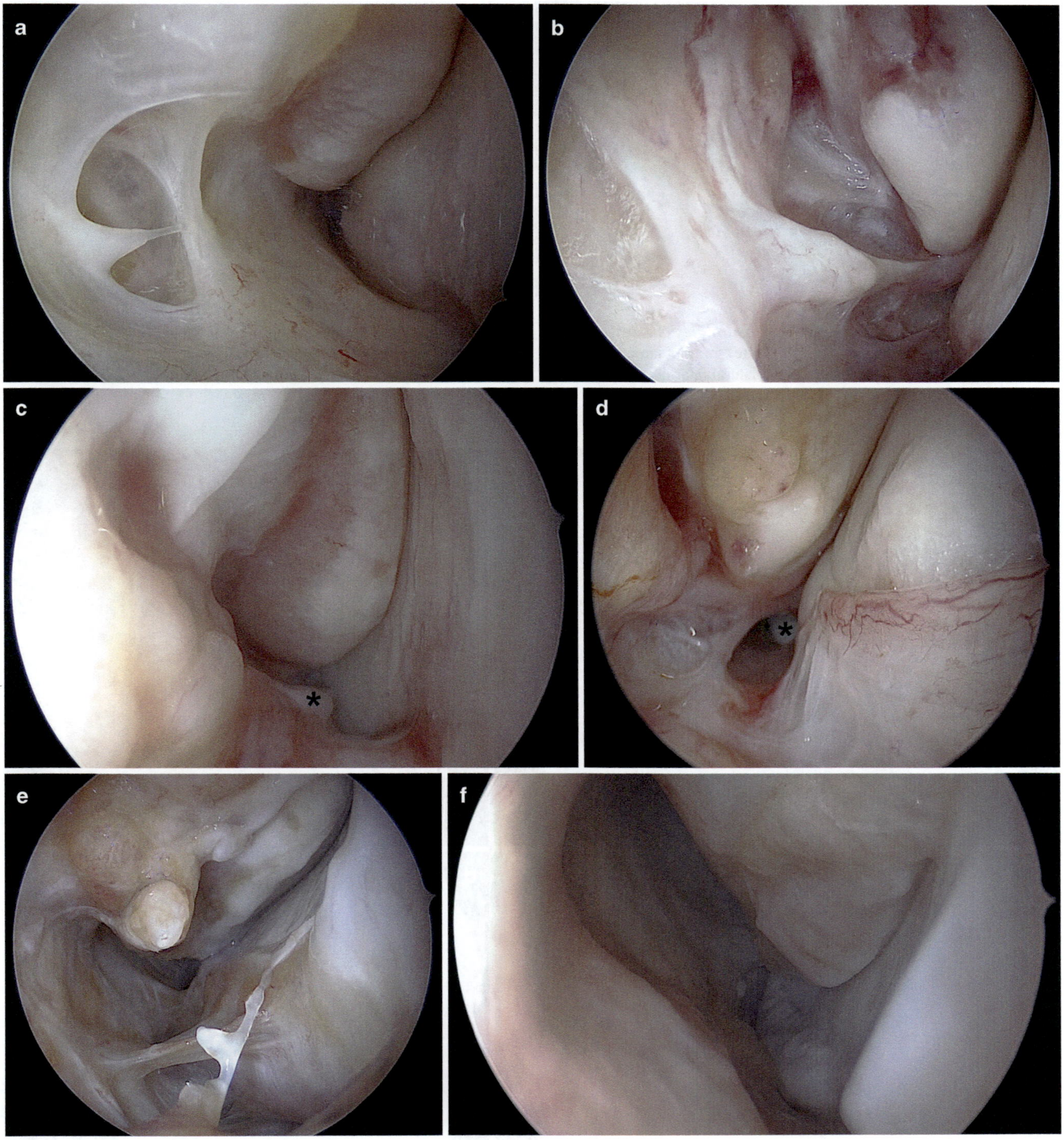

Fig. 2.25 *Surgical Technique: Arthroscopic findings from different patients suffering from chronic ankle instability*. (**a**) A normal and continuous ATFL without tearing, normal in thickness and taut between the lateral malleolus and the talar neck. (**b**) A thin ATFL with fibular avulsion and decreased tension. Some remaining fibrous tissue can be seen, and the superficial layers are still connected to the periosteum. (**c**) Avulsion of the ATFL and CFL with a small bony fragment (asterisk) resulting in no mechanical resistance. (**d**) Complete avulsion of the ATFL and CFL with some scars left, with visible peroneal tendons (asterisk) in their disrupted sheath. (**e**) Complete absence of the ATFL and CFL with some scar tissue left at the fibular insertion in a severely unstable ankle. (**f**) Scar tissue with no residual ligament, leaving a bald malleolus in a severely unstable ankle

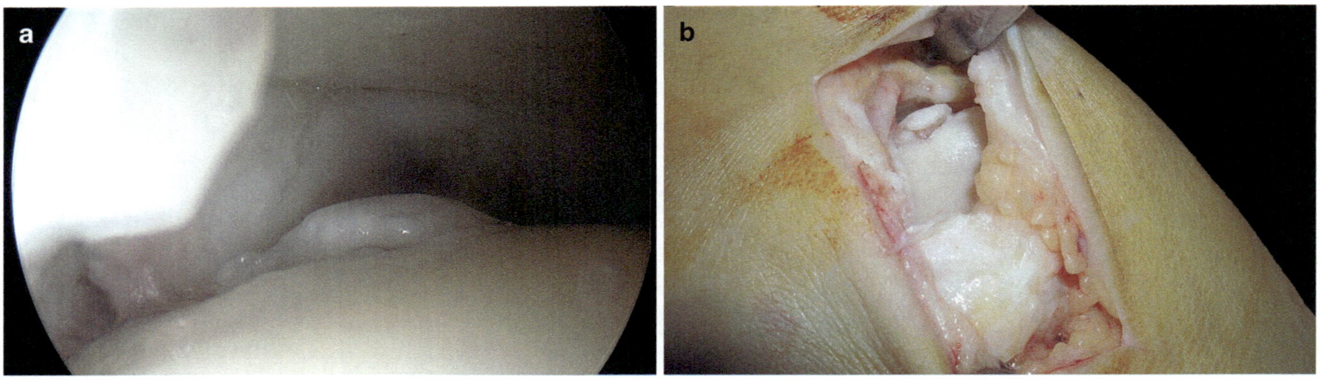

Fig. 2.26 *Surgical Technique: Osteochondral lesion.* Arthroscopic findings in a painful ankle after an acute sprain (same patient as Fig. 2.22). (**a**) A chondral fragment at the lateral talar dome is detected, there exists an inflammatory response of the anterolateral capsular. (**b**) Surgical exposure in the same patient of open ligament reconstruction shows the partially detached chondral fragment

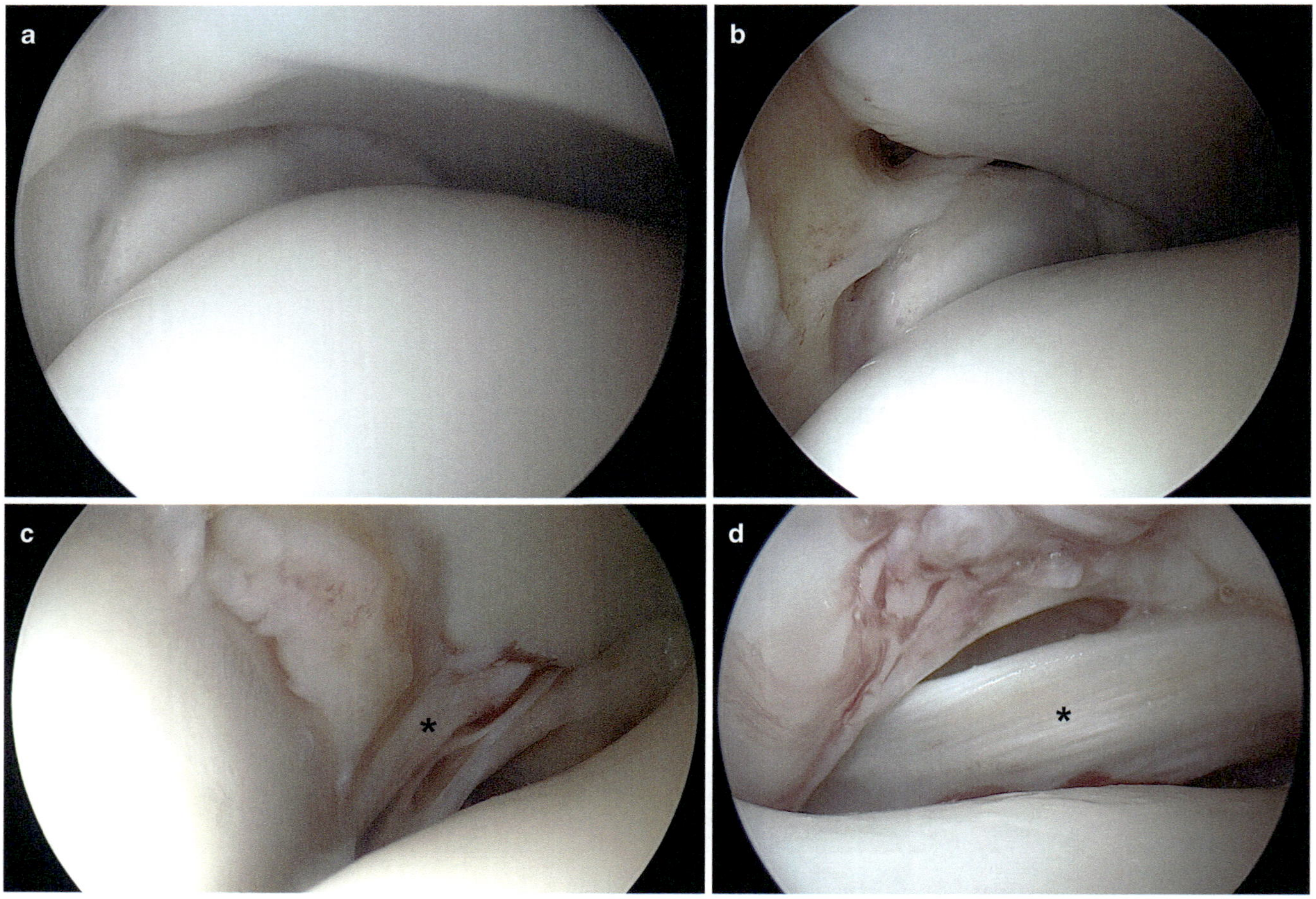

Fig. 2.27 *Surgical Technique: Mechanical testing of the lateral ankle stability under arthroscopy.* (**a**) A stable ankle with some translocation of the talus, but not allowing to introduce the 4.5-mm arthroscope into the tibiotalar space. (**b**) Moderate lateral ankle instability with enough translocation of the talus to insert the 4.5-mm arthroscope into the anterior tibiotalar space, but not enough to get insight of the posterior ankle. (**c**) Severe lateral ankle instability with substantial translocation of the talus, allowing to insert the 4.5-mm arthroscope deeper in the tibiotalar joint and to visualize the posterolateral structures (asterisk, posterior inferior tibiofibular (syndesmotic) ligament). (**d**) Severe global ankle instability involving also the medial side with significant talar extrusion out of the mortise, thus allowing to insert the 4.5-mm arthroscope all the way to the posterior aspect of the tibiotalar joint and to visualize overall posterior structures from laterally to medially (asterisk, intermalleolar ligament)

Table 2.1 Arthroscopic classification of chronic lateral ankle instability ([107], modified)

Grade	Arthroscopic findings	Figure
Stable ankle	when there is some translocation of the talus, but not enough to introduce the 4.5-mm arthroscope into the tibiotalar space	Figure 2.27a
Moderate lateral ankle instability	when there is enough translocation of the talus to introduce the 4.5-mm arthroscope into anterior tibiotalar space, but not enough to visualize the posterolateral structures	Figure 2.27b
Severe lateral ankle instability	when there is substantial translocation of the talus, typically allowing to insert the 4.5-mm arthroscope deeper into tibiotalar joint and to visualize the posterolateral structures	Figure 2.27c
Severe global ankle instability	When there is significant extrusion of the talus out of the mortis, typically allowing to insert the 4.5-mm arthroscope into the posterior aspect of the tibiotalar joint and to visualize overall structures from lateral to medial	Figure 2.27d

Table 2.2 French classification of chronic ATFL lesions [111]

Grade	Arthroscopic findings	Figure
Grade 0	normal and continuous ligament without tearing, normal in thickness and taut between the lateral malleolus and the talar neck	Fig. 2.25a
Grade 1	distended ligament without tearing, normal in thickness but with decreased tension by hook palpation	
Grade 2	fibular or talar avulsion (with fibrous tissue) of the ATFL, normal thickness, but decreased tension by hook palpation	Fig. 2.25b
Grade 3	thin ATFL ligament with no mechanical resistance by hook palpation, with or without scar tissue	Fig. 2.25d
Grade 4	scar tissue with no residual ligament, leaving a bald malleolus	Fig. 2.25f

2.8 Conservative Treatment and Rehabilitation

- Conservative treatment is indicated in the great majority of acute lateral ankle ligament injuries.
- Rehabilitation should include strengthening of the peroneal muscles as well as proprioception and coordination training.
- Despite conservative treatment, up to 40% of the patients complain about persistent pain and/or instability.

2.8.1 Acute Ankle Sprains

Treatment is usually nonoperative, with immobilization and/or rest, ice, elevation, physical therapy, and bracing. Initially, non-weight-bearing may be advised until pain and swelling are gone.

A grade III acute lateral ankle ligament injury can be treated by cast immobilization, which usually entails a brief period (≤3 weeks) in a below-knee walking cast, followed by up to 12 weeks of proprioceptive rehabilitation. Although immobilization may not be advantageous in the high-performance athlete, it should be accepted by the low-demand patient, who is unable to bear weight through the affected limb immediately following a severe acute sprain.

2.8.2 Chronic Ankle Instability

A recurrent acute ankle sprain in a patient with chronic ankle instability is first treated like an acute ankle sprain with immobilization and bracing. The local symptoms are usually less, and local pain will disappear within a few days which may motivate for early return to sports activities.

However, the patient may benefit from a structured program of functional and prophylactic rehabilitation, which may be supplemented with external splinting. The patient with functional instability is more likely to benefit than is the patient with mechanical instability [114].

2.8.3 Rehabilitation

Functional management implies early mobilization with external support and a protocol of rest, ice, compression, and elevation. This is followed by a rehabilitation program consisting of ROM exercises, strengthening, proprioception, and activity-specific training. Proprioception training, which is essential for the recovery of balance and postural control, consists of a series of progressive drills on devices such as wobble boards and trampolines. In addition to providing mechanical stability, external support also provides proprioceptive feedback and thus aids rehabilitation.

2.9 Surgical Management of Lateral Ankle Instability

- Primary surgical treatment of acute lateral ankle ligament injuries may be considered in high-level athletes.
- In chronic lateral ankle instability, reconstruction by reattachment of the anterior talofibular and calcaneofibular ligaments to the fibula is the primary choice.
- If the remaining ligaments are deficient, an augmentation with the use of an auto- or allograft tendon may be considered; however, meticulous reconstruction of isometricity is mandatory for normal joint motion.
- Surgical techniques using the peroneal tendons should be strictly avoided, as they alter functional control.
- Tenodesis techniques should be abandoned.
- First results with newer arthroscopic techniques are promising; but there is need to show their efficacy over time.
- Additional bony corrections might be considered in a preexistent varus deformity.

2.9.1 Acute Ankle Sprain

In some instances, especially in high-level athletes, surgical treatment may be indicated, as is also the case for the presence of concomitant osteochondral lesions.

Primary surgical repair is considered in high-performance athletes (Fig. 2.28) or in the case of associated injuries that need surgical reconstruction (Fig. 2.29).

2.9.2 Avulsion Fractures of the Fibula

In the majority of the cases, avulsion fractures of the fibula (Fig. 2.11) should be treated by primary repair with reattachment of the fragment (Fig. 2.30) or, if it too small, with ligament reattachment after excision of the fragment (Fig. 2.31). This has been mainly proposed since several authors have observed that nonoperative treatment does not yield satisfactory results [73, 74, 115, 116]. As much as 66% of the patients who underwent lateral ankle ligament repair or reconstruction due to symptomatic lateral ankle instability had the presence of an osseous pathology consisting of accessory ossicles or avulsion fractures of the lateral malleolus [117].

2.9.3 Chronic Lateral Ankle Instability

The clinical management of patients with chronically unstable ankles should include identifying symptoms of both mechanical and functional instabilities. Once specific insufficiencies have been identified, treatment efforts should focus on addressing these impairments and emphasis should be placed on reducing the risk of recurrent ankle sprains.

Chronic ankle instability is initially treated nonoperatively, with surgical management reserved for those who have failed to improve after 3–6 months of bracing and functional rehabilitation [118]. Anatomic repair using a modified Broström procedure is the preferred technique for initial surgery with enough ligament quality (Fig. 2.32) [19]. Especially the modification as proposed by Gould [119] has been very popular, even though the effect of side-to-side suture of the inferior extensor retinaculum to the anterior fibula must be questioned (Fig. 2.33) [120]. Anatomic reconstruction with a tendon graft should be considered when repair is not possible anymore, as it maintains the physiological joint kinematics. The author's preference is the use of a free autologous plantaris tendon graft which meets the thickness and mechanical properties of the ATFL best [36] (Fig. 2.34). Usually the graft is long enough to be used as a doubled graft when only the ATFL is reconstructed (Fig. 2.35). If additionally the CFL needs reconstruction (Fig. 2.36), the graft must have a length of 17–19 cm. Very satisfying results have been reported with this technique, and no ankle has had to be revised for impingement or restraint motion [21, 121]. Others prefer the use of a free semitendinosus graft which is stronger, but also thicker than ATFL and CFL. In fear of breaking the bone when pulling through bony tunnels, interference screws are mostly used for fixation [122]. Recently, the use of internal braces has been found to be effective to protect the repaired ligaments from elongation and thus enable the patients to recover earlier and go back to pre-injury sport levels (Fig. 2.37) [123–125].

Nonanatomic reconstructions should be avoided, as the nonanatomic ATFL repair state demonstrated significant inversion and internal rotation kinematics and internal rota-

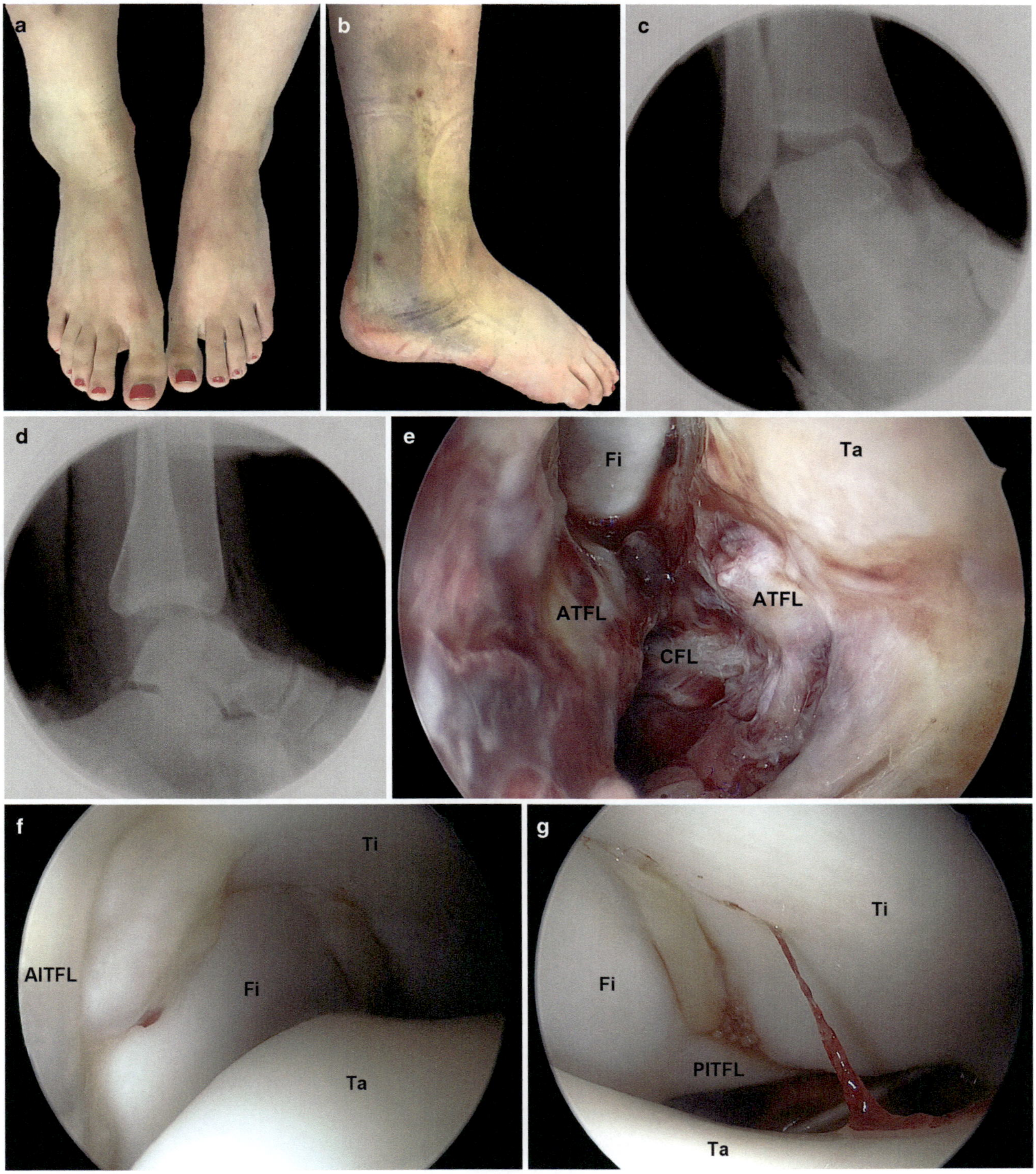

Fig. 2.28 *Surgical Technique: Arthroscopic assessment and primary repair of the lateral ankle ligaments*. Acute severe ankle sprain in a 22-year-old female high-level uni-hockey player after previous conservatively treated sprains. (**a**) Swelling over the lateral ankle ligaments immediately after the accident. (**b**) After 4 days, extension of the hematoma with pain on palpation over the lateral ankle ligaments, but not at the syndesmotic ligaments. Analogously, some hematoma and tenderness over the deltoid ligament (not visible). (**c**) Preoperatively, when applying manual stress, a varus tilt of 18° can be seen. (**d**) The drawer test shows a significant extrusion of the talus. (**e**) Arthroscopy shows an intraligamentary tear of the scarred ATFL involving the CFL. (**f**) Under moderate varus stress, an important gapping of the lateral joint space is seen, while the anterior inferior tibiofibular (syndesmotic) ligament (AITFL) is intact. (**g**) The posterior inferior tibiofibular (syndesmotic) ligament (PITFL) is also found to be intact. (**h**) Medially an acute rupture of the superficial deltoid ligament (asterisk) at its proximal insertion is seen. (**i**) Exploration of the lateral ankle ligaments shows the intraligamentary rupture of the scarred ATFL extending towards the CFL posteriorly. (**j**) The ATFL and CFL ligaments after reattachment by an anchor suture and additional superficial sutures. The peroneal tendon sheath is also reconstructed. (**k**) On the medial side, surgical exposure confirms the proximal rupture of the superficial deltoid ligament, with partial detachment typically seen at the anterior colliculus of the medial malleolus (see Fig. 5.49). Ligament repair was done by reattachment through a suture anchor (not shown). (**l**) postoperative testing under fluoroscopy demonstrates a stable position of the talus within the ankle mortise. *F* fibula, *Ti* tibia, *Ta* talus, *MM* medial malleolus

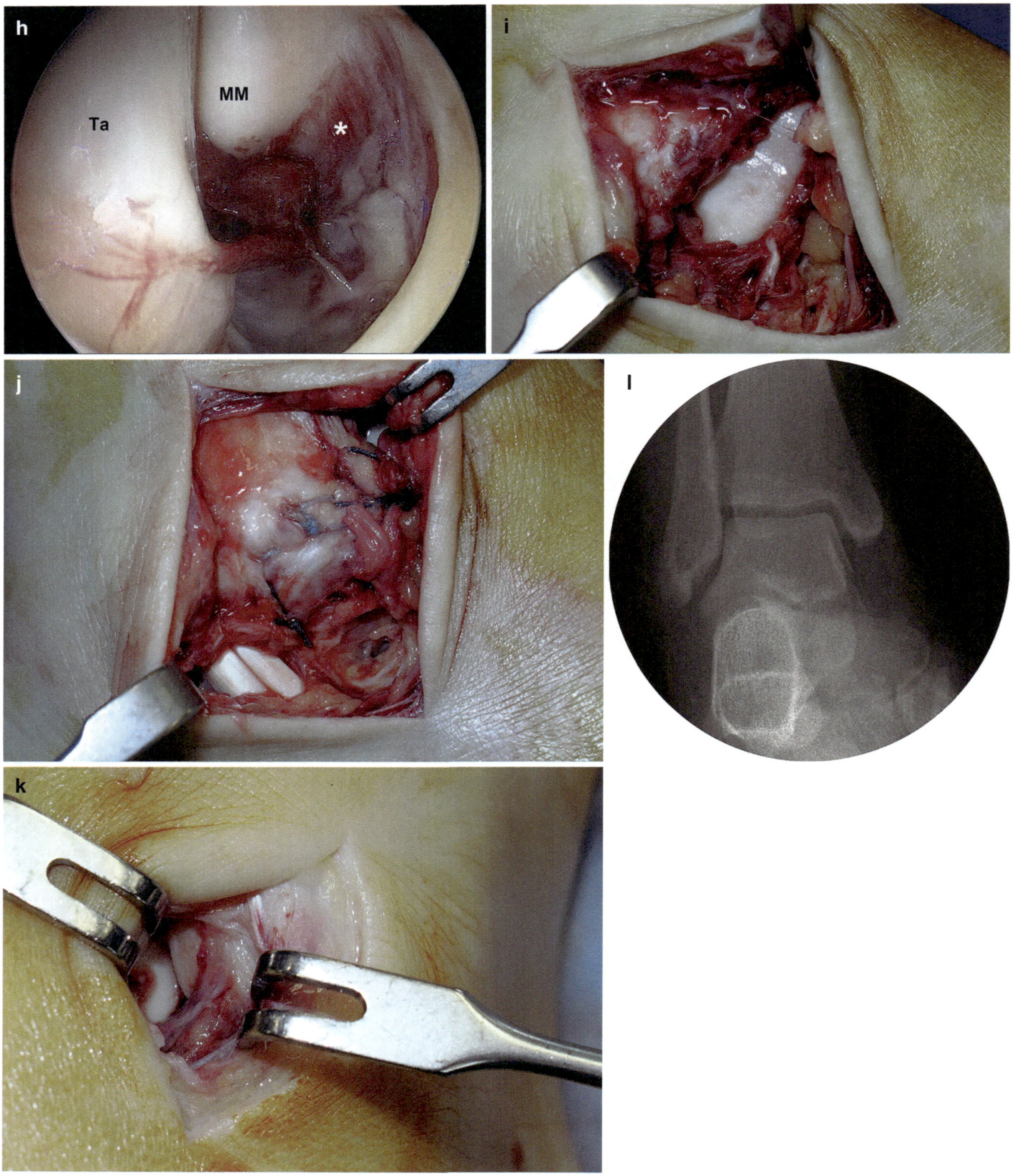

Fig. 2.28 (continued)

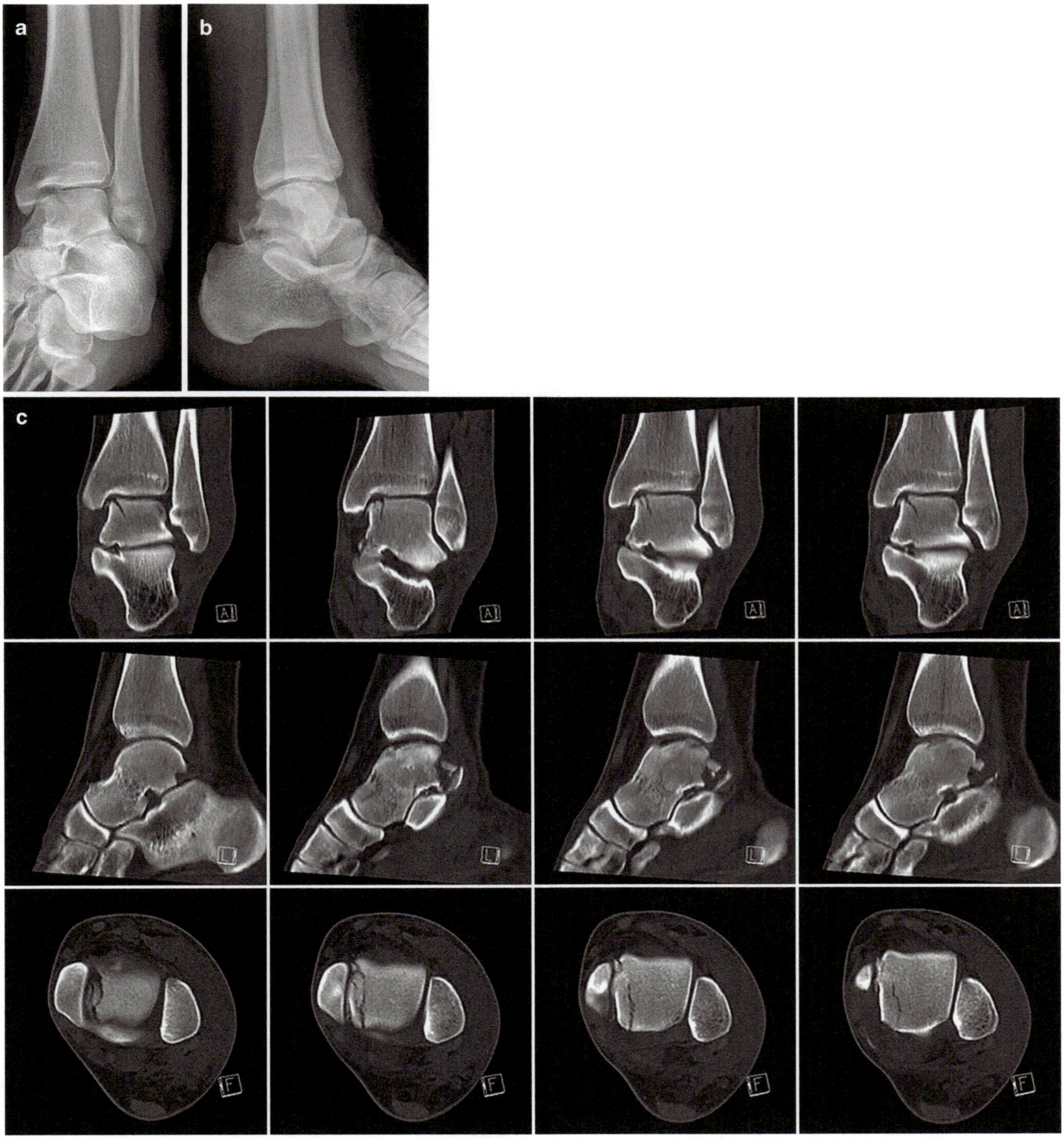

Fig. 2.29 *Surgical Technique: Arthroscopic ORIF talus and repair of lateral ankle ligaments.* Acute inversion trauma in a 16-year-old female athlete after falling while bouldering. (**a**) AP view showing an impression fracture of the medial shoulder of the talus and soft tissue swelling over the lateral malleolus. (**b**) Lateral view. (**c**) CT scans showing the extent of the multi-fragmentary talar fracture. (**d**) Arthroscopic view of the medial talar shoulder showing the main fragment that is impressed and dislocated. (**e**) The fragment is mobilized and reduced by aid of a hook. (**f**) A K-wire is inserted percutaneously for preliminary fixation (arrow). (**g**) A cannulated 3.0-mm screw is inserted for final fixation. (**h**) An AP and (**i**) lateral fluoroscopic view after final fixation of the fracture by three screws. (**j**) Exploration of the lateral ankle ligaments evidences a distal avulsion of the ATFL from the talar neck. (**k**) A suture anchor fixed to the talar neck is used for surgical repair of the ATFL. (**l**) Final repair. (**m**) CT scan 8 weeks after surgery showing complete healing of the fracture. (**n**) AP- and (**o**) lateral radiograph showing the healing of the fracture after 8 weeks

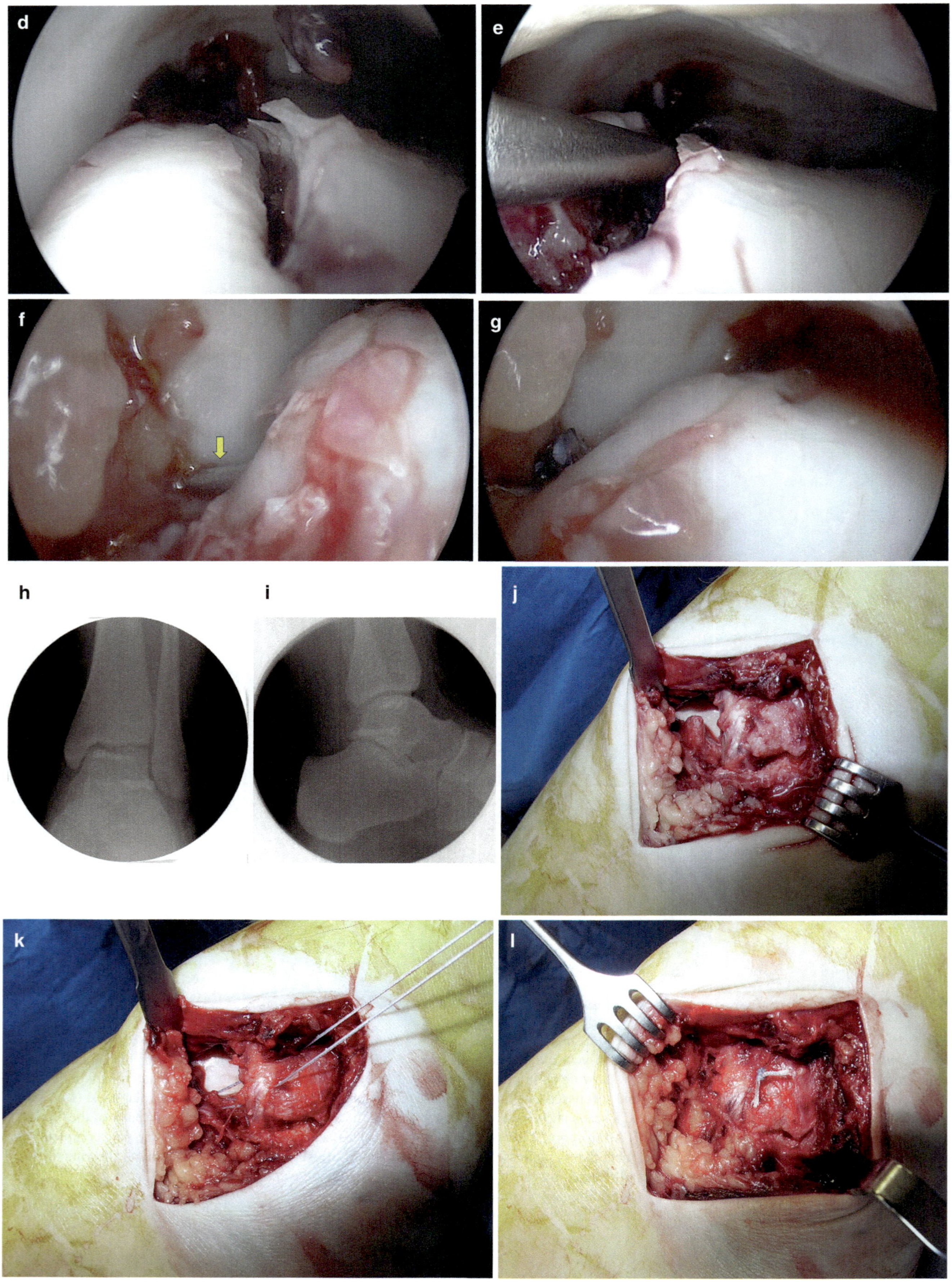

Fig. 2.29 (continued)

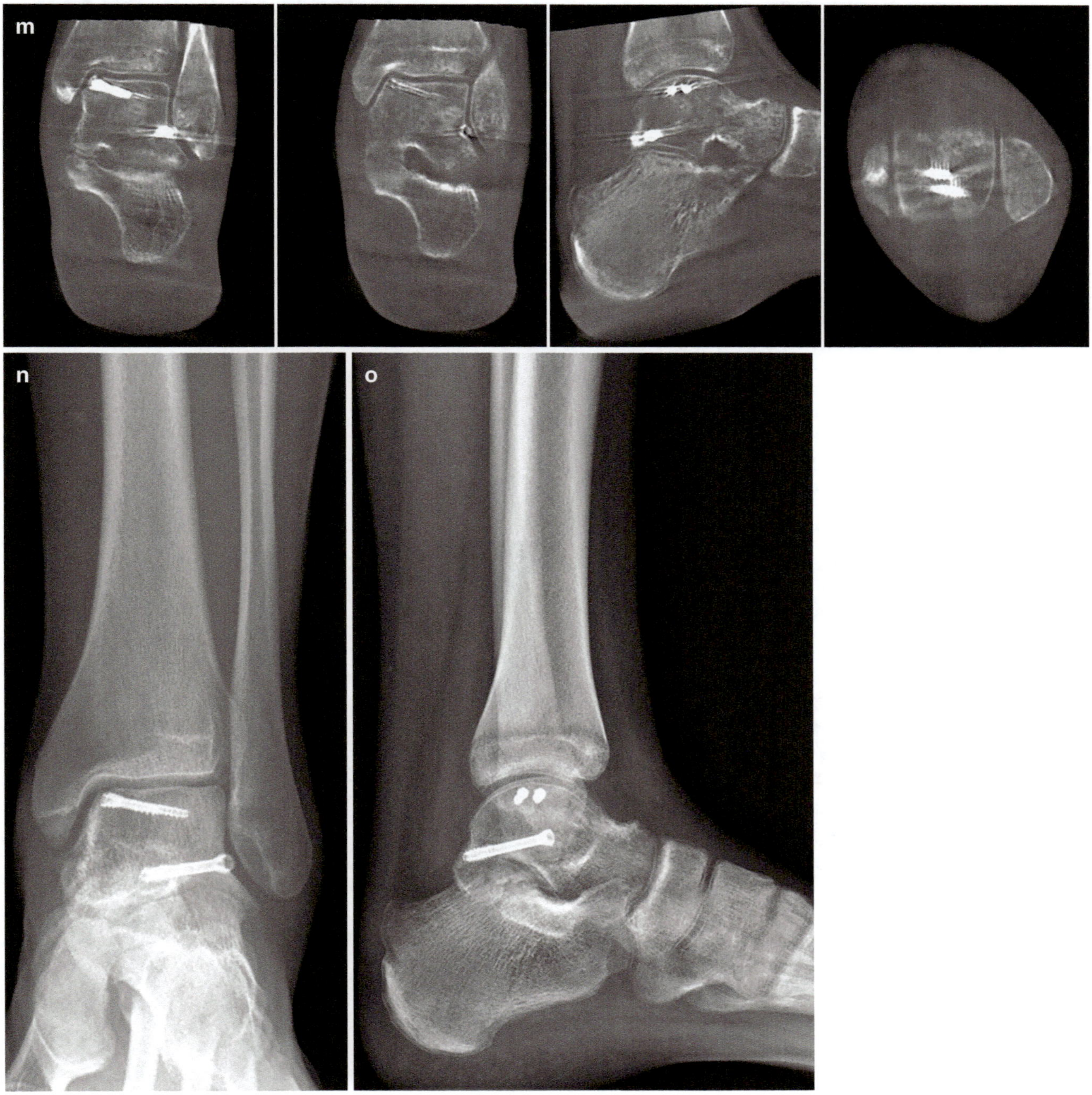

Fig. 2.29 (continued)

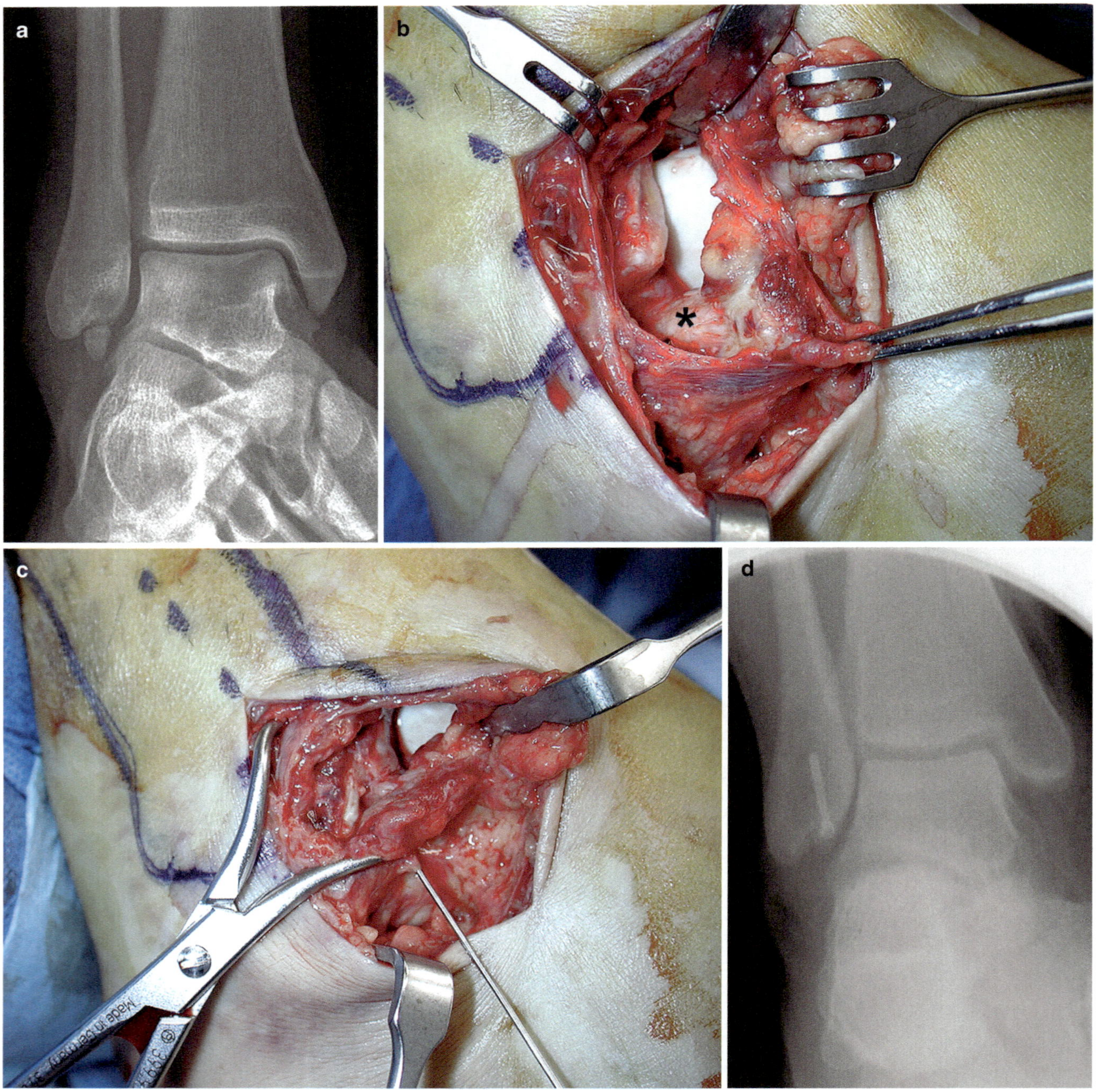

Fig. 2.30 *Surgical Technique: Repair of the lateral ankle ligaments after bony avulsion with fragment refixation*. Acute ankle sprain after previously experiencing a sprain 3 months earlier in a 16-year-old female soccer player. (**a**) AP view showing a big bony fragment and soft tissue swelling indicating a bony avulsion of the lateral ankle ligaments. (**b**) Surgical exploration shows the fragment (asterisk); additionally, showing a complete detachment of the ATFL and CFL thus not leaving any connection to the fibula. (**c**) After debridement of the articular surface of both, the fibular and fragment side, the fragment is reduced and held by a reduction clamp, allowing to insert a K-wire and, thereafter, to insert a cannulated screw. (**d**) Fluoroscopic control shows the fragment reattached to the fibula

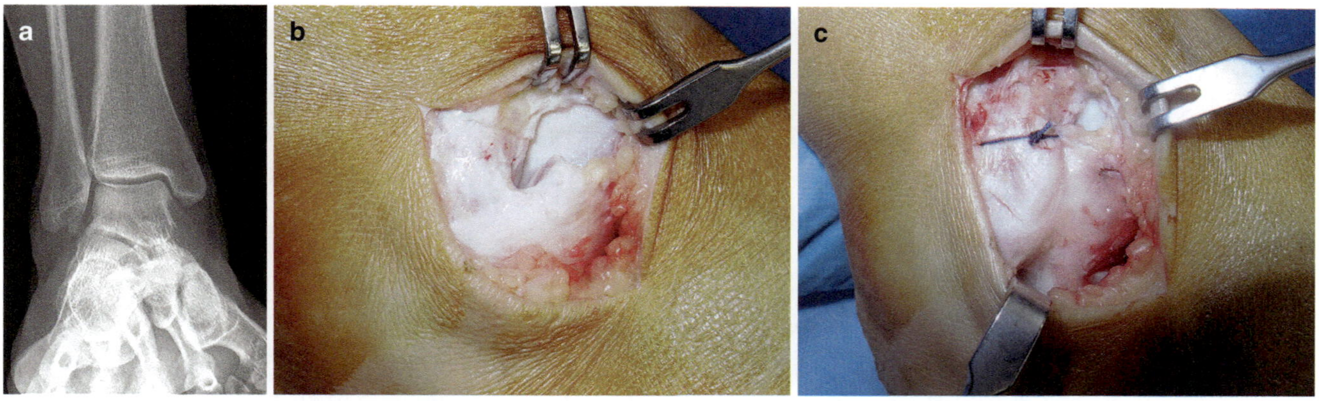

Fig. 2.31 *Surgical Technique: Repair of the lateral ankle ligaments after bony avulsion by excision of the fragment.* Eight weeks after an ankle sprain in a 17-year-old female volleyball player who complains about continuous local pain and instability. (**a**) AP view showing a small subfibular fragment indicating a complete avulsion of the lateral ankle ligaments, thus indicating surgical repair. (**b**) Surgical exploration shows the scared superficial layers of the ATFL and CFL, while the main substances of both ligaments are detached from the fibula. (**c**) As the fragment is very small, it is excised, and the ligaments are reattached to the fibula by transosseous sutures

tion laxity when compared with the intact state (Fig. 2.38) [120, 126]. Minimally invasive surgical treatment [127, 128] and arthroscopic repair or reconstruction [128–134] of the lateral ankle ligaments is a promising new technique with results similar to those of open surgery (Fig. 2.39), with the advantage of earlier recovery [128]. However, the evidence supporting this technique is still limited [135, 136]. The near future will show whether these new minimally invasive and arthroscopic techniques are capable of reproducing the same stability in the long term as open reconstruction surgery has.

2.9.4 Concomitant Injuries and Pathologies

2.9.4.1 Peroneal Tendon Injuries

The incidence of peroneal tendon injuries after acute ankle sprains has been reported to be as high as 15% and, in most instances, is accompanied by incomplete tears of the peroneus brevis tendon (Fig. 2.40). If conservative treatment fails, surgical reconstruction is advised. If partially ruptured, the tendon is debrided, and tubular sutures are done to obtain a solid tendon (Fig. 2.41). If less than one-third of the tendon remains intact, a transfer of the peroneal longus tendon to the peroneal brevis tendon is considered (Fig. 2.42) [137].

2.9.4.2 Osteochondral Lesions (OCL)

Osteochondral fractures after an acute ankle sprain can typically be found at the anterolateral talar dome (Fig. 2.43) or also on the medial talar dome [84]. There is general agreement that if the bony fragment is thicker than 3 mm, it should be reattached by solid screw fixation. However, the treatment of chronic OCL remains controversial. Debridement with microfracturing is mostly preferred for superficial lesions of up to 15 mm in diameter [138–140], filling of the defect by osteochondral plugs (mosaicoplasty) or cancellous bone is used for greater defects and cystic lesions [141, 142]. For deep cystic lesions, allografts are used for reconstruction of the talar surface [143, 144]. A promising alternative is the use of a vascularized cortical-periosteal graft from the medial femur condyle [145].

2.9.4.3 Inframalleolar Misalignment

In a varus deformity of the heel originating from a calcaneus varus (inframalleolar deformity), a closing wedge osteotomy with an angle of 45° to the ground was proposed by Dwyer to realign the heel (Fig. 2.44) [146]. However, its capacity for heel valgization is limited, and in addition, it shortens the heel which may have an adversary effect in athletic patients. In contrast, the Italian Z-shaped osteotomy with removal of a wedge in the horizontal plane permits more extended valgization of the heel without shortening it [147, 148].

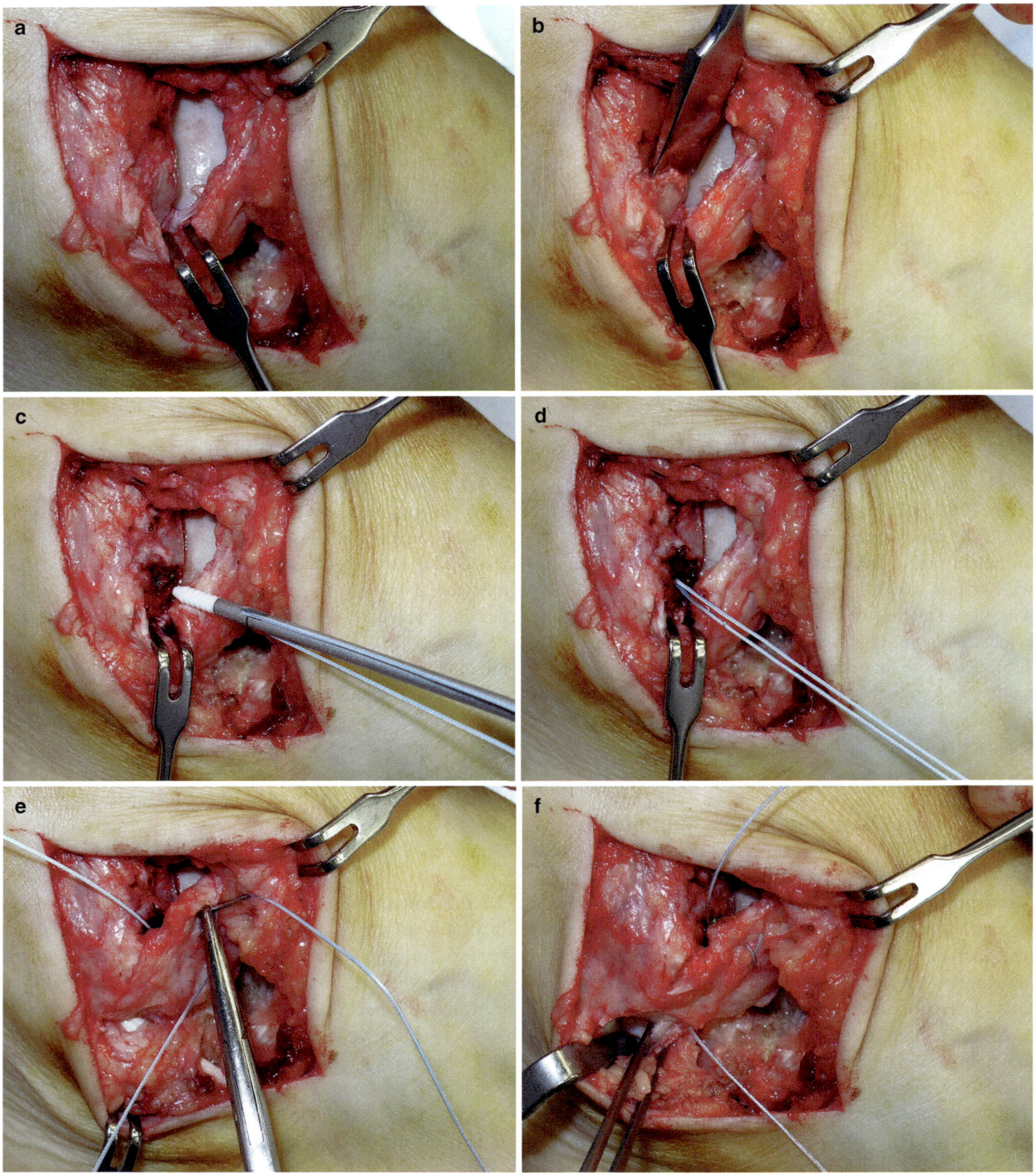

Fig. 2.32 *Surgical Technique: Primary reconstruction of lateral ankle ligaments*. This 44-year-old former handball player suffers from severe chronic ankle instability with progressive valgus and abductus deformity of his right foot. Thus, a moderate lateral column lengthening osteotomy was performed prior to lateral ligament reconstruction, and a medial ligament reconstruction was done thereafter. This figure series shows the lateral ligament reconstruction. (**a**) The ATFL/CFL ligament complex is detached from the anterior aspect of the distal fibula, with only some superficial connecting soft tissue left. (**b**) The insertion area on the fibula is debrided with the use of a chisel. (**c**) A suture anchor is placed 10 mm above the tip of the fibula, close to the articular surface. (**d**) Thigh fit is checked by pulling on suture. (**e**) With one suture end, first the ATFL is taken, (**f**) thereafter, the other end is brought to the CFL which is then taken with one or two slings. (**g**) When pulling on both sutures, the ATFL/CFL complex is seen to be tightened. (**h**) Each of the sutures is now brought, with a transosseous stitch, to the lateral aspect of the fibula. (**i**) While the foot is held in a neutral position, pull is applied on both sutures until overall lateral ankle ligaments are seen tightened. (**j**) The suture is secured by a knot. (**k**) As the insertion area of the ATFL is large (Fig. 2.1), the superficial fibers of the ATFL are still loose. (**l**) With a continuous resorbable suture, this part of the ligament is reattached to the periosteum, which is usually very strong. Transosseous sutures can also be used if necessary

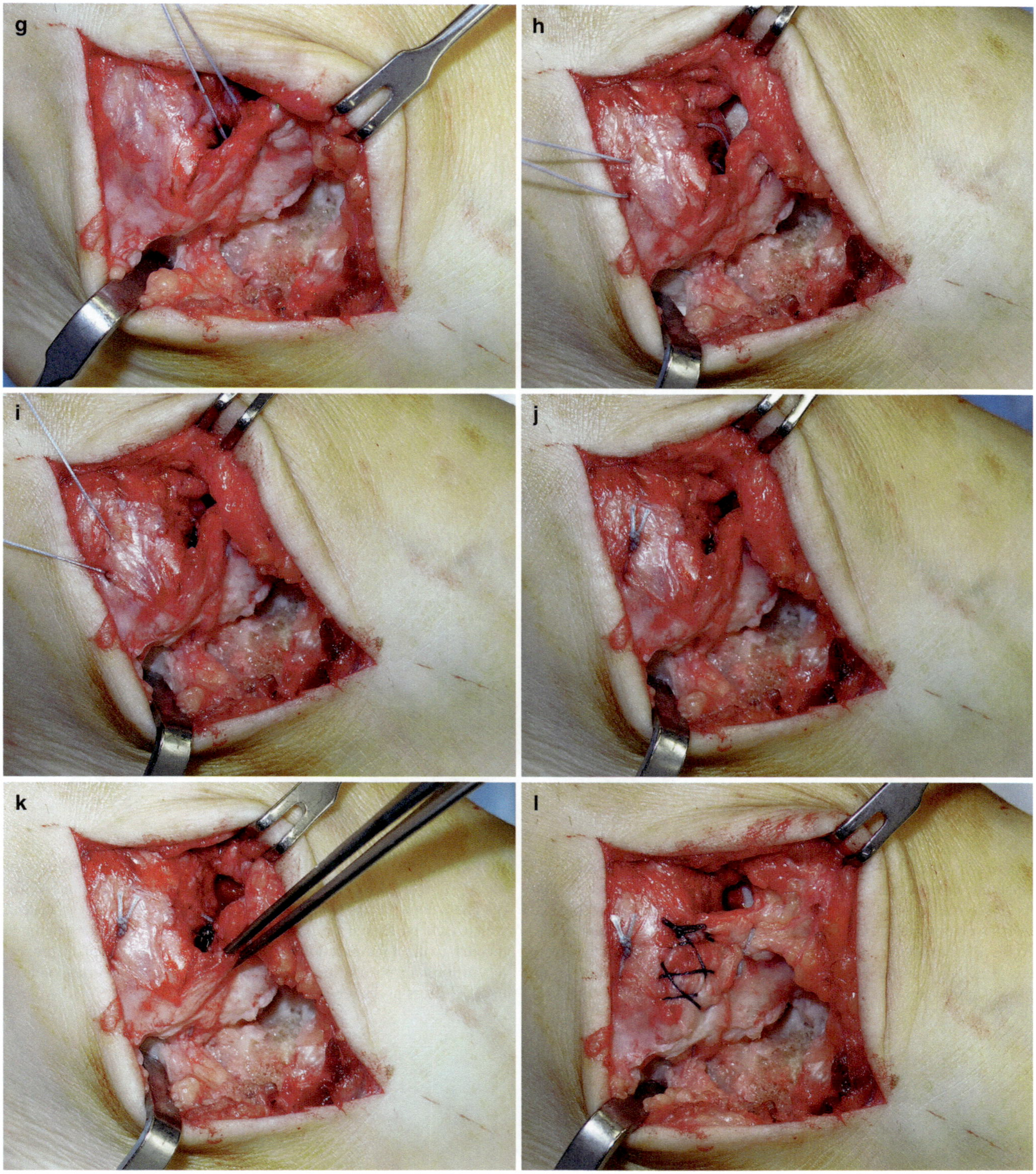

Fig. 2.32 (continued)

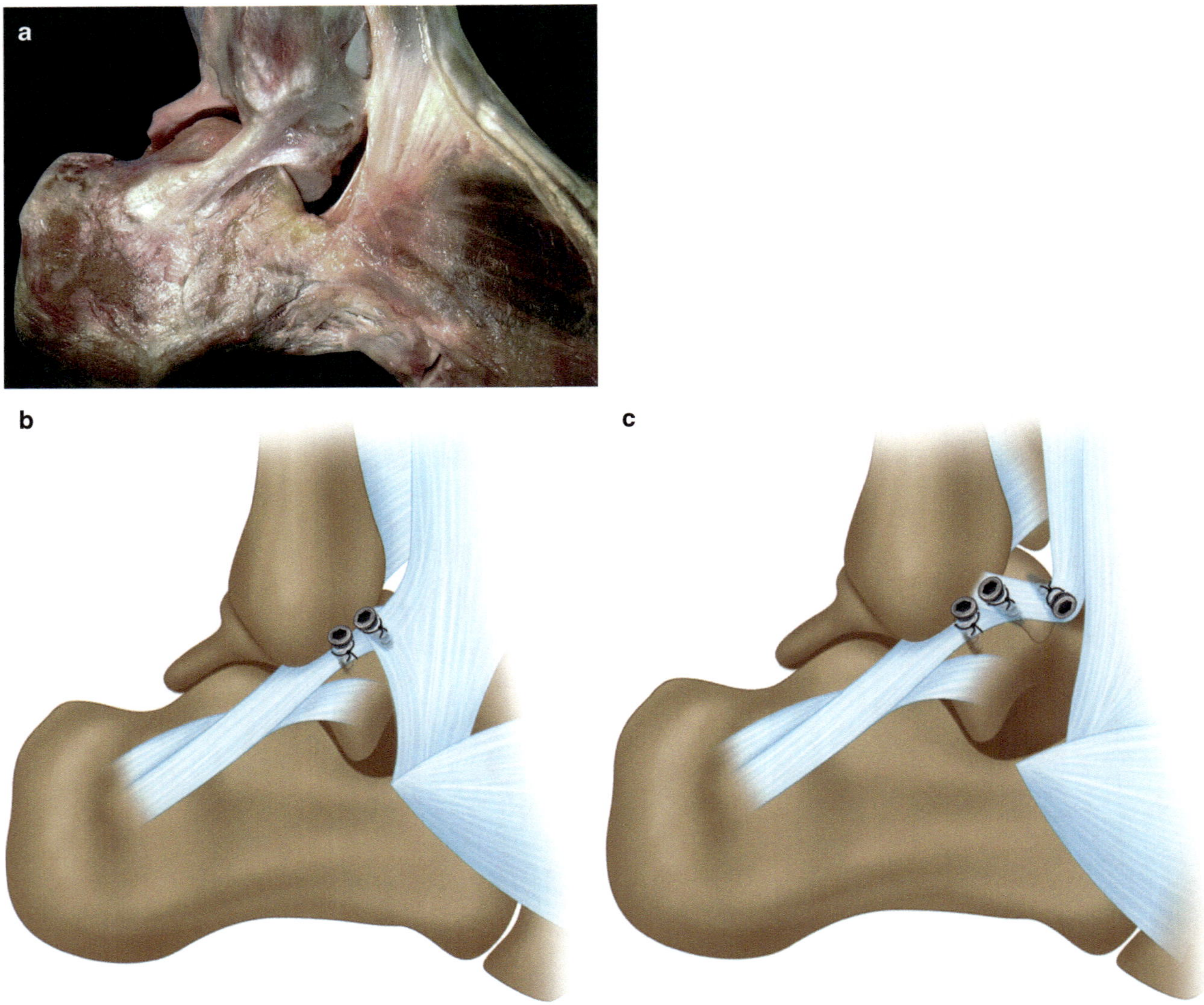

Fig. 2.33 *Surgical Technique: The modified Gould procedure.* (**a**) Anatomic preparation of the inferior extensor retinaculum showing that its fibers run perpendicular to the direction of the ATFL fibers. The inferior extensor retinaculum runs close to the distal insertion of the ATFL at the talar neck. In chronically unstable ankles, these two layers are usually completely separated and some connective tissue can be found in between. (**b**) The original procedure of Gould [119] uses a shift of the intact retinaculum that is fixed to the proximal insertion of the ATFL at the anterior fibula, thereby reinforcing the repaired ATFL. (**c**) The author prefers to modify the technique and use a strip instead which is fixed first at the talar neck and then to the anterior fibula, thereby giving it the direction of the ATFL. With this, the tensile properties of the transferred strip of the inferior retinaculum corresponds to the load stress of the reconstructed and reinforced ATFL

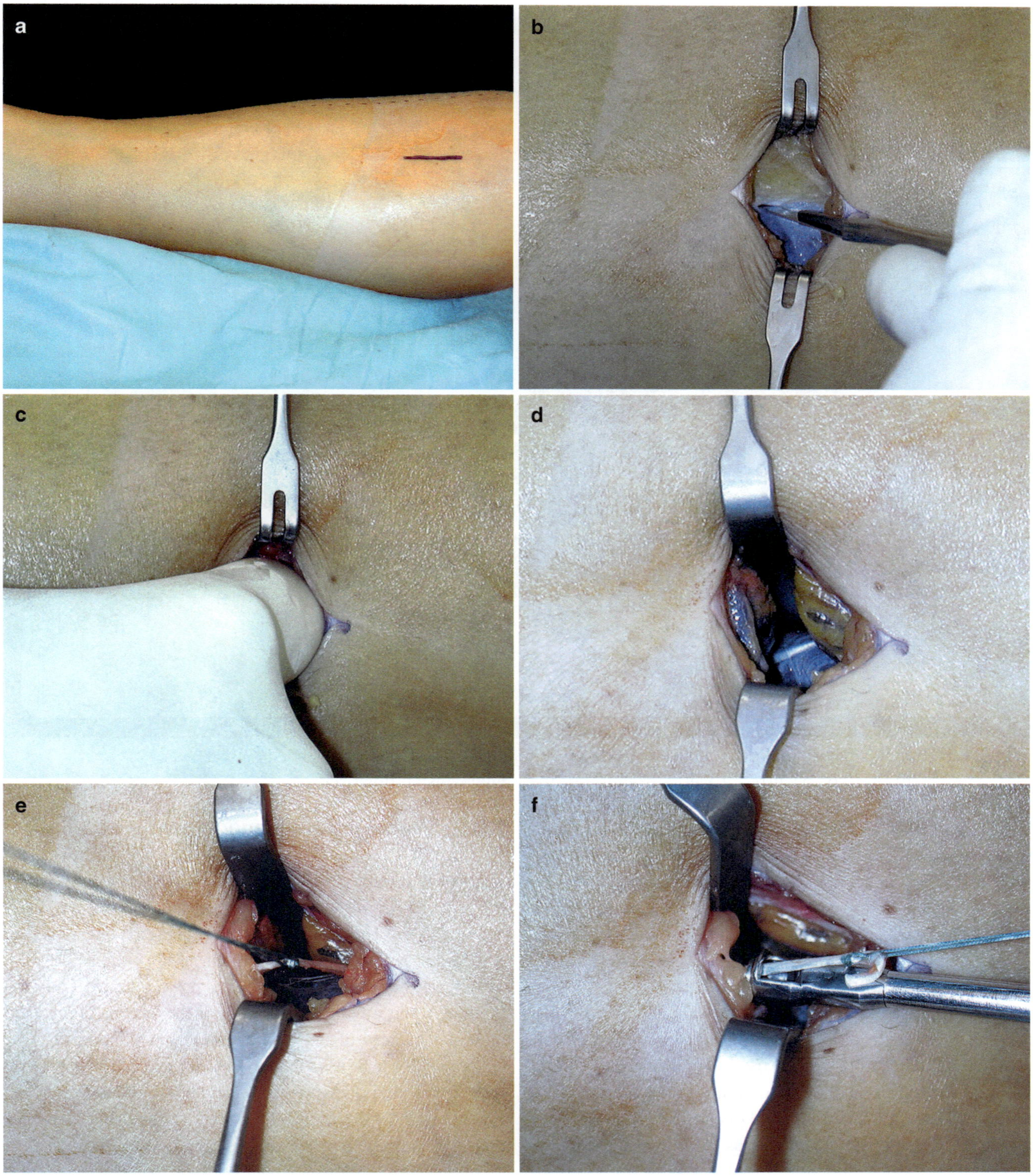

Fig. 2.34 *Surgical Technique: Harvesting a free plantaris tendon graft*. (**a**) A 3–4 cm long longitudinal incision is done approximately 2 cm posterior to the posteromedial tibia and starting proximately at the level of the tibia curvature. (**b**) The fascia is exposed by careful dissection, taking care not to injure the saphenal nerve. A longitudinal dissection is done. (**c**) The gap between the soleus and gastrocnemius muscles is identified and mobilized with the aid of the index finger, a maneuver that is facilitated by wiping movements of the finger. (**d**) The plantaris tendon can be exposed by insertion of two Langenbeck hooks. (**e**) A suture is made to the plantaris tendon as proximal as possible, typically where the distal end of the tiny muscle belly is seen. (**f**) After dissection of the tendon proximal to the suture, the stripper is introduced. (**g**) The stripper is carefully pushed distally following the direction to the medial aspect of the heel until it reaches the area of the cranial aspect of the calcaneus. The tendon is cut by the special feature of the stripper and then harvested by pulling the stripper back. (**h**) The fascia is closed paying attention not to catch the saphenal nerve and the skin is closed thereafter. (**i**) The harvested plantaris tendon graft is usually 20–30 cm long and 2–4 mm thick. Alternatively, the plantaris tendon graft can be harvested from distally; however, the author believes that identification of the plantaris tendon distally is often critical as it is connected to the Achilles tendon

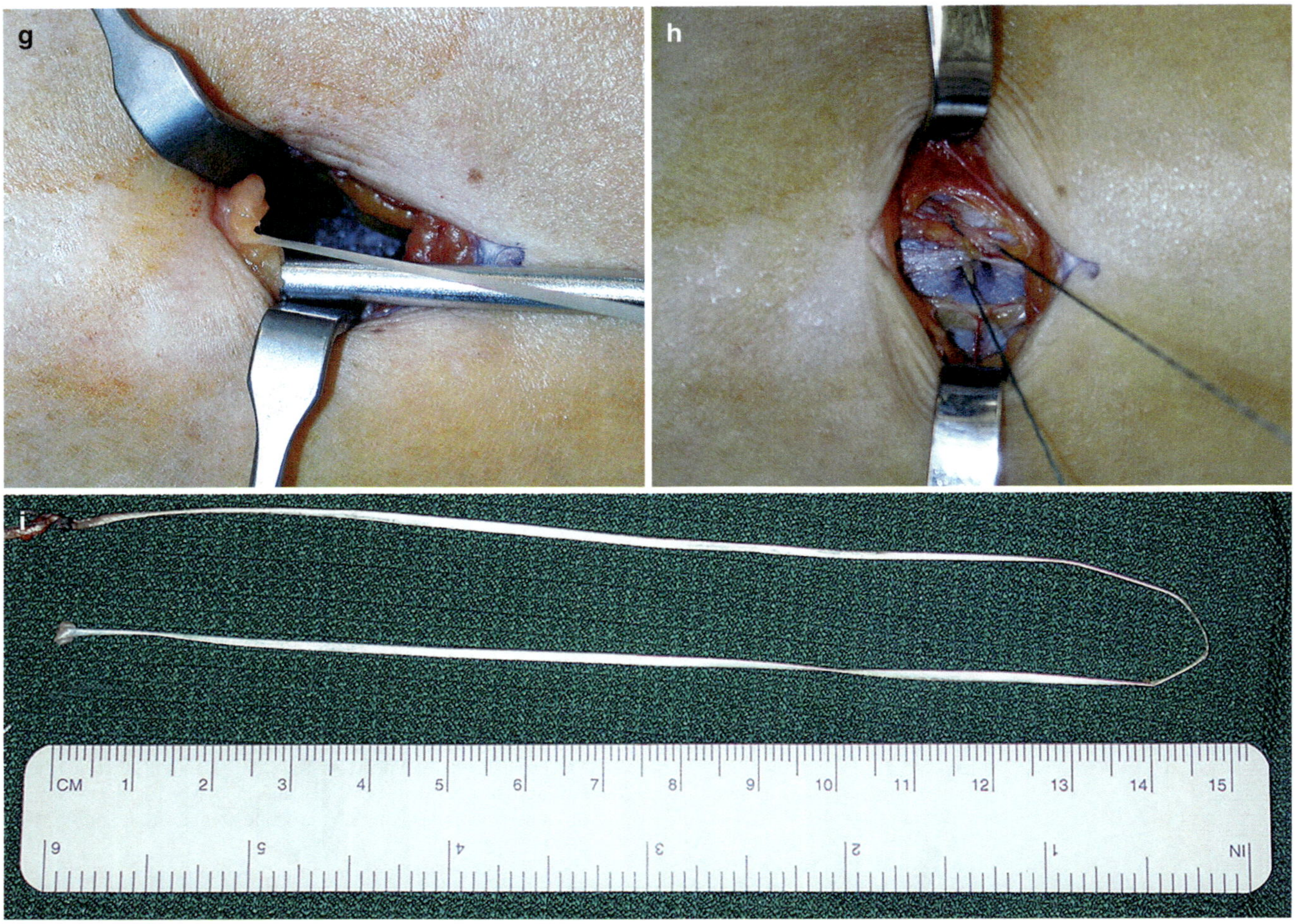

Fig. 2.34 (continued)

Furthermore, its effect in realigning the heel can be increased by an additional lateral shift (Fig. 2.45) [149]. In a cavovarus foot, additional bone removal in the horizontal part of the Z-shaped osteotomy may be beneficial to decrease the height of the calcaneus (Fig. 2.46).

2.9.4.4 Supramalleolar Misalignment

In a varus misaligned hindfoot originating from a varus deformity of the distal tibia (Fig. 2.47), a correcting osteotomy of the distal tibia can be used to normalize the tibial articular surface angle (TAS) and to move the loading axis of the ankle laterally. While a medial open wedge osteotomy of the distal tibia may be advantageous for minor angular corrections (Fig. 2.48), a dome osteotomy may be preferred for greater corrections to avoid critical prolonged bone healing (Fig. 2.49). This technique is especially beneficial for an angular correction of varus deformities while the congruency of the tibiotalar joint is preserved.

2.9.5 Postoperative Management

The foot is protected by a boot or stabilizing shoe for 6 weeks and allowed for full weight-bearing as soon as pain-free loading is possible. The rehabilitation program starts after 2 weeks. It includes passive and active mobilization of the ankle joint, training of the muscular strength and protection, by a stabilizing shoe when walking. Depending on the amount of regained muscular balance of the hindfoot, a brace or taping may be recommended to be used for 4–6 weeks after boot or stabilizing shoe removal. Following this, the author recommends the patient to further use the brace for walks on uneven ground, for high-risk sports activities and for professional work outside.

In the case of additional surgeries such as supramalleolar correcting osteotomies or osteochondral fracture fixation, the ankle is always protected by a boot or plaster for 6–8 weeks with partial weight-bearing being permitted during this period of time.

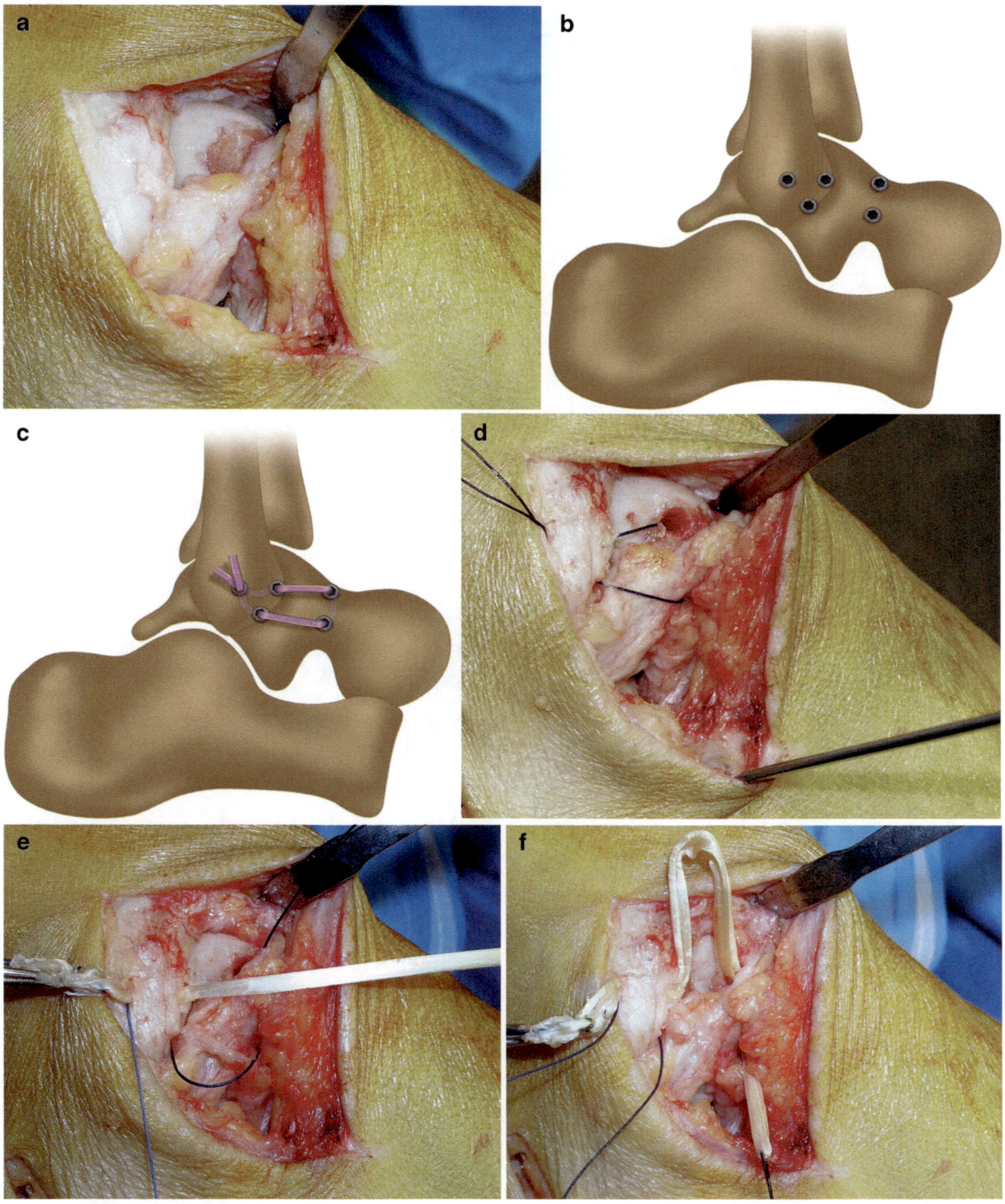

Fig. 2.35 *Surgical Technique: Reconstruction of ATFL with a free plantaris tendon graft.* This 38-year-old former volleyball player sustained multiple sprains. After a Broström procedure 6 years earlier, he is complaining of an instability feeling and recurrent sprains. To address the varus position of the heel, a calcaneal closing wedge osteotomy was performed before the ligament reconstruction. (**a**) Surgical exposure of lateral ankle ligaments shows some scarred ATFL tissue left that has little superficial connection to the fibula and the insertion area to talar neck. (**b**) Two 3.5-mm drill holes are made in the talus and three holes in the fibula; on the talar side, the first hole is done 3–4 mm below the tibiotalar articular surface, and the second hole is done in an oblique direction on the upper border of the sinus tarsi. Putting a K-wire in the first hole can help to guide the second drill precisely to meet the hole. The bony tunnel can be smoothened with the insertion of a small reduction clamp. On the fibula, the first hole is drilled from the lateral aspect in the center of the fibula 10–12 mm above its tip, slightly in an oblique direction towards anterior. A K-wire is inserted. This allows to drill a first hole from the anterior aspect of the fibula starting 14–15 mm above its tip, and a second hole 8–9 mm above its tip, while aiming to meet the K-wire. Both tunnels can be smoothened by the small reduction clamp. (**c**) A drawing showing the pathway of the plantaris tendon. (**d**) A suture is now brought from the fibula through the upper tunnel to the talar neck, from where, after having passed the tunnel, it is directed back through the lower tunnel. (**e**) The plantaris tendon graft is passed through the sling so that both ends have the same length before they are fixed together by a clamp. The graft is now brought through the upper tunnel by pulling on the suture. (**f**) Analogously it is passed through the tunnel at the talar neck. (**g**) Finally, it is brought through the lower tunnel. (**h**) While the foot is held in neutral position, the tendon graft is tightened by pulling on both ends. (**i**) Sutures through both ends of the graft to the periosteum are used to fix the graft in this position. Notice the oblique position of the superior loop of the graft that corresponds to the original direction of the ATFL (Fig. 2.1). (**j**) Additional resorbable sutures are used to reattach the remaining ligament tissue to the fibula. Notice the strong CFL ligament that crosses the subtalar joint in a perpendicular direction when the foot is held in a neutral position. (**k**) After having finished the reconstruction, functional testing shows no constraints when the foot is brought into supination and (**l**) pronation position, respectively

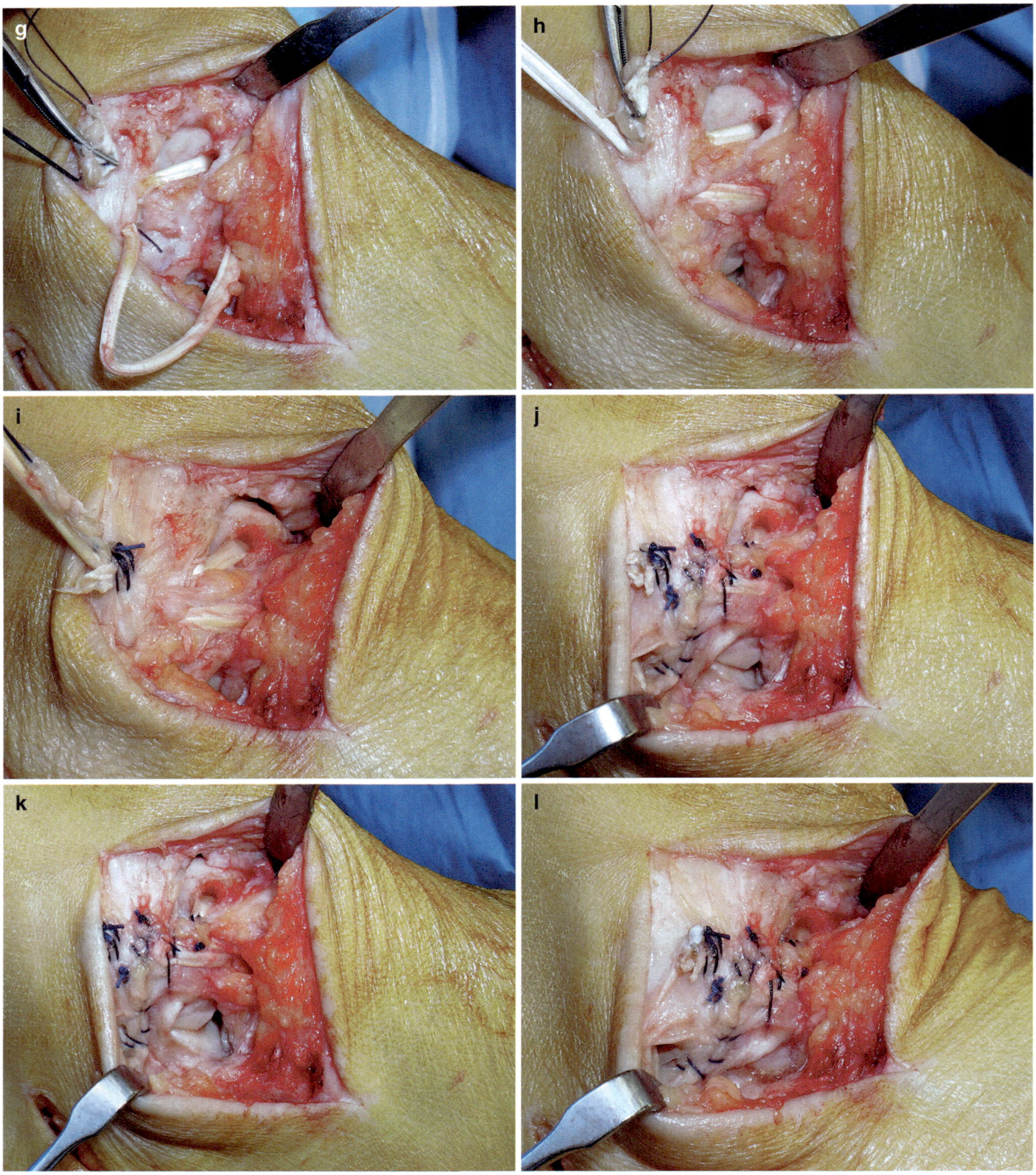

Fig. 2.35 (continued)

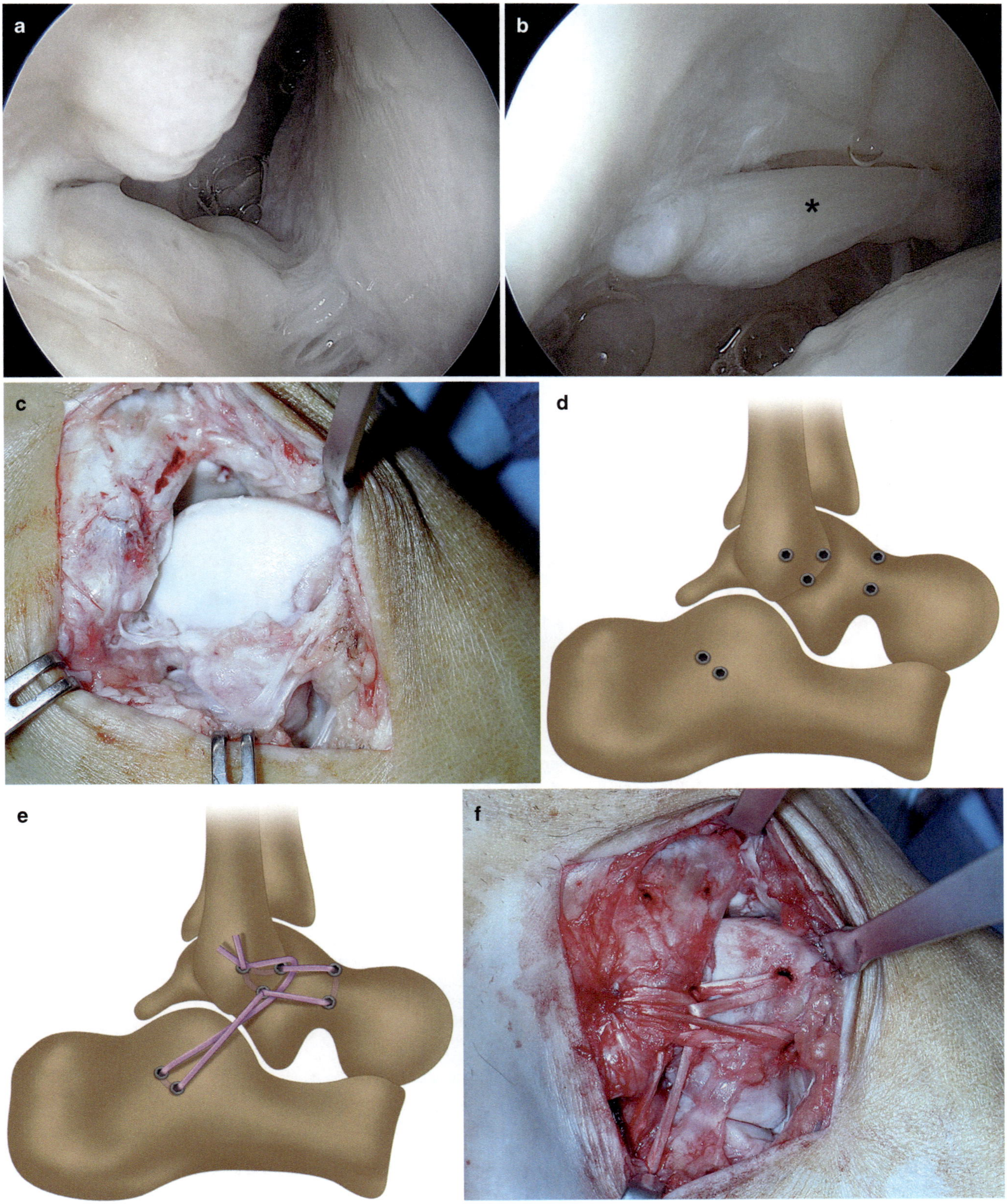

Fig. 2.36 *Surgical Technique: Reconstruction of ATFL and CFL with a free plantaris tendon graft.* This 48-year-old former male soccer player sustained several ankle sprains in the past before complaining about instability feeling and pain. (**a**) Arthroscopy showed the distal fibula completely free from the lateral ankle ligaments and the PTFL could no longer be detected. (**b**) The highly unstable ankle allowed to insert the arthroscope easily into the posterolateral joint. The partially detached and retracted PTFL (asterisk) is visible. (**c**) Surgical exposure confirms that lateral ankle ligaments are mostly gone, and only some scarred connective tissue is left. Notice the anterolateral extrusion of the talus. (**d**) Therefore, a free plantaris tendon graft is used for reconstruction of both, the ATFL and CFL. For the latter, two drill holes were made 13 mm caudally to the subtalar point so that the constructed ligament could cross the subtalar joint perpendicularly. (**e**) After having done the sling to reconstruct the ATFL, the plantaris graft was routed over this sling before being directed to the calcaneus and then brought through the inferior tunnel in the fibula, thereby ensuring for a strictly anatomical course of the reconstructed CFL. (**f**) Final situation showing the anatomical position of both the reconstructed ATFL and CFL

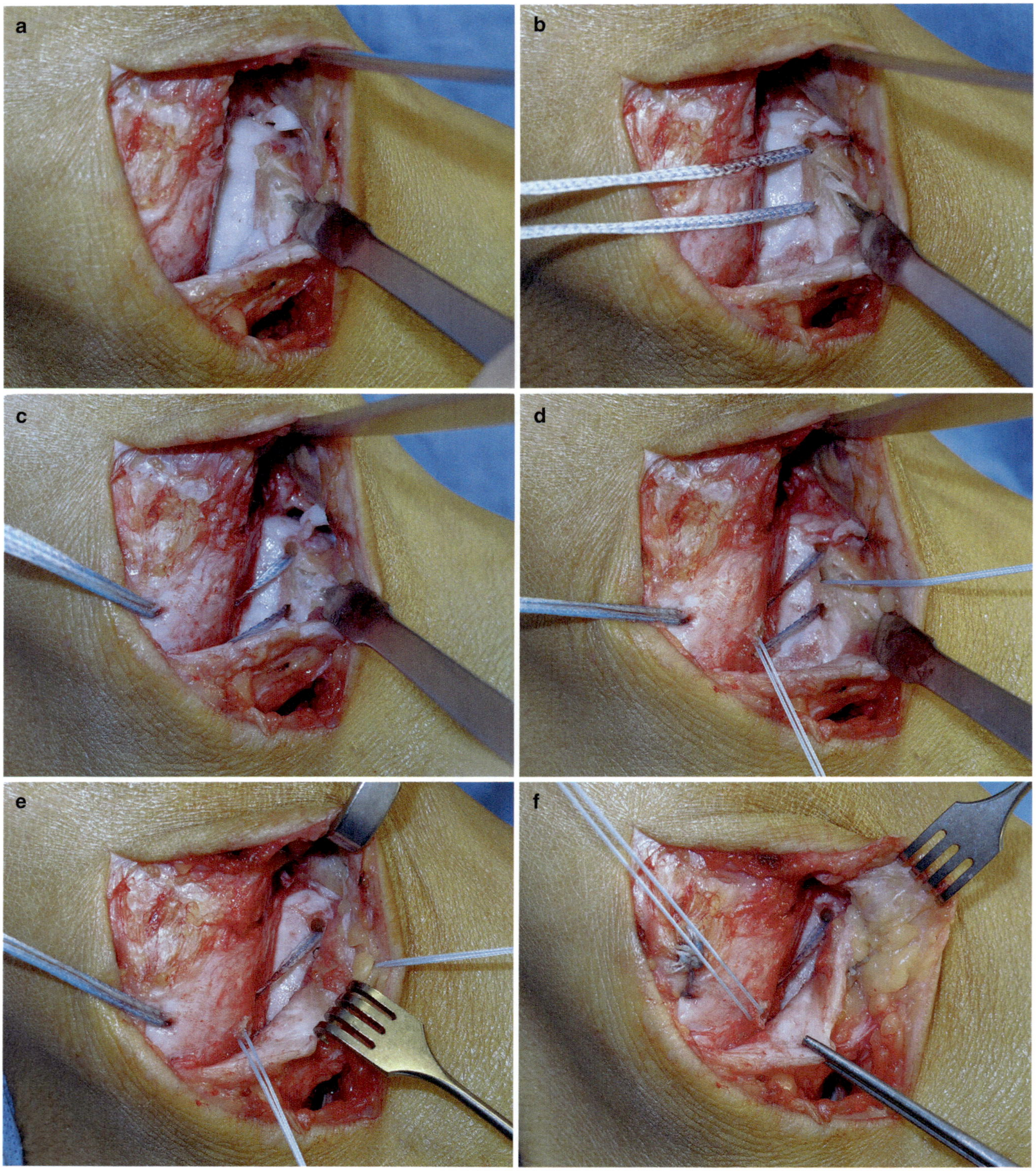

Fig. 2.37 *Surgical Technique: Reconstruction of ATFL with augmentation with an internal brace.* This 28-year-old active high-level soccer player could not resume his activity after experiencing a severe sprain with a history of recurrent sprains. (**a**) Surgical exposure reveals a rather strong, but scarred ligament complex that is completely detached from the fibula and from the talar neck. (**b**) An internal brace is routed through the talar tunnel made by a 2.5-mm drill on the talar neck. (**c**) One end is brought through the proximal and one through the distal tunnel of the distal fibula; after having tightened the internal brace by pulling, the talus is well centralized in the mortise and joint motion is not constrained. (**d**) A bony suture anchor is fixed to the talar neck and another to the fibula between the tunnels. (**e**) First, the scarred ATFL is taken by the suture at the talar neck. (**f**) The suture is secured by a knot. (**g**) The ATFL/CFL complex is reduced. (**h**) This allows to catch both parts of these ligaments by the anchor suture. (**i**) The sutures are tightened and secured by a knot. (**j**) After final sutures of the superficial layers, the anatomic reconstruction of lateral ligaments evidences high lateral stability without disturbing the motion at the ankle and subtalar joint

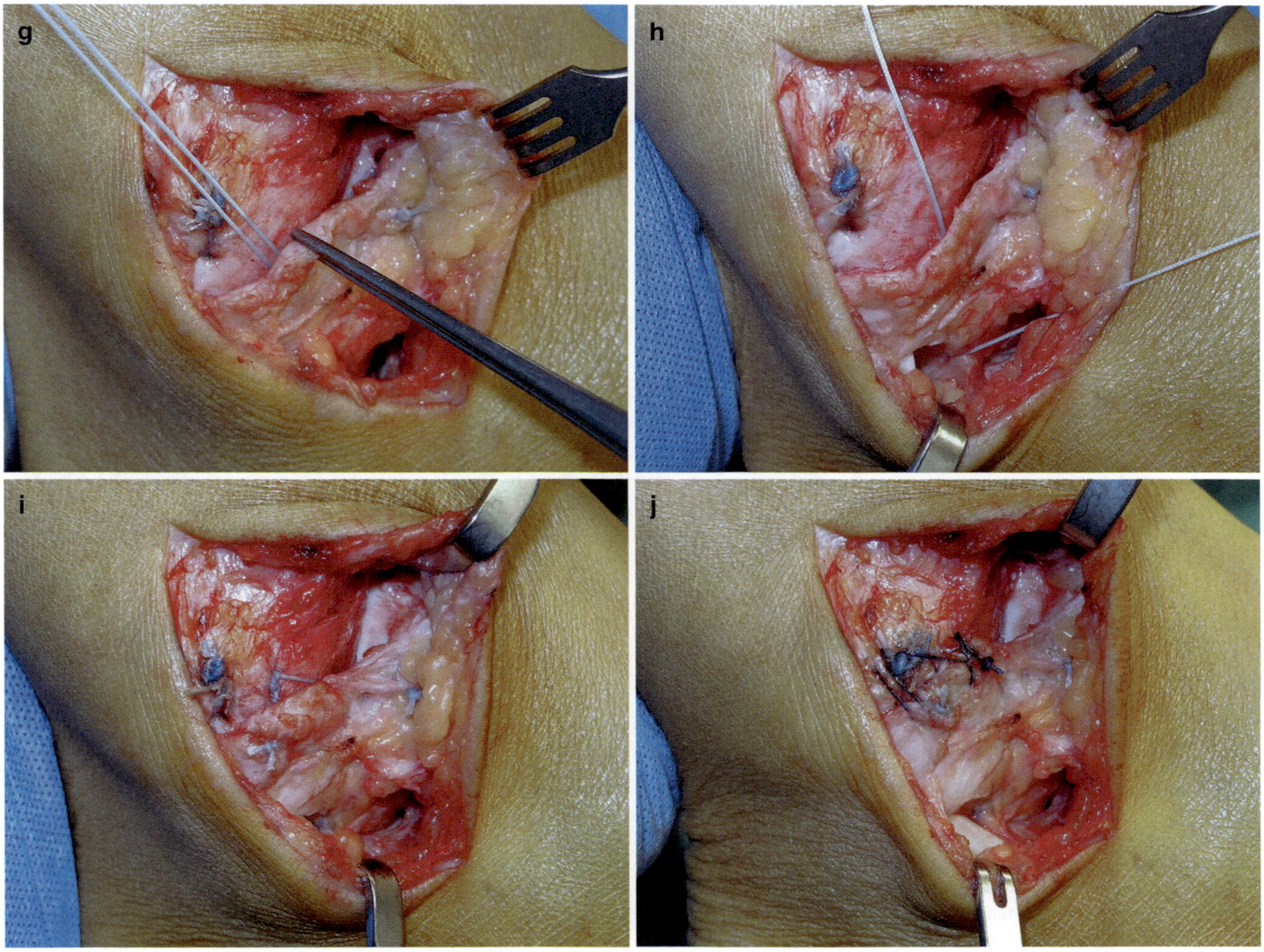

Fig. 2.37 (continued)

2.10 Outcome

- The outcome of surgical reconstruction is good to excellent in the majority of cases, as long as the physiological position of reconstructed ligaments is respected.
- An adjuvant rehabilitation program is mandatory for success.
- A high rate of return to former activity level has been reported.

Though conservative treatment is generally accepted as the primary treatment after an acute ankle sprain [2, 150], approximately 10–30% of the patients fail conservative treatment and exhibit chronic lateral ankle instability, which may require surgical treatment [4, 14, 36, 151]. In patients with chronic ankle instability, excellent and good results have been reported for a great majority of the cases after lateral ligament reconstruction [8, 21, 101, 120, 136, 152, 153]. Lateral ankle repair and anatomic allograft reconstruction were found to produce similarly favorable outcomes, including high patient satisfaction, high function and activity levels as well as very few revision surgeries [154].

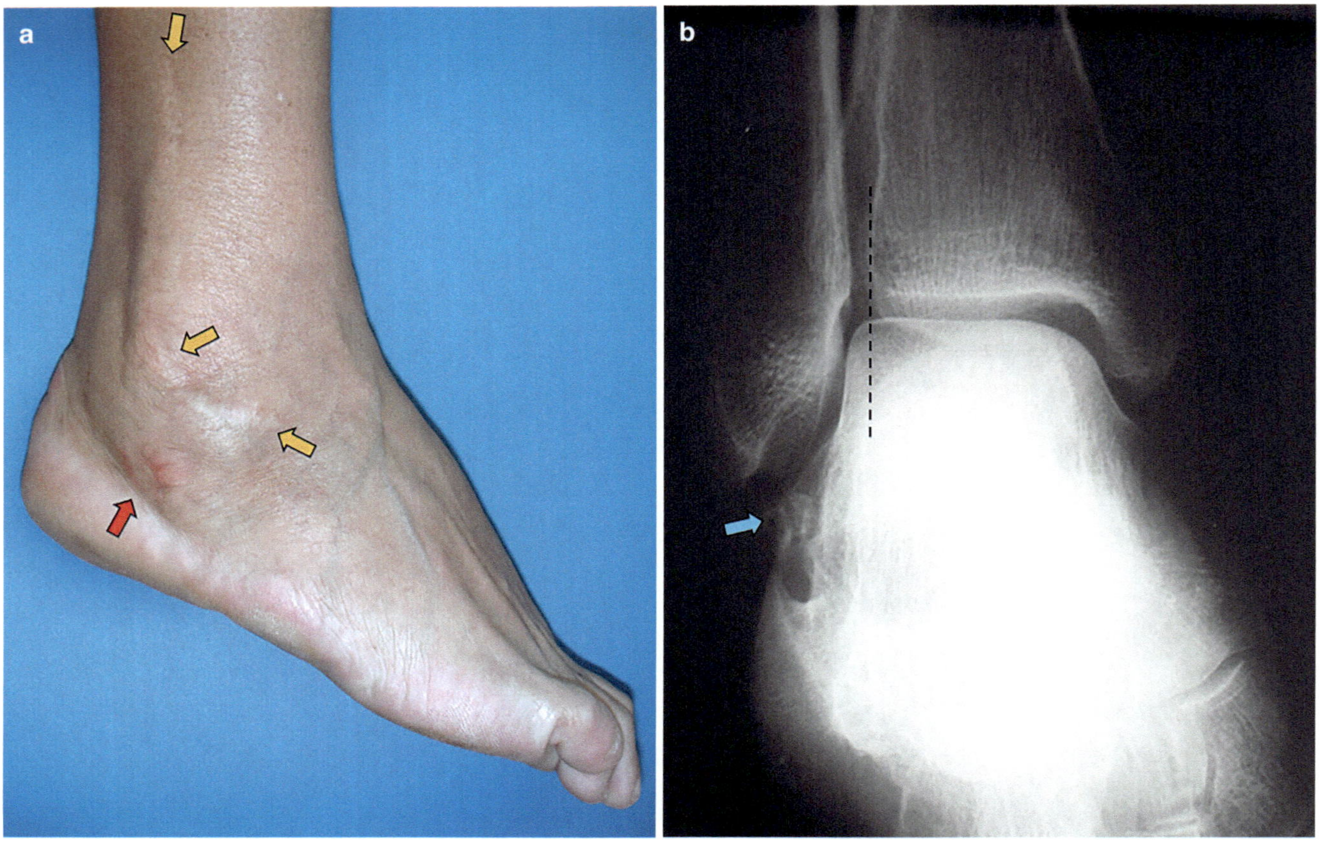

Fig. 2.38 A 33-year-old female former badminton player who was unable to return to sports after suffering from painful stiffening secondary to lateral ligament reconstruction by a tenodesis procedure with the use of the peroneus brevis tendon 6 years earlier. (**a**) The foot was blocked in slight pronation and abduction and the peroneal tendon sheath was swollen and painful upon palpation. Notice the long scar of the surgery (yellow arrows) and the skin irritation on the lateral aspect of the calcaneus (red arrow). (**b**) The non-weight-bearing X-ray shows the talus lateralized in the ankle mortise due to the lateral contracture and exostosis formation in the peroneal tendon sheath (blue arrow) explaining the skin irritation. Notice the lateral offset of the talus about the tibia, the bony response of the distal fibula due to the increased pressure with trabecular formation and the tibiotalar gapping of the medial ankle joint

Among the various arthroscopic techniques for repairing chronic lateral ankle instability, most patients have been treated successfully using the arthroscopic Broström–Gould procedure [128, 135], with an AOFAS score of 94.5 points at short term (14 months) [129] and 90 points at long term (9.8 years) [131]. Similar results were reported following arthroscopic Broström anatomical repair without reinforcement of the inferior extensor retinaculum (Gould procedure) [130, 133], using an all-inside knotless suture anchor technique.

The question however still remains, whether an acute rupture of the lateral ankle ligaments should be treated nonoperatively or operatively. In general, the recurrence of lateral ankle instability has been shown to be lower when treated operatively and gained stability has been found to be higher after surgical reconstruction. Furthermore, patients were able to go back to pre-injury sports level earlier after operative treatment.

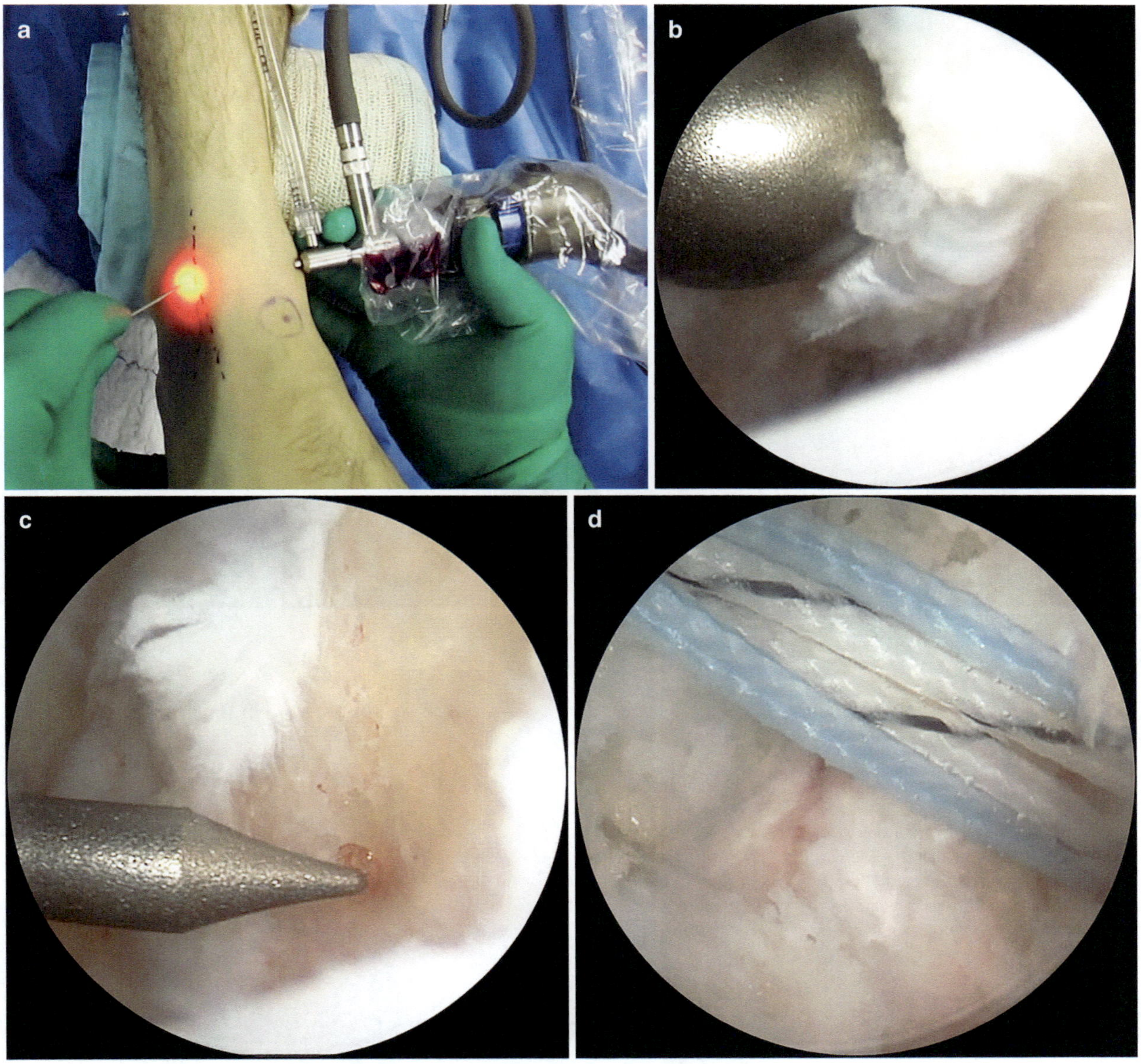

Fig. 2.39 *Surgical Technique: Arthroscopic-assisted Broström–Gould for chronic ankle instability by Caio Nery* [131]. (**a**) The anteromedial portal is the best location for the anterolateral portal, avoiding the neural branches. It is determined by trans-illumination and marked with a needle. After having inserted the arthroscope, (**b**) the scar tissue and ligament rests are removed from the anterior surface of the distal fibula in order to prepare the "foot-print" for the ligament repair. (**c**) A bone anchor is introduced through the portal and its tip is directed to the prepared anterior surface of the distal fibula. (**d**) After having inserted the anchor, the insertion instrument is removed, and the sutures become visible. (**e**) A curved suture passer with a nitinol loop inside is introduced through the portal and directed with a smooth movement to the lateral ankle groove to embrace the ligament rests and the joint capsule. The suture passer is then introduced deep enough to reach the proximal border of the inferior extensor retinaculum to reinforce the construct. (**f**) The nitinol loop is used to pull out each of the suture arms. (**g**) The nitinol loop is inserted again with the suture passer that is then to be removed. While pulling the nitinol loop, the suture is brought through the tissues until it externalizes it through the skin. (**h**) With the help of an arthroscopic probe inserted through one of the skin holes through which the sutures were externalized, the other portion of the same suture is taken and brought outside so that both ends will occupy the same skin hole. This maneuver is repeated for the other suture. (**i**) While the foot is held in neutral position, a slipping knot (Duncan) is made first in the most posterior suture, and thereafter in the anterior suture. *(Courtesy of Prof. Caio Nery, Sao Paolo, Brazil)*

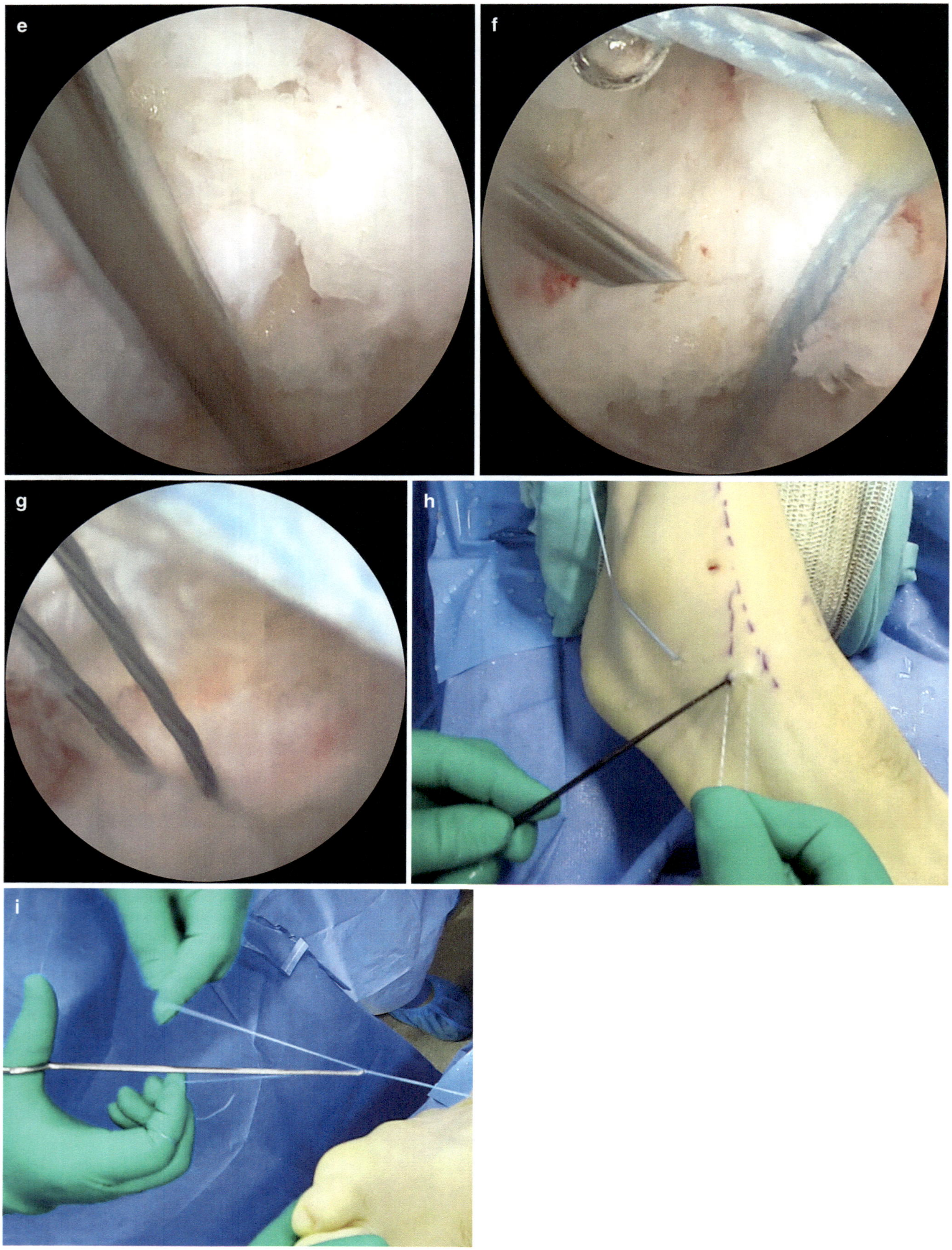

Fig. 2.39 (continued)

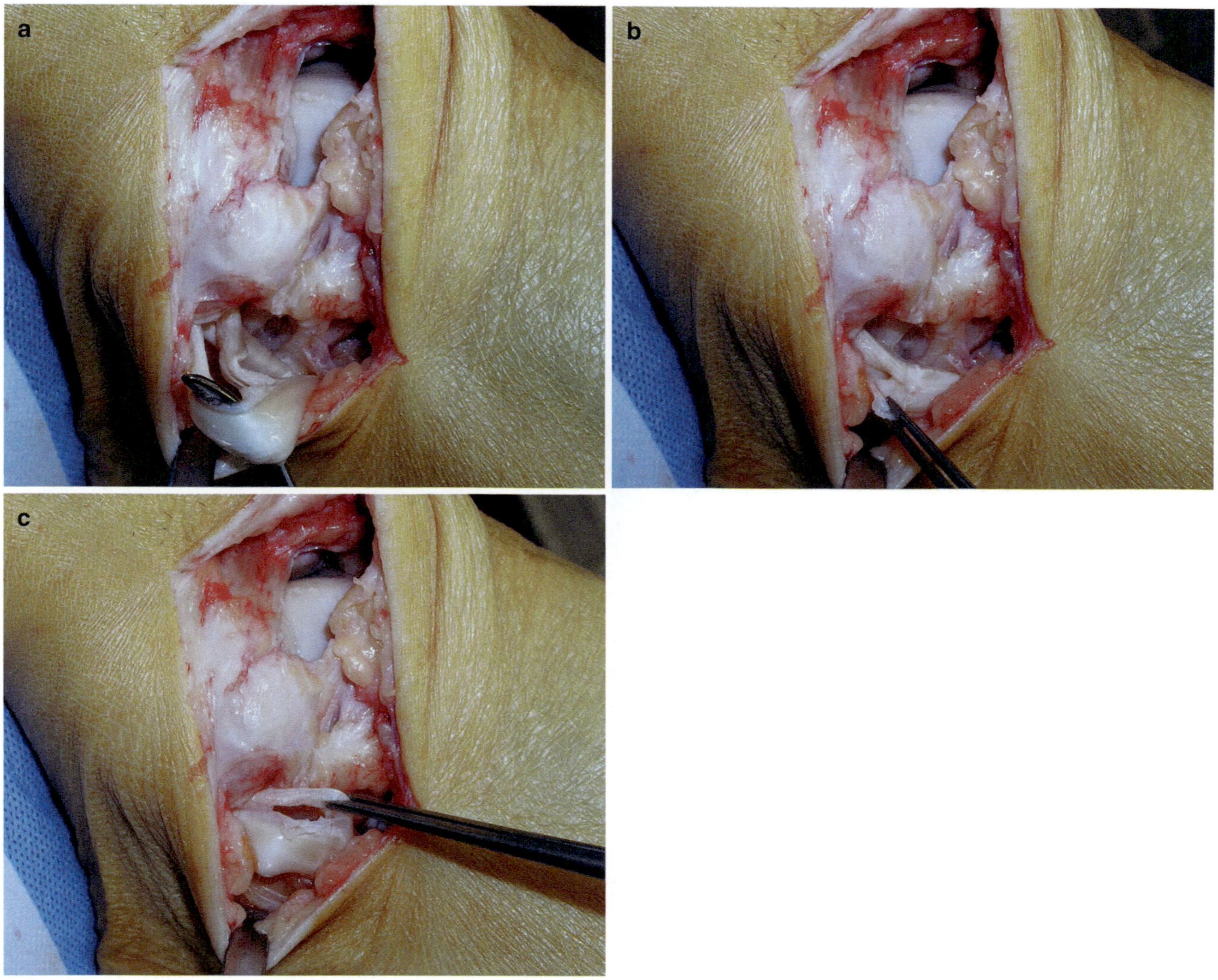

Fig. 2.40 *Surgical Technique: Tear of peroneal brevis tendon in chronic ankle instability*. This 36-year-old former soccer player suffered from recurrent sprains after a severe ankle sprain 13 years earlier. (**a**) Surgical exploration evidenced a longitudinal tear of the peroneus brevis tendon with scarring and degeneration of the tendon tissue (**b**, **c**). Notice the scarred and incompetent lateral ankle ligaments

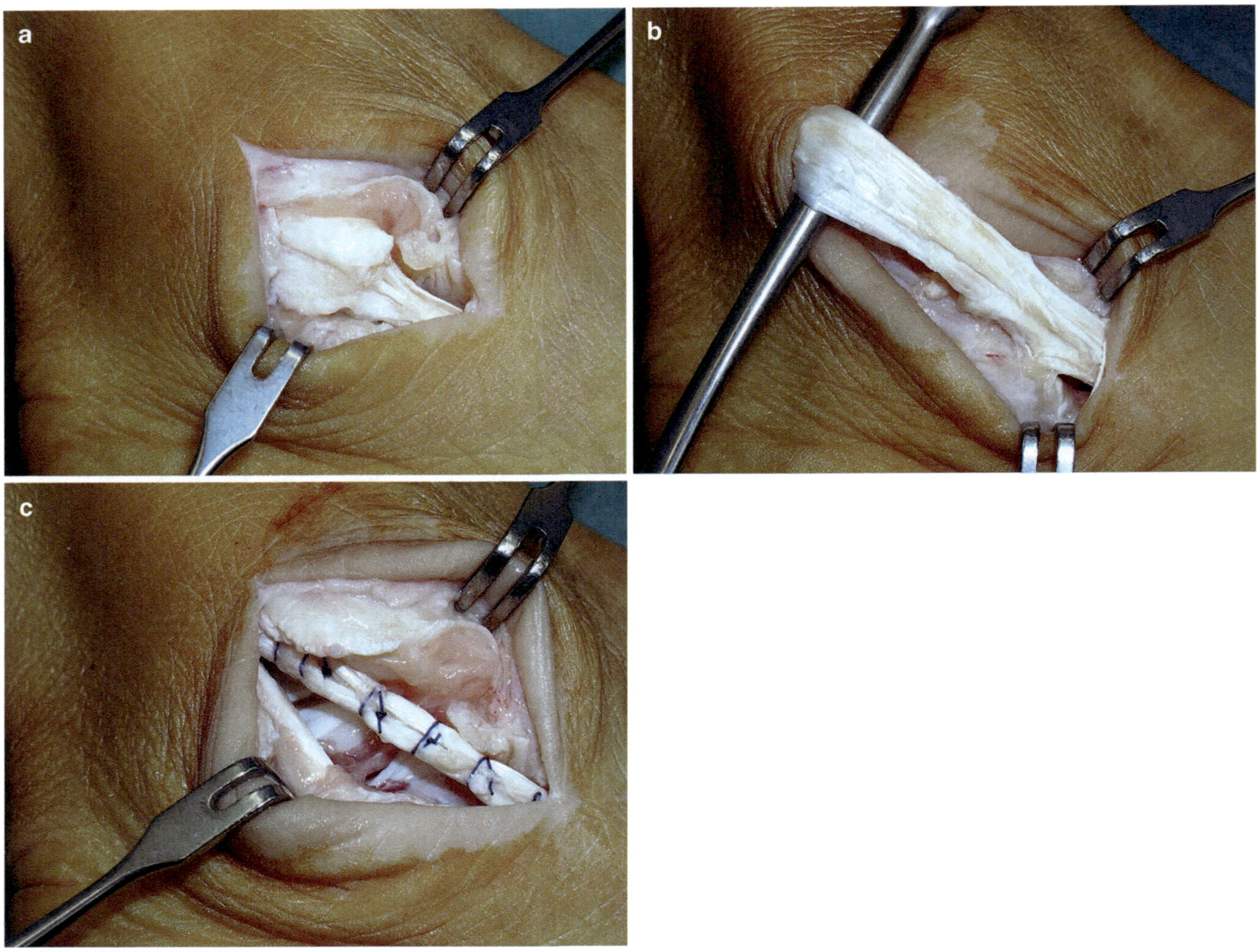

Fig. 2.41 *Surgical Technique: Partial rupture with longitudinal tears of the peroneal brevis tendon in chronic ankle instability*. This 48-year-old female physiotherapist suffered from chronic ankle instability. After a sprain some months ago, she complained about persistent pain in the peroneal tendons and eversion power was significantly decreased. (**a**) Surgical exposure showed the scarred proximal stump of a partially ruptured peroneus brevis tendon. (**b**) The tendon was first meticulously debrided from scarred and degenerated tissue. (**c**) Then, the tendon was reconstructed by imbricating sutures. Afterwards, the lateral ankle ligaments were reconstructed (not shown)

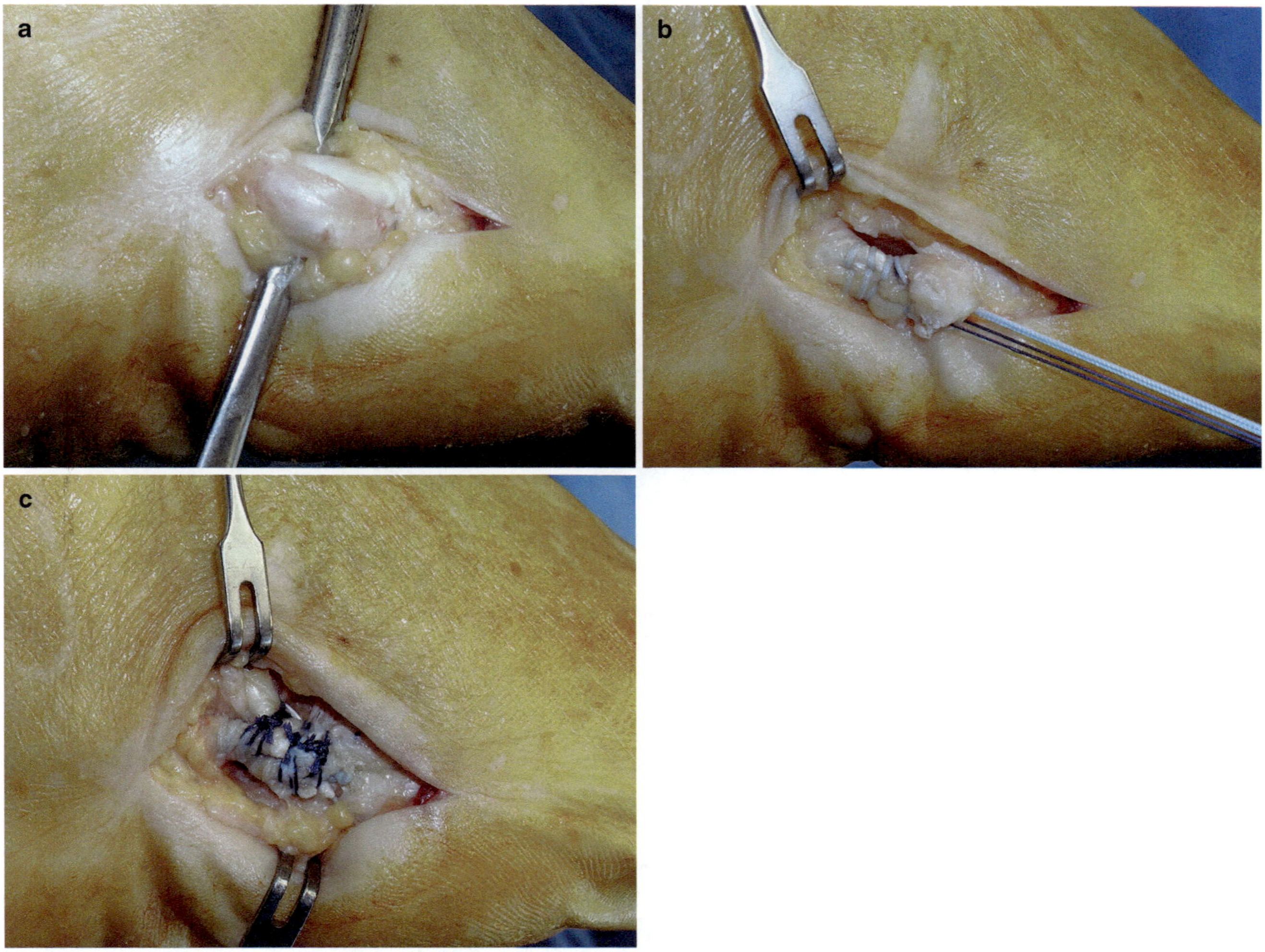

Fig. 2.42 *Surgical Technique: Peroneus longus to peroneus brevis transfer*. This 45-year-old former basketball player underwent lateral ligament reconstruction with partial use of the peroneus brevis tendon 16 years earlier. After another sprain he was suffering from recurrent sprains and persistent instability feeling. Clinical investigation revealed distinct varus alignment of the heel, a highly unstable ankle and no eversion power. While lateral ligament reconstruction was performed, the peroneus brevis tendon was found to be completely absent. Therefore, a peroneus longus to peroneus brevis transfer was indicated. (**a**) A 3–4 cm longitudinal incision was made starting proximal to the base of fifth metatarsal and exposing 1 cm of the bone. An incision was made along the inferior border of the peroneus brevis tendon which allowed exposure and grabbing of the peroneus longus tendon with an elevatorium. (**b**) After having dissected the peroneus longus tendon as distal as possible, the proximal stump was taken by a non-resorbable suture. (**c**) While the foot was held in maximal eversion, the tendon was fixed to the base of fifth metatarsal by transosseous suture. Finally, side-to-side sutures were used to fix the tendon to the distal peroneus brevis tendon

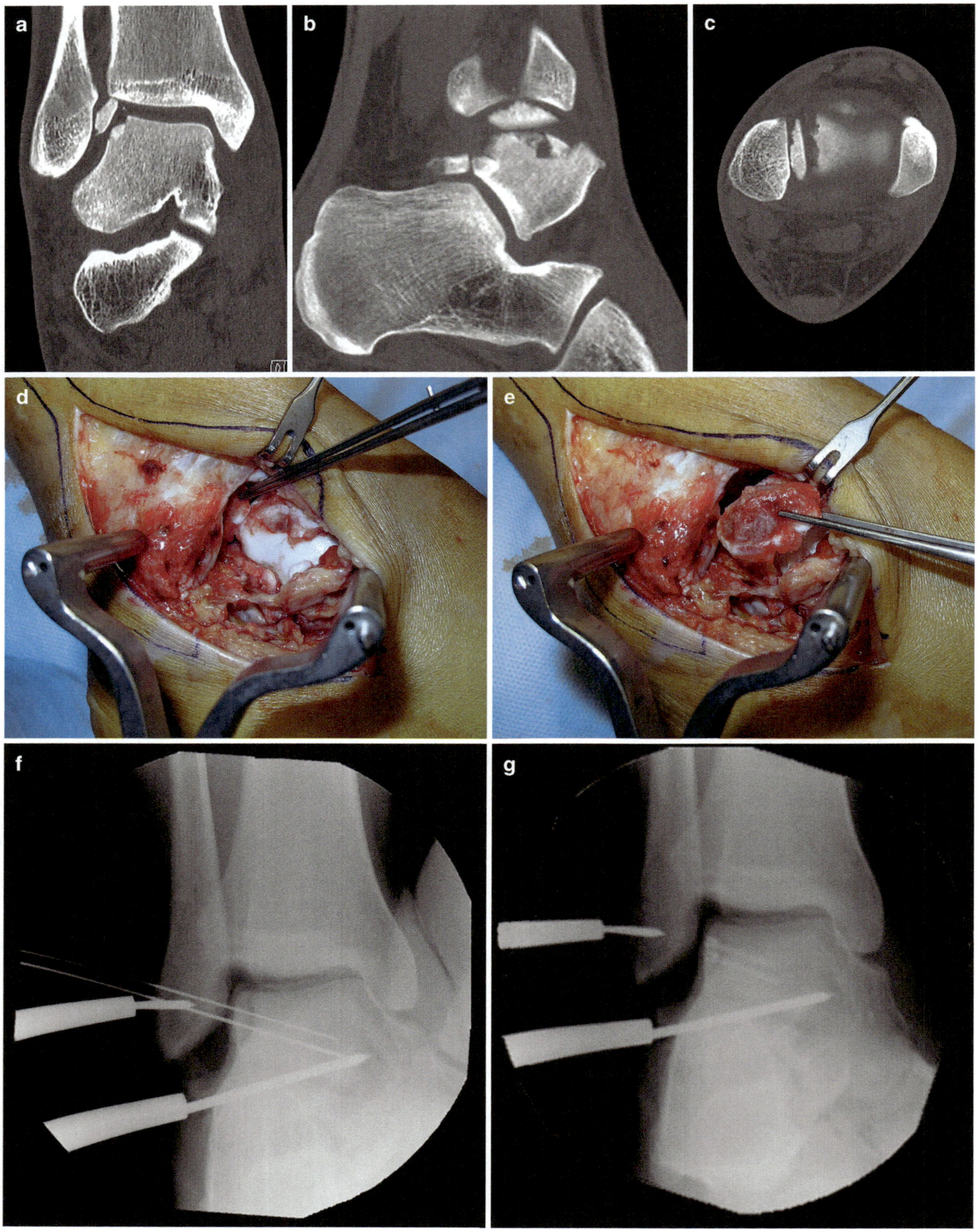

Fig. 2.43 *Surgical Technique: Reconstruction of lateral talar dome for an osteochondral fracture*. This 19-year-old gymnast sustained a severe supination trauma while landing. (**a**) The CT scan showed a big osteochondral fracture of the lateral talar dome which was dislocated and rotated. (**b**) In the sagittal view, a smaller fragment could be seen. (**c**) The horizontal view showed the extent of the fracture and the fragment rotation of 180°. (**d**) Surgical exploration showed the complete rupture of the lateral ankle ligaments, the lesion on the lateral talar dome, and the dislocated rotated fragment. (**e**) The fragment was solid and measured >20 mm in diameter. (**f**) The fragment was repositioned to the talus and preliminarily fixed by two K-wires. (**g**) Final fixation was carried out with two 3-mm cannulated screws. (**h**) The lateral talar dome was anatomically restored. (**i–k**) CT scans after 8 weeks show complete healing with full reintegration of the bone and anatomical restoration of lateral talar dome. Full recovery allowed this gymnast to return to high-level sports with attendance of Olympic Games

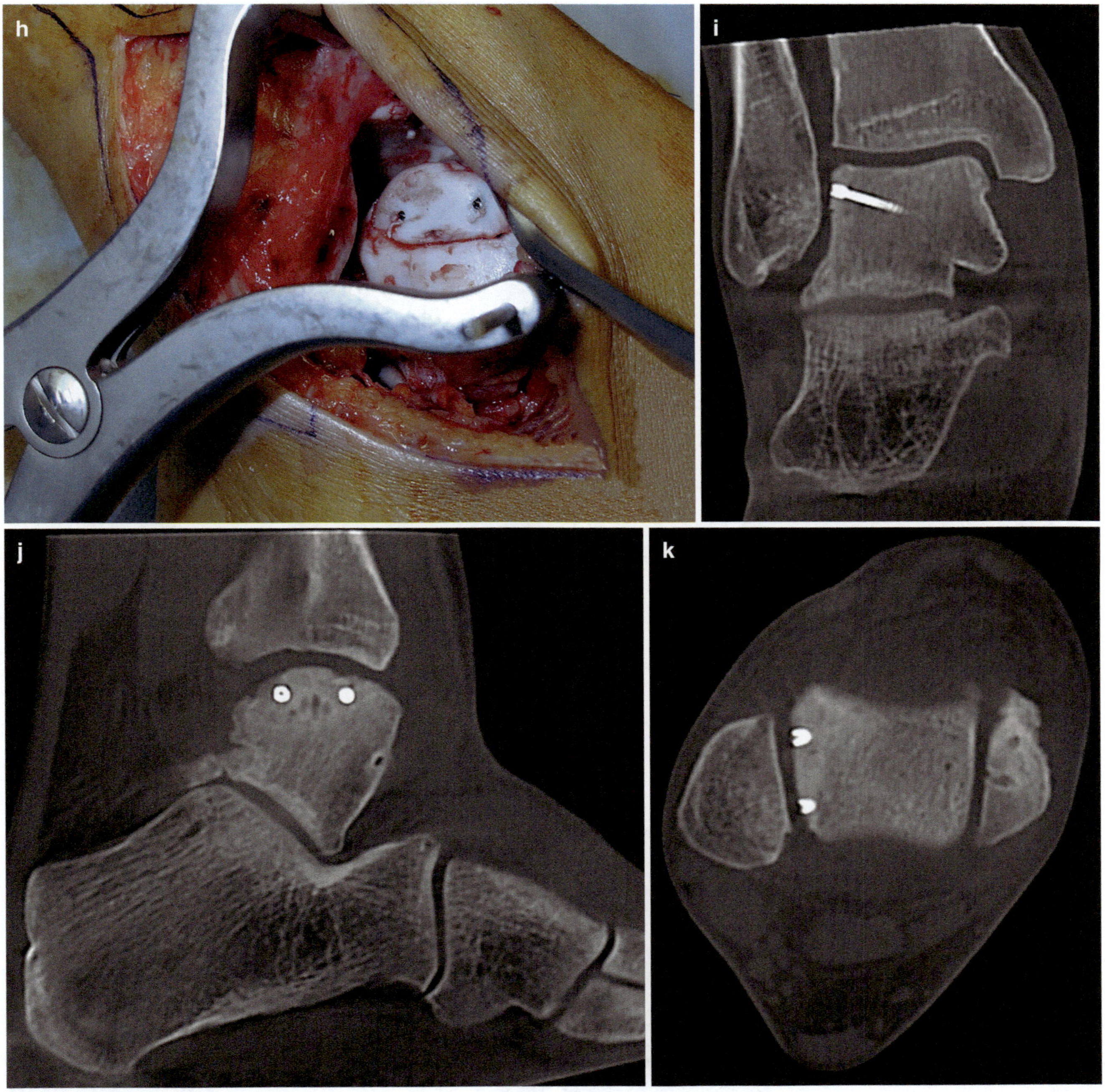

Fig. 2.43 (continued)

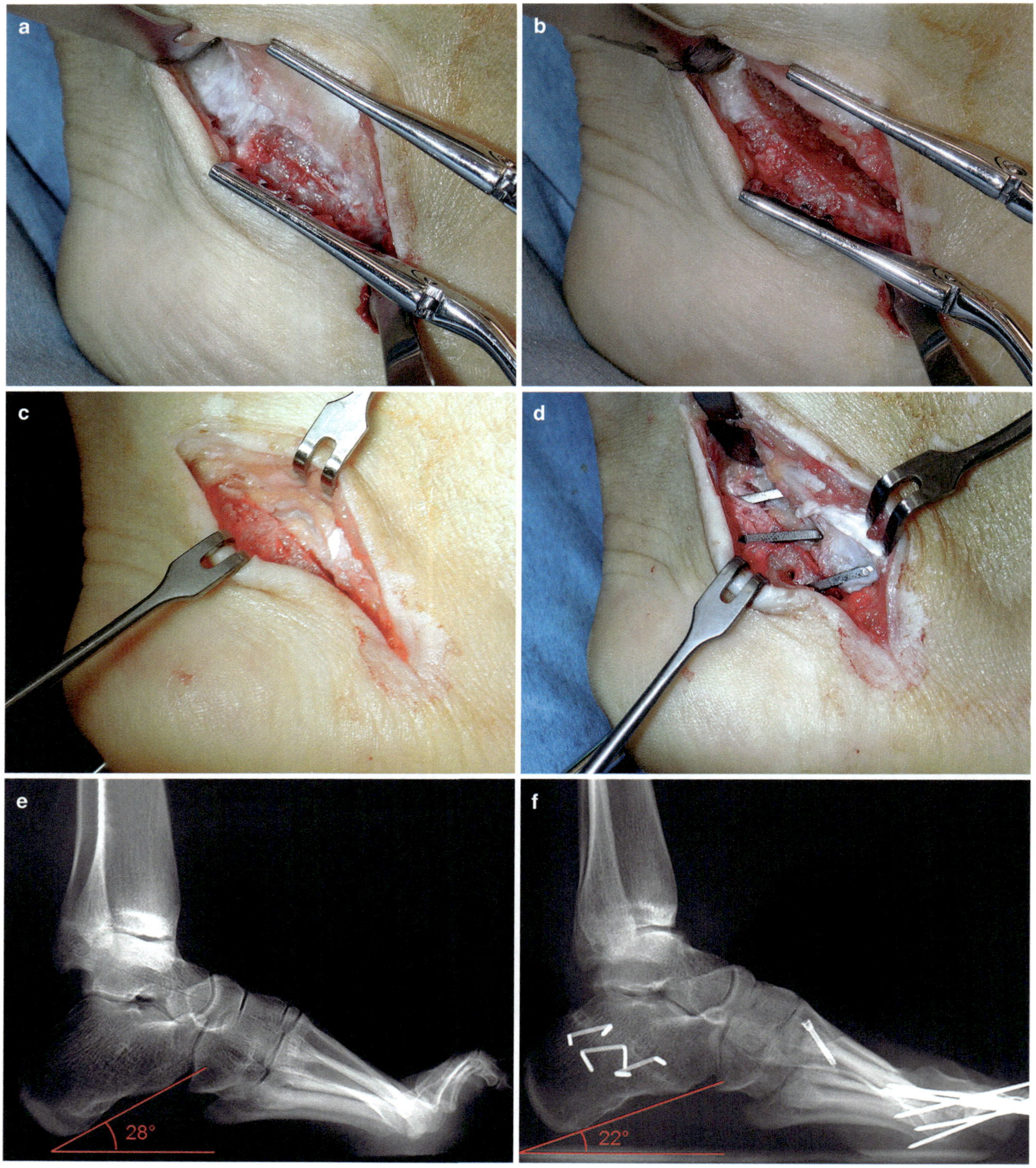

Fig. 2.44 *Surgical Technique: Dwyer osteotomy of the calcaneus to correct a heel varus*. (**a**) The tuber of the calcaneus was exposed by an oblique incision. (**b**) A double osteotomy with two convergent cuts was made with the saw with an inclination to the ground of 45° to remove a wedge with a base measuring 8–12 mm, depending on the wanted amount of correction. The medial cortex is aimed to remain intact. (**c**) The osteotomy was closed manually by valgization force applied to the heel and preliminary fixed by a K-wire inserted from the heel. (**d**) In this case, three staples were used for fixation; alternatively, one or two screws can be used, instead. (**e**) Preoperative lateral view showing the cavovarus deformity with a calcaneal pitch angle of 28°. (**f**) Eight weeks after surgical correction including a dorsiflexion osteotomy of the first ray and claw toe correction, the osteotomy is healed, and the calcaneal pitch angle has improved to 22°

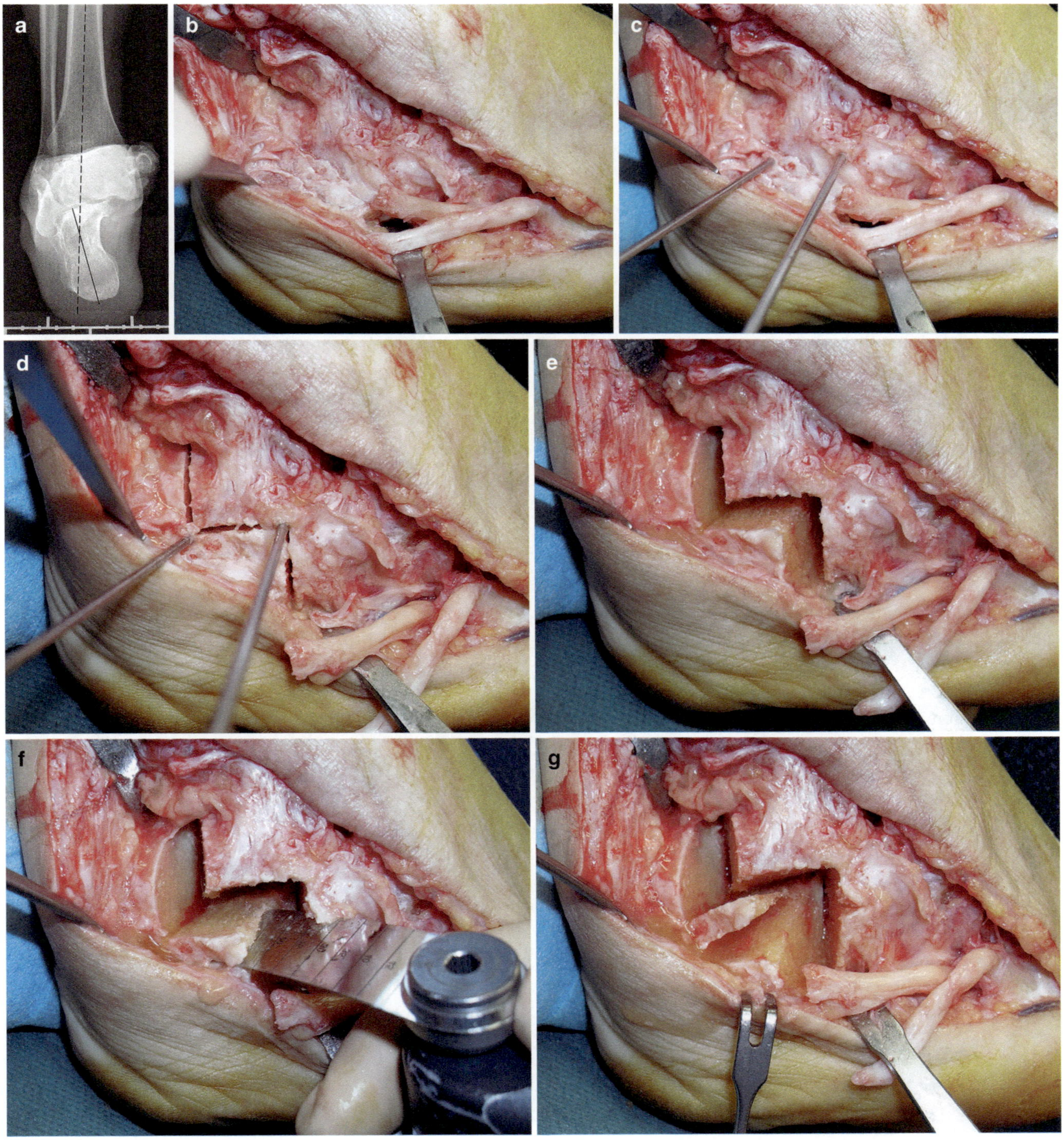

Fig. 2.45 *Surgical Technique: Z-osteotomy of calcaneus for correction of heel varus (modified Italian osteotomy).* This 64-year-old female patient sustained an injury to the lateral leg 5 cm above the ankle by a knife at the age of 14 years. The soft tissues were closed remaining the peroneal tendons with a simple readaptation suture, leaving the patient with limited function of her foot. In the last years, she noticed a progressive supination deformity with a subsequent instability feeling and experiencing recurrent sprains. Clinical investigation showed a significant varus deformity of the heel and no active eversion. (**a**) The Saltzman alignment view showed the significant varus malalignment of the heel. (**b**) Surgical exploration showed the distal stumps of the atrophic peroneal tendons. One Hohmann retractor was positioned over the top of tuberosity, and a second one was positioned on the bottom opposite to sinus tarsi. (**c**) Two K-wires were inserted parallel in all plane in the center of calcaneal body. (**d**) A Z-shaped osteotomy is made with the saw using the two K-wires as a guide. (**e**) The tuberosity fragment was mobilized. (**f**) An additional osteotomy was made in the horizontal plane to remove a wedge to achieve the planned valgization of the heel. (**g**) Through the wedge removal, (**h**) the heel is shifted lateral; a small Hohmann retractor can be used to push the heel lateral. The osteotomy was closed with the foot in a dorsiflexed position, and a screw was used for percutaneous fixation of the tuberosity fragment. (**i**) Lateral fluoroscopy showing the osteotomy and the screw fixation. (**j**) Achieved correction was seen in the axial view. (**k**) A reconstruction of the ATFL and CFL was made with the use of a free plantaris tendon graft (Fig. 2.36) and augmentation with an internal brace (Fig. 2.37). (**l**) Finally, a PTT transfer was then performed to reconstruct the peroneal tendons

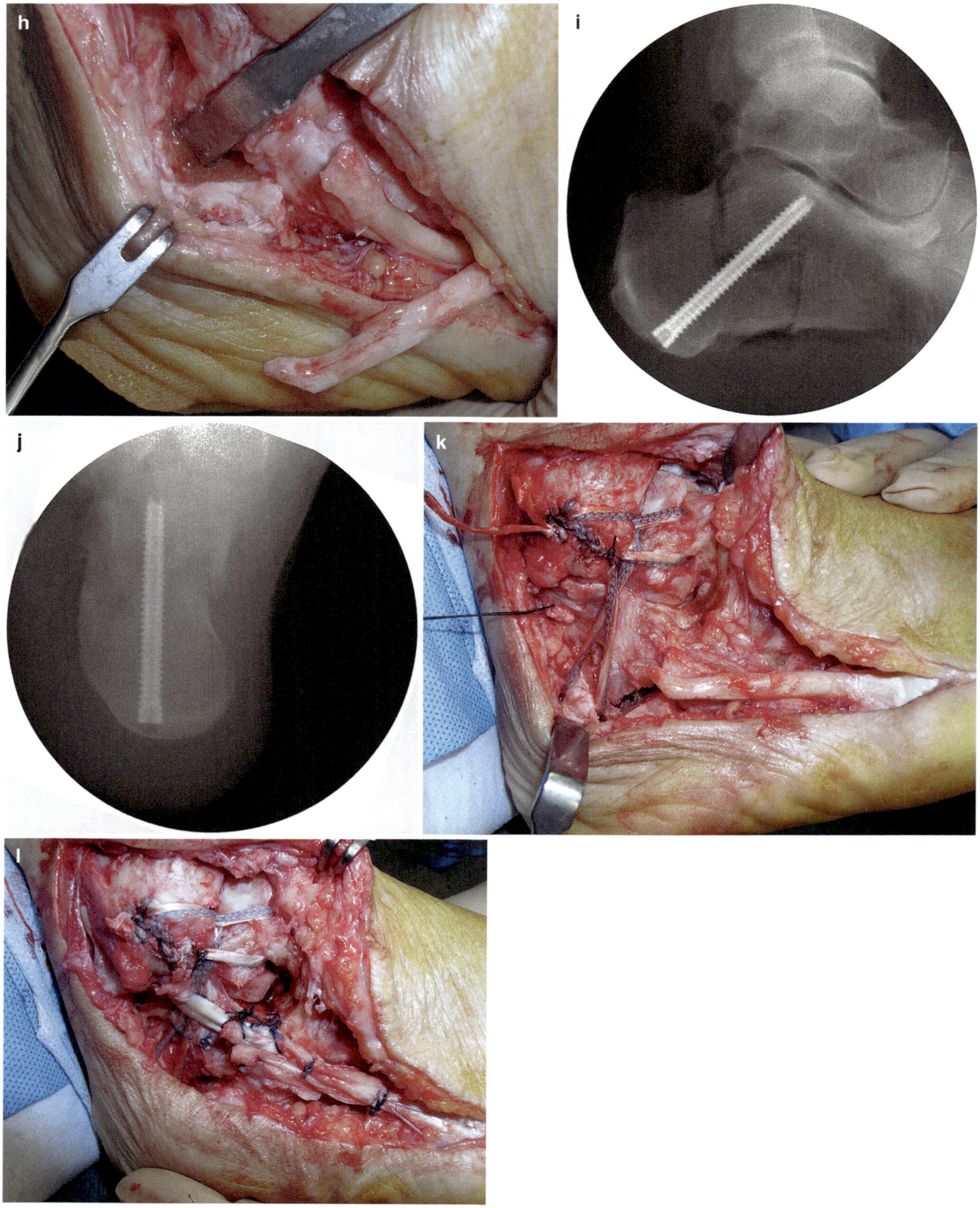

Fig. 2.45 (continued)

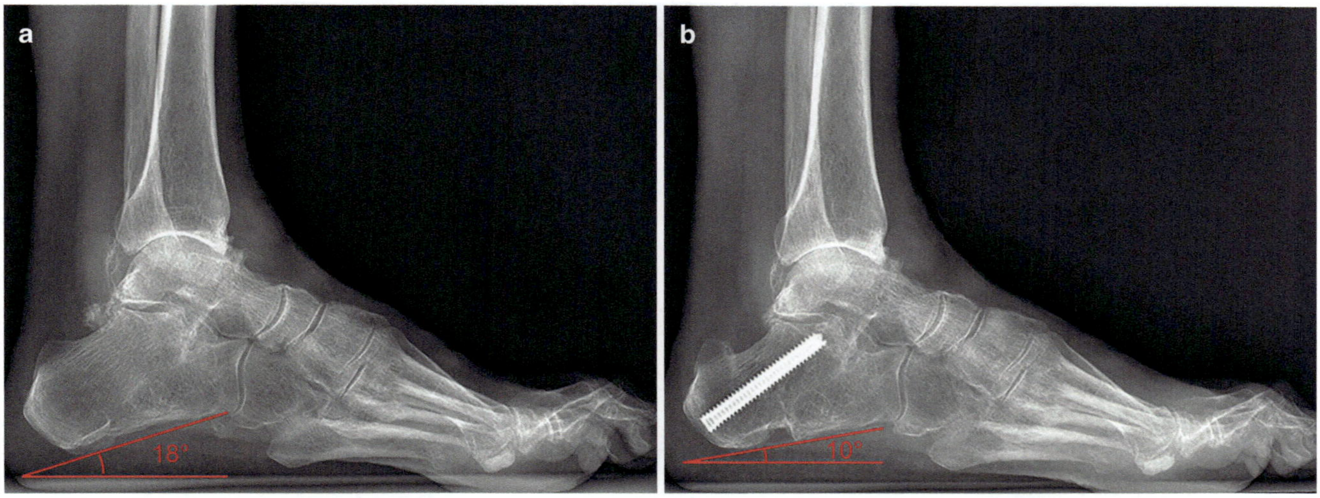

Fig. 2.46 *Surgical Technique: Z-osteotomy of the calcaneus for correcting a varus heel and the height of the calcaneus.* This osteotomy also permits to decrease the height of the calcaneus by resecting a horizontal bone slice. (**a**) Preoperative situation. (**b**) The decrease of height and the calcaneal pitch angle respectively is seen 4 months after surgery

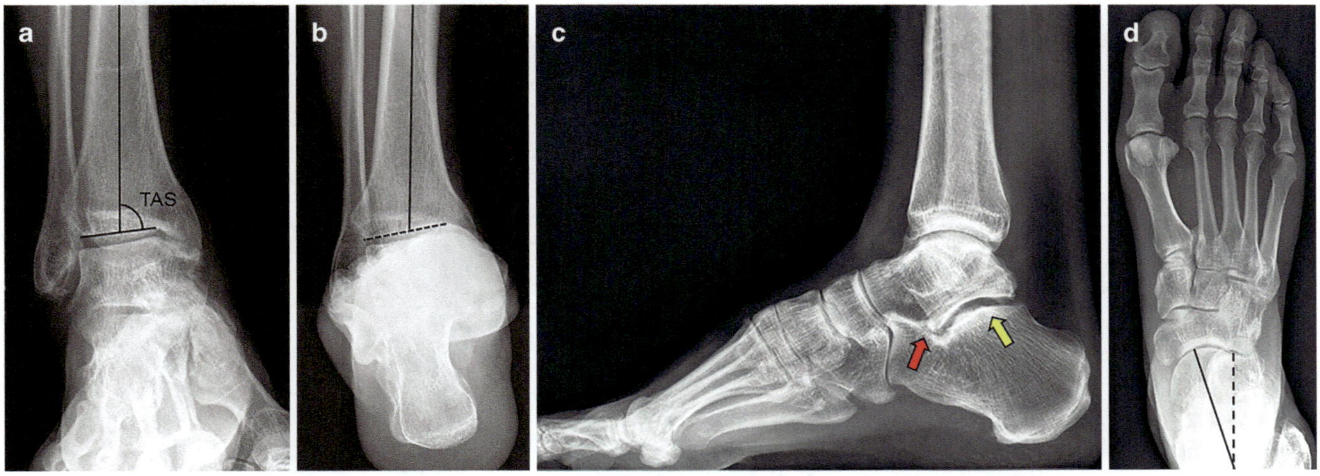

Fig. 2.47 This patient was complaining about feeling progressive instability after recurrent ankle sprains and pain mainly in his medial ankle. (**a**) Standard weight-bearing radiographs showed a varus deformity of the distal tibia in the coronal plane (tibia-articular surface angle [TAS] = 7°) with talar tilt and narrowing of the medial tibiotalar joint. (**b**) The hindfoot alignment view confirmed that the main varus deformity originated from supramalleolar. (**c**) The lateral view evidenced a peritalar instability as seen by asymmetric joint space of the subtalar joint with gapping (yellow arrow) and sinus tarsi impingement (red arrow) due to exorotation of the talus. (**d**) The exorotation position of the talus can also be seen in the horizontal plane with a decreased talocalcaneal angle

2.11 Complications

- Non-isometric positioning of the reconstructed ligaments may result in pain and stiffness.
- The use of bulky tendon grafts may result in painful impingement and disturbance of motion.
- Too tight ligament reconstructions may result in progression of the degenerative disease, especially when using tendon grafts and nonanatomic tenodesis procedures.

Besides the cases that have persistent instability, most complications experienced during or after lateral ankle ligament treatment are a consequence of nonanatomical reconstruction. This is especially the case when tendon autografts and allografts have been used [31]. There are several reasons for this. Tenodesis procedures may change the biomechanics of the ankle joint complex, resulting in increased joint load, limited motion, subsequent pain, and progression of the degenerative disease (Fig. 2.50) [34, 126]. The use of bulky tendon grafts may result in painful soft tissue impingement and stiffening of the joint (Fig. 2.51). Furthermore, failure to reattach the ligaments or reroute the used grafts or internal

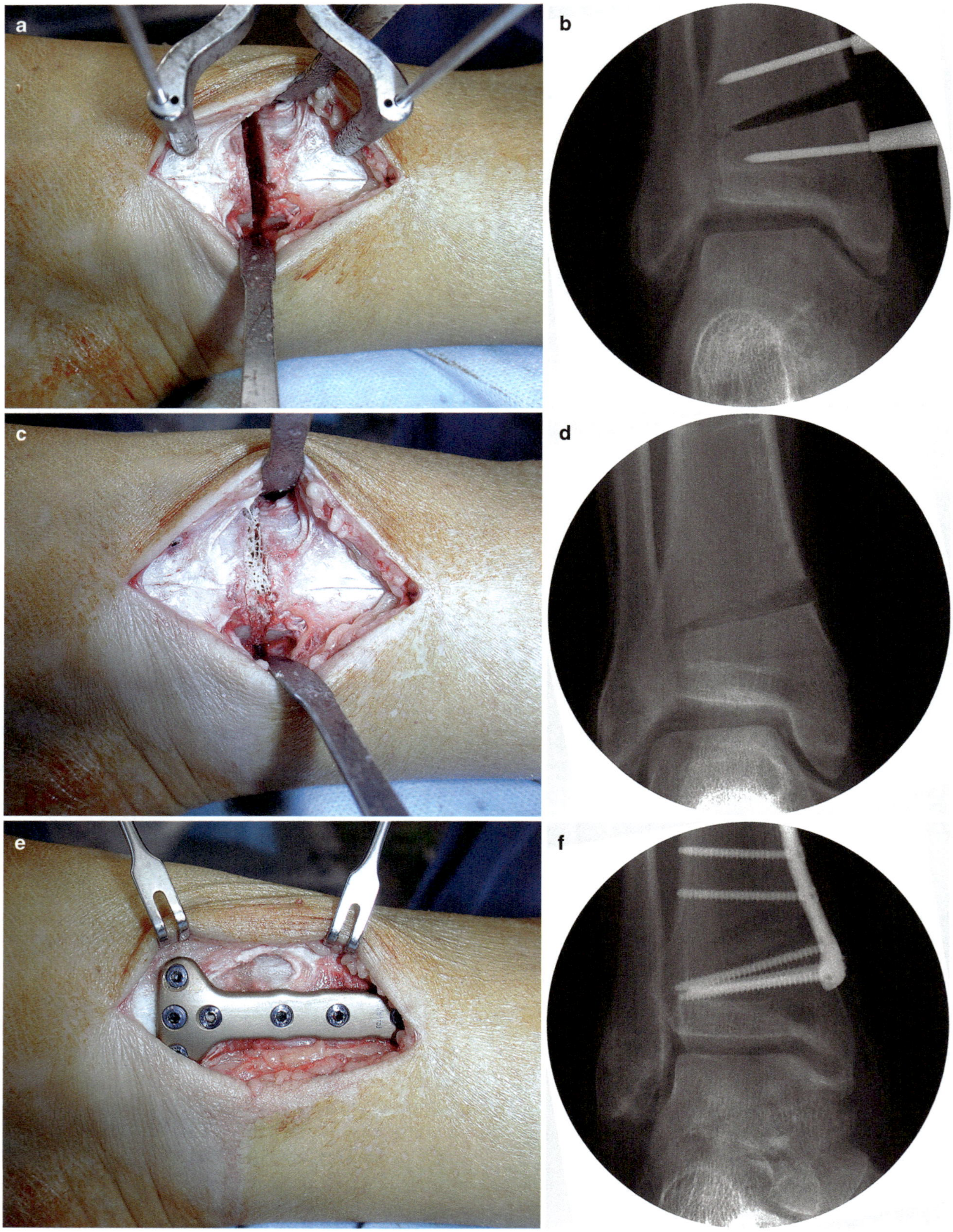

Fig. 2.48 *Surgical Technique: Open wedge osteotomy of the distal tibia*. The procedure is shown on the same patient as Fig. 2.47. (**a**, **b**) After exposure of the distal tibia through a 5–6 cm long incision, the osteotomy was performed perpendicular to the tibial surface in an oblique way, while attention was paid to preserve the lateral cortex intact. The osteotomy was then gradually opened by a Hintermann distractor mounted over two K-wires until the TAS angle was slightly overcorrected to approximately 2° of valgus. (**c**, **d**) An autologous or allograft was shaped accordingly and inserted; then the distractor was removed. (**e**, **f**) A plate was used for fixation. (**g**–**j**) Radiographs taken 8 weeks postoperative, showing the osteotomy healed. The procedure was able to normalize the TAS angle and the hindfoot alignment was well corrected. Notice the changes of the angles and talar position

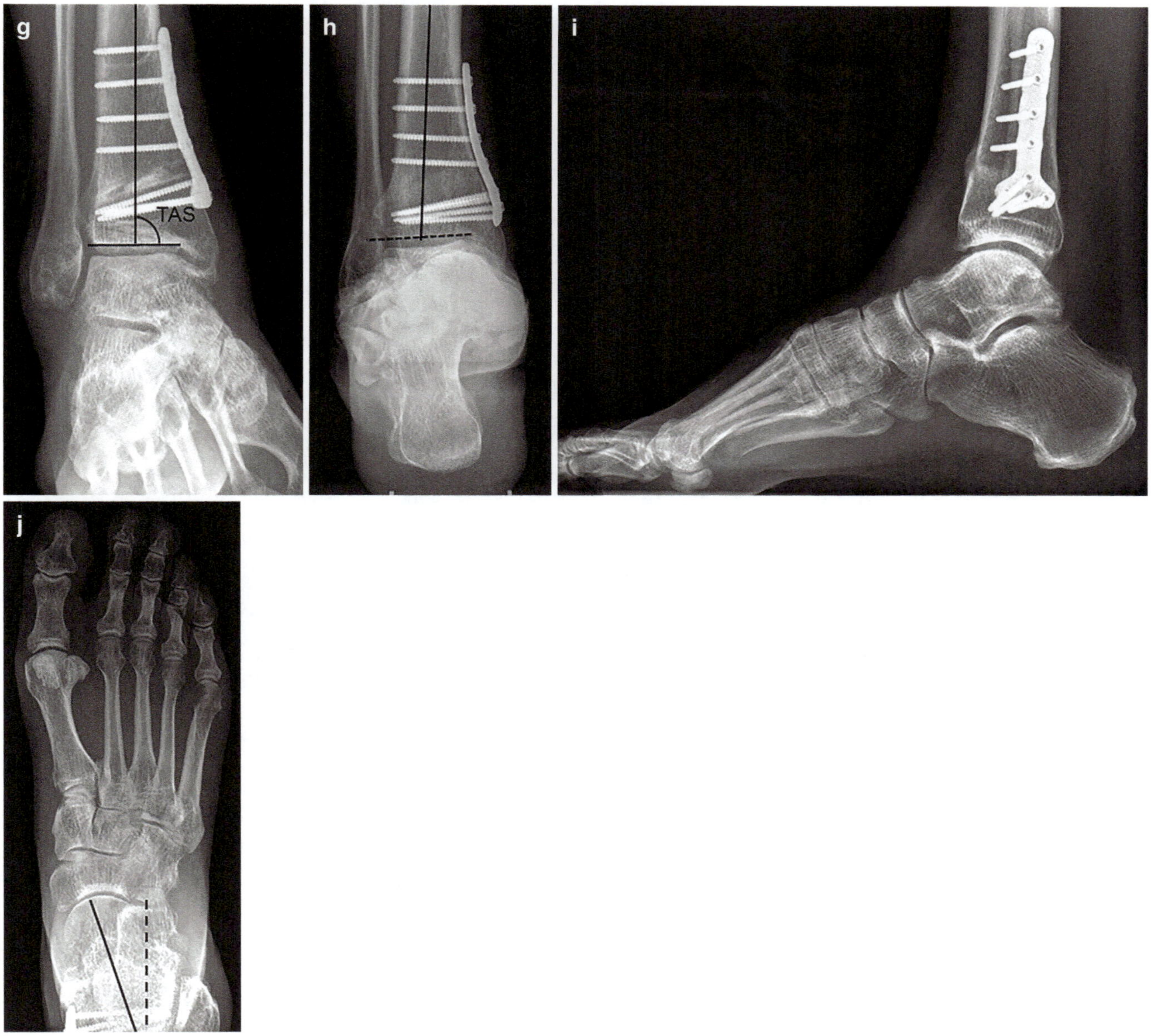

Fig. 2.48 (continued)

braces on the anatomic insertion area of the fibula, talus, and calcaneus may result in restriction of motion and laxity at the ankle and subtalar joint, depending on the foot position, pain, and secondary osteoarthritis (Fig. 2.52).

2.12 Conclusions and Future Evolution

- Injuries to the lateral ankle ligaments are not harmless.
- Conservative treatment should not mean neglecting the injury.
- There is need for better criteria to define lateral ankle ligament injuries that need primary surgical repair.
- Specific studies are necessary to define the potential risks for developing secondary osteoarthritis, and how it can be prevented.

Though there has been a better understanding of lateral ankle instability and subsequent biomechanical changes in last two decades, the question remains how an acute injury to the lateral ankle ligaments should be best treated [118]. Data has shown that after physical rehabilitation and nonoperative

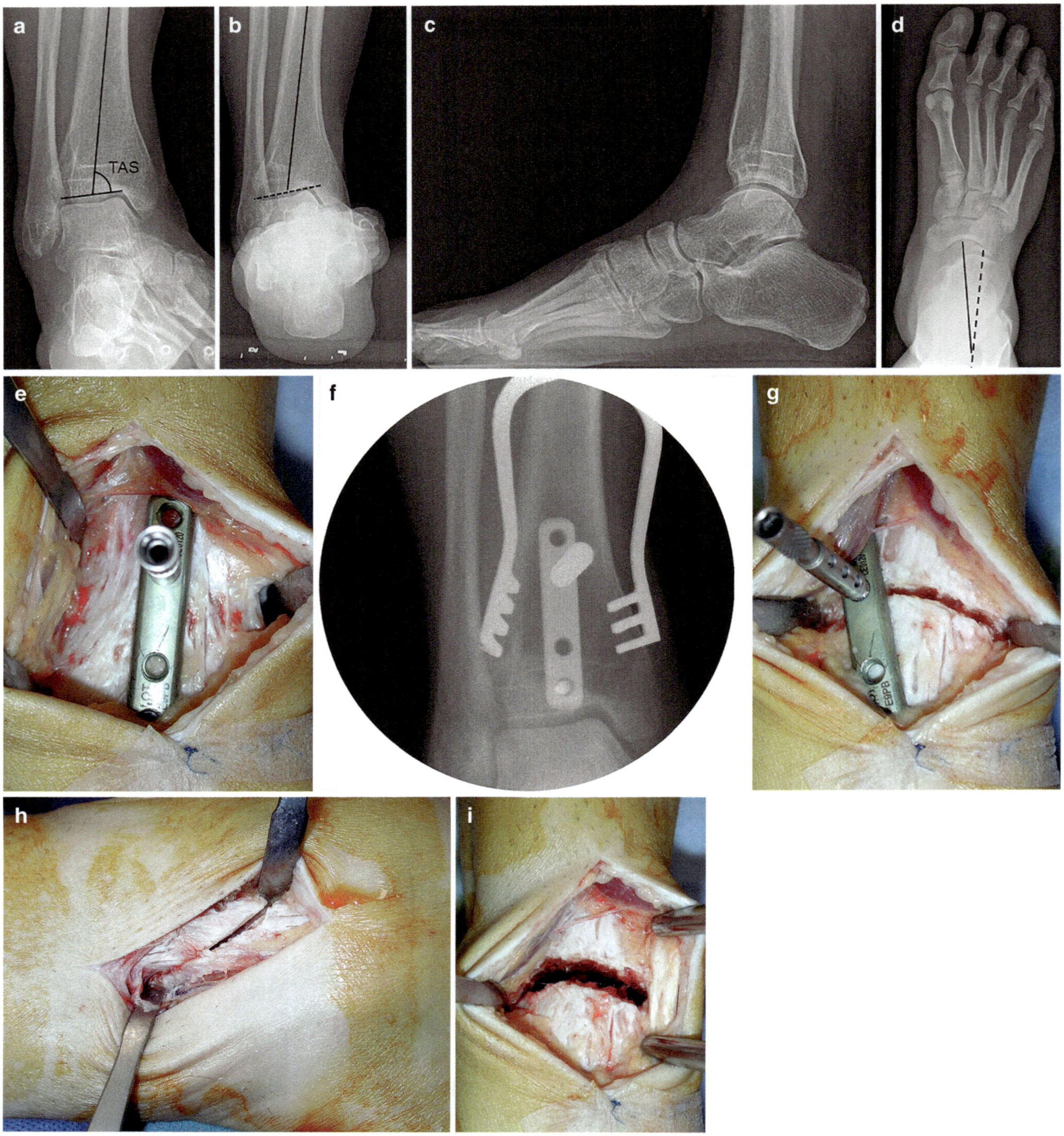

Fig. 2.49 *Surgical Technique: Dome osteotomy of distal tibia*. This 48-year-old male patient was suffering from lateral ankle pain and a feeling of instability since a sprain some months earlier. (**a–d**) Standard weight-bearing radiographs showing a major varus deformity of the distal tibia with a congruent ankle joint, a significant varus malalignment of the heel, and a supination position of the midfoot. (**e**) After exposure of distal tibia through an anterior approach without opening the ankle joint, a small plate was fixed to the center of tibia close to the tibiotalar joint, as verified under fluoroscopy (**f**). (**g**) The osteotomy was done by multiple drillings through the mounted drill guide, while the plate was rotated step-by-step. (**h**) The fibula was exposed through a longitudinal incision at the same level, and an oblique osteotomy was made from proximal-posterior to distal-anterior. (**i**) The distal tibia was mobilized by the Hintermann distractor mounted over two K-wires at the anteromedial aspect of tibia. This allows to rotate the distal tibia and then to close the osteotomy. (**j**) A K-wire inserted percutaneously from the medial malleolus was used for preliminary fixation. (**k**) Two plates were used to fix the tibial osteotomy. (**l**) Another plate was used to fix the fibular osteotomy. (**m**) Finally, the correct alignment and the ankle joint congruency were checked under fluoroscopy. As the ankle joint was considered stable by manual testing, no additional soft tissue reconstruction work was done. (**n–q**) Radiographs taken after 8 weeks show that the osteotomies have healed. The TAS angle has been normalized and the hindfoot was well aligned. Though no ligament reconstruction was done, the patient was able to return to full sports activities without any instability feelings or sprains

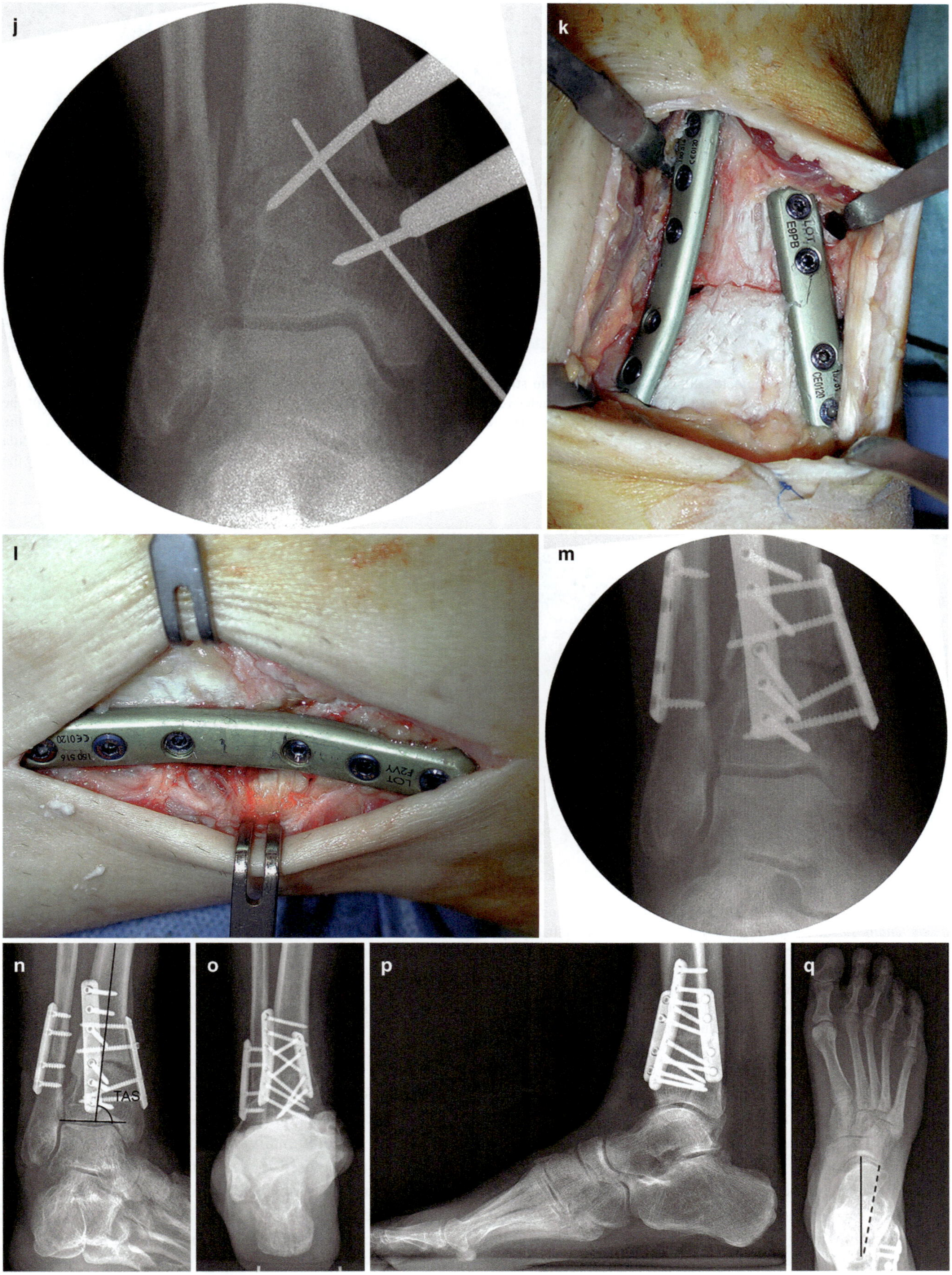

Fig. 2.49 (continued)

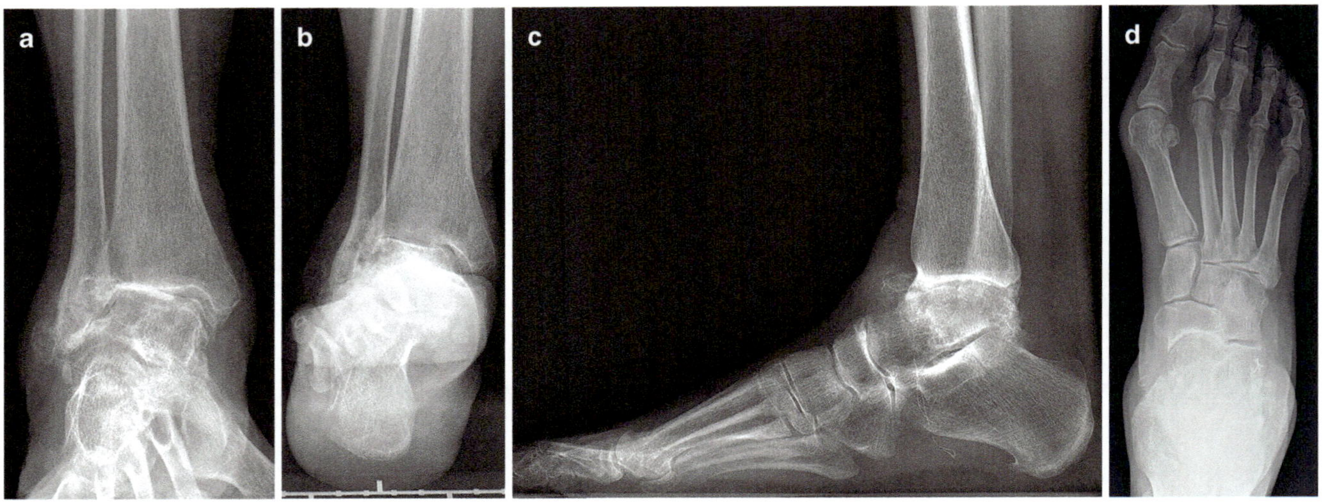

Fig. 2.50 This 54-year-old female patient was suffering from strong ankle pain due to end-stage osteoarthritis 22 years after she underwent a tenodesis procedure for treatment of chronic ankle instability. (**a**) The AP radiograph showed the valgus tilted talus with destroyed lateral tibiotalar and talofibular joints and a lateral gapping at the subtalar joint, resulting in a zigzag deformity. (**b**) The zigzag deformity can also be seen in the hindfoot alignment view. (**c**) The lateral view showed the advanced stage of ankle osteoarthritis and degenerative disease of the subtalar joint that has become flattened over the years due to the changed mechanics. (**d**) As the tenodesis was made between the fibula and anterior calcaneus, the calcaneocuboid joint was not affected by the osteoarthritis process

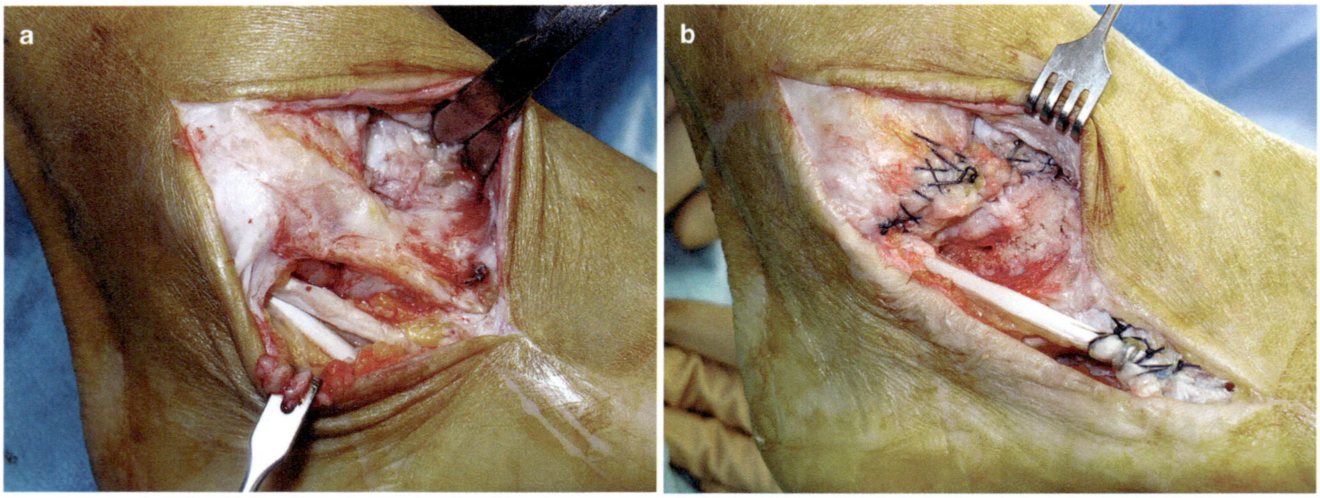

Fig. 2.51 *Surgical Technique: Salvage of a failed reconstruction with a semitendinosus allograft.* This 28-year-old female basketball player underwent lateral ligament reconstruction with the use of a semitendinosus allograft. As she was left with pain and a dysfunctional ankle since the surgery, she did not return to sports. (**a**) Surgical exposure evidenced the bulky tendon graft that ran from distal fibula parallel to the atrophic peroneal tendons to the anterolateral calcaneus and the bottom of talar neck. The subtalar joint was destroyed, and only very little motion was left. The peroneus brevis tendon was scarred and did not show any excursion. (**b**) After having fused the subtalar joint, the tendon allograft was revised by partial resection and rerouting to the anatomical insertion area of the ATFL on the talar neck. Finally, the peroneus longus tendon was transferred to the peroneus brevis tendon and the base of the fifth metatarsal, respectively

treatment, 20–40% of the patients with injuries to the lateral ligaments will go on to experience chronic instability and subsequent disability. A high incidence of persistent instability is related to bony avulsion injuries with subsequent disconnection of both the ATF and CF ligaments from the fibula. Therefore, reattachment of the fragment or excision thereof with reattachment of the ligaments to the fibula is generally recommended [73, 74, 116].

There is no doubt that surgical reconstruction must respect the anatomy. Nonanatomic tenodesis procedures should no longer be used. Additionally, data suggests that peroneal tendons should not be used for reconstruction either, due to the compromising functional stabilization of the ankle joint complex when used [71].

The role of associated lesions and pathologies in patients with lateral ankle instability is still not fully understood [17,

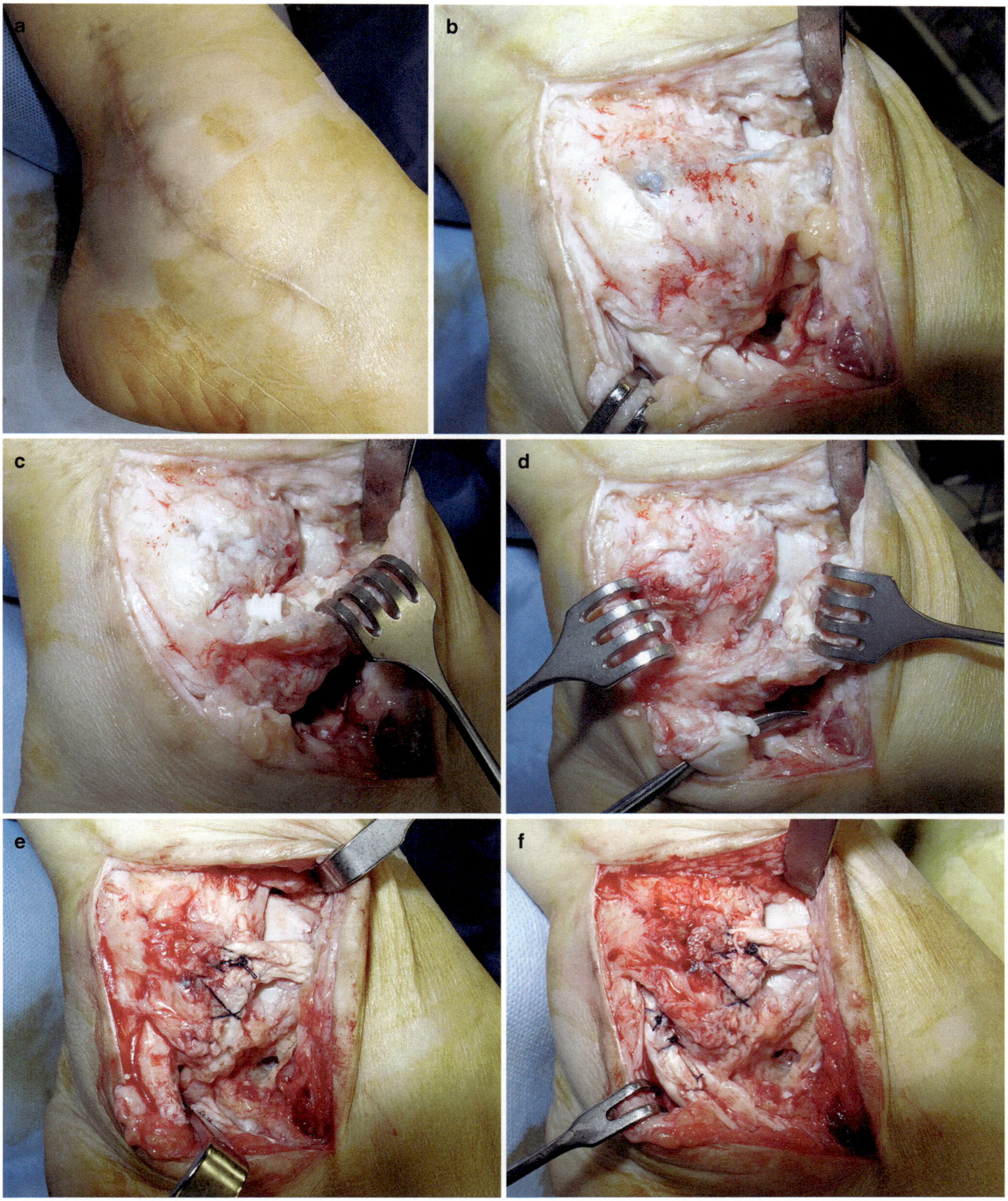

Fig. 2.52 *Surgical Technique: Salvage of a failed reconstruction with the peroneus brevis tendon and internal brace augmentation*. This 26-year-old female soccer player was complaining about strong pain in her lateral ankle after she underwent a lateral ligament reconstruction 7 months earlier. The foot was found fixed in equinus position and stiff without any supination. There was marked pain on palpation over the swollen peroneal tendon sheath and the lateral ankle. (**a**) Lateral view of the swollen ankle. (**b**) Surgical exposure evidenced a hypertrophic scar formation over the distal fibula as well as a bulky and scarred ATFL and CFL. The internal brace could be seen running in a nonanatomic course. Also, the peroneal tendons were scarred. (**c**) While dissecting the scars from the fibula, the loose interference screw from the internal brace was found. (**d**) Further dissection showed the peroneus brevis tendon connected to the scarred ligaments. (**e**) First, the scarred ligaments and remaining tendon grafts were shaped to normal size and then reattached to the fibula and talar neck for anatomic reconstruction of the ATFL and CFL. (**f**) Second, the peroneal tendon sheath was debrided and the distal stump of the peroneus brevis tendon was transferred with side-to-side sutures to the peroneus longus tendon

110]. The question often remains whether surgical reconstruction of the ligaments will be sufficient to restore ankle joint mechanics, treating the symptoms of associated pathologies, or whether pain and disability will continue due to the unaddressed pathologies [108]. Furthermore, to which extent secondary osteoarthritis of the ankle joint has its origin in untreated instability or in neglected associated pathologies is still not clear [15, 35].

The tremendous increase of available imaging tools over the last two decades and progress made in arthroscopy have renewed surgeons' interests for the unstable ankle. Many new arthroscopic techniques have been developed to reconstruct the ligaments, for which mostly high success rates have been reported at short term. However, mid- to long-term results are still outstanding. The use of internal braces has been popularized as a single reconstruction measure or as an augmentation of ligament repair [124, 125, 155] without long-term follow-up data being available yet. Furthermore, especially for arthroscopic ligament reconstruction, some worries exist in how accurate the surgeons can restore anatomy of the lateral ankle ligaments.

More studies are therefore necessary to further answer open questions and improve not only the reconstruction techniques, but also to determine when conservative treatment is adequate and when surgical reconstruction is necessary to restore ankle stability and gain a pain-free functioning ankle joint again.

References

1. Boruta PM, Bishop JO, Braly WG, Tullos HS. Acute lateral ankle ligament injuries: a literature review. Foot Ankle. 1990;11(2):107–13.
2. Doherty C, Delahunt E, Caulfield B, Hertel J, Ryan J, Bleakley C. The incidence and prevalence of ankle sprain injury: a systematic review and meta-analysis of prospective epidemiological studies. Sports Med. 2014;44(1):123–40.
3. Garrick JG. Sports medicine. Pediatr Clin N Am. 1977; 24(4):737–47.
4. Herzog MM, Kerr ZY, Marshall SW, Wikstrom EA. Epidemiology of ankle sprains and chronic ankle instability. J Athl Train. 2019;54(6):603–10.
5. Mack RP. Ankle injuries in athletics. Clin Sports Med. 1982;1(1):71–84.
6. Garrick JG, Requa RK. The epidemiology of foot and ankle injuries in sports. Clin Sports Med. 1988;7(1):29–36.
7. Hintermann B. Bandverletzung der Sprunggelenke (Teil1) [Ligament injury of the ankle joint (I)]. Sportverletz Sportschaden. 1996;10(3):47.
8. Hsu AR, Ardoin GT, Davis WH, Anderson RB. Intermediate and long-term outcomes of the modified brostrom-evans procedure for lateral ankle ligament reconstruction. Foot Ankle Spec. 2016;9(2):131–9.
9. Mauntel TC, Wikstrom EA, Roos KG, Djoko A, Dompier TP, Kerr ZY. The epidemiology of high ankle sprains in national collegiate athletic association sports. Am J Sports Med. 2017;45(9):2156–63.
10. Baumhauer JF, Alosa DM, Renstrom AF, Trevino S, Beynnon B. A prospective study of ankle injury risk factors. Am J Sports Med. 1995;23(5):564–70.
11. Brand RL, Collins MD, Templeton T. Surgical repair of ruptured alteral ankle ligaments. Am J Sports Med. 1981;9(1):40–4.
12. Brostrom L. Sprained ankles. V. Treatment and prognosis in recent ligament ruptures. Acta Chir Scand. 1966;132(5):537–50.
13. Cass JR, Morrey BF, Chao EY. Three-dimensional kinematics of ankle instability following serial sectioning of lateral collateral ligaments. Foot Ankle. 1984;5(3):142–9.
14. Freeman MA. Instability of the foot after injuries to the lateral ligament of the ankle. J Bone Joint Surg (Br). 1965;47(4):669–77.
15. Harrington KD. Degenerative arthritis of the ankle secondary to long-standing lateral ligament instability. J Bone Joint Surg Am. 1979;61(3):354–61.
16. Karlsson J, Bergsten T, Lansinger O, Peterson L. Reconstruction of the lateral ligaments of the ankle for chronic lateral instability. J Bone Joint Surg Am. 1988;70(4):581–8.
17. Renstrom PA. Persistently painful sprained ankle. J Am Acad Orthop Surg. 1994;2(5):270–80.
18. Staples OS. Ruptures of the fibular collateral ligaments of the ankle. Result study of immediate surgical treatment. J Bone Joint Surg Am. 1975;57(1):101–7.
19. Brostrom L. Sprained ankles. VI. Surgical treatment of "chronic" ligament ruptures. Acta Chir Scand. 1966;132(5):551–65.
20. Colville MR, Marder RA, Zarins B. Reconstruction of the lateral ankle ligaments. A biomechanical analysis. Am J Sports Med. 1992;20(5):594–600.
21. Hintermann B, Renggli P. Anatomische Rekonstruktion der lateralen Sprunggelenkbänder mit der Plantarissehne zur Behandlung der chronischen Instabilität [Anatomic reconstruction of the lateral ligaments of the ankle using a plantaris tendon graft in the treatment of chronic ankle joint instability]. Orthopade. 1999;28(9):778–84.
22. Knupp M, Lang TH, Zwicky L, Lotscher P, Hintermann B. Chronic ankle instability (medial and lateral). Clin Sports Med. 2015;34(4):679–88.
23. Rudert M, Wulker N, Wirth CJ. Reconstruction of the lateral ligaments of the ankle using a regional periosteal flap. J Bone Joint Surg (Br). 1997;79(3):446–51.
24. Sammarco GJ, DiRaimondo CV. Surgical treatment of lateral ankle instability syndrome. Am J Sports Med. 1988;16(5):501–11.
25. Snook GA, Chrisman OD, Wilson TC. Long-term results of the Chrisman-Snook operation for reconstruction of the lateral ligaments of the ankle. J Bone Joint Surg Am. 1985;67(1):1–7.
26. St Pierre R, Allman F Jr, Bassett FH III, Goldner JL, Fleming LL. A review of lateral ankle ligamentous reconstructions. Foot Ankle. 1982;3(2):114–23.
27. Trichine F, Friha T, Boukabou A, Belaid L, Bouzidi T, Bouzitouna M. Surgical treatment of chronic lateral ankle instability using an inferior extensor retinaculum flap: a retrospective study. J Foot Ankle Surg. 2018;57(2):226–31.
28. Valderrabano V, Wiewiorski M, Frigg A, Hintermann B, Leumann A. Chronische Instabilität des oberen Sprunggelenks [Chronic ankle instability]. Unfallchirurg. 2007;110(8):691–9.
29. Valderrabano V, Wiewiorski M, Frigg A, Hintermann B, Leumann A. Direkte anatomische Rekonstruktion des lateralen Bandapparats bei chronischer lateralen Instabilität des oberen Sprunggelenks [Direct anatomic repair of the lateral ankle ligaments in chronic lateral ankle instability]. Unfallchirurg. 2007;110(8):701–4.
30. Rosenbaum D, Becker HP, Sterk J, Gerngross H, Claes L. Functional evaluation of the 10-year outcome after modified Evans repair for chronic ankle instability. Foot Ankle Int. 1997;18(12):765–71.
31. Sammarco VJ. Complications of lateral ankle ligament reconstruction. Clin Orthop Relat Res. 2001;391:123–32.
32. Barg A, Tochigi Y, Amendola A, Phisitkul P, Hintermann B, Saltzman CL. Subtalar instability: diagnosis and treatment. Foot Ankle Int. 2012;33(2):151–60.
33. Kjaersgaard-Andersen P, Wethelund JO, Helmig P, Soballe K. The stabilizing effect of the ligamentous structures in the sinus and

canalis tarsi on movements in the hindfoot. An experimental study. Am J Sports Med. 1988;16(5):512–6.
34. Becker HP, Rosenbaum D. [Functional disorders of the foot after tenodeses: is the method still currently acceptable?]. Sportverletz Sportschaden 1996;10(4):94–9.
35. Valderrabano V, Horisberger M, Russell I, Dougall H, Hintermann B. Etiology of ankle osteoarthritis. Clin Orthop Relat Res. 2009;467(7):1800–6.
36. Burks RT, Morgan J. Anatomy of the lateral ankle ligaments. Am J Sports Med. 1994;22(1):72–7.
37. Kakegawa A, Mori Y, Tsuchiya A, Sumitomo N, Fukushima N, Moriizumi T. Independent attachment of lateral ankle ligaments: anterior talofibular and calcaneofibular ligaments - a cadaveric study. J Foot Ankle Surg. 2019;58(4):717–22.
38. Matsui K, Takao M, Tochigi Y, Ozeki S, Glazebrook M. Anatomy of anterior talofibular ligament and calcaneofibular ligament for minimally invasive surgery: a systematic review. Knee Surg Sports Traumatol Arthrosc. 2017;25(6):1892–902.
39. Milner CE, Soames RW. Anatomical variations of the anterior talofibular ligament of the human ankle joint. J Anat. 1997;191(Pt 3):457–8.
40. Milner CE, Soames RW. Anatomy of the collateral ligaments of the human ankle joint. Foot Ankle Int. 1998;19(11):757–60.
41. Prins JG. Diagnosis and treatment of injury to the lateral ligament of the ankle. A comparative clinical study. Acta Chir Scand Suppl. 1978;486:3–149.
42. Sarrafian SK. Anatomy of foot and ankle. 2nd ed. Philadelphia, PA: Lippincott Williams and Wilkins; 1993.
43. Hintermann B. Biomechanics of the unstable ankle joint and clinical implications. Med Sci Sports Exerc. 1999;31(7 Suppl):S459–69.
44. Inman VT. The joints of the ankle. Baltimore, MD: Williams & Wilkins; 1976.
45. Colville MR, Marder RA, Boyle JJ, Zarins B. Strain measurement in lateral ankle ligaments. Am J Sports Med. 1990;18(2): 196–200.
46. Rasmussen O. Stability of the ankle joint. Analysis of the function and traumatology of the ankle ligaments. Acta Orthop Scand Suppl. 1985;211:1–75.
47. Johnson EE, Markolf KL. The contribution of the anterior talofibular ligament to ankle laxity. J Bone Joint Surg Am. 1983;65(1): 81–8.
48. Hollis JM, Blasier RD, Flahiff CM, Hofmann OE. Biomechanical comparison of reconstruction techniques in simulated lateral ankle ligament injury. Am J Sports Med. 1995;23(6):678–82.
49. Bulucu C, Thomas KA, Halvorson TL, Cook SD. Biomechanical evaluation of the anterior drawer test: the contribution of the lateral ankle ligaments. Foot Ankle. 1991;11(6):389–93.
50. Cawley PW, France EP. Biomechanics of the lateral ligaments of the ankle: an evaluation of the effects of axial load and single plane motions on ligament strain patterns. Foot Ankle. 1991;12(2):92–9.
51. McCullough CJ, Burge PD. Rotatory stability of the load-bearing ankle. An experimental study. J Bone Joint Surg (Br). 1980;62-B(4):460–4.
52. Michelson JD, Clarke HJ, Jinnah RH. The effect of loading on tibiotalar alignment in cadaver ankles. Foot Ankle. 1990;10(5):280–4.
53. Nigg BM, Skarvan G, Frank CB, Yeadon MR. Elongation and forces of ankle ligaments in a physiological range of motion. Foot Ankle. 1990;11(1):30–40.
54. Sommer C, Hintermann B, Nigg BM, van den Bogert AJ. Influence of ankle ligaments on tibial rotation: an in vitro study. Foot Ankle Int. 1996;17(2):79–84.
55. Stormont DM, Morrey BF, An KN, Cass JR. Stability of the loaded ankle. Relation between articular restraint and primary and secondary static restraints. Am J Sports Med. 1985;13(5):295–300.
56. Larsen E. Experimental instability of the ankle. A radiographic investigation. Clin Orthop Relat Res. 1986;204:193–200.
57. Stephens MM, Sammarco GJ. The stabilizing role of the lateral ligament complex around the ankle and subtalar joints. Foot Ankle. 1992;13(3):130–6.
58. Cass JR, Settles H. Ankle instability: in vitro kinematics in response to axial load. Foot Ankle Int. 1994;15(3):134–40.
59. Hunt KJ, Pereira H, Kelley J, Anderson N, Fuld R, Baldini T, et al. The role of calcaneofibular ligament injury in ankle instability: implications for surgical management. Am J Sports Med. 2019;47(2):431–7.
60. Hintermann B, Nigg BM, Sommer C, Cole GK. Transfer of movement between calcaneus and tibia in vitro. Clin Biomech. 1994;9(6):349–55.
61. Laurin CA, Ouellet R, St-Jacques R. Talar and subtalar tilt: an experimental investigation. Can J Surg. 1968;11(3):270–9.
62. Lundberg A, Svensson OK, Nemeth G, Selvik G. The axis of rotation of the ankle joint. J Bone Joint Surg (Br). 1989;71(1):94–9.
63. Lundberg A, Svensson OK, Bylund C, Goldie I, Selvik G. Kinematics of the ankle/foot complex--Part 2: Pronation and supination. Foot Ankle. 1989;9(5):248–53.
64. Hintermann B, Sommer C, Nigg BM. Influence of ligament transection on tibial and calcaneal rotation with loading and dorsi-plantarflexion. Foot Ankle Int. 1995;16(9):567–71.
65. Clanton TO. Instability of the subtalar joint. Orthop Clin North Am. 1989;20(4):583–92.
66. Kjaersgaard-Andersen P, Wethelund JO, Helmig P, Nielsen S. Effect of the calcaneofibular ligament on hindfoot rotation in amputation specimens. Acta Orthop Scand. 1987;58(2):135–8.
67. Cass JR, Morrey BF, Katoh Y, Chao EY. Ankle instability: comparison of primary repair and delayed reconstruction after long-term follow-up study. Clin Orthop Relat Res. 1985;198:110–7.
68. Chrisman OD, Snook GA. Reconstruction of lateral ligament tears of the ankle. An experimental study and clinical evaluation of seven patients treated by a new modification of the Elmslie procedure. J Bone Joint Surg Am. 1969;51(5):904–12.
69. Evans DL. Recurrent instability of the ankle; a method of surgical treatment. Proc R Soc Med. 1953;46(5):343–4.
70. Lee HG. Surgical repair in recurrent dislocation of the ankle joint. J Bone Joint Surg Am. 1957;39-A(4):828–34.
71. Purevsuren T, Batbaatar M, Khuyagbaatar B, Kim K, Kim YH. Comparative evaluation between anatomic and non-anatomic lateral ligament reconstruction techniques in the ankle joint: a computational study. J Biomech Eng. 2018.
72. Hertel J. Functional anatomy, pathomechanics, and pathophysiology of lateral ankle instability. J Athl Train. 2002;37(4):364–75.
73. Haraguchi N, Toga H, Shiba N, Kato F. Avulsion fracture of the lateral ankle ligament complex in severe inversion injury: incidence and clinical outcome. Am J Sports Med. 2007;35(7):1144–52.
74. Diallo J, Wagener J, Schweizer C, Lang TH, Ruiz R, Hintermann B. Intraoperative findings of lateral ligament avulsion fractures and outcome after refixation to the fibula. Foot Ankle Int. 2018;39(6):669–73.
75. Kumai T, Takakura Y, Rufai A, Milz S, Benjamin M. The functional anatomy of the human anterior talofibular ligament in relation to ankle sprains. J Anat. 2002;200(5):457–65.
76. Cho JH, Lee DH, Song HK, Bang JY, Lee KT, Park YU. Value of stress ultrasound for the diagnosis of chronic ankle instability compared to manual anterior drawer test, stress radiography, magnetic resonance imaging, and arthroscopy. Knee Surg Sports Traumatol Arthrosc. 2016;24(4):1022–8.
77. Gehring D, Li L, Bonsignore G, Dorn-Lange N, Gollhofer A, Lohrer H. Detecting ankle instability with an instrumented ankle arthrometer: an experimental study. J Orthop Res. 2019;37(9):2019–26.
78. Kikumoto T, Akatsuka K, Nakamura E, Ito W, Hirabayashi R, Edama M. Quantitative evaluation method for clarifying ankle plantar flexion angles using anterior drawer and inversion stress tests: a cross-sectional study. J Foot Ankle Res. 2019;12:27.

79. Kim YS, Kim YB, Kim TG, Lee SW, Park SH, Lee HJ, et al. Reliability and validity of magnetic resonance imaging for the evaluation of the anterior talofibular ligament in patients undergoing ankle arthroscopy. Arthroscopy. 2015;31(8):1540–7.
80. Li Q, Tu Y, Chen J, Shan J, Yung PS, Ling SK, et al. Reverse anterolateral drawer test is more sensitive and accurate for diagnosing chronic anterior talofibular ligament injury. Knee Surg Sports Traumatol Arthrosc. 2020;28(1):55–62.
81. Miller AG, Myers SH, Parks BG, Guyton GP. Anterolateral drawer versus anterior drawer test for ankle instability: a biomechanical model. Foot Ankle Int. 2016;37(4):407–10.
82. Fujii T, Luo ZP, Kitaoka HB, An KN. The manual stress test may not be sufficient to differentiate ankle ligament injuries. Clin Biomech (Bristol, Avon). 2000;15(8):619–23.
83. Coleman SS, Chesnut WJ. A simple test for hindfoot flexibility in the cavovarus foot. Clin Orthop Relat Res. 1977;123:60–2.
84. Ikoma K, Kido M, Maki M, Imai K, Hara Y, Ikeda R, et al. Early stage and small medial osteochondral lesions of the talus in the presence of chronic lateral ankle instability: a retrospective study. J Orthop Sci. 2020;25(1):178–82.
85. Tohyama H, Yasuda K, Ohkoshi Y, Beynnon BD, Renstrom PA. Anterior drawer test for acute anterior talofibular ligament injuries of the ankle. How much load should be applied during the test? Am J Sports Med. 2003;31(2):226–32.
86. Brooks SC, Potter BT, Rainey JB. Treatment for partial tears of the lateral ligament of the ankle: a prospective trial. Br Med J (Clin Res Ed). 1981;282(6264):606–7.
87. Seligson D, Gassman J, Pope M. Ankle instability: evaluation of the lateral ligaments. Am J Sports Med. 1980;8(1):39–42.
88. Rijke AM. MR imaging versus stress radiography in the evaluation of chronic ankle instability. Radiology. 1995;196(2):580–1.
89. Campbell DG, Menz A, Isaacs J. Dynamic ankle ultrasonography. A new imaging technique for acute ankle ligament injuries. Am J Sports Med. 1994;22(6):855–8.
90. Chandnani VP, Harper MT, Ficke JR, Gagliardi JA, Rolling L, Christensen KP, et al. Chronic ankle instability: evaluation with MR arthrography, MR imaging, and stress radiography. Radiology. 1994;192(1):189–94.
91. Lee KT, Park YU, Jegal H, Park JW, Choi JP, Kim JS. New method of diagnosis for chronic ankle instability: comparison of manual anterior drawer test, stress radiography and stress ultrasound. Knee Surg Sports Traumatol Arthrosc. 2014;22(7):1701–7.
92. Khor YP, Tan KJ. The anatomic pattern of injuries in acute inversion ankle sprains: a magnetic resonance imaging study. Orthop J Sports Med. 2013;1(7):2325967113517078.
93. Roemer FW, Jomaah N, Niu J, Almusa E, Roger B, D'Hooghe P, et al. Ligamentous injuries and the risk of associated tissue damage in acute ankle sprains in athletes: a cross-sectional MRI study. Am J Sports Med. 2014;42(7):1549–57.
94. Elkaim M, Thes A, Lopes R, Andrieu M, Cordier G, Molinier F, et al. Agreement between arthroscopic and imaging study findings in chronic anterior talo-fibular ligament injuries. Orthop Traumatol Surg Res. 2018;104(8S):S213–S8.
95. Li HY, Li WL, Chen SY, Hua YH. Increased ATFL-PTFL angle could be an indirect MRI sign in diagnosis of chronic ATFL injury. Knee Surg Sports Traumatol Arthrosc. 2020;28(1):208–12.
96. Morvan A, Klouche S, Thes A, Hardy P, Bauer T. Reliability and validity of preoperative MRI for surgical decision making in chronic lateral ankle instability. Eur J Orthop Surg Traumatol. 2018;28(4):713–9.
97. Cha SD, Kim HS, Chung ST, Yoo JH, Park JH, Kim JH, et al. Intra-articular lesions in chronic lateral ankle instability: comparison of arthroscopy with magnetic resonance imaging findings. Clin Orthop Surg. 2012;4(4):293–9.
98. Hintermann B. What the orthopaedic foot and ankle surgeon wants to know from MR Imaging. Semin Musculoskelet Radiol. 2005;9(3):260–71.
99. Staats K, Sabeti-Aschraf M, Apprich S, Platzgummer H, Puchner SE, Holinka J, et al. Preoperative MRI is helpful but not sufficient to detect associated lesions in patients with chronic ankle instability. Knee Surg Sports Traumatol Arthrosc. 2018;26(7):2103–9.
100. Jung HG, Kim TH, Park JY, Bae EJ. Anatomic reconstruction of the anterior talofibular and calcaneofibular ligaments using a semitendinosus tendon allograft and interference screws. Knee Surg Sports Traumatol Arthrosc. 2012;20(8):1432–7.
101. Vega J, Montesinos E, Malagelada F, Baduell A, Guelfi M, Dalmau-Pastor M. Arthroscopic all-inside anterior talo-fibular ligament repair with suture augmentation gives excellent results in case of poor ligament tissue remnant quality. Knee Surg Sports Traumatol Arthrosc. 2020;28(1):100–7.
102. Biercevicz AM, Miranda DL, Machan JT, Murray MM, Fleming BC. In Situ, noninvasive, T2*-weighted MRI-derived parameters predict ex vivo structural properties of an anterior cruciate ligament reconstruction or bioenhanced primary repair in a porcine model. Am J Sports Med. 2013;41(3):560–6.
103. Fleming BC, Vajapeyam S, Connolly SA, Magarian EM, Murray MM. The use of magnetic resonance imaging to predict ACL graft structural properties. J Biomech. 2011;44(16):2843–6.
104. Li H, Hua Y, Feng S, Li H, Chen S. Lower signal intensity of the anterior talofibular ligament is associated with a higher rate of return to sport after ATFL repair for chronic lateral ankle instability. Am J Sports Med. 2019;47(10):2380–5.
105. Zanetti M, De Simoni C, Wetz HH, Zollinger H, Hodler J. Magnetic resonance imaging of injuries to the ankle joint: can it predict clinical outcome? Skelet Radiol. 1997;26(2):82–8.
106. Ferkel RD, Chams RN. Chronic lateral instability: arthroscopic findings and long-term results. Foot Ankle Int. 2007;28(1):24–31.
107. Hintermann B, Boss A, Schafer D. Arthroscopic findings in patients with chronic ankle instability. Am J Sports Med. 2002;30(3):402–9.
108. Okuda R, Kinoshita M, Morikawa J, Yasuda T, Abe M. Arthroscopic findings in chronic lateral ankle instability: do focal chondral lesions influence the results of ligament reconstruction? Am J Sports Med. 2005;33(1):35–42.
109. Taga I, Shino K, Inoue M, Nakata K, Maeda A. Articular cartilage lesions in ankles with lateral ligament injury. An arthroscopic study. Am J Sports Med. 1993;21(1):120–6; discussion 6–7.
110. Lee J, Hamilton G, Ford L. Associated intra-articular ankle pathologies in patients with chronic lateral ankle instability: arthroscopic findings at the time of lateral ankle reconstruction. Foot Ankle Spec. 2011;4(5):284–9.
111. Thes A, Odagiri H, Elkaim M, Lopes R, Andrieu M, Cordier G, et al. Arthroscopic classification of chronic anterior talo-fibular ligament lesions in chronic ankle instability. Orthop Traumatol Surg Res. 2018;104(8S):S207–S11.
112. Komenda GA, Ferkel RD. Arthroscopic findings associated with the unstable ankle. Foot Ankle Int. 1999;20(11):708–13.
113. Schafer D, Hintermann B. Arthroscopic assessment of the chronic unstable ankle joint. Knee Surg Sports Traumatol Arthrosc. 1996;4(1):48–52.
114. Maffulli N, Ferran NA. Management of acute and chronic ankle instability. J Am Acad Orthop Surg. 2008;16(10):608–15.
115. Chun TH, Park YS, Sung KS. The effect of ossicle resection in the lateral ligament repair for treatment of chronic lateral ankle instability. Foot Ankle Int. 2013;34(8):1128–33.
116. Yamaguchi S, Akagi R, Kimura S, Sadamasu A, Nakagawa R, Sato Y, et al. Avulsion fracture of the distal fibula is associated with recurrent sprain after ankle sprain in children. Knee Surg Sports Traumatol Arthrosc. 2019;27(9):2774–80.

117. Reiner MM, Sharpe JJ. The role of the accessory malleolar ossicles and malleolar avulsion fractures in lateral ankle ligament reconstruction. Foot Ankle Spec. 2018;11(4):308–14.
118. Song Y, Li H, Sun C, Zhang J, Gui J, Guo Q, et al. Clinical guidelines for the surgical management of chronic lateral ankle instability: a consensus reached by systematic review of the available data. Orthop J Sports Med. 2019;7(9):2325967119873852.
119. Gould N, Seligson D, Gassman J. Early and late repair of lateral ligament of the ankle. Foot Ankle. 1980;1(2):84–9.
120. Cao Y, Hong Y, Xu Y, Zhu Y, Xu X. Surgical management of chronic lateral ankle instability: a meta-analysis. J Orthop Surg Res. 2018;13(1):159.
121. Pagenstert GI, Hintermann B, Knupp M. Operative management of chronic ankle instability: plantaris graft. Foot Ankle Clin. 2006;11(3):567–83.
122. Jung HG, Park JT, Eom JS, Jung MG, Lee DO. Reconstruction of superficial deltoid ligaments with allograft tendons in medial ankle instability: a technical report. Injury. 2016;47(3):780–3.
123. Kirk KL, Campbell JT, Guyton GP, Parks BG, Schon LC. ATFL elongation after Brostrom procedure: a biomechanical investigation. Foot Ankle Int. 2008;29(11):1126–30.
124. Schuh R, Benca E, Willegger M, Hirtler L, Zandieh S, Holinka J, et al. Comparison of Brostrom technique, suture anchor repair, and tape augmentation for reconstruction of the anterior talofibular ligament. Knee Surg Sports Traumatol Arthrosc. 2016;24(4): 1101–7.
125. Yoo JS, Yang EA. Clinical results of an arthroscopic modified Brostrom operation with and without an internal brace. J Orthop Traumatol. 2016;17(4):353–60.
126. Shoji H, Teramoto A, Sakakibara Y, Kamiya T, Watanabe K, Fujie H, et al. Kinematics and laxity of the ankle joint in anatomic and nonanatomic anterior talofibular ligament repair: a biomechanical cadaveric study. Am J Sports Med. 2019;47(3):667–73.
127. Matsui K, Takao M, Miyamoto W, Innami K, Matsushita T. Arthroscopic Brostrom repair with Gould augmentation via an accessory anterolateral port for lateral instability of the ankle. Arch Orthop Trauma Surg. 2014;134(10):1461–7.
128. Matsui K, Takao M, Miyamoto W, Matsushita T. Early recovery after arthroscopic repair compared to open repair of the anterior talofibular ligament for lateral instability of the ankle. Arch Orthop Trauma Surg. 2016;136(1):93–100.
129. Cottom JM, Baker JS, Richardson PE. The "All-Inside" arthroscopic brostrom procedure with additional suture anchor augmentation: a prospective study of 45 consecutive patients. J Foot Ankle Surg. 2016;55(6):1223–8.
130. Kim ES, Lee KT, Park JS, Lee YK. Arthroscopic anterior talofibular ligament repair for chronic ankle instability with a suture anchor technique. Orthopedics. 2011;34(4).
131. Nery C, Raduan F, Del Buono A, Asaumi ID, Cohen M, Maffulli N. Arthroscopic-assisted Brostrom-Gould for chronic ankle instability: a long-term follow-up. Am J Sports Med. 2011;39(11):2381–8.
132. Song YJ, Hua YH. Similar outcomes at early term after arthroscopic or open repair of chronic ankle instability: a systematic review and meta-analysis. J Foot Ankle Surg. 2019;58(2):312–9.
133. Vega J, Golano P, Pellegrino A, Rabat E, Pena F. All-inside arthroscopic lateral collateral ligament repair for ankle instability with a knotless suture anchor technique. Foot Ankle Int. 2013;34(12):1701–9.
134. Wang J, Hua Y, Chen S, Li H, Zhang J, Li Y. Arthroscopic repair of lateral ankle ligament complex by suture anchor. Arthroscopy. 2014;30(6):766–73.
135. Brown AJ, Shimozono Y, Hurley ET, Kennedy JG. Arthroscopic repair of lateral ankle ligament for chronic lateral ankle instability: a systematic review. Arthroscopy. 2018;34(8):2497–503.
136. Yasui Y, Shimozono Y, Kennedy JG. Surgical procedures for chronic lateral ankle instability. J Am Acad Orthop Surg. 2018;26(7):223–30.
137. Kilger R, Knupp M, Hintermann B. Peroneus longus to peroneus brevis tendon transfer. Tech Foot Ankle Surg. 2009;8(3):146–9.
138. Choi GW, Choi WJ, Youn HK, Park YJ, Lee JW. Osteochondral lesions of the talus: are there any differences between osteochondral and chondral types? Am J Sports Med. 2013;41(3):504–10.
139. Chuckpaiwong B, Berkson EM, Theodore GH. Microfracture for osteochondral lesions of the ankle: outcome analysis and outcome predictors of 105 cases. Arthroscopy. 2008;24(1):106–12.
140. van Bergen CJA, Zwiers R, van Dijk CN. Arthroscopic treatment of osteochondral talar defects. JBJS Essent Surg Tech. 2014;3(2):e10.
141. Hangody L, Kish G, Modis L, Szerb I, Gaspar L, Dioszegi Z, et al. Mosaicplasty for the treatment of osteochondritis dissecans of the talus: two to seven year results in 36 patients. Foot Ankle Int. 2001;22(7):552–8.
142. Valderrabano V, Leumann A, Rasch H, Egelhof T, Hintermann B, Pagenstert G. Knee-to-ankle mosaicplasty for the treatment of osteochondral lesions of the ankle joint. Am J Sports Med. 2009;37(Suppl 1):105S–11S.
143. Ahmad J, Jones K. Comparison of osteochondral autografts and allografts for treatment of recurrent or large talar osteochondral lesions. Foot Ankle Int. 2016;37(1):40–50.
144. Berlet GC, Hyer CF, Philbin TM, Hartman JF, Wright ML. Does fresh osteochondral allograft transplantation of talar osteochondral defects improve function? Clin Orthop Relat Res. 2011;469(8):2356–66.
145. Hintermann B, Wagener J, Knupp M, Schweizer C, Schaefer D. Treatment of extended osteochondral lesions of the talus with a free vascularised bone graft from the medial condyle of the femur. Bone Jt J. 2015;97-B(9):1242–9.
146. Dwyer FC. Osteotomy of the calcaneum for pes cavus. J Bone Joint Surg (Br). 1959;41-B(1):80–6.
147. Malerba F, De Marchi F. Calcaneal osteotomies. Foot Ankle Clin. 2005;10(3):523–40, vii.
148. Pisani G. Subtalar osteotomy for correction of deformities of the calcaneus in the frontal plane. Paris: Expansion Scientifique Française; 1985.
149. Knupp M, Horisberger M, Hintermann B. A new Z-shaped calcaneal osteotomy for 3-plane correction of severe varus deformity of the hindfoot. Tech Foot Ankle Surg. 2008;7(2):90–5.
150. Evans GA, Hardcastle P, Frenyo AD. Acute rupture of the lateral ligament of the ankle. To suture or not to suture? J Bone Joint Surg (Br). 1984;66(2):209–12.
151. Takao M, Miyamoto W, Matsui K, Sasahara J, Matsushita T. Functional treatment after surgical repair for acute lateral ligament disruption of the ankle in athletes. Am J Sports Med. 2012;40(2):447–51.
152. Bell SJ, Mologne TS, Sitler DF, Cox JS. Twenty-six-year results after Brostrom procedure for chronic lateral ankle instability. Am J Sports Med. 2006;34(6):975–8.
153. Lee KT, Park YU, Kim JS, Kim JB, Kim KC, Kang SK. Long-term results after modified Brostrom procedure without calcaneofibular ligament reconstruction. Foot Ankle Int. 2011;32(2):153–7.
154. Matheny LM, Johnson NS, Liechti DJ, Clanton TO. Activity level and function after lateral ankle ligament repair versus reconstruction. Am J Sports Med. 2016;44(5):1301–8.
155. Mackay GM, Blyth MJ, Anthony I, Hopper GP, Ribbans WJ. A review of ligament augmentation with the InternalBrace: the surgical principle is described for the lateral ankle ligament and ACL repair in particular, and a comprehensive review of other surgical applications and techniques is presented. Surg Technol Int. 2015;26:239–55.

Lateral Ankle Instability Including Chopart Joint

3

Injuries involving the Chopart joint complex are relatively rare and frequently missed or misdiagnosed, often leading to a poor functional outcome [1, 2]. Typically, midtarsal sprains result from low-energy inversion-type ankle trauma. They are distinct from Chopart joint fracture-dislocations, which result from high-energy trauma such as motor vehicle crashes.

Midtarsal sprains may affect the supporting ligaments along the talocalcaneonavicular and calcaneocuboid joints. The most commonly injured ligaments are the dorsal calcaneocuboid, bifurcate, and dorsal talonavicular ligaments and the spring ligament complex, with plantar ligament injuries thought to be significantly less frequent [3, 4]. The range of osseous injuries includes contusions, avulsions, or impaction fractures of the anterior process of the calcaneus, talar head, cuboid bone, and navicular bone [3–5].

It is reported that 40.5% of the patients with chronic lateral ankle instability have clinical signs of damage to the ligamentum bifurcatum (LB) of the midfoot [6].

3.1 Anatomy of the Chopart Joint Ligaments

- The transverse tarsal joints have a complex ligament apparatus.
- The spring ligament complex plays a significant role in stabilizing the foot.

The transverse tarsal joint complex includes two movable calcaneocuboid and talocalcaneonavicular joints:

3.1.1 The Calcaneocuboid Joint

The calcaneocuboid joint is formed by the quadrilateral facets of the calcaneus and cuboid bones and its capsule, which is reinforced by ligaments [7]. The four ligaments connecting the calcaneus and cuboid are the medial calcaneocuboid ligament, a component of the bifurcate ligament; the dorsolateral calcaneocuboid ligament; the plantar calcaneocuboid ligament, or short plantar ligament; and the long plantar ligament (Fig. 3.1) [3, 7, 8]. The bifurcate ligament also designated as the "ligament of Chopart" is formed by two ligaments, the medial cal-

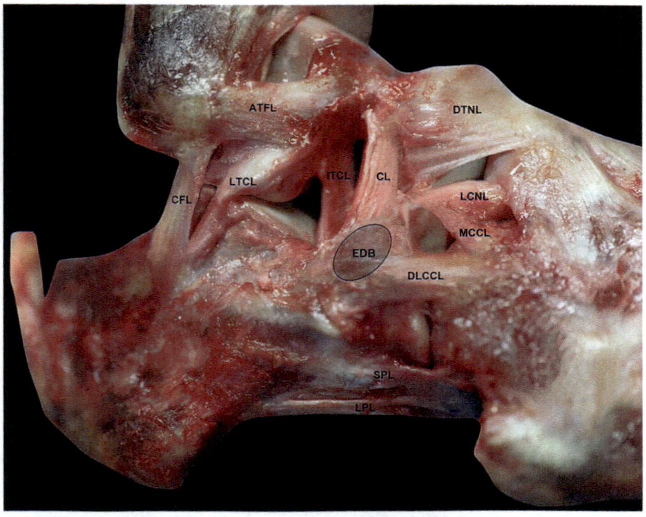

Fig. 3.1 The bifurcate ligament is formed by the medial calcaneocuboid ligament (MCCL) and the lateral calcaneonavicular ligament (LCNL). It has an origin as the cervical ligament (CL) and the origin of the extensor digitorum brevis muscle (EDB), on the intermediary tubercle of the calcaneus, just slightly more anterior. While the LCNL runs to the posterosuperior aspect of the lateral margin of the navicular, the MCCL runs slightly more lateral to the dorsum of the cuboid, inserting approximately 15 mm anterior to the calcaneocuboid joint. The dorsolateral calcaneocuboid ligament (DLCCL) extends from the lateral calcaneus to the cuboid. The inferior calcaneocuboid ligament is formed by the long (LPL) and short plantar ligaments (SPL). The LPL originates from the inferior surface of the calcaneus between the posterior and anterior tubercles and divides distally into at least two bands that attach to the cuboid (lateral band) and variably to the metatarsal bases (medial band). The SPL originates at the plantar surface of the calcaneus, anterior to the long plantar ligament. It extends anteromedially to the plantar surface of the cuboid, proximal to the peroneus longus tunnel. *ATFL* anterior talofibular ligament, *CFL* calcaneofibular ligament, *LTCL* lateral talocalcaneal ligament, *ITCL* interosseous talocalcaneal ligament, *DTNL* dorsal talonavicular ligament

B. Hintermann, R. Ruiz, *Foot and Ankle Instability*, https://doi.org/10.1007/978-3-030-62926-7_3

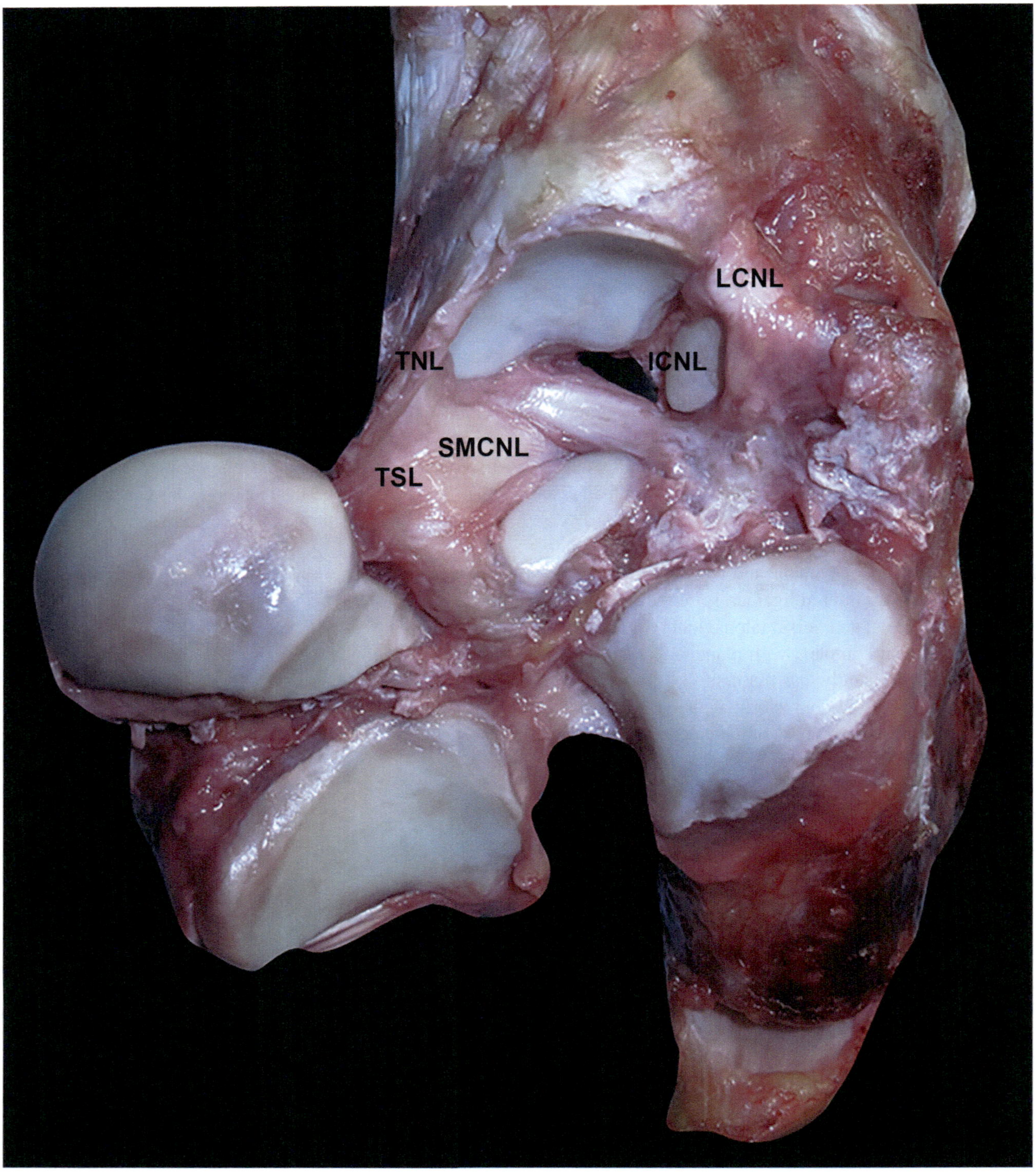

Fig. 3.2 The talonavicular joint has a ball-and-socket configuration, formed by the rounded head of the talus, the concave posterior articular surface of the navicular, and the anterior and the middle articular surface of the calcaneus. Its stability is provided by the inferior (ICNL), medioplantar oblique (MPOCNL) and superomedial (SMCNL) calcaneonavicular ligament (spring ligament), the tibiospring ligament (TSL), the tibionavicular ligament (TNL), and the lateral calcaneonavicular ligament (LCNL)

caneocuboid ligament and lateral calcaneonavicular ligament, thus supporting the talonavicular and calcaneocuboid joints [7]. It is located anterior to the cervical ligament and the origin site of the extensor digitorum brevis muscle. The lateral calcaneonavicular ligament extends between the intermediary tubercle of the calcaneus and the posterosuperior aspect of the lateral margin of the navicular. The medial calcaneocuboid ligament extends between the intermediary tubercle, slightly lateral to the lateral calcaneonavicular ligament, and the dorsum of the cuboid, inserting approximately 15 mm anterior to the calcaneocuboid joint [9–11]. The long and short plantar ligaments form the superficial and deep components of the inferior calcaneocuboid ligament, respectively. The long plantar ligament originates from the inferior surface of the calcaneus between the posterior and anterior tubercles and divides distally into at least two bands that attach to the cuboid (lateral band) and variably to the metatarsal bases (medial band) (Fig. 3.1). When present, the medial band forms the roof of the peroneus longus tunnel [8, 11]. The short plantar ligament originates at the plantar surface of the calcaneus, anterior to the long plantar ligament. It extends anteromedially to the plantar surface of the cuboid and proximal to the peroneus longus tunnel.

3.1.2 The Talocalcaneonavicular Joint

The talocalcaneonavicular joint comprises the rounded head of the talus; concave posterior surface of the navicular; anterior articular surface of the calcaneus; and upper surface of the calcaneonavicular ligament, or spring ligament (Fig. 3.2) [7, 11, 12]. Injuries of the spring ligament complex are typically seen in patients after a pronation-abduction trauma and subsequent to an acquired flatfoot deformity; therefore, special focus to the spring ligament is given in Chap. 5.

The capsule of the talonavicular joint, which is defective anteriorly, is reinforced superolaterally by both the dorsal talonavicular ligament and the lateral calcaneonavicular ligament, which is the other component of the bifurcate ligament (Fig. 3.3). The dorsal talonavicular ligament is a capsular thickening connecting the dorsal aspect of the talar neck and the dorsal surface of the navicular bone [10]. It runs from proximal lateral to distal medial, being the continuation of the anterior talofibular ligament.

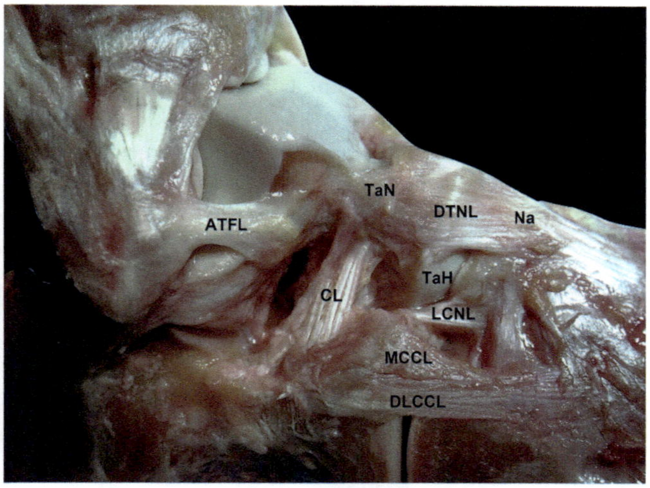

Fig. 3.3 The capsule of talonavicular joint is reinforced superolaterally by the dorsal talonavicular ligament (DTNL) and laterally by the lateral calcaneonavicular ligament (LCNL). The DTNL is a capsular thickening connecting the dorsal aspect of the talar neck (TaN) to the dorsal surface of the navicular (Na) bone. It runs from proximal lateral to distal medial, being the continuation of the anterior talofibular ligament (ATFL). *TaH* talar head, *CL* cervical ligament, *MCCL* medial calcaneocuboid ligament, *DLCCL* dorsolateral calcaneocuboid ligament

3.2 Biomechanics of the Chopart joint

- The Chopart joint complex has a crucial function in adapting the foot to the ground.
- With its locking mechanism, it allows load transfer to the metatarsal heads during push-off.

The Chopart complex has a high degree of mobility, which allows the hindfoot to pivot while the forefoot remains stationary on the ground. This joint complex, together with the subtalar joint, functions as a unit to invert and evert the foot. When the heel is everted, the calcaneocuboid and talonavicular joints are parallel, allowing for motion across the Chopart complex [13]. When the heel is inverted, the two joints are not parallel and are "locked," becoming immobile and thus stabilizing the midfoot during the push-off phase of gait. Furthermore, a windlass mechanism is provided by the plantar aponeurosis which locks the midfoot and stiffens the longitudinal arch. During push-off, dorsiflexion of the first metatarsophalangeal joint tightens the aponeurosis and plantar fascia, elevating the arch and inverting the calcaneus [14].

Loss of talonavicular motion results in loss of complex hindfoot circumduction. It is therefore extremely important to retain talonavicular function as even a small amount of motion has a protective function on the adjacent joints [13]. Loss of talonavicular motion leads to adjacent joint degeneration. Due to its extensive range of motion, the talonavicular joint is also known as the "coxa pedis" [15].

3.3 Injuries to the Midtarsal Joints

- Injuries to the midtarsal joints occur mainly subsequent to an eversion or inversion trauma.
- Fractures are seen mostly in high-energy trauma.

Although midtarsal sprains most commonly result from ankle inversion, eversion injuries are also a possible mechanism. Each mechanism results in a distinct injury pattern at the Chopart joint complex, and recognition of these patterns is mandatory for accurate diagnosis and adequate treatment.

3.3.1 Inversion Midtarsal Sprains

Most midtarsal sprains occur as a result of an inversion injury, resulting in distraction forces across the lateral and dorsolateral aspects of calcaneocuboid joint [3, 4, 16]. Distraction injuries often result in avulsion fractures of the extensor digitorum brevis origin in combination with a tear or sprain of the ligaments stabilizing the joint, including the dorsal calcaneocuboid ligament, calcaneocuboid component of the bifurcate ligament (Fig. 3.4). When ankle inversion is accompanied by plantar flexion, distraction forces propagate dorsally through the talonavicular joint, often causing dorsal talonavicular ligament avulsion (Fig. 3.5) [17].

3.3.2 Eversion Midtarsal Sprains

Although a less common injury mechanism, ankle eversion can also result in midtarsal sprains [1]. The distinguishing feature of this injury is the compressive impaction force of the lateral aspect of the calcaneocuboid joint, producing impaction fractures of the anterior process of the calcaneus

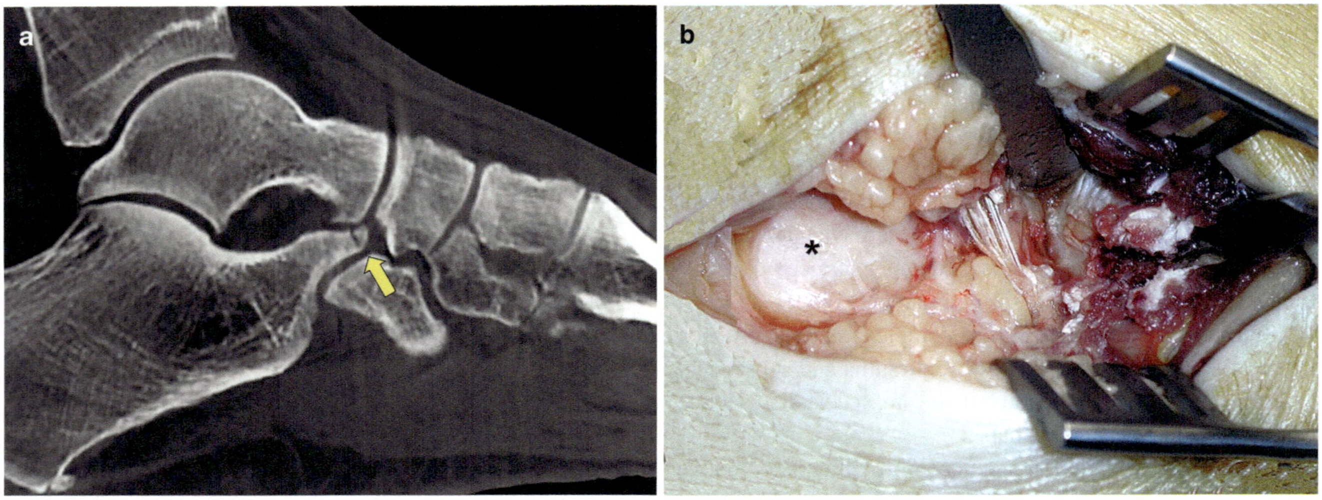

Fig. 3.4 The most common inversion injuries result in distraction forces across the lateral and dorsolateral aspects of the calcaneocuboid joint, often associated with avulsion fractures in combination with a tear or sprain of the ligament stabilizing the joint. This may include the dorsal calcaneocuboid ligament and calcaneocuboid component of the bifurcate ligament as well as the origin of the extensor digitorum brevis. (**a**) A CT scan showing the bony avulsion of the bifurcate ligament on the calcaneus (arrow). (**b**) Surgical exposure evidenced a much higher extent of injury, showing an involvement of the origin of the extensor digitorum brevis and the base of the cervical ligament. *Asterisk* subtalar joint capsula

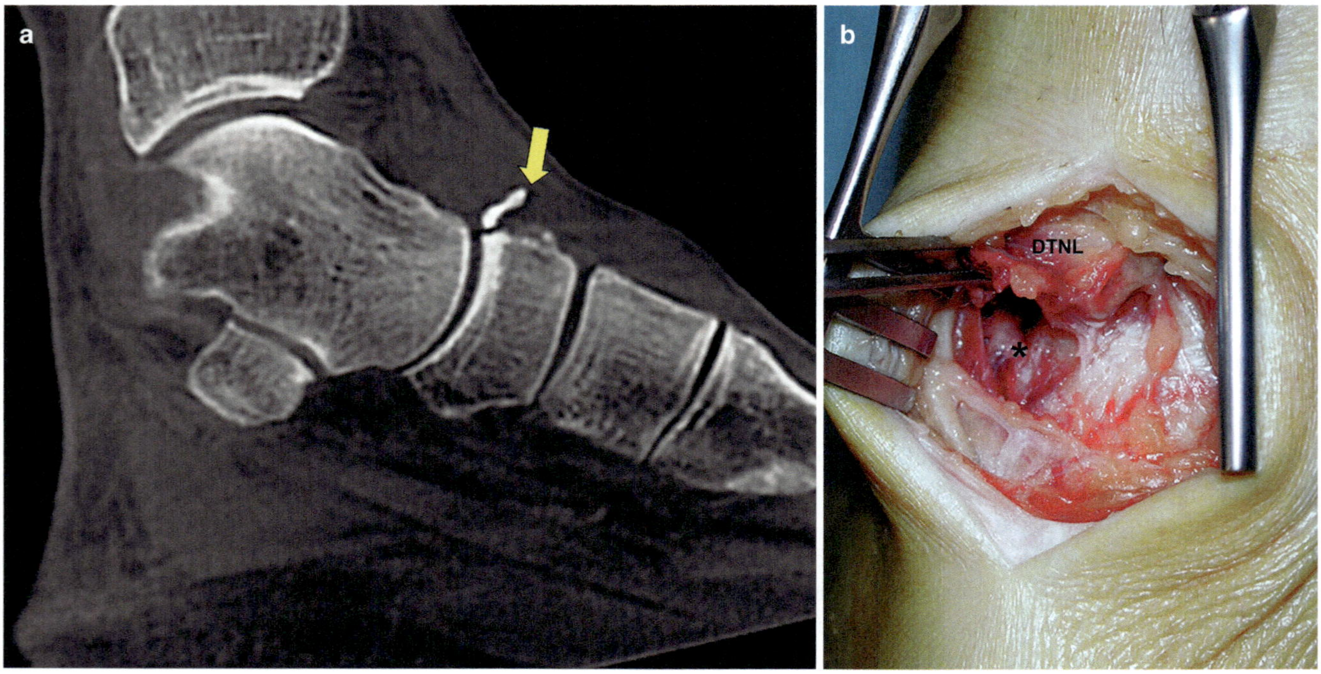

Fig. 3.5 When the trauma is accompanied by plantar flexion, distraction forces propagate dorsally through the talonavicular joint, often causing dorsal talonavicular ligament avulsion, which can be at the talar or navicular side. (**a**) CT scan showing a major dorsal avulsion of the dorsal talonavicular ligament (arrow). (**b**) Surgical exposure through a longitudinal incision on the dorsal aspect of the foot evidencing the complete avulsion of the broad insertion area of the dorsal talonavicular ligament (DTNL). Asterisk = avulsion area on navicular

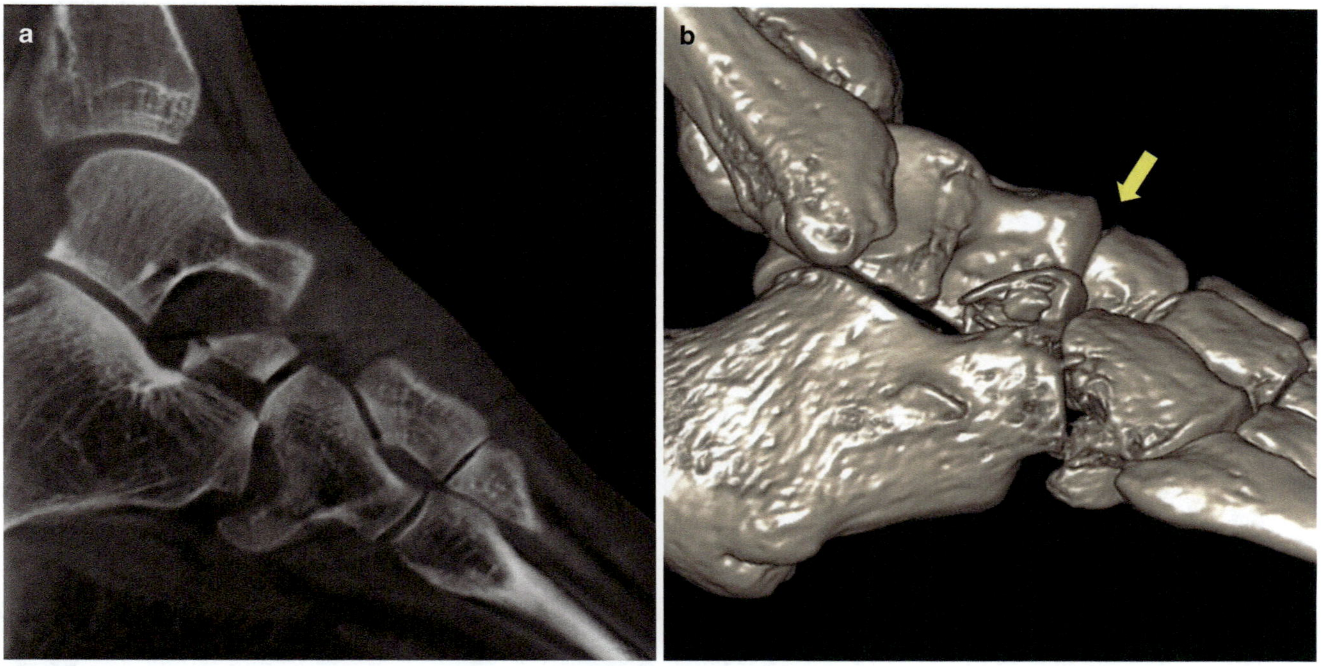

Fig. 3.6 The less common injury mechanism are the eversion injuries, resulting in compressive impaction force on the lateral aspect of the calcaneocuboid joint, producing impaction fractures of the anterior process of the calcaneus and posterolateral cuboid. (**a**) A sagittal plane CT scan showing the impaction fracture on both the calcaneus and cuboid. (**b**) 3D shows the effect of these impaction fractures, resulting in an abduction deformity of the mid- and forefoot. Furthermore, a gapping of the talonavicular joint, as a result of associated ligament injuries, can be seen (arrow)

and posterolateral cuboid (Fig. 3.6). Distraction forces medially can cause navicular tuberosity avulsion fractures due to the pull of the posterior tibial tendon (Fig. 3.7).

3.3.3 High-Energy Midtarsal Injuries

Direct longitudinal forces propagating along the metatarsal axes from a blow to the forefoot may cause complex compressive forces at the midtarsal joints and result in crash injuries [1]. Midtarsal fracture dislocations also occur usually in high-energy lower extremity trauma [18, 19], though also seen among low-energy traumas [20]. Isolated dislocations were found in up to 25% of cases [21]. Chopart joint injuries may also occur subsequently to subtalar dislocations, given that the stabilizing ligaments of the talonavicular joint are not as strong as those of the talocalcaneal joint (Fig. 3.8) [22].

3.4 History and Clinical Presentation

- The presumptive clinical diagnosis is often mistaken as an ankle sprain and thus definitive diagnosis is delayed or overlooked entirely.

Because midtarsal sprains most commonly occur with inversion-type injuries, the presumptive clinical diagnosis is often mistaken as an ankle sprain and thus definitive diagnosis is delayed or overlooked entirely [23, 24]. Diagnostic accuracy is further confounded by the fact that most midtarsal sprains are accompanied by lateral collateral ligament sprains or occur in the setting of chronic anterolateral ankle instability.

Pain, swelling, and point tenderness over the calcaneocuboid or talonavicular joints are suggestive of a Chopart joint injury. Varus stress applied at the lateral calcaneocuboid joint may show joint laxity. Prolonged lateral foot pain after an acute ankle injury, reflecting failure of conservative management, may be the first sign of a missed midtarsal sprain. Persistent instability specifically involving the calcaneocuboid joint is thought to be the most likely cause [25].

3.5 Imaging

- Besides radiographs, CT scans are the main imaging tools used in diagnosing injuries to the Chopart joint and recognizing associated bony injuries.
- MRI may play a certain role in detecting isolated ligament injuries.

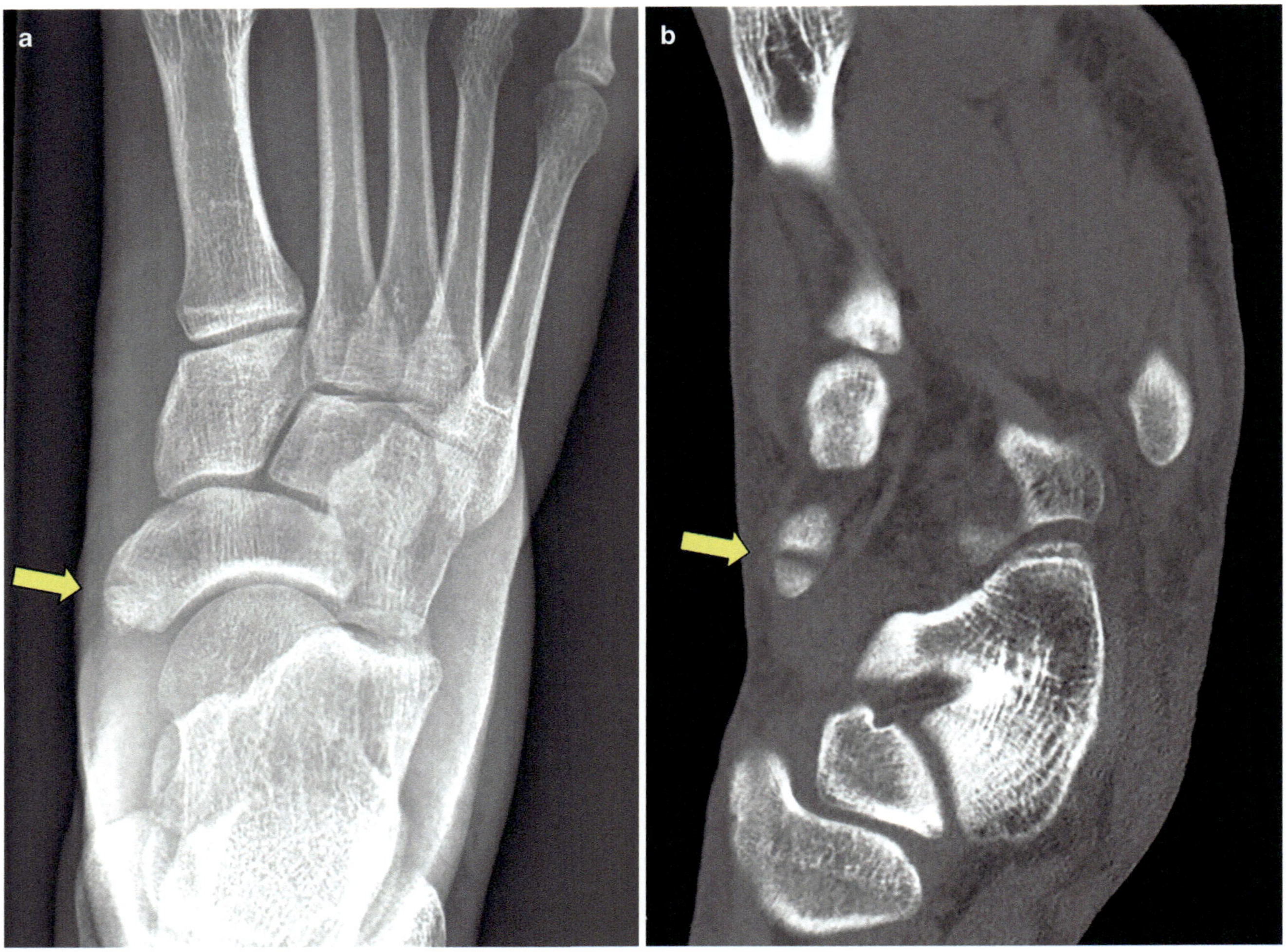

Fig. 3.7 Distraction forces on the medial side of the foot can cause navicular tuberosity avulsion fractures due to the pull by the posterior tibial tendon during injury. (**a**) Radiograph showing the minimally displaced avulsion fracture of the navicular tuberosity (arrow). (**b**) A CT scan in the same patient, showing the avulsion fracture (arrow)

Radiography should be the initial imaging modality for making the diagnosis of a Chopart joint injury. Radiographic or CT evaluation is especially useful for detecting fractures of the Chopart joint that are frequently associated with midtarsal sprains. The lateral ankle or foot views are optimal for detecting a dorsal talonavicular ligament avulsion fracture (Fig. 3.9a). An oblique view of the foot is optimal for visualizing the anterior process of the calcaneus (Fig. 3.9b), although a displaced fracture of the anterior process of the calcaneus may also be detected on lateral views. Stress radiographs may help to quantify the instability resulting from injuries to the calcaneocuboid ligament (Fig. 3.10) [3]. Under normal circumstances, the calcaneocuboid angle is <5°.

CT is a sensitive (Figs. 3.4, 3.5, 3.6, and 3.7), confirmatory examination and may reveal fractures not otherwise detected on radiography, so the Chopart joint should again be scrutinized. Overall, radiographic detection of midtarsal injuries is thought to be insensitive, missing up to 33% of cases with fractures [26].

MRI is superior to conventional radiography in the detection of soft tissue injuries and sometimes also in osseous injuries of the Chopart joint (Fig. 3.11). In one recent study, calcaneocuboid avulsion fractures were evident in 48% of radiographs and 100% of MR images and talonavicular joint injuries were evident in 38% of radiographs and 76% of MR images [5]. Since midtarsal sprains are predominantly ligamentous injuries, the superior soft tissue contrast of MRI is optimal for establishing a comprehensive, accurate diagnosis of a Chopart joint injury. While the MRI appearance of acute or subacute injuries will be ligamentous edema, discontinuity, irregularity, waviness, and laxity [5], old injuries are a common cause of increased ligament conspicuity [4].

Ultrasound evaluation of the midtarsal ligaments is of great utility in experienced hands, particularly suited for evaluating the superficial dorsal and lateral soft tissues about the joint, including the dorsal calcaneocuboid, dorsal talonavicular, and calcaneocuboid joint capsules [27].

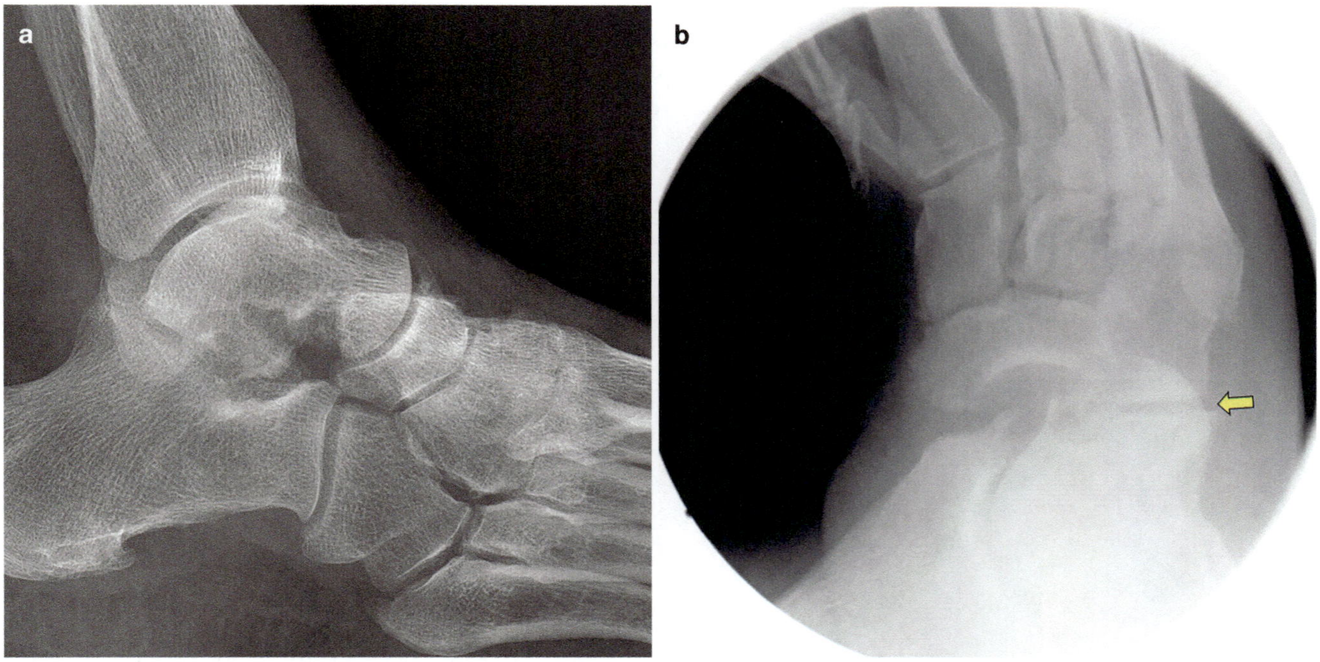

Fig. 3.8 Chopart joint injuries may also occur subsequently to subtalar dislocation. As the dorsolateral ligaments of the talonavicular joint are not as strong as the medioplantar structures, the head dislocates typically dorsolaterally. (**a**) Radiograph showing the subtalar dislocation with involvement of the talonavicular joint. (**b**) Under fluoroscopy, the dorsolateral instability of the Chopart joint can be confirmed as the talar head is seen to dislocate dorsolaterally out of the talonavicular joint. A gapping of the lateral calcaneocuboid joint can also be seen (arrow)

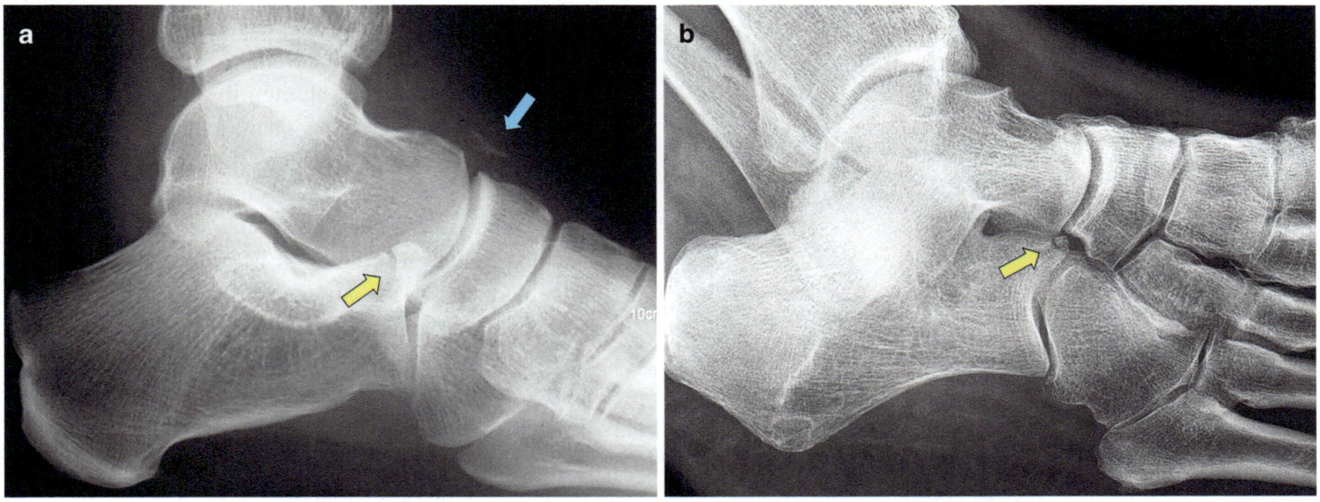

Fig. 3.9 (**a**) The lateral ankle or foot views are optimal for detecting a dorsal talonavicular ligament avulsion fracture (blue arrow) and visualizing an avulsion of the anterior process of the calcaneus (yellow arrow). (**b**) Smaller avulsion of the anterior process of the calcaneus (yellow arrow) can often be seen better in an oblique view of the foot

3.6 Treatment

- Purely ligamentous injuries are managed conservatively; however, they need more aggressive immobilization than ankle sprains.
- Ligament injuries with bony avulsions and fractures need surgical treatment.

Most midtarsal sprains, especially purely ligamentous injuries, are managed conservatively, but they need more aggressive immobilization using below-knee cast for 6–8 weeks followed by a soft brace and rehabilitation program [1, 28]. In active patients however, surgical treatment should be considered for bony avulsion injuries [1]. Small avulsion fragments of the bifurcate ligament may be excised, and the ligament then reattached with the use of transosseous sutures or an anchor suture (Fig. 3.12). Bigger avulsion fragments

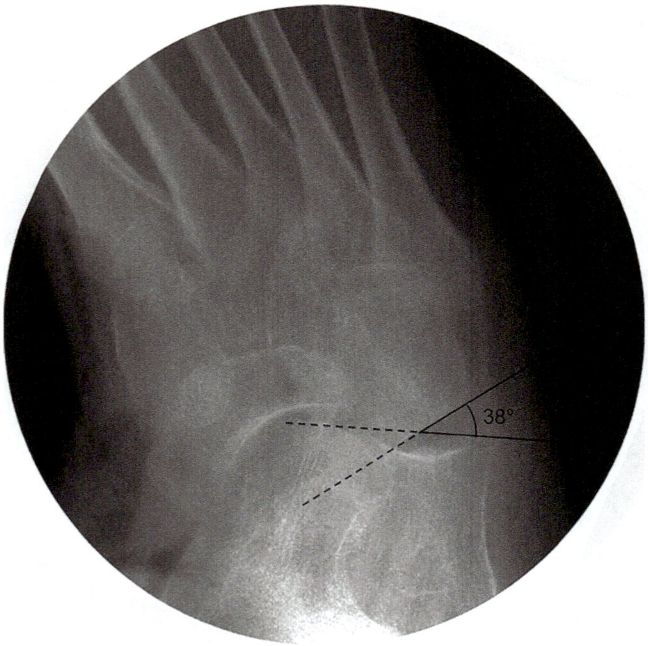

Fig. 3.10 Stress testing of the calcaneocuboid ligament under fluoroscopy showing a calcaneocuboid angle of 38°

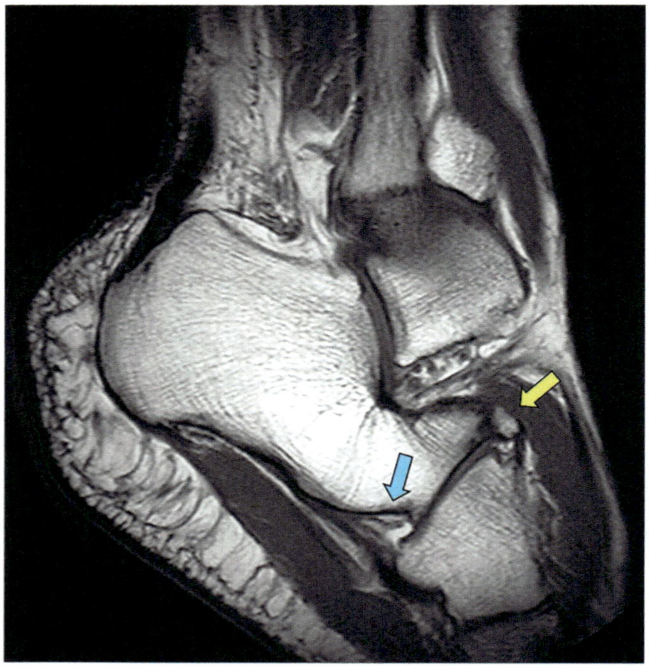

Fig. 3.11 MRI may be helpful to detect soft tissue injuries and sometimes also osseous injuries at the Chopart joint. In this case, it evidences a bony avulsion of the bifurcate ligament (yellow arrow) and a partial rupture of the inferior calcaneocuboid ligament, especially of the short plantar ligament (blue arrow)

are reattached by one or two screws (Fig. 3.13). Displaced avulsion fractures of the dorsal talonavicular ligament need to be reattached by screw fixation and/or sutures (Fig. 3.14).

Ankle eversion injuries that are typically associated with midfoot abduction can result in a compressive impaction force at the lateral aspect of the calcaneocuboid joint, pro-

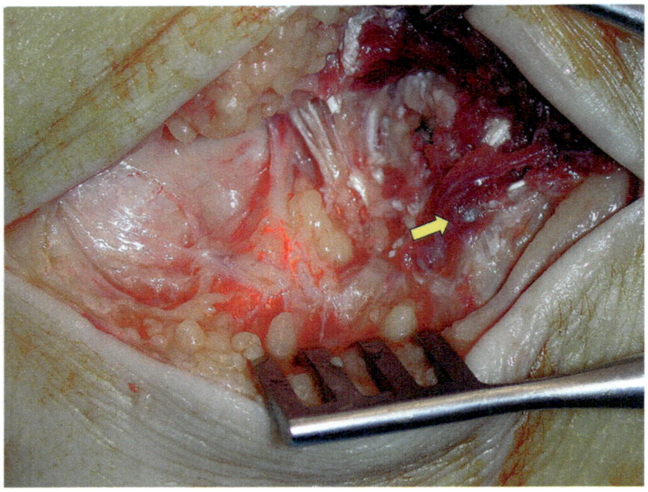

Fig. 3.12 *Surgical Technique: Repair of bifurcate ligament.* This 58-year-old male passionate tennis player sustained a severe supination injury (same patient as Fig. 3.4). The bony avulsion is too small to be reattached; therefore, it is removed, and the bifurcate ligament is reattached to the intermediary tubercle of the anterior calcaneus by using an anchor. The figure shows the final reconstruction (arrow = knot of the suture). The patient was able to return to his level of sports activity after recovery

ducing impaction fractures of the anterior process of the calcaneus (Fig. 3.15) or nutcracker-type impaction fractures occurring at the opposing surfaces of the calcaneus and cuboid (Fig. 3.16). Both injury types require surgical reconstruction to restore the lateral column of the foot. Fractures along the talonavicular joint shorten the medial column of the midfoot, causing adduction malalignment that requires surgical reduction as well [29].

Some patients will not improve with conservative treatment [2, 30, 31] and may require surgical intervention [32–34]. Traditionally, midtarsal arthrodesis is performed for chronic instability, pain, and secondary Chopart osteoarthrosis [1, 35, 36]. New operative techniques have been developed to address soft tissue injuries with or without significant osseous injuries, particularly in young athletes, including reconstruction of the dorsolateral ligament complex of the calcaneocuboid joint with a periosteal flap [30, 31], extensor digitorum brevis tendon [5], plantaris tendon graft or internal brace (Fig. 3.17).

3.7 Outcome

- Delayed or neglected treatment results in bad outcome with persistent pain.

In a retrospective analysis of 27 patients, functional treatment of fractures to the anterior process of the calcaneus yielded good to excellent results and a fast return to work in most patients [28]. Yet, a prolonged return to sports was noted. No significant differences regarding the outcome were observed when comparing the different fracture types.

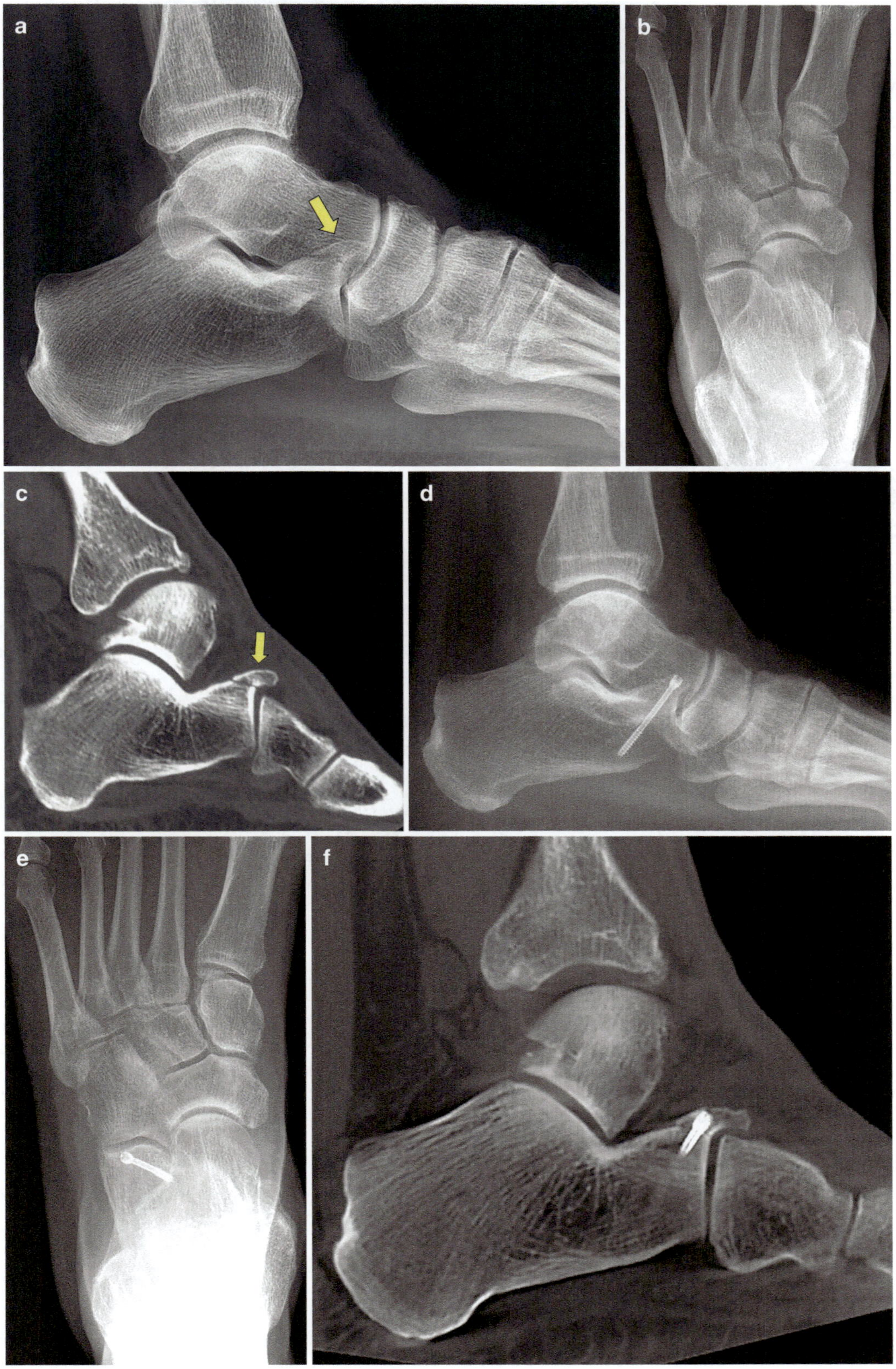

Fig. 3.13 *Surgical Technique: Repair of bifurcate ligament avulsion by bony fixation.* This 55-year-old active patient sustained a severe supination injury while walking in the forest. (**a**) The lateral radiograph evidences an 8 mm long avulsion of the bifurcate ligament on the anterior process of the calcaneus (arrow). This is also the area where the most pain on palpation is found in the clinical investigation. (**b**) The DP view of the foot does not show the fragment, nor any other bony lesion. (**c**) The CT scan confirms the bony avulsion (arrow). The fragment is first fixed by a percutaneous inserted K-wire under fluoroscopic control (not shown), and then fixed by a 3-mm cannulated screw. (**d**) Lateral radiograph taken 6 weeks after surgery, showing screw fixation. (**e**) The DP view shows a congruent calcaneocuboid joint. (**f**) Eight weeks later, the CT scan confirms complete healing of fracture in an anatomic position

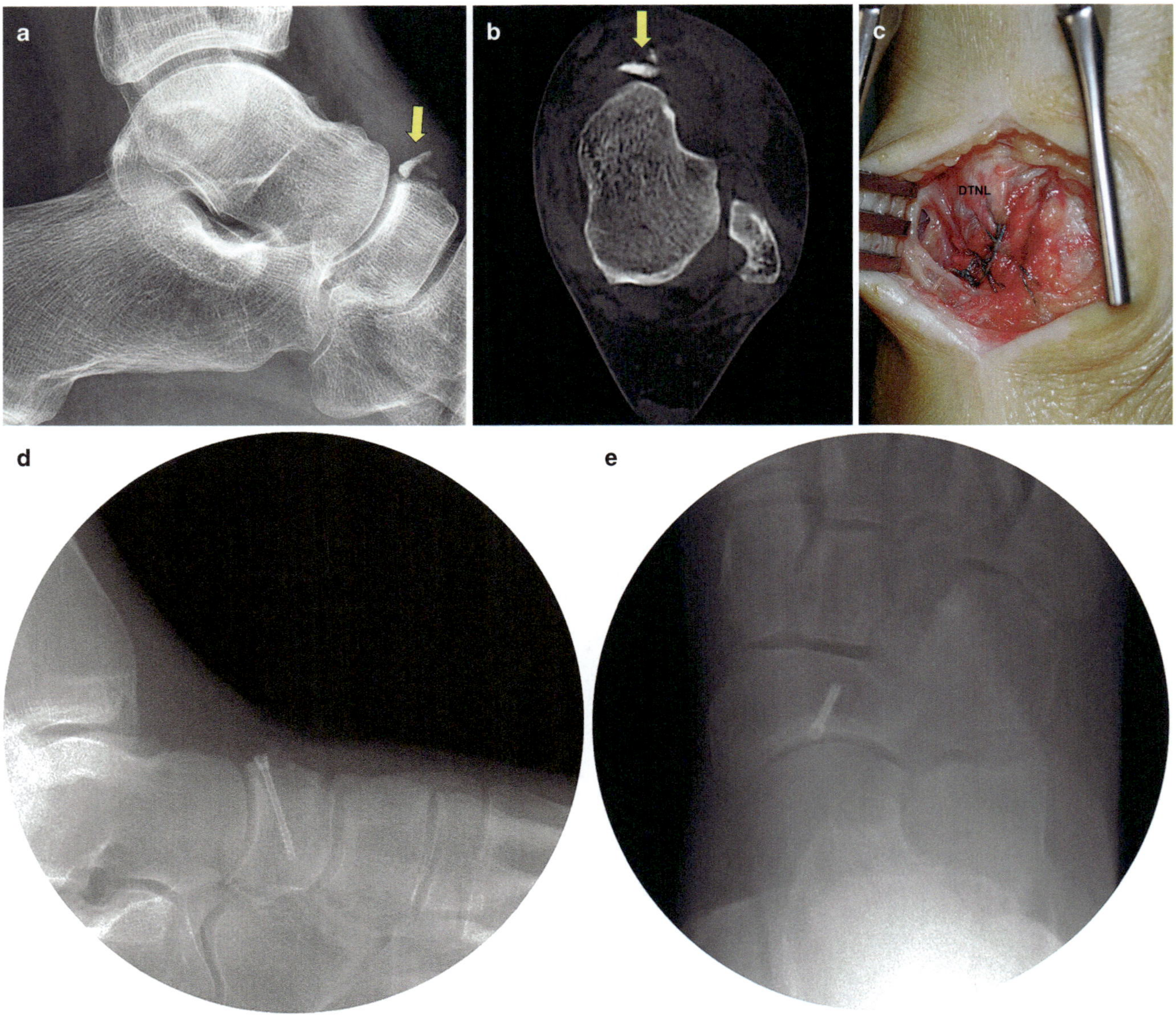

Fig. 3.14 *Surgical Technique: Repair of dorsal talonavicular ligament avulsion by bony fixation*. This 47-year-old female runner sustained a sever supination injury after previously experiencing an ankle sprain that left her with some instability feeling (same patient as Fig. 3.5). (**a**) The lateral radiograph evidences an avulsion fracture of the dorsal talonavicular ligament (DTNL) that includes the articular surface of the navicular bone (arrow). (**b**) The DP view on the CT scan shows the size of the fragment (arrow). (**c**) An intraoperative picture showing the fragment was first reduced and fixed by a 2.5-mm screw and thereafter, the ligament was additionally reattached by multiple sutures to the periosteum. Intraoperative fluoroscopic control shows the anatomically reduced and fixed fragment in the (**d**) lateral and (**e**) DP view

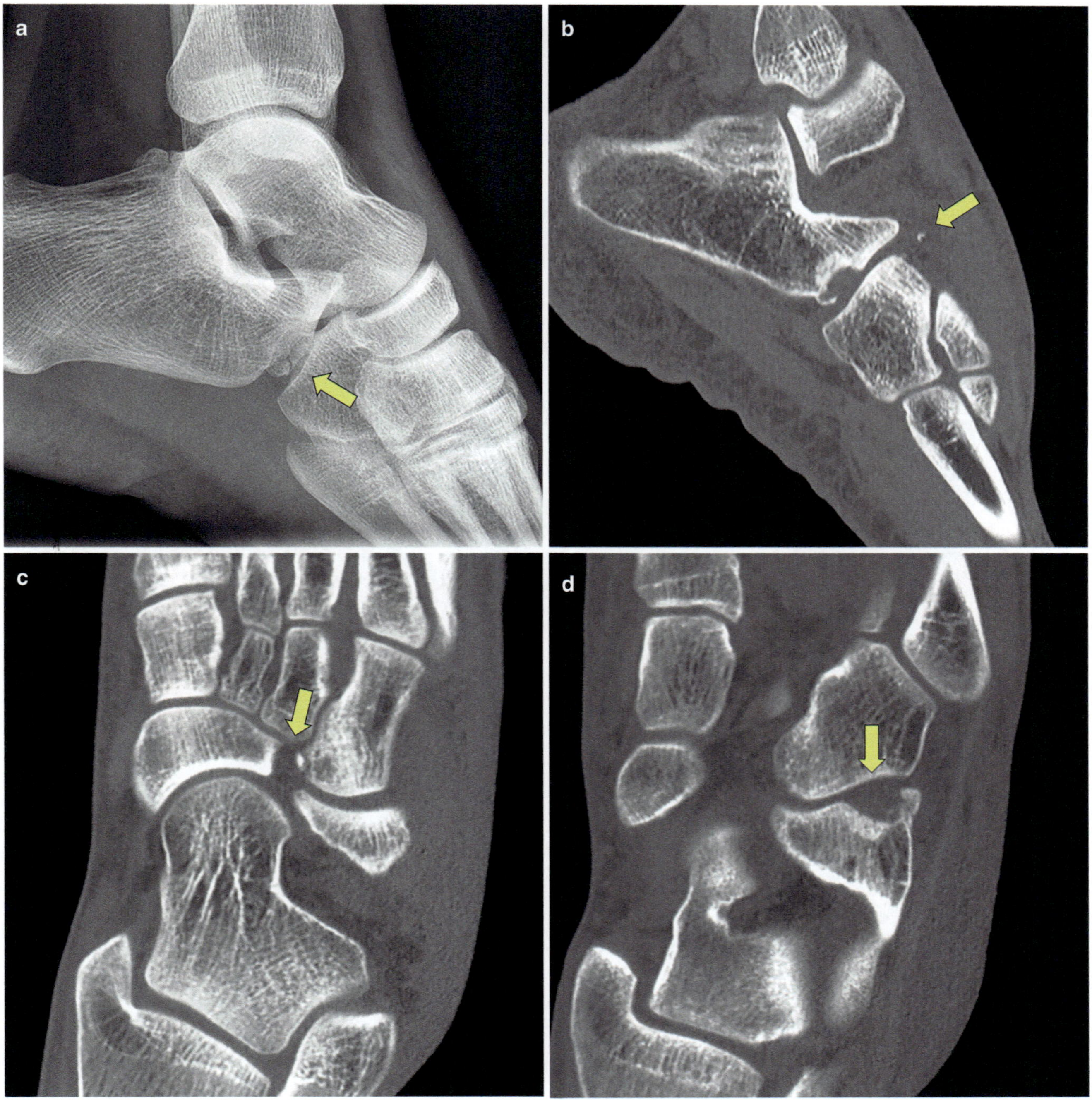

Fig. 3.15 *Surgical technique: reconstruction of articular impaction fracture of calcaneus*. This 19-year-old high-level gymnast sustained an acute eversion trauma when landing after a jump. (**a**) The non-weight-bearing lateral radiograph shows an impaction fracture of the anterior calcaneus (arrow) and some gapping at the dorsal talonavicular joint. (**b**) The CT scan shows the impaction fracture on the inferior part of the articular surface and it also shows a small bony avulsion of the distal medial calcaneocuboid ligament (arrow). (**c**) In the horizontal view, the fragment can be identified as an avulsion from the lateral navicular, thereby creating an increased gap between the calcaneus and navicular (arrow). Notice also the moderate gapping of the calcaneocuboid joint. (**d**) The impaction fracture of the articular surface of the calcaneus is seen in the central part (arrow), while the lateral cortex remained intact. (**e**) After surgical exposure, the calcaneocuboid joints are distracted over two K-wires. The central impaction fracture is visible. (**f**) A hole is made in the lateral cortex with a 4.5-mm drill (arrow). (**g**) This allows to tap an allograft (arrow) through this hole to lift the articular surface. (**h**) The fracture is stabilized by a 2.4-mm plate. The medial calcaneocuboid ligament is then reattached by a suture anchor to the lateral navicular (not shown). Intraoperative fluoroscopy is used to check the reduction of the fracture in the (**i**) lateral and (**j**) dorsal view. The implants were removed after 8 months. The CT scan shows the anatomic restoration of the calcaneocuboid joint after 18 months in the (**k**) lateral and (**l**) dorsal view. The athlete returned to full sports activity after 9 months, and 2.5 years later he participated at Olympic games

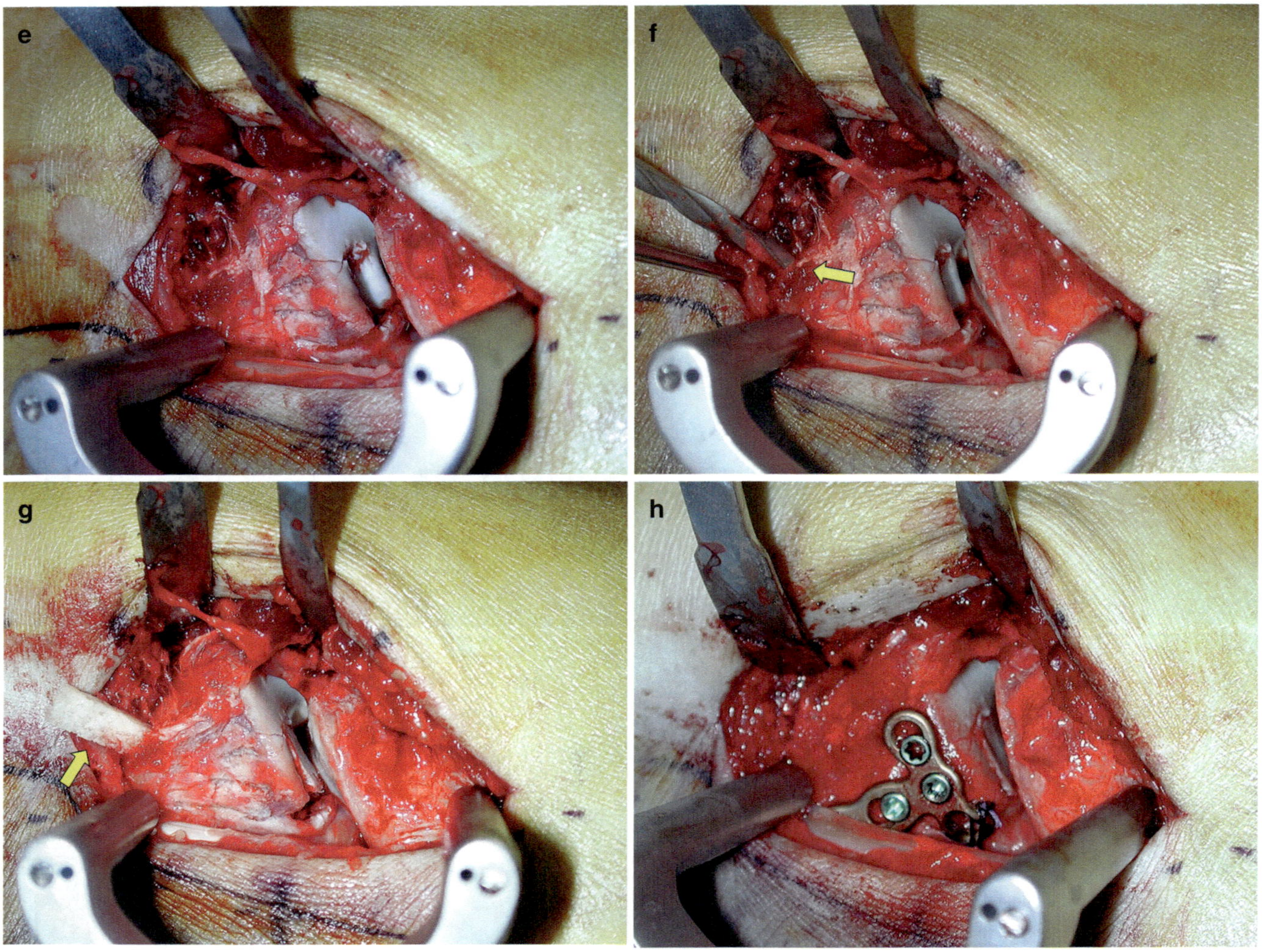

Fig. 3.15 (continued)

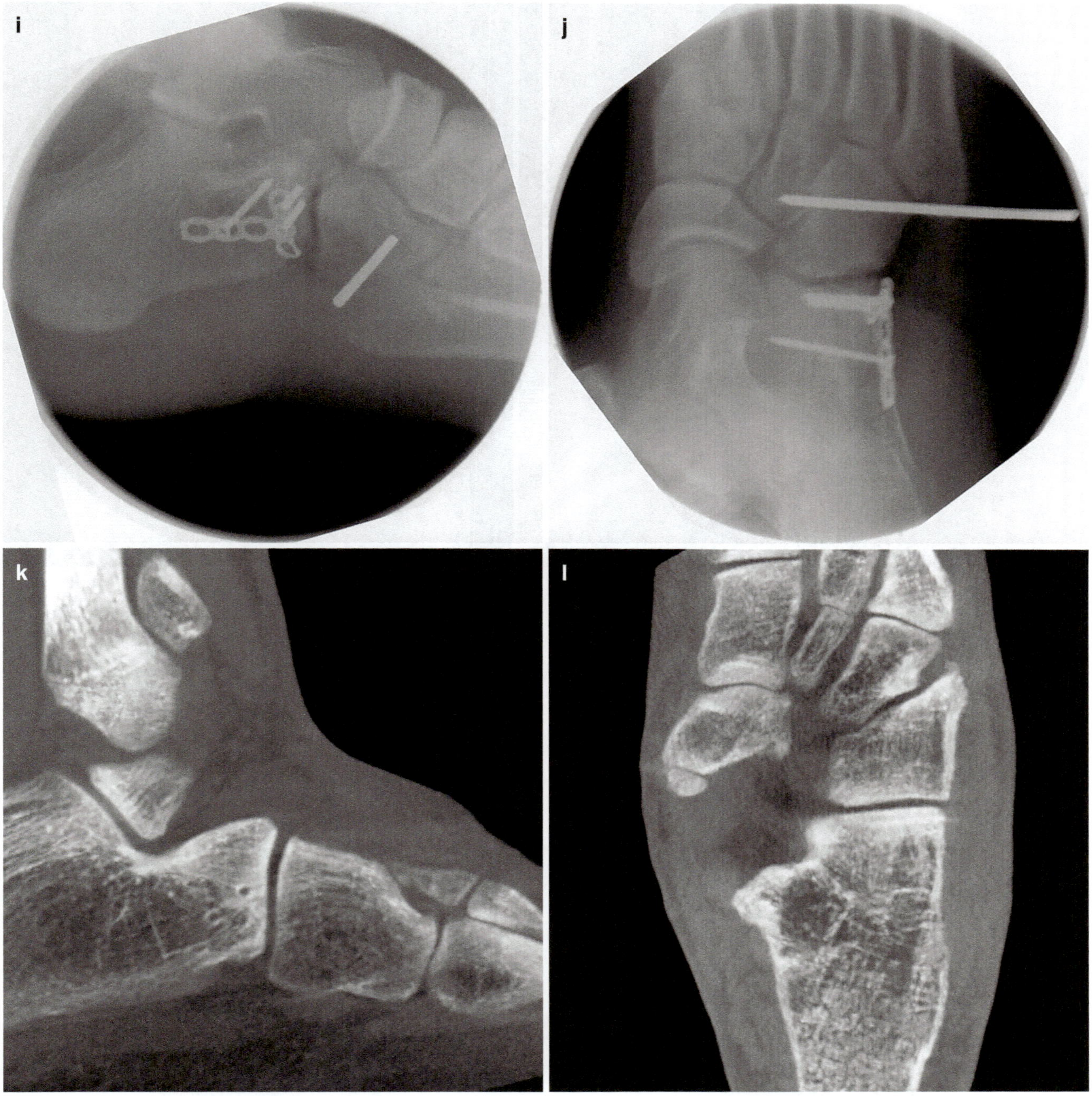

Fig. 3.15 (continued)

In the case of surgical treatment, no improvements in VAS pain score, AOFAS score, and/or mean calcaneocuboid angle were found after excision of the fracture, whereas patients who underwent repair or reconstruction of the bifurcate ligament showed significant improvements in VAS pain score and AOFAS score at the last follow-up [37]. These results indicate that simple excision of the fracture fragment is not an ideal way to treat bifurcate ligament injuries. Analogously, avulsion of the dorsal talonavicular ligament may result in a better outcome than after excision, particularly in patients with a larger distal fragment that involves the talonavicular joint (Fig. 3.14).

3.8 Complications

Besides feeling some tenderness and swelling over the reconstructed ligaments, persistent pain in the foot while weight-bearing which increases with supination of the foot is the main complication and particularly seen in primarily missed and thus not adequately treated injuries of midtarsal joints. In chronic settings, persistent instability can additionally be found over the bifurcate ligament (Fig. 3.18).

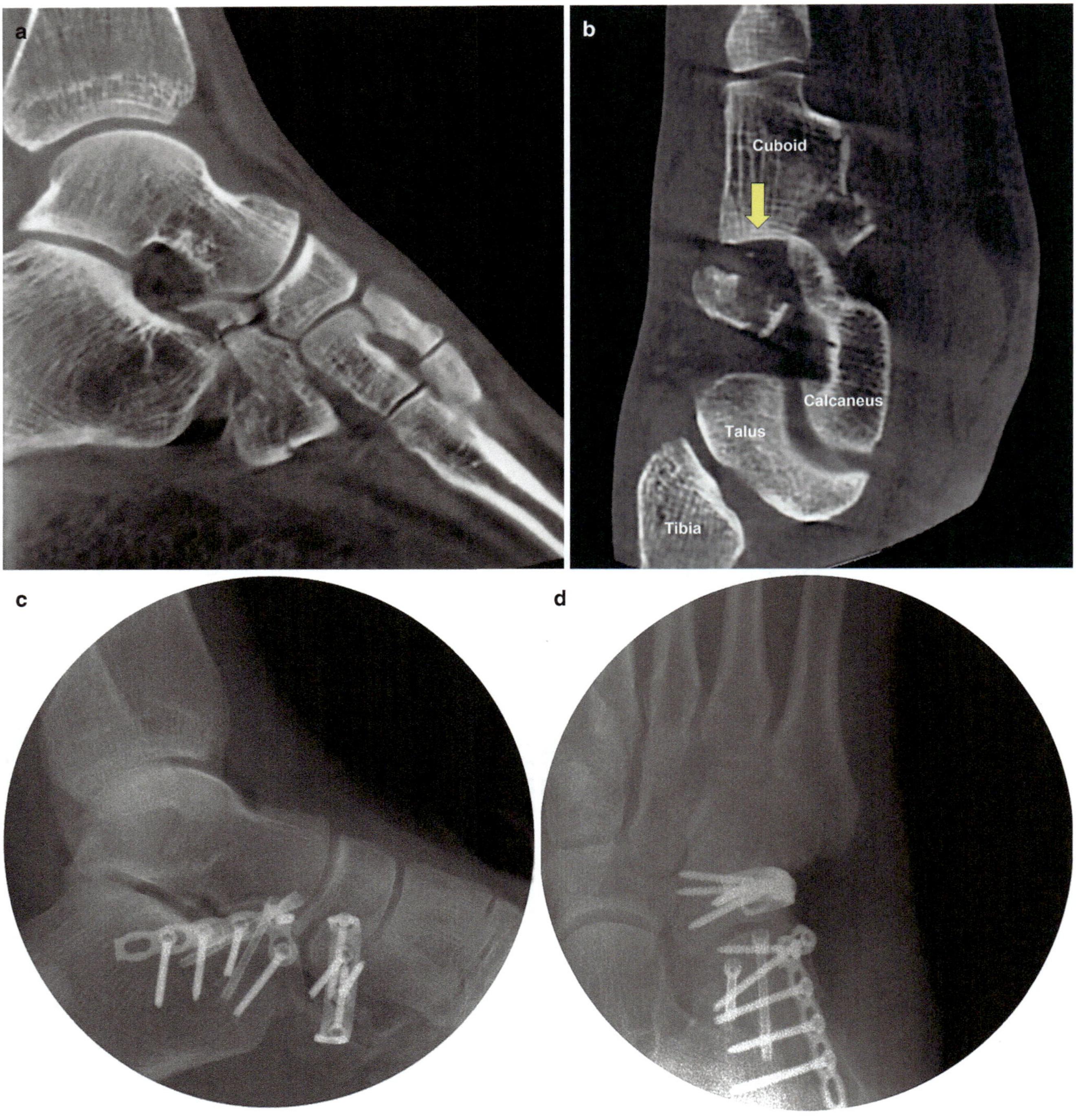

Fig. 3.16 *Surgical technique: reconstruction of intra-articular fracture of calcaneocuboid joint*. This 28-year-old motocross driver sustained an acute eversion trauma that resulted in a high compressive impaction force at the lateral aspect of the calcaneocuboid joint (same patient as Fig. 3.6). (**a**) The CT scan shows the impaction fractures of the anterior process of the calcaneus and posterolateral cuboid, with shortening of the lateral column. (**b**) The direction of the compressive forces and resulting fractures can be visualized in the AP view (arrows). The calcaneocuboid joint is exposed through a lateral longitudinal approach, and the fractures are reduced and fixed by plates and screws. Intraoperative fluoroscopy shows the achieved reduction of articular surfaces and restoration of bony geometry in the (**c**) lateral and (**d**) DP view

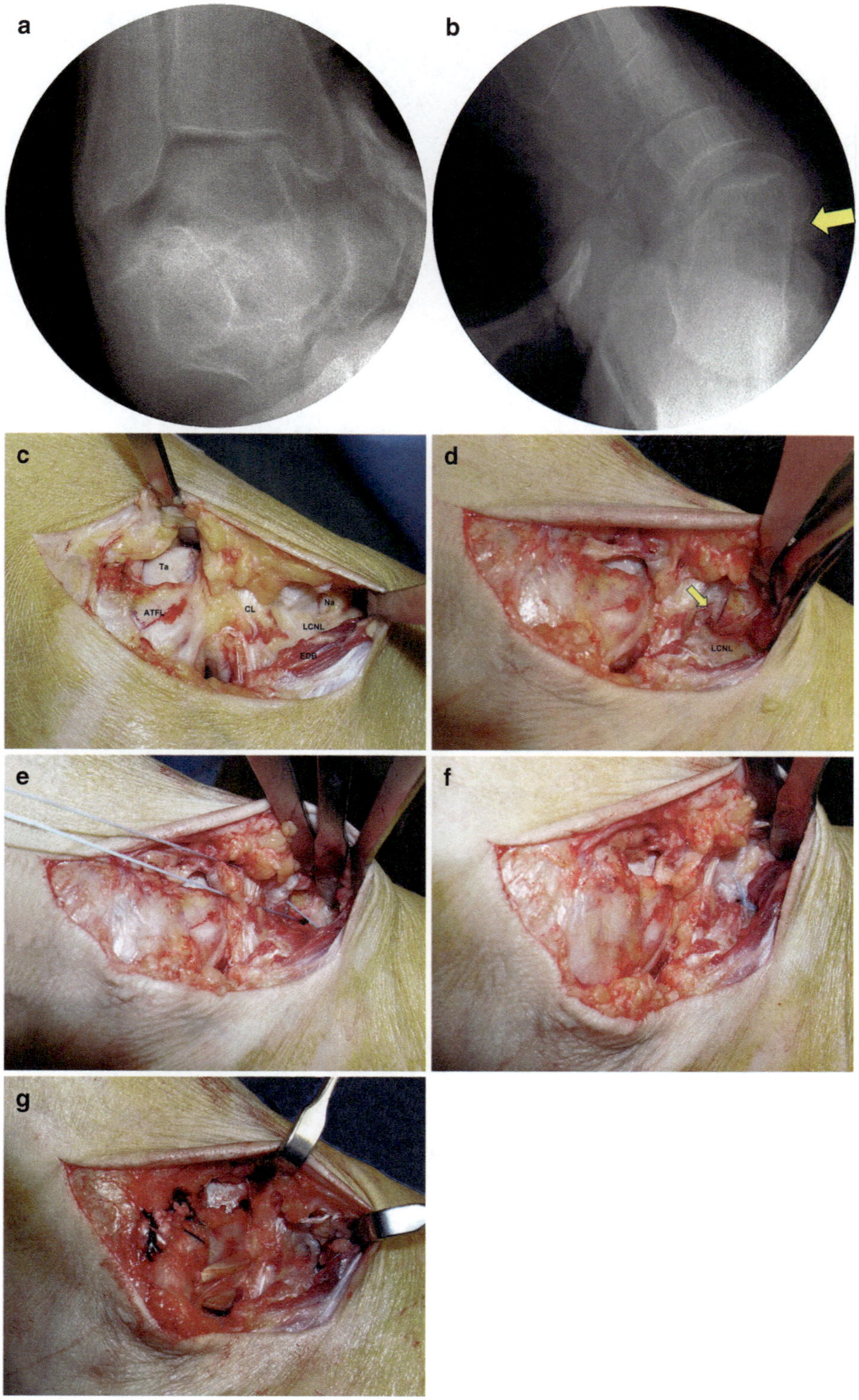

Fig. 3.17 *Surgical technique: reconstruction of bifurcate ligament with a free plantaris tendon graft.* This 51-year-old female tennis player suffered from recurrent ankle sprains over many years. Two years ago, she sustained a heavy supination trauma with subsequent persisting pain at the lateral Chopart joint. Clinically, pain on palpation is found over the lateral ankle ligament and, more pronounced, over the anterior process of the calcaneus. Pain can also be provoked at the same areas with manual inversion and adduction stress to the foot. (**a**) Preoperative testing under fluoroscopy evidences lateral instability at the tibiotalar joint. (**b**) Adduction stress to the foot shows gapping of the calcaneocuboid joint accounting for an angulation of >20° (arrow). (**c**) Surgical exploration evidences a scarred and incompetent anterior talofibular ligament (ATFL) with anterolateral subluxation of talus (Ta). The lateral calcaneonavicular ligament (LCNL) is very weak and lax, and the lateral border of the navicular (Na) can be seen. *CL* cervical ligament, *EDB* extensor digitorum brevis muscle. (**d**) After further exposure and debridement of the lateral border of the navicular, the remaining LCNL can be seen detached from the navicular (arrow). (**e**) Two drill holes are made into the lateral navicular to create a tunnel into which a fiber wire is inserted. (**f**) The LCNL is now firmly fixed to the navicular while the foot is held in eversion. (**g**). The ATFL is finally reconstructed with the use of a free plantaris tendon graft and further reinforced by additional sutures to reattach the remaining ligament structures. This patient was able to play tennis again 6 months postoperative

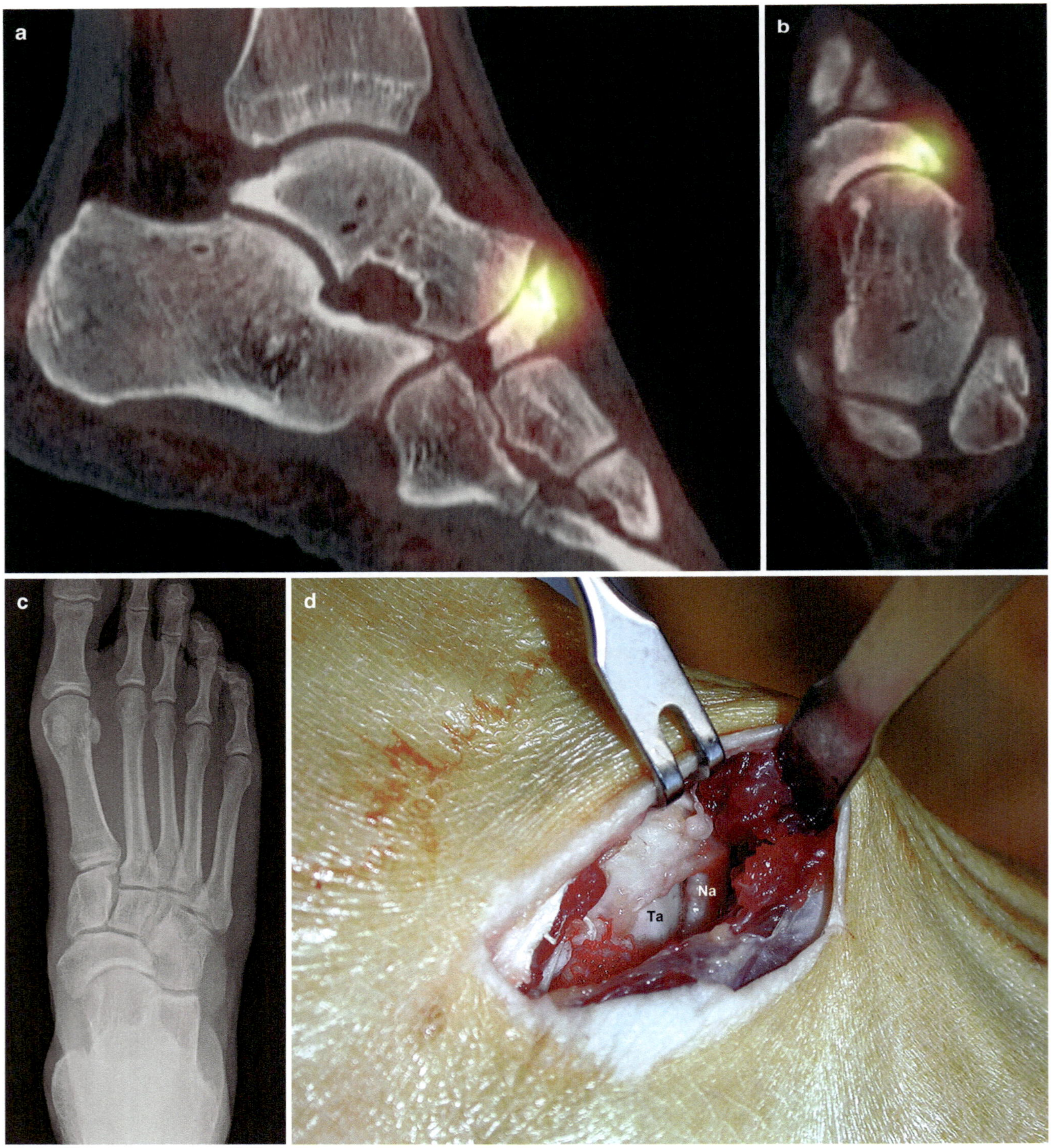

Fig. 3.18 *Surgical Technique: Delayed reconstruction of bifurcate ligament with a free plantaris tendon graft.* This 52-year-old orienteer complained about increasing pain in his midfoot after having sustained multiple sprains. Three years ago, he underwent surgical reconstruction of the lateral ankle ligament which allowed him to return to sports activities at his former level. However, since a few months, he senses severe midfoot pain not permitting him to run anymore. Clinical investigation reveals a stable ankle joint, but severe pain over the lateral navicular and bifurcate ligament. Pain can be provoked at the same locations while applying supination-adduction stress to the foot and, to a lesser extent, when applying eversion-abduction stress to the foot. The Spect CT shows increased activity at dorsolateral navicular in both the (**a**) lateral and (**b**) DP views. (**c**) Weight-bearing foot DP radiograph shows some tilting of the navicular towards medial as a potential consequence of the incompetent lateral calcaneonavicular ligament. (**d**) This is confirmed by open exploration where additionally, a defect of the lateral talonavicular joint capsule is found. *Ta* talar head, *Na* navicular. Subsequentially, a reconstruction of the lateral calcaneonavicular ligament with the use of a plantaris tendon graft was performed (not shown). This patient was able to regain sports activities with some limitations

3.9 Conclusions

- Understanding midtarsal joint anatomy, the mechanisms of injury, and the implications for management is important for successful treatment.
- Healing time is longer than after ankle sprains.

Midtarsal sprains are relatively common in inversion-type ankle injuries and typically present as avulsion injuries across the calcaneocuboid joint and impaction injuries at the talonavicular joint. Conversely, an eversion mechanism will cause impaction injuries at the calcaneocuboid joint and medial avulsion fractures, typically at the navicular tuberosity. Understanding midtarsal joint anatomy, the mechanisms of injury, and the implications for management is important for successful treatment. Healing time after Chopart joint injuries is longer than after an ankle sprain and it needs 6–8 weeks of immobilization in a below-knee cast.

References

1. Kutaish H, Stern R, Drittenbass L, Assal M. Injuries to the Chopart joint complex: a current review. Eur J Orthop Surg Traumatol. 2017;27(4):425–31.
2. van Dorp KB, de Vries MR, van der Elst M, Schepers T. Chopart joint injury: a study of outcome and morbidity. J Foot Ankle Surg. 2010;49(6):541–5.
3. Andermahr J, Helling HJ, Maintz D, Monig S, Koebke J, Rehm KE. The injury of the calcaneocuboid ligaments. Foot Ankle Int. 2000;21(5):379–84.
4. Walter WR, Hirschmann A, Alaia EF, Garwood ER, Rosenberg ZS. JOURNAL CLUB: MRI evaluation of midtarsal (Chopart) sprain in the setting of acute ankle injury. AJR Am J Roentgenol. 2018;210(2):386–95.
5. Hirschmann A, Walter WR, Alaia EF, Garwood E, Amsler F, Rosenberg ZS. Acute fracture of the anterior process of calcaneus: does it herald a more advanced injury to Chopart joint? AJR Am J Roentgenol. 2018;210(5):1123–30.
6. Agnholt J, Nielsen S, Christensen H. Lesion of the ligamentum bifurcatum in ankle sprain. Arch Orthop Trauma Surg. 1988;107(5):326–8.
7. Sarrafian SK. Anatomy of foot and ankle. 2nd ed. Philadelphia: Lippincott Williams and Wilkins; 1993.
8. Ward KA, Soames RW. Morphology of the plantar calcaneocuboid ligaments. Foot Ankle Int. 1997;18(10):649–53.
9. Dorn-Lange NV, Nauck T, Lohrer H, Arentz S, Konerding MA. Morphology of the dorsal and lateral calcaneocuboid ligaments. Foot Ankle Int. 2008;29(9):942–9.
10. Kelikian AS. Sarrafian's anatomy of the foot and ankle: descriptive, topographic, funtional. 3rd ed. Philadelphia: Lippincott Williams & Wilkins; 2011.
11. Melao L, Canella C, Weber M, Negrao P, Trudell D, Resnick D. Ligaments of the transverse tarsal joint complex: MRI-anatomic correlation in cadavers. AJR Am J Roentgenol. 2009;193(3):662–71.
12. Sammarco VJ. The talonavicular and calcaneocuboid joints: anatomy, biomechanics, and clinical management of the transverse tarsal joint. Foot Ankle Clin. 2004;9(1):127–45.
13. Rammelt S. Chopart and Lisfranc Joint Injuries. In: Bentley G, editor. European surgical orthopaedics and traumatology the EFORT textbook. Berlin: Springer; 2014. p. 3835–57.
14. Benirschke SK, Meinberg E, Anderson SA, Jones CB, Cole PA. Fractures and dislocations of the midfoot: Lisfranc and Chopart injuries. J Bone Joint Surg Am. 2012;94(14):1325–37.
15. Pisani G. "Coxa pedis" today. Foot Ankle Surg. 2016;22(2):78–84.
16. Sondergaard L, Konradsen L, Holmer P, Jorgensen LN, Nielsen PT. Acute midtarsal sprains: frequency and course of recovery. Foot Ankle Int. 1996;17(4):195–9.
17. De Dea M, LL C, Allen GM, Wilson DJ, Athanasou N, Uchihara Y, et al. Talonavicular ligament: prevalence of injury in ankle sprains, histological analysis and hypothesis of its biomechanical function. Br J Radiol. 2017;90(1071):20160816.
18. Richter M, Wippermann B, Krettek C, Schratt HE, Hufner T, Therman H. Fractures and fracture dislocations of the midfoot: occurrence, causes and long-term results. Foot Ankle Int. 2001;22(5):392–8.
19. Wilson LS Jr, Mizel MS, Michelson JD. Foot and ankle injuries in motor vehicle accidents. Foot Ankle Int. 2001;22(8):649–52.
20. Harris AP, Johnson J, Waryasz GR. Isolated dorsal dislocations of the talonavicular and calcaneocuboid articulations (Chopart joints) from a low-energy mechanism. Am J Emerg Med. 2016;34(8):1733.e1–4.
21. Richter M, Thermann H, Huefner T, Schmidt U, Goesling T, Krettek C. Chopart joint fracture-dislocation: initial open reduction provides better outcome than closed reduction. Foot Ankle Int. 2004;25(5):340–8.
22. Saltzman C, Marsh JL. Hindfoot dislocations: when are they not benign? J Am Acad Orthop Surg. 1997;5(4):192–8.
23. Lee SW, Kim DD, Buskanets A, Oh-Park M. Midtarsal sprain misdiagnosed as ankle sprain: role of ultrasonography in diagnosis. Am J Phys Med Rehabil. 2016;95(3):e44–5.
24. Zwipp H, Rammelt S, Grass R. Ligamentous injuries about the ankle and subtalar joints. Clin Podiatr Med Surg. 2002;19(2):195–229, v.
25. Durall CJ. Examination and treatment of cuboid syndrome: a literature review. Sports Health. 2011;3(6):514–9.
26. Haapamaki VV, Kiuru MJ, Koskinen SK. Ankle and foot injuries: analysis of MDCT findings. AJR Am J Roentgenol. 2004;183(3):615–22.
27. Sconfienza LM, Orlandi D, Lacelli F, Serafini G, Silvestri E. Dynamic high-resolution US of ankle and midfoot ligaments: normal anatomic structure and imaging technique. Radiographics. 2015;35(1):164–78.
28. Massen FK, Baumbach SF, Herterich V, Bocker W, Waizy H, Polzer H. Fractures to the anterior process of the calcaneus - clinical results following functional treatment. Injury. 2019;50(10):1781–6.
29. Swords MP, Schramski M, Switzer K, Nemec S. Chopart fractures and dislocations. Foot Ankle Clin. 2008;13(4):679–93, viii.

30. Lohrer H, Arentz S. Calcaneocuboid joint instability: a novel operative technique for anatomic reconstruction. Foot Ankle Int. 2004;25(5):349–56.
31. Lohrer H, Nauck T. Augmented periosteal flap repair of the chronically unstable calcaneocuboid joint. A series of six cases. J Bone Joint Surg Am. 2006;88(7):1596–601.
32. Degan TJ, Morrey BF, Braun DP. Surgical excision for anterior-process fractures of the calcaneus. J Bone Joint Surg Am. 1982;64(4):519–24.
33. Dhinsa BS, Latif A, Walker R, Abbasian A, Back D, Singh S. Fractures of the anterior process of the calcaneum; a review and proposed treatment algorithm. Foot Ankle Surg. 2019;25(1):94.
34. Halm JA, Schepers T. Resection of small avulsion fractures of the anterior process of the calcaneus for refractory complaints. J Foot Ankle Surg. 2017;56(1):135–41.
35. Main BJ, Jowett RL. Injuries of the midtarsal joint. J Bone Joint Surg Br. 1975;57(1):89–97.
36. Rammelt S, Schepers T. Chopart injuries: when to fix and when to fuse? Foot Ankle Clin. 2017;22(1):163–80.
37. Sun Y, Wang H, Tang Y, Qin S, Zhao M, Zhang F. Diagnosis and treatment of chronic lateral ankle instability with ligamentum bifurcatum injury: an observational study. Medicine (Baltimore). 2018;97(9):e0028.

The Unstable Syndesmosis

4

For the bony anatomy, the medial rough convex surface of the distal fibula articulates with the lateral triangular fibular notch of the distal tibia to form a fibrous joint, which is linked by strong ligaments. Although the syndesmosis is a joint, in the literature the term syndesmotic injury is used to describe injuries of the syndesmotic ligaments.

Syndesmotic injuries account for 1–10% of all ankle sprains [1]. They are more common in ankle fractures, found in about 10% of all ankle fractures and 25% of ankle fractures that require surgery [2, 3].

Forty percent of patients still have complaints of ankle instability 6 months after an ankle sprain [1, 4, 5]. This could be due to the widening of the ankle mortise as a result of the increased length of the syndesmotic ligaments after an acute ankle sprain. Widening of the ankle mortise by 1 mm decreases the contact area of the tibiotalar joint by 42% [6, 7], this could lead to instability and hence early osteoarthritis of the tibiotalar joint.

As the syndesmosis of the ankle plays an important role in the stability of the talocrural joint, understanding of the exact anatomy of both the osseous and ligamentous structures is essential for interpretation of plain radiographs, CT and MR images as well as understanding findings of ankle arthroscopy and deciding on the best therapeutic management.

4.1 Anatomy of Syndesmosis

- The ligamentous complex ensures the integrity of the highly congruent ankle joint that is formed by the tibia, fibula, and talus.
- The stability of the distal fibula is provided by the contours of the fibula and tibia and the syndesmotic ligaments.

4.1.1 Bony Configuration

The distal tibiofibular syndesmosis is formed by two bones and four ligaments. The convex shape of the distal fibula matches the concave incisura tibialis (Fig. 4.1). The size and

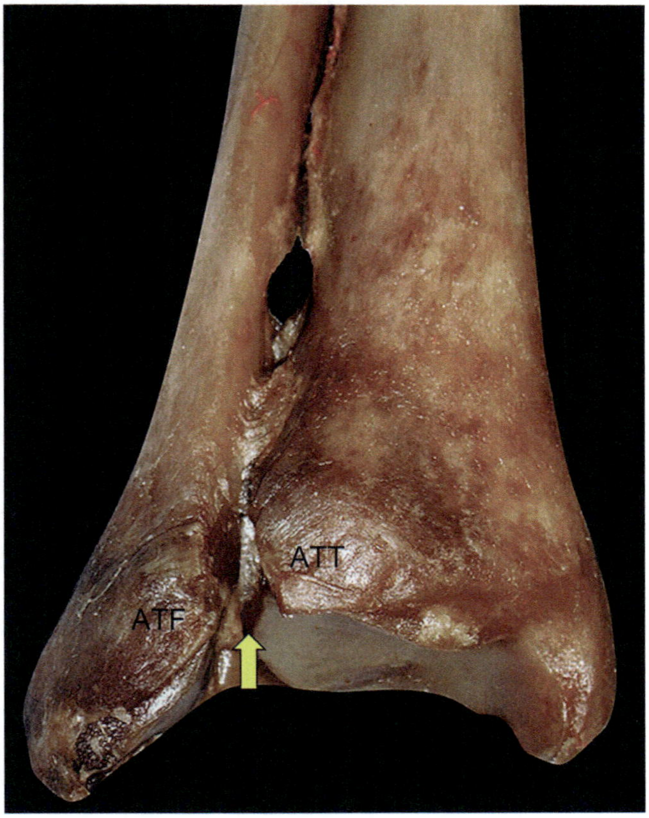

Fig. 4.1 Anterior view of the ankle mortise. In this specimen, there is a shallow incisura tibialis (arrow) which can be seen after having dissected the anterior inferior tibiofibular ligament (AITFL). *ATT* anterior tibial tubercle (Chaput's tubercle), *ATF* anterior fibular tubercle (Wagstaffe–Le Fort tubercle)

B. Hintermann, R. Ruiz, *Foot and Ankle Instability*, https://doi.org/10.1007/978-3-030-62926-7_4

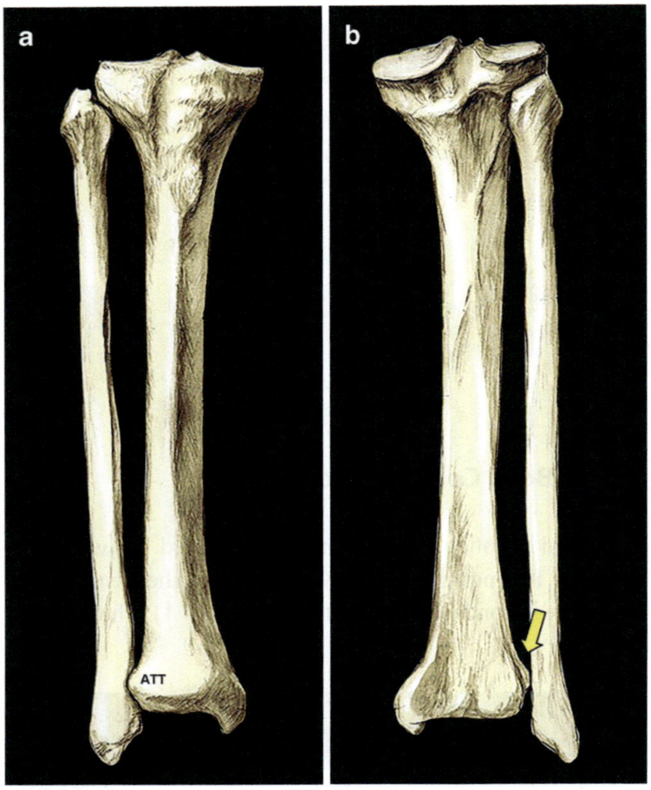

Fig. 4.2 The anterior tibial tubercle (ATT) is larger than the posterior tubercle (arrow) and prevents forward slipping of the distal fibula, while the diminutive posterior tubercle allows backward dislocation of the distal fibula. (**a**) anterior view; (**b**) posterior view

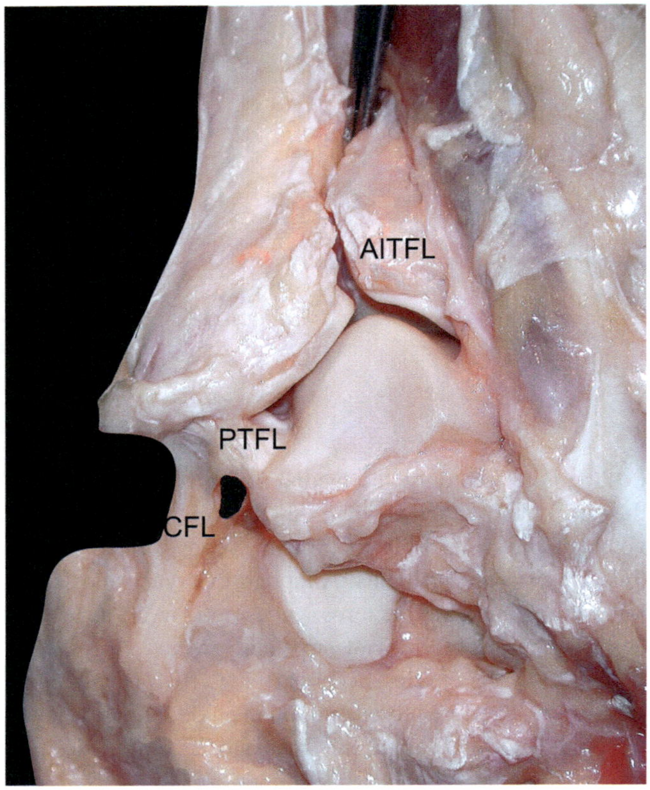

Fig. 4.3 Anterolateral view of the ankle with the anterior inferior tibiofibular ligament (AITFL) dissected. As the posterior tubercle functions as a fulcrum and the distal fibula spins around its longitudinal axis in a lateral direction, external rotation forces have resulted in a disruption of anterior inferior tibiofibular ligament (AITFL). *CFL* calcaneofibular ligament, *PTFL* posterior talofibular ligament

shape of the incisura tibialis plays an important role in ankle injury (Fig. 4.2). A shallow incisura tibialis may predispose to recurrent ankle sprains [8] or syndesmotic injury with fracture-dislocation [9]. The anterior tibial tubercle (Chaput's tubercle) is larger than the posterior tubercle and prevents forward slipping of the distal fibula, while the diminutive posterior tubercle allows backward dislocation of the distal fibula (Fig. 4.3). In fibula fractures caused by external rotation, the posterior tubercle functions as a fulcrum and the distal fibula spins around its longitudinal axis in a lateral direction [10].

The fibular part of the syndesmosis is congruent with its tibial counterpart. The crista interossea fibularis forms a convex triangle that is located above the articular facet on the lateral malleolus. The base of the fibular triangle is formed by the anterior tubercle (Wagstaffe–Le Fort tubercle) and the, almost negligible, posterior tubercle.

4.1.2 The Syndesmotic Ligaments

Four ligaments form the syndesmotic ligament complex: anterior inferior tibiofibular ligament (AITFL), posterior inferior tibiofibular ligament (PITFL), tibiofibular interosseous ligament (TFIL), and transverse tibiofibular ligament (TTFL). These ligaments work together with the bony restraints to maintain the integrity between the distal tibia and the fibula by resisting the axial, rotational, and translational forces. There is also a synovial-lined plica which extends from the tibiotalar joint, called the syndesmotic recess. It attaches to the distal tibia medially and the distal fibula laterally with an interposing fat-containing synovial fold [11, 12]. In acute syndesmotic injuries, this recess can tear causing leakage of contrast into the incisura tibialis when using arthrography [13]. In chronic syndesmotic injuries, the synovial lining may become irregular due to inflammation.

4.1.2.1 The Anterior Inferior Tibiofibular Ligament

The anterior inferior tibiofibular ligament (AITFL) extends in an oblique way from the anterior tubercle of the distal tibia, on average 5 mm above the articular surface, to the anterior tubercle of the distal fibula (Fig. 4.4). The AITFL has a multifascicular aspect, caused by fatty tissue interposed between the multiple collagen bundles.

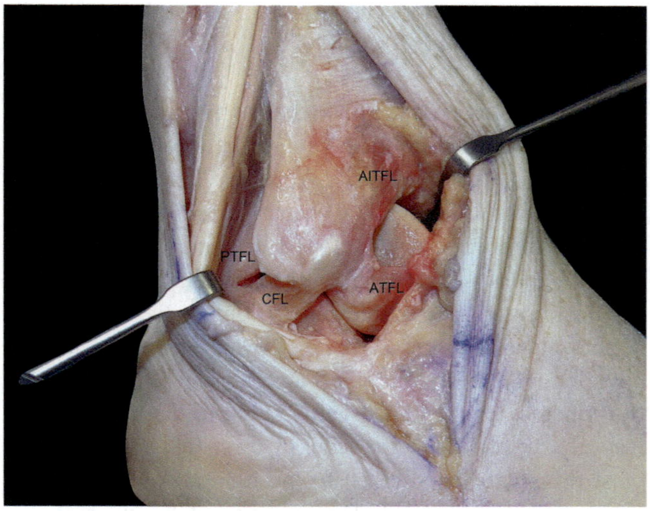

Fig. 4.4 Anterolateral view of the ankle showing the anterior inferior tibiofibular ligament (AITFL) with its multifascicular aspect, caused by fatty tissue interposed between the multiple collagen bundles. *ATFL* anterior talofibular ligament, *PTFL* posterior talofibular ligament, *CFL* calcaneofibular ligament

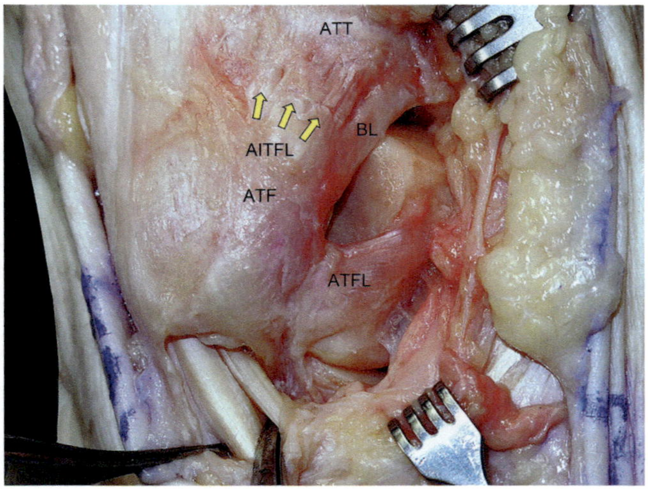

Fig. 4.5 Anterolateral view of the ankle. The anterior inferior tibiofibular ligament (AITFL) is divided into three parts: the most proximal and shortest part, originates just above the anterior tubercle of the tibia (ATT) and is attached just above the anterior tubercle of the fibula (ATF). The middle and strongest part runs between the anterior tubercle of the tibia (ATT) and fibula (ATF). The most distal and longest part extends just below the anterior tubercles. An accessory antero-inferior tibiofibular ligament, also called the Bassett's ligament (BL), runs inferior and parallel to the AITFL. It is not covered by synovial tissue, is intra-articular, crosses the proximo-lateral margin of the ankle and meets the lateral talar trochlea during dorsiflexion. *ATFL* anterior talofibular ligament

The AITFL is divided into three parts of which the upper part is the shortest one (Fig. 4.5). It originates just above the anterior tubercle of the tibia and is attached just above the anterior tubercle of the fibula. The middle and strongest part runs between the anterior tubercle of the tibia and fibula. The lower part, which is the longest, extends just below the anterior tubercles.

An accessory antero-inferior tibiofibular ligament, also called Bassett's ligament (BL), which runs inferior and parallel to the AITFL, can be identified in 21–92% of dissected ankles of human anatomic specimen or MRI studies (Fig. 4.5) [14–16]. It is not covered by synovial tissue, is intra-articular, crosses the proximo-lateral margin of the ankle and comes into contact with the lateral talar trochlea during dorsiflexion.

The AITFL is the weakest of the four syndesmotic ligaments and is the first to yield to forces that create an external rotation of the fibula around its longitudinal axis (Fig. 4.3) [10].

4.1.2.2 The Posterior Inferior Tibiofibular Ligament

The posterior inferior tibiofibular ligament (PITFL) is a strong ligament that extends from the posterior tibial malleolus to the posterior tubercle of the fibula and runs from proximal-medial to distal-lateral (Fig. 4.6). Its lower part, or transverse ligament (TTFL), runs more horizontally than the PITFL [11]. The PITFL has a similar shape and structure as the AITFL. The PITFL, like the AITFL, is multifascicular and consists of multiple collagen bundles interspersed with fat. Its most distal fibers are in close contact with the transverse ligament and fibers from the fibular insertion sometimes even appear to be continuous with the latter [17].

As the PITFL is a thick and strong ligament, excessive stress results more often in a posterior malleolus avulsion fracture than in a rupture of the ligament [18].

4.1.2.3 The Transverse Tibiofibular Ligament

The transverse tibiofibular ligament (TTFL) runs horizontally between the proximal margin of the fibular malleolar fossa and the dorso-distal rim of the tibia and may extend as far as the dorsal aspect of the medial malleolus (Fig. 4.6). It is a thick, round ligament that deepens the postero-inferior rim of the tibia and forms a labrum analogue [15, 17]. Some fibers of the posterior talofibular ligament coalesce with the most distal fibers of the transverse ligament and form the so-called tibial slip, or intermalleolar ligament (IML).

4.1.2.4 The Intermalleolar Ligament

The intermalleolar ligament (IML) is a separate anatomic entity and has been shown to be almost invariably present in 81.8% of 77 specimens [19, 20]. The IML arises slightly proximal to the origin of the posterior talofibular ligament in the malleolar fossa and distal to the origin of the transverse ligament (Fig. 4.6) [21]. The IML runs parallel to the transverse ligament, from which it is always separated by a triangular- or quadrilateral-shaped soft tissue space. During plantar flexion, the IML becomes less taut and approximates

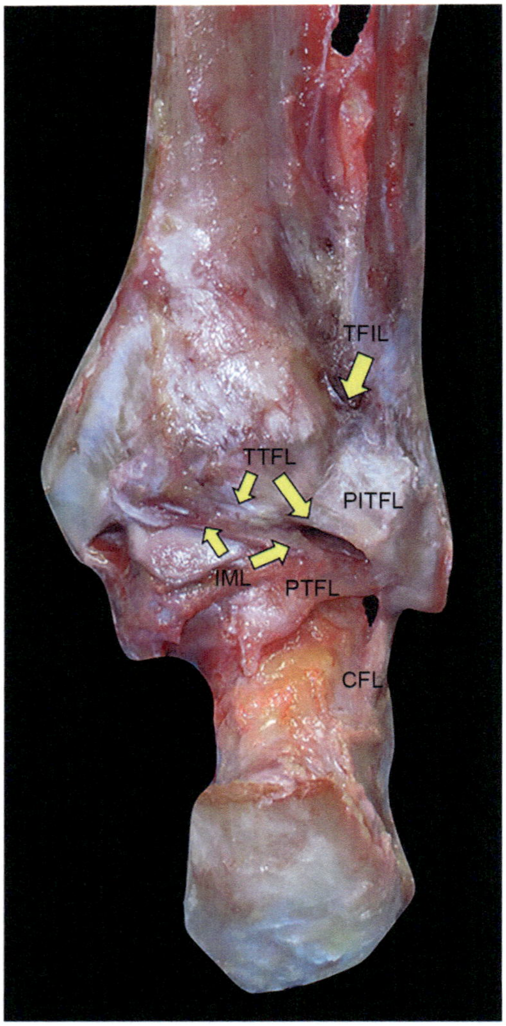

Fig. 4.6 Posterior view of the ankle joint complex. The posterior inferior tibiofibular ligament (PITFL) is a strong ligament that extends from the posterior tibial malleolus to the posterior tubercle of the fibula. It runs from proximal-medial to distal-lateral. The PITFL, like the AITFL, is multifascicular and consists of multiple collagen bundles interspersed with fat. Its deep component or transverse (tibiofibular) ligament (TTFL) runs more horizontal than the superficial component of the PITFL. The TTFL is a thick, round ligament that deepens the postero-inferior rim of the tibia and forms a labrum analogue. The intermalleolar ligament (IML) runs parallel to the transverse ligament, from which it is always separated by a triangular- or quadrilateral-shaped soft tissue space. The tibiofibular interosseous ligament (TFIL) is the most distal part of the tibiofibular membrane. The area underneath the interosseous ligament is generally filled with the synovial plica from the tibiotalar joint. *PTFL* posterior talofibular ligament, *CFL* calcaneofibular ligament

the transverse ligament [19]. The space between the transverse ligament and IML makes the posterolateral approach in ankle arthroscopy the most suitable for avoiding ligamentous structures. The IML can be the cause of posterior impingement syndrome in ballet dancers, where in extreme plantar flexion, entrapment or even a bucket handle tear of the ligament can occur [20, 21].

4.1.2.5 The Interosseous Membrane

The interosseous membrane extends between the tibia and fibula, and at its lowermost end thickens and gives rise to a spatial network of pyramidal shape (Fig. 4.7). This network is filled with fatty tissue and steep running fascicles which form the interosseous ligament. Most fibers run in a latero-distal and anterior direction from the tibia to the fibula, some fibers on the anterior aspect, however, run in the reverse direction. The most distal fibers attach to the tibia at the anterior tubercle level and descend straight to the fibula, where they attach just above the level of the talocrural joint. The most proximal fibers attach to the tibia at the apex of the incisura tibialis [11, 17]. The presence of the interosseous ligament is variable. In some individuals it is absent, whereas in others it is markedly present, especially in those with a flattened incisura of the tibia and fibula. The area underneath the interosseous ligament is generally filled with the synovial plica from the tibiotalar joint [11, 17].

4.2 Biomechanics of Syndesmotic Instability

- Loss of the lateral buttress for the ankle mortise joint permits the axial, rotational, and translational forces to separate the fibula and tibia, thus destroying the integrity of the ankle joint.
- The syndesmotic ligaments and the deltoid ligament form a functional unit.

In anatomical specimens, the relative importance of the individual syndesmotic ligaments for syndesmotic stability was found to be 35% for the AITFL, 33% for the TTFL, 22% for the TFIL, and 9% for the PITFL (Fig. 4.8) [22].

The distal tibiofibular syndesmosis is an important functional structure to maintain ankle stability during weight-bearing and walking. The distal fibula and tibia with the syndesmotic ligaments form a stable articulation. The syndesmosis provides a strong lateral buttress for the ankle mortise joint and resists the axial, rotational, and translational forces that attempt to separate these two bones [2, 17]. The relative motion of the syndesmosis correlates to the ankle position and loading patterns [23]. While moving the foot from plantar flexion to dorsiflexion, 1.25-mm lateral translation and 2° external rotation of the fibula have been reported [24].

Fig. 4.7 The interosseous membrane extends between the tibia and fibula (see text). (**a**) Anterior view and (**b**) posterior view

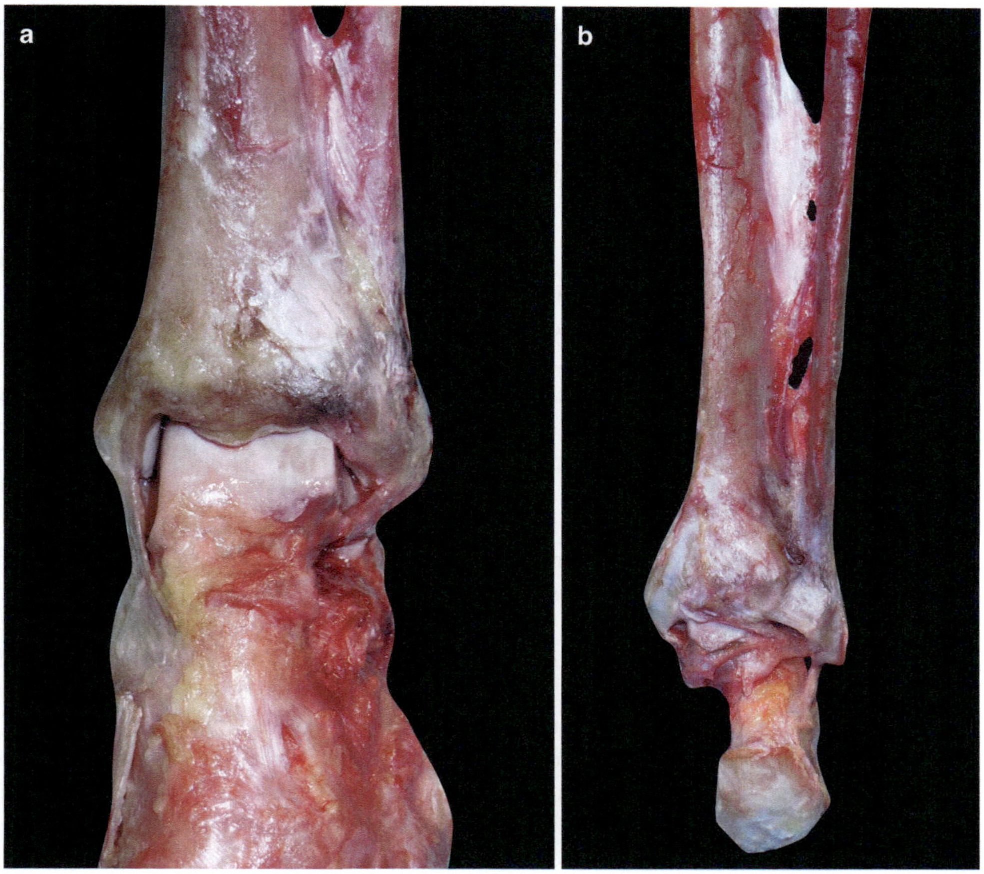

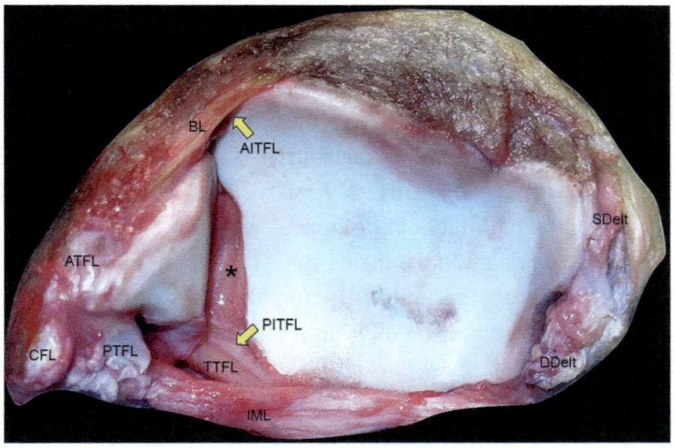

Fig. 4.8 Caudal view of the ankle mortise after resection of the talus showing the articular surfaces of the distal tibia and fibula. While the anterior inferior tibiofibular ligament (AITFL) accounts for approximately 35% of syndesmotic stability, the posterior ligaments provide 65% of syndesmotic stability. *BL* Basset ligament, *PITFL* posterior inferior tibiofibular ligament, *TTFL* transverse ligament, *IML* untermalleolar ligament, *PTFL* posterior talofibular ligament, *CFL* calcaneofibular ligament, *ATFL* anterior talofibular ligament, *DDelt* deep deltoid ligament, *SDelt* superficial deltoid ligament, *Asterisk* synovial-lined plica filling the syndesmotic recess. The intermalleolar and the tibiofibular interosseous ligaments are not shown

The load transfer of the fibula is reduced by 30% when the interosseous membrane is injured, thus resulting in irregular load and dynamic changes in the ankle joint when the continuity of the fibula is not restored [25]. Changes in ankle load, in turn, will cause articular cartilage damage and subsequently arthritis [26].

A fibular fracture higher than 7 cm above the tip of the lateral malleolus has previously been considered not to affect the rotational stability of the ankle joint [27] and good outcome was reported without internal fixation of the fibula fracture [28, 29]. However, the middle fibular fracture, which injures the interosseous membrane, often results in a shortening of the distal fibula [30] which makes a restoration of the congruity at the ankle joint impossible without fixation of the fibular fracture. If the fibular fracture is not fixed, the distal tibiofibular syndesmosis may fail due to shear stress.

The distal tibiofibular syndesmosis and the interosseous membrane are important factors in maintaining the stability of the ankle joint. When injured, the talus will shift lateralwards. A lateral displacement of the talus of 1 mm reduces the tibia contact surface by 40%. The displacement of the talus of >1.5 mm will result in a concentration of stress in the ankle such that articular surface degeneration will occur in the ankle in the long run [7, 30, 31].

4.3 Conclusions and Clinical Implications

- The distal tibiofibular syndesmosis and the interosseous membrane are important factors in maintaining the stability of the ankle joint.
- They co-work with the deltoid ligament to maintain coronal plane stability of talus within the ankle mortise.

Although the AITFL is weaker than the PITFL [11], it acts as the primary constraint to excessive fibular motion relative to the tibia and talar external rotation within the ankle mortise [32]. Mechanical disruption of the interosseous ligament and membrane may result in increased compressive stress within the tibia, increased likelihood of lateral dislocation of the distal fibula and incongruent ankle joint articulating surfaces [5]. Dynamic ankle joint motion and relative joint position of the talus within the mortise would be altered under these circumstances, resulting in abnormal distribution of contact pressure and thus increased likelihood of developing joint arthritis [7, 30, 31].

4.4 Injury Mechanism

- External rotation of the foot will cause external rotation and external displacement of the fibula, resulting in a gradual increase in the tension of the syndesmotic and interosseous ligament, until the ligament tears.
- Eversion of the talus within the ankle mortise and excessive dorsiflexion can also cause injuries to the syndesmotic ligaments.

External rotation stress is the most potent mechanism for spreading the distal tibiofibular syndesmosis [1, 5, 22]. External rotation of the foot will cause external rotation and external displacement of the fibula, resulting in a gradual increase in the tension of the AITFL and interosseous ligament, until the ligament tears. The injury will lead to interosseous membrane damage once the fibula is moved outward beyond the extent of the interosseous membrane [33–35]. When the external rotation stress is large enough and continues to be transmitted to the proximal fibula, it may result in stress concentration on the fibula due to the limitation of the superior tibiofibular syndesmosis. If the fibula has not been shifted to the outside, a fracture of the fibula will occur under excessive stress [36]. The tension on the interosseous membrane injury site is simultaneously increased due to the swelling, which, in turn, often leads to shortening of the lower part of fibula. This will further lead to ankle instability and induce traumatic arthritis if the injury is not treated properly.

Other mechanisms for syndesmotic injuries can be eversion of the talus within the ankle mortise [37] and excessive dorsiflexion [1, 37, 38]. The latter is due to the attribution of the anterior portion of the talar dome being wider. This anatomical feature can contribute to spreading the distal tibiofibular articulation during extreme dorsiflexion [39]. The talus tends to act as a wedge within the ankle mortise in extremes of dorsiflexion. Extreme dorsiflexion, therefore, may be involved in the mechanism of injury to the ligamentous structures that stabilize the distal tibia and fibula.

Syndesmotic injuries usually are associated with ankle fractures, most commonly the Weber C type [40], but also Weber B type fractures [41]. Syndesmotic injuries can also occur after trauma to the ankle without a fracture of the osseous part [1]. Several cases of distal tibiofibular dislocations with an intact fibula have been reported in the past [42]. All of these injuries involved a twisting load with a traumatic supination injury [38]. These cases were usually missed since there was no high index of suspicion that the syndesmosis could have been injured.

4.5 History and Clinical Findings

- Most patients report an external rotation trauma of the foot.
- Pain at the ankle syndesmosis which may extend proximally, inability to bear weight, and swelling are the hallmarks after an acute injury.
- As syndesmotic injuries may be accompanied by injuries to the deltoid ligament, evaluation of the involvement of the deltoid ligament is needed.
- As none of the syndesmotic stress tests are sensitive or specific, the diagnosis of syndesmotic injuries should not be made based on the medical history and physical examination alone.

Although a syndesmotic ankle sprain may have various mechanisms of injury, external rotation of the foot is most often reported by patients. Pain at the ankle syndesmosis which may extend proximally [43], inability to bear weight, and swelling are typical symptoms following syndesmotic injury. The pain is usually localized over the AITFL [38, 44, 45], furthermore, pain can be induced by active or passive external rotation of the foot or forced dorsiflexion. A normal heel-toe walking gait pattern may be replaced by a heel raise gait pattern to avoid excessive ankle dorsiflexion and to avoid pain during push-off [43, 46].

Specific clinical tests (Fig. 4.9) are commonly used to triage ankle injuries as a referral for confirmatory imaging tests. These clinical tests assess the integrity of the anatomical structures and generally aim to reproduce symptoms or test function by applying stress to the injured structure: palpatory tenderness of the inferior tibiofibular ligaments (Fig. 4.9a) [47, 48], squeeze test (Fig. 4.9b) [1, 48, 49], external rotation stress test (Fig. 4.9c) [4, 38, 48], cross-leg test (Fig. 4.9d) [50], dorsiflexion test (Fig. 4.9e) [50], and the heel thump test (Fig. 4.9f) [50]. However, it has been shown that none of the syndesmotic stress tests were sensitive or specific [48], therefore the diagnosis of syndesmotic injuries should not be made based on the medical history and physical examination alone.

Syndesmotic injuries are traditionally graded from I to III in the same manner as lateral ankle sprains. Grade I refers to mild stretching, grade II represents incomplete tear, and grade III is a complete disruption of the syndesmosis [51]. A new anatomic classification system for syndesmosis diastasis was also suggested dividing the diastasis into frank or occult, which were further subdivided into coronal, sagittal, rotational, or longitudinal pattern [52].

Because injury of the deltoid ligament may accompany syndesmotic injuries, a differential diagnosis is needed to evaluate the involvement of the deltoid ligament and to develop a more effective rehabilitation program for patients. Significant swelling, tenderness, and ecchymosis over the medial ankle, combined with more than 4 mm of radiologically confirmed widening of the syndesmosis, may indicate involvement of the deltoid ligament [53]. Injury to the deltoid ligament in combination with injury to the syndesmotic ligament usually results in very significant ankle mortise instability.

4.6 Imaging

- Weight-bearing radiographs and CT scans of the suspected injured diastasis should be compared with images of the contralateral intact ankle to assess the presence and severity of injuries to the diastasis.
- CT scans are the more sensitive diagnostic tool for assessing syndesmotic integrity and are capable of detecting syndesmotic malreduction, which are otherwise difficult to visualize on plain radiographs, especially in subtle cases.
- In acute injuries, MRI was found to provide higher diagnostic accuracy over conventional radiographs or CT scans with a sensitivity of up to 91% and specificity of 100%.

Standard radiography with a true anteroposterior (AP) view and a mortise view can be used to evaluate the tibiofibular clear space (TFCS), tibiofibular overlap (TFO), and medial clear space (MCS) (Fig. 4.10) [54]. TFCS in the AP and mortise views should be less than 6 mm with an intact syndesmosis. Normal TFO for the AP view is more than 6 mm or more than 42% of the fibular width; for the mortise view, it should be more than 1 mm [54]. MCS should be less than or equal to the clear space between the talar dome and the tibial plafond. A mortise view taken with weight-bearing is the most accurate way to assess syndesmotic instability radiographically, but many patients with mortise instability may not be able to tolerate unilateral standing due to pain [37]. Imaging of the suspected injured diastasis should be compared with imaging of the contralateral intact ankle to assess the presence and severity of its involvement. Attention should also be paid to a potential shortening of the fibula associated with the syndesmotic injury [37, 55]. However, these classic radiographic measurements of the syndesmosis can be unreliable when assessing the distal tibiofibular relationship (Fig. 4.11) [56–58].

Intraoperative stress radiography may help assess the distal tibiofibular syndesmosis (Fig. 4.12) [5, 59, 60]. Widening of the TFCL and the MCL by more than 2 mm during external rotation stress indicates injury of the syndesmosis [5]; however, the evidence for stress views as the principal assessment for syndesmotic injuries is weak, especially in the case of chronic injuries.

Intraoperative lateral hook testing (LHT) has effectively diagnosed an unstable syndesmosis in the coronal plane, although the degree of diastasis necessary to define instability remains controversial (Fig. 4.13) [60, 61]. Instability was defined when the TFCS exceeded 5 mm using an LHT during radiographic examination [60] or when widening of the ankle syndesmosis of more than 2 mm was seen intraoperatively [59].

Computed tomography (CT) scans are a more sensitive diagnostic tool for assessing syndesmotic integrity and are capable of detecting syndesmotic malreduction, which are otherwise difficult to visualize on plain radiographs, especially in subtle cases [57, 62]. The ability to review both ankles makes the CT scan a preferred noninvasive method for the evaluation of syndesmotic reduction. The CT scan of the distal tibiofibular syndesmosis is usually measured and analyzed by scanning the most prominent level of the anterior tibial tuberosity. It is generally believed that an ankle syndesmosis injury is present when the gap is >6 mm or wider than 2 mm compared with the contralateral side (Fig. 4.14). In addition, ankle syndesmosis injury with a separation of 2–3 mm can be confirmed on the coronal plane in CT images (Fig. 4.15) [63, 64]. Though questioned in a cadaveric study [65], weight-bearing CT scans (WBCT) have the specific additional advantage of dynamic evaluation of the syndesmosis, as shown by significant lateral fibular translation and fibular external rotation relative to the incisura during weight-bearing vs non-weight-bearing imaging [66–68]. Of note, application of torque to the tibia impacts 2D measurements and may be useful when diagnosing syndesmotic injuries by digitally reconstructed radiographs or axial CT images [69].

Magnetic resonance imaging (MRI) was found to provide higher diagnostic accuracy over conventional radio-

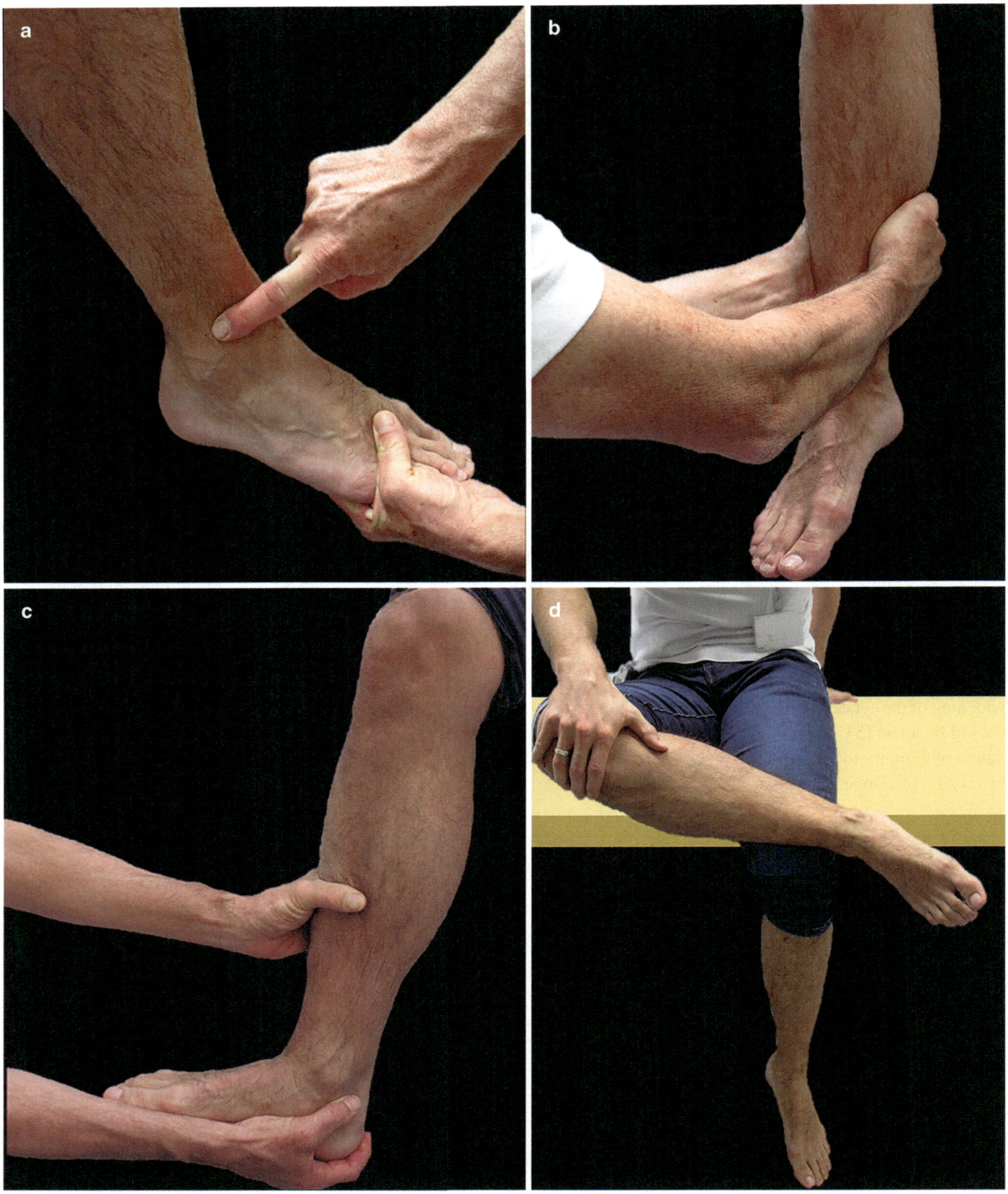

Fig. 4.9 Common clinical tests used to diagnose syndesmotic injury; if pain can be provoked at the distal tibiofibular syndesmosis through one of these tests, the presence of an injury is highly likely. (**a**) The point test: The examiner applies pressure directly over the anterior aspect of the distal tibiofibular syndesmosis. (**b**) The squeeze test: The examiner cups both hands around the distal tibia and fibula and imposes compression. (**c**) The external rotation stress test. The examiner stabilizes the leg with one hand and applies an external rotation load to the foot, with the ankle in neutral flexion. (**d**) The crossed-leg test: The patient is sitting with the injured leg resting across the knee of the uninjured leg. The patient then applies a gentle force on the medial knee of the injured leg. (**e**) The dorsiflexion test: The examiner stabilizes the leg with one hand and passively moves the foot towards dorsiflexion with the other hand to impose possible widening of the mortise. (**f**) The heel thump test: The examiner holds the patient's leg with one hand and with the other hand applies a gentle but firm thump on the heel with the fist. This force is applied at the center of the heel and in line with the long axis of the tibia

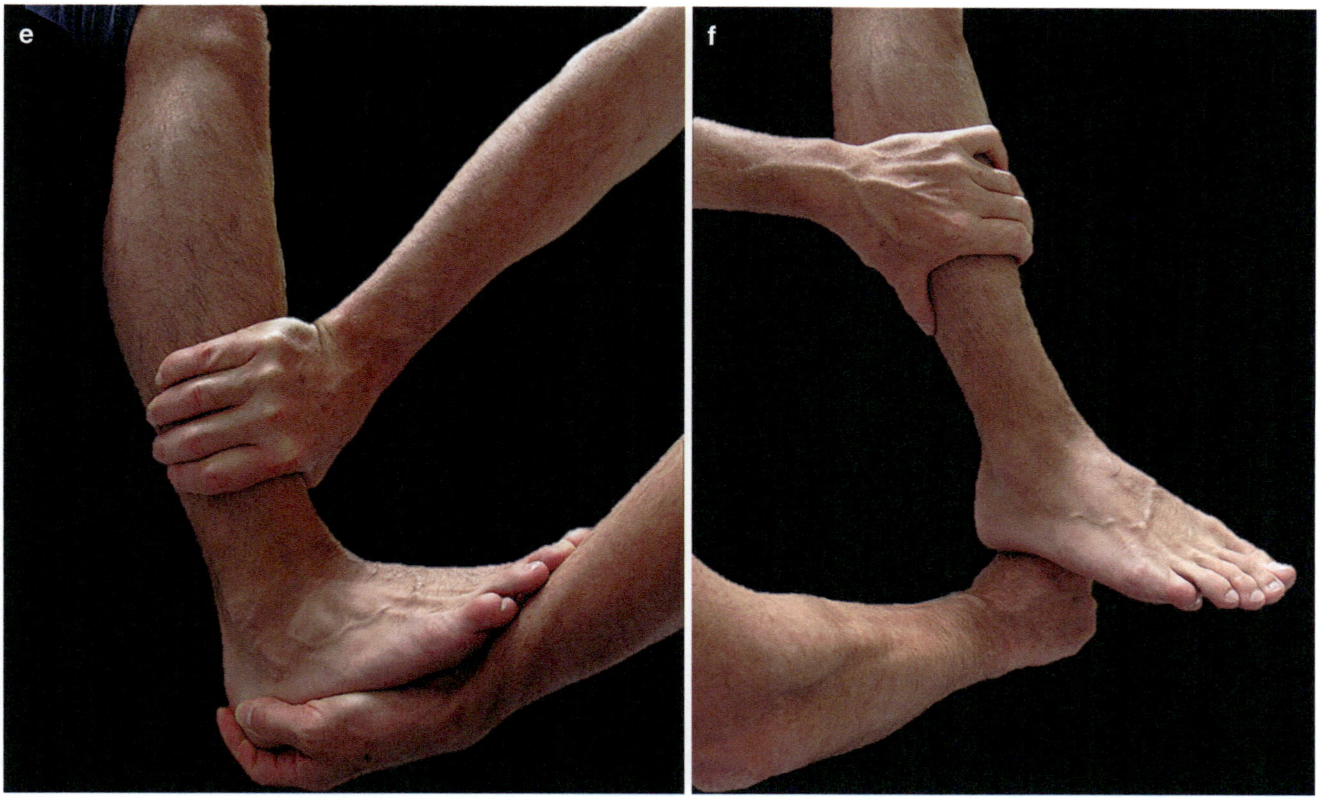

Fig. 4.9 (continued)

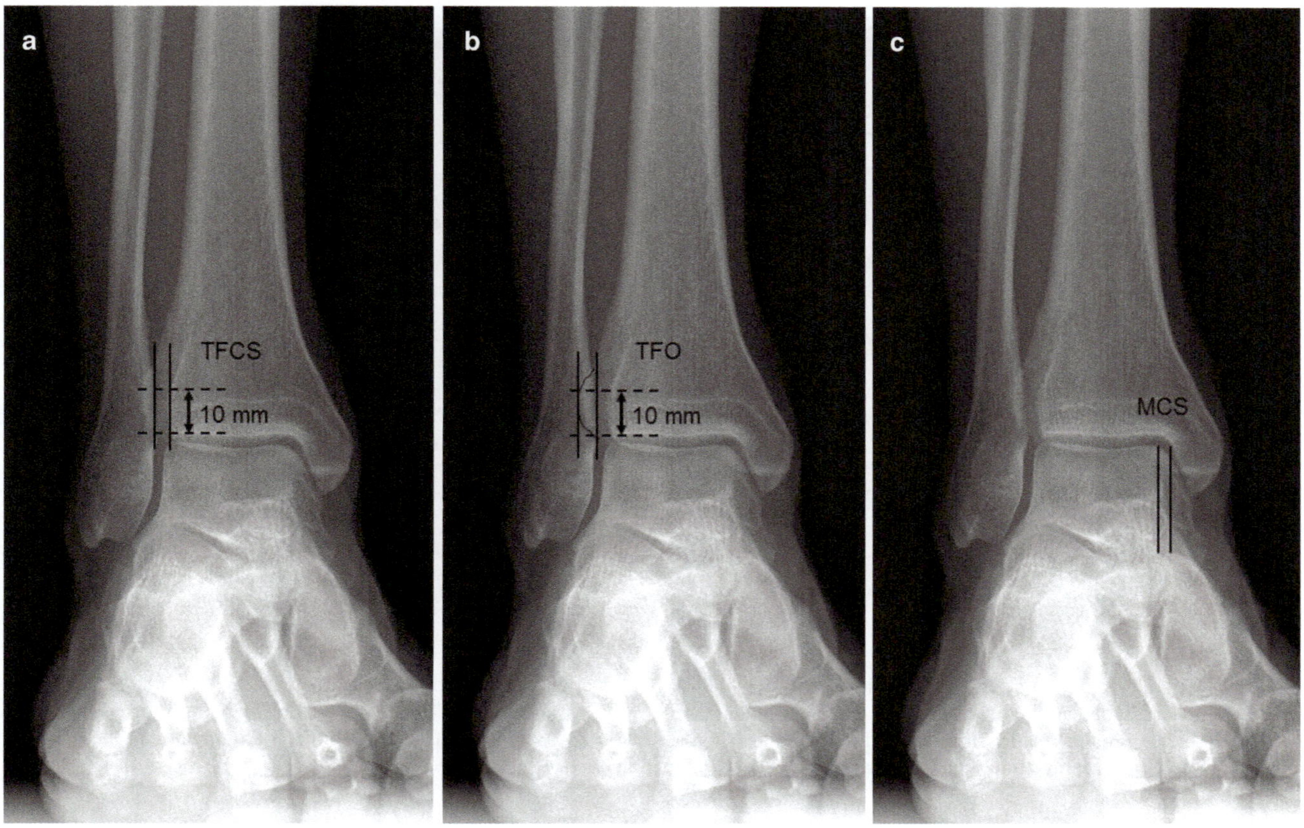

Fig. 4.10 The three most frequently used measurements to assess the distal tibiofibular syndesmosis using plain radiographs. (**a**) Measurement of the tibiofibular clear space (TFCS) 1 cm above the tibia plafond; in an intact syndesmosis, it should be less than 6 mm. (**b**) Measurement of the tibiofibular overlap (TFO) 1 cm above the tibia plafond; in the AP-view, it should be more than 6 mm or more than 42% of the fibular width. (**c**) Measurement of the medial clear space (MCS); it should be less than or equal to the clear space between the talar dome and the tibial plafond

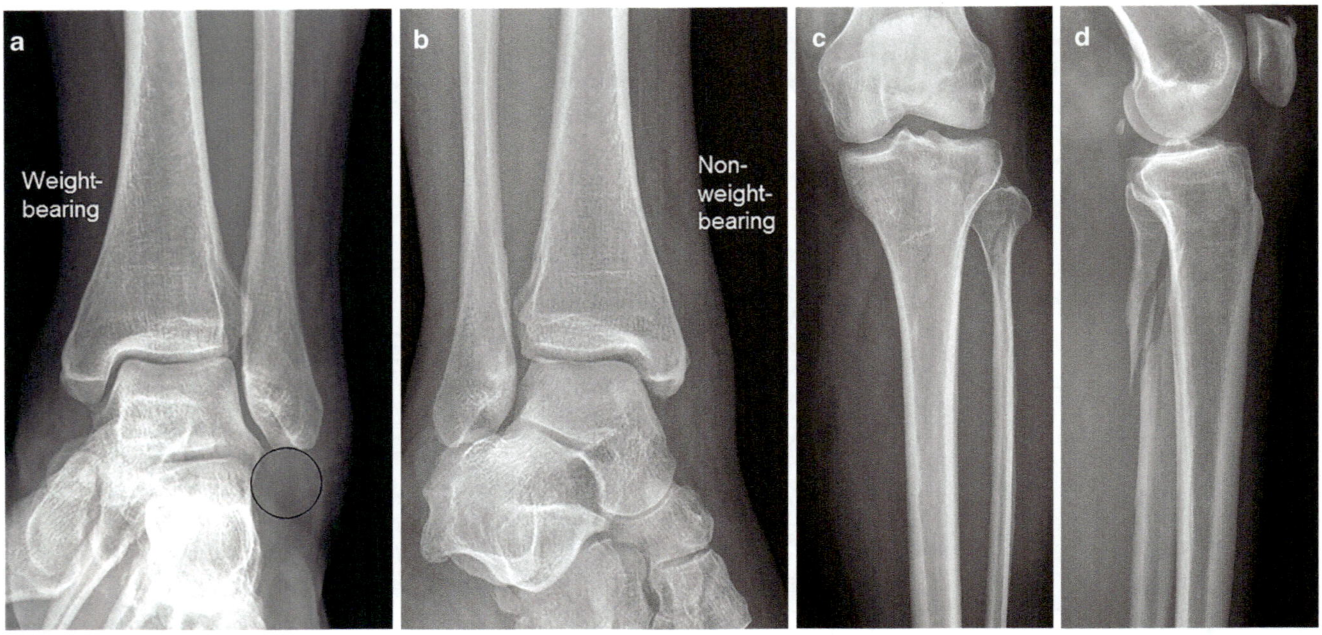

Fig. 4.11 A 47-year-old female patient with an acute syndesmotic injury of her right ankle following a high fibular fracture. (**a**) AP view of the contralateral ankle under weight-bearing showing a regular distal tibio-fibular relationship. (**b**) The plain radiograph of the injured right ankle without weight-bearing does not show a syndesmotic injury. Missing tibiofibular overlap (TFO) may be a result of exposure with some increased internal rotation of the ankle. The tibiofibular clear space (TFCS) does not evidence a widening, and the circle formed by lateral talus and fibular groove of the fibula cannot be reconstructed. (**c**, **d**) Plan radiograph of proximal tibia shows the Maisonneuve-type fracture of high fibula

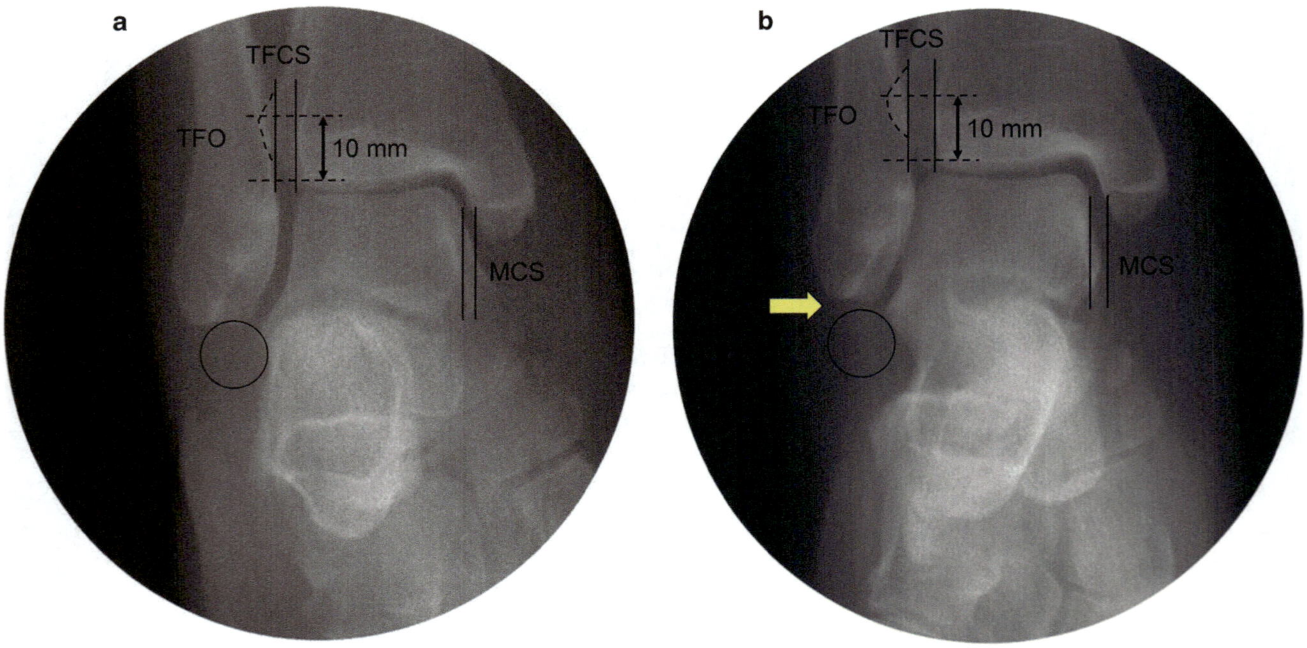

Fig. 4.12 Intraoperative stress test (same patient as Fig. 4.11). (**a**) Lateral tibiotalar alignment, medial clear space (MCS), and length of the fibula indicate regular relationship of the distal tibia and fibula; however, there is a missing tibiofibular overlap (TFO). (**b**) Under abduction and eversion stress of the foot, the tibiofibular clear space (TFCS) and the MCS widen and the fibula is shortened (arrow). Notice the interrupted lateral tibiotalar alignment and the increased TFO

graphs or CT scans (Fig. 4.16) [70–72]. Furthermore, contrast media and/or a 3 T MRI improve diagnostic accuracy of MRI [12, 73]. While direct assessment of the tibiofibular syndesmosis is possible by MRI, assessment of syndesmotic injury by X-ray or CT scans must rely on recognition of secondary signs [64]. Sensitivity of up to 91.0% and specificity of 100% have been reported for syndesmotic injuries. Sensitivity of 84.0% and specificity of 93.5% have been reported for additional deltoid ligament tears using MRI [73].

4.6.1 Conclusion

In conclusion, conventional radiographs cannot predict syndesmotic injuries reliably [64]. CT outperforms conventional X-rays in detecting syndesmotic malreduction. Additionally, the syndesmotic interval can be assessed in greater detail by CT scans. Using MRI, sensitivity and specificity of nearly 100% can be achieved. However, correlating MRI findings with patients' complaints can be difficult, and utility hereof in patients with subtle syndesmotic instability needs further investigation.

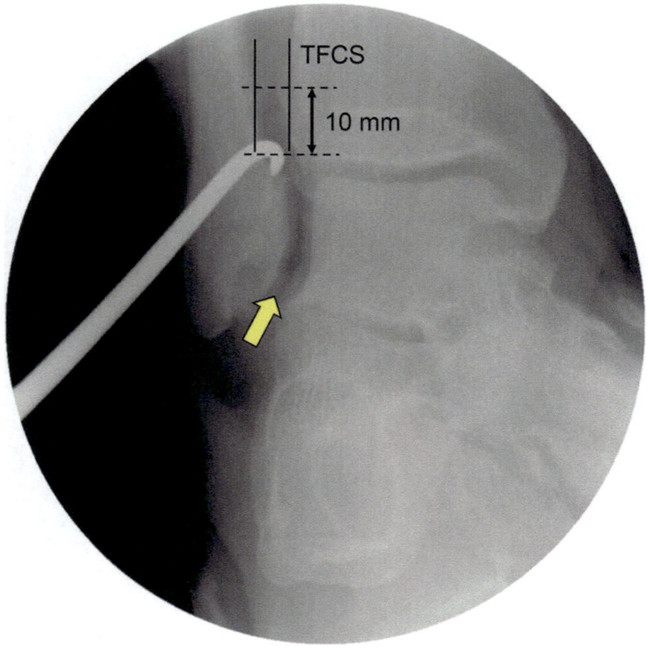

Fig. 4.13 When applying lateral hook test (LHT) intraoperatively, the tibiofibular clear space (TFCS) is widened to more than 6 mm (same patient as Fig. 4.11). Notice the gapping of the tibiofibular joint space (arrow)

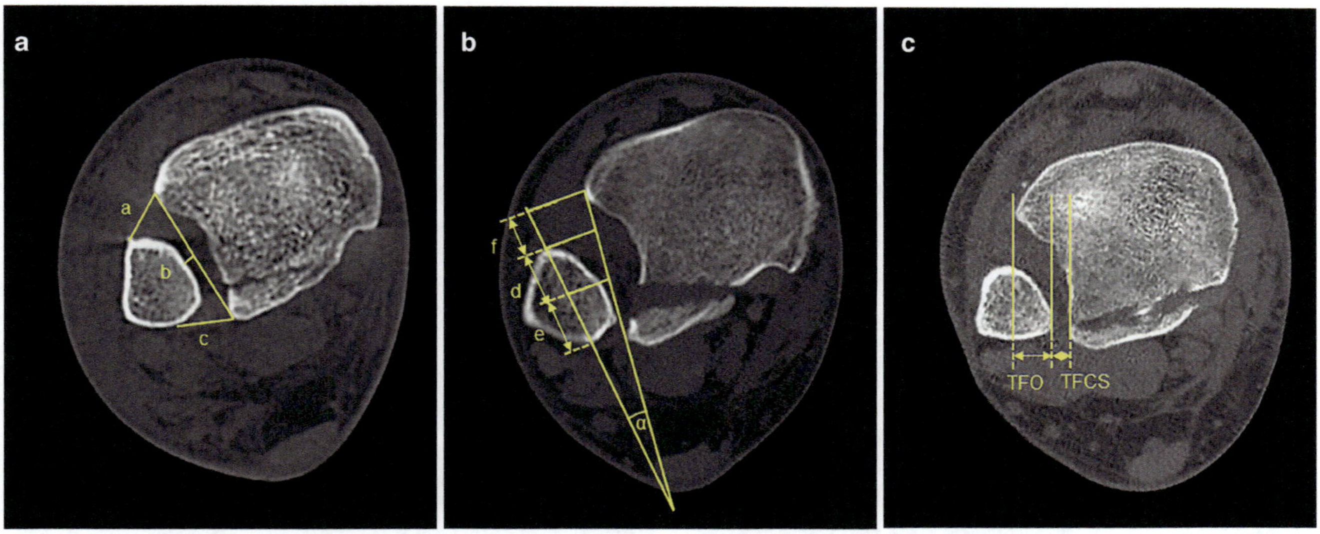

Fig. 4.14 Frequently used measurement methods to assess the distal tibiofibular syndesmosis using computed tomography (CT) scans. Measurements were performed 1 cm above the distal tibial plafond. (**a**) Measurement of the tibiofibular width anterior (a), middle (b), and posterior (c). (**b**) Measurement of the antero-posterior translation (d, e, f) and the rotation (angle α) of the distal fibula. (**c**) Measurement of the tibiofibular clear space (TFCS) and tibiofibular overlap (TFO)

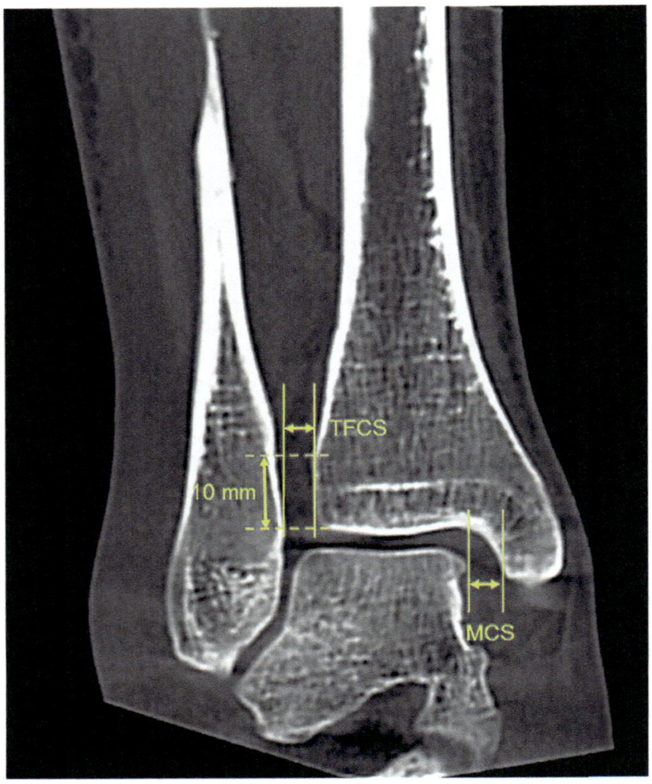

Fig. 4.15 Ankle syndesmosis injury, with a separation of 2–3 mm, confirmed by a coronal plane CT image

4.7 Arthroscopy

- In acute injuries, the torn parts of the anterior syndesmotic ligament and the resulting instability of the fibula can be seen, allowing to understand the injury and to determine appropriate treatment.
- In chronic injuries, arthroscopy permits to assess the position of the fibula in the incisura and the stability of the ankle joint provided by the syndesmotic ligaments.

Arthroscopic assessment of the syndesmosis has emerged as a useful technique to evaluate stability of the ankle ligamentous complex, allowing both direct visualization of the tibiofibular articulation and the ability to assess stability in multiple planes (coronal, transverse, sagittal) under simulated loading conditions [52, 70, 71, 74–77]. Diagnosis of syndesmosis disruption can be made by ankle arthroscopy with a 100% accuracy [76].

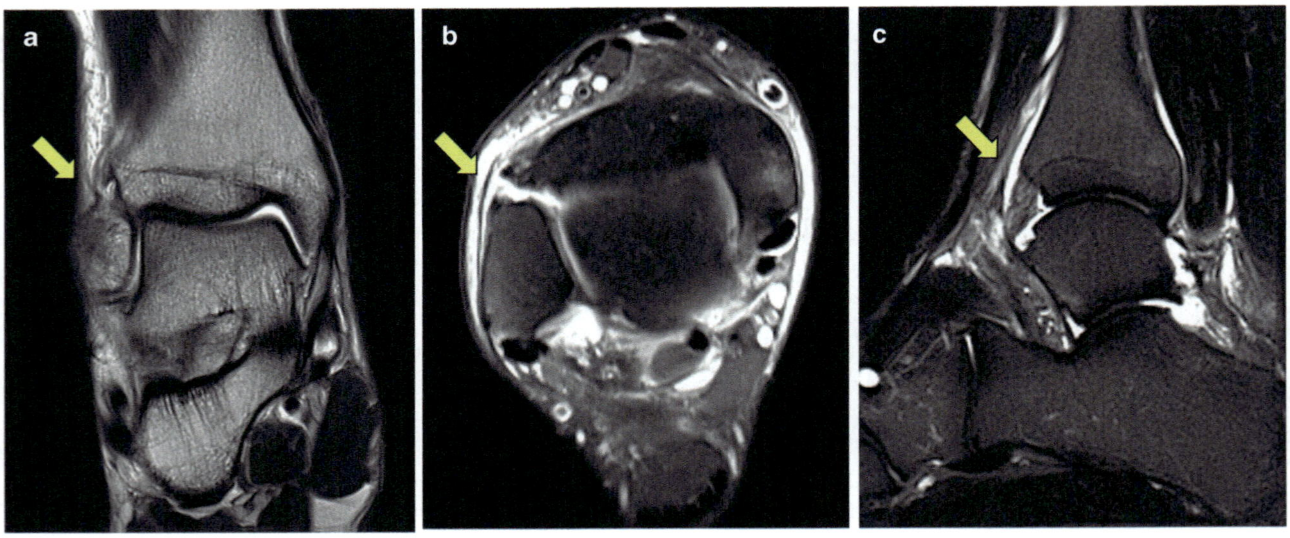

Fig. 4.16 In contrast to X-ray or CT scans, a 3 T MRI permits direct assessment of the distal tibiofibular syndesmosis ligaments. The AITFL is seen ruptured (arrow) best in the (**a**) coronal plane and (**b**) horizontal plane; whereas in the (**c**) sagittal plane, the hematoma along the lateral border of the fibula is seen as an indirect sign

4.7.1 Acute Injuries

In acute injuries, the torn parts of the anterior syndesmotic ligament and the resulting instability of fibula can be seen, allowing to understand the injury and to determine appropriate treatment: partial rupture of the AITFL (Fig. 4.17), complete rupture of the AITFL without dislocation (Fig. 4.18), complete rupture of the AITFL with dislocation (Fig. 4.19), and complete rupture of the AITFL and avulsion of the PITFL (Fig. 4.20). Besides the injury to the lateral ankle, injuries to the deltoid ligament and resulting instability of the whole ankle mortise can also be assessed using arthroscopy.

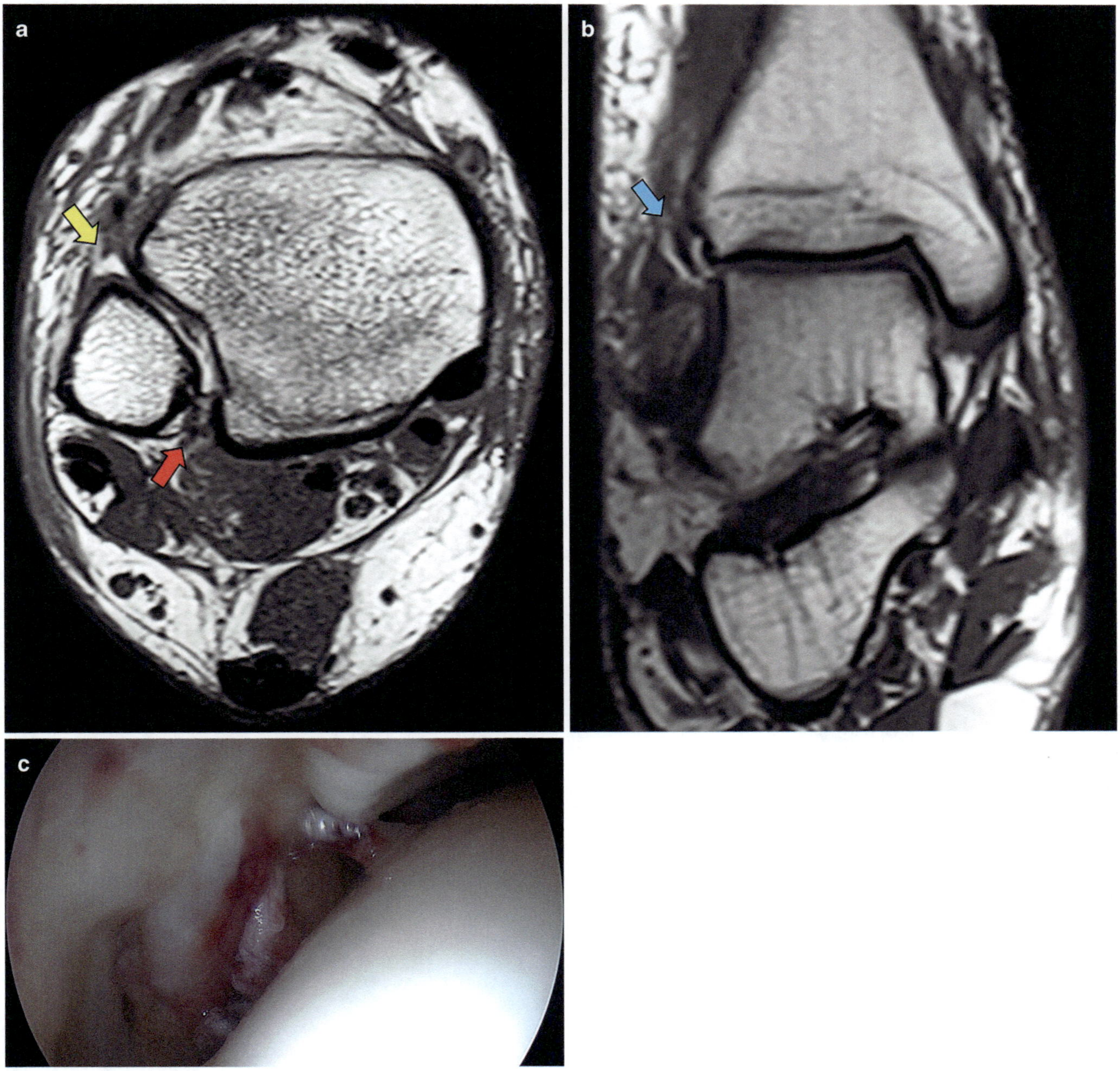

Fig. 4.17 This is a 45-year-old female tennis player who sustained an acute ankle sprain. (**a**) In the MRI, the AITFL is ruptured (yellow arrow), whereas the PITFL is seen to be avulsed with a slightly dislocated posterior malleolar (Volkman) fragment (red arrow). (**b**) The coronal view shows the ruptured AITFL (blue arrow). (**c**) Under arthroscopic visualization, the continuity of the AITFL seems to be intact despite the main part of the ligament being ruptured. Manual testing by external rotation of the foot evidenced the instability of the fibula. This was also seen when a 3-mm probe was inserted in tibiofibular space and twisted (not shown). Percutaneous fixation with a suture button was performed to stabilize the syndesmosis. The outcome was uneventful

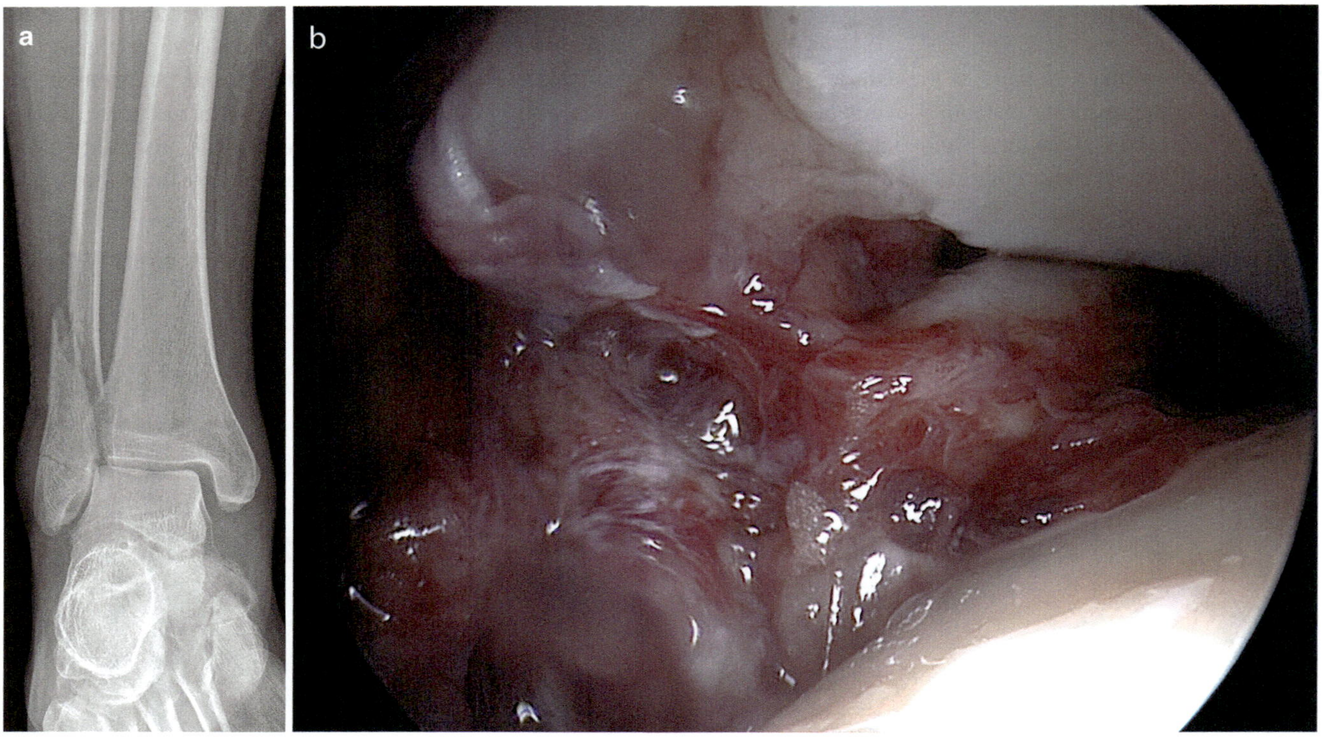

Fig. 4.18 Complete rupture of the AITFL in a 26-year-old male gardener who sustained a complex supination-external rotation trauma. (**a**) The AP plain radiograph shows a Weber Type C-fracture in combination with a minimally dislocated horizontal fracture at the height of the tibiotalar joint associated with a deltoid ligament injury resulting in a lateral shift of the talus within the mortise. (**b**) Arthroscopy shows the extended injury to the anterolateral capsular and the AITFL, of which some fibers are interposed in the talofibular joint. The fibula is minimally displaced in the incisura. The fibula fractures were reduced and fixed by a plate and the deltoid ligament was repaired. After this, the syndesmosis was found to be stable as tested by the lateral hook test

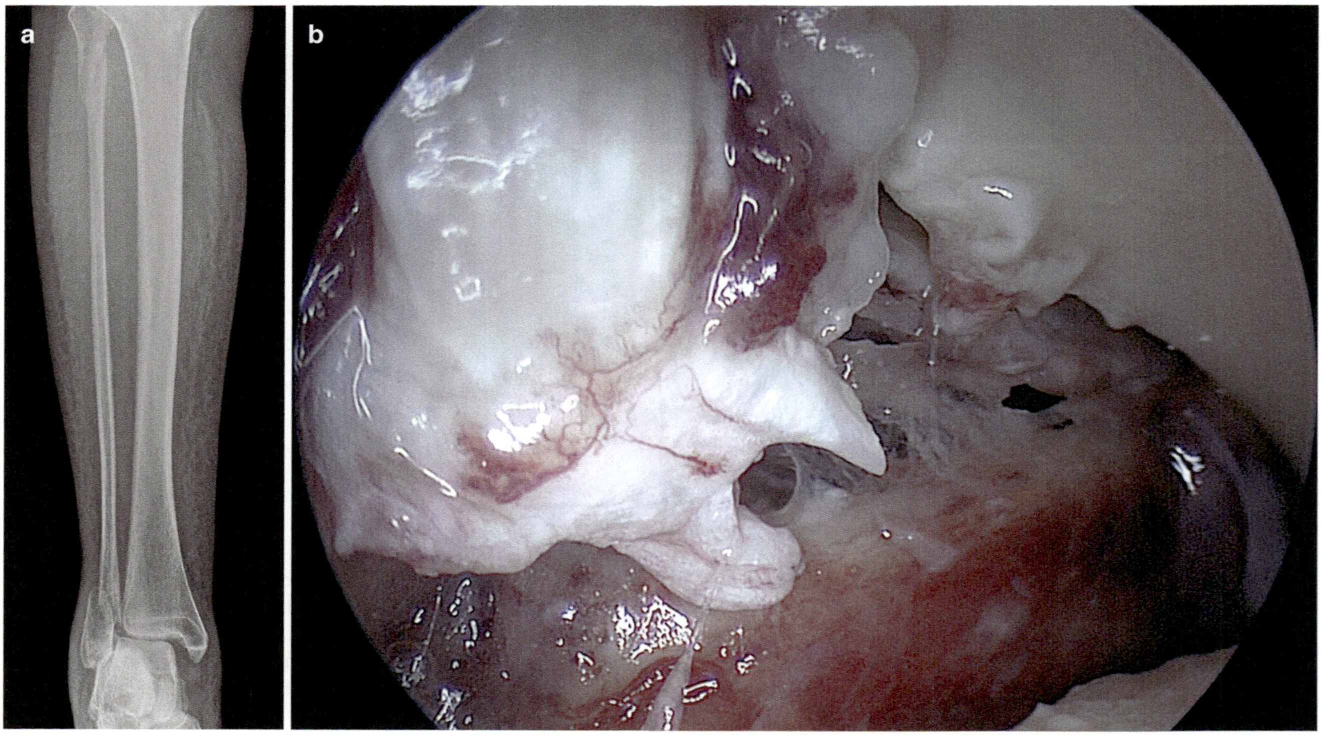

Fig. 4.19 This 61-year-old very sportive female patient sustained a complex injury of her right ankle after slipping on ice. (**a**) The AP plain radiograph shows a 2-level fracture of the fibula with a widened medial clear space, suggesting a complete rupture of the deltoid ligament. (**b**) Arthroscopy evidences a complete rupture of the distal AITFL, seen by the presence of a proximal stump. Furthermore, interposed soft tissue in the talofibular joint and the distal fracture of the fibula can be seen. The treatment and evolution are shown in Fig. 4.26

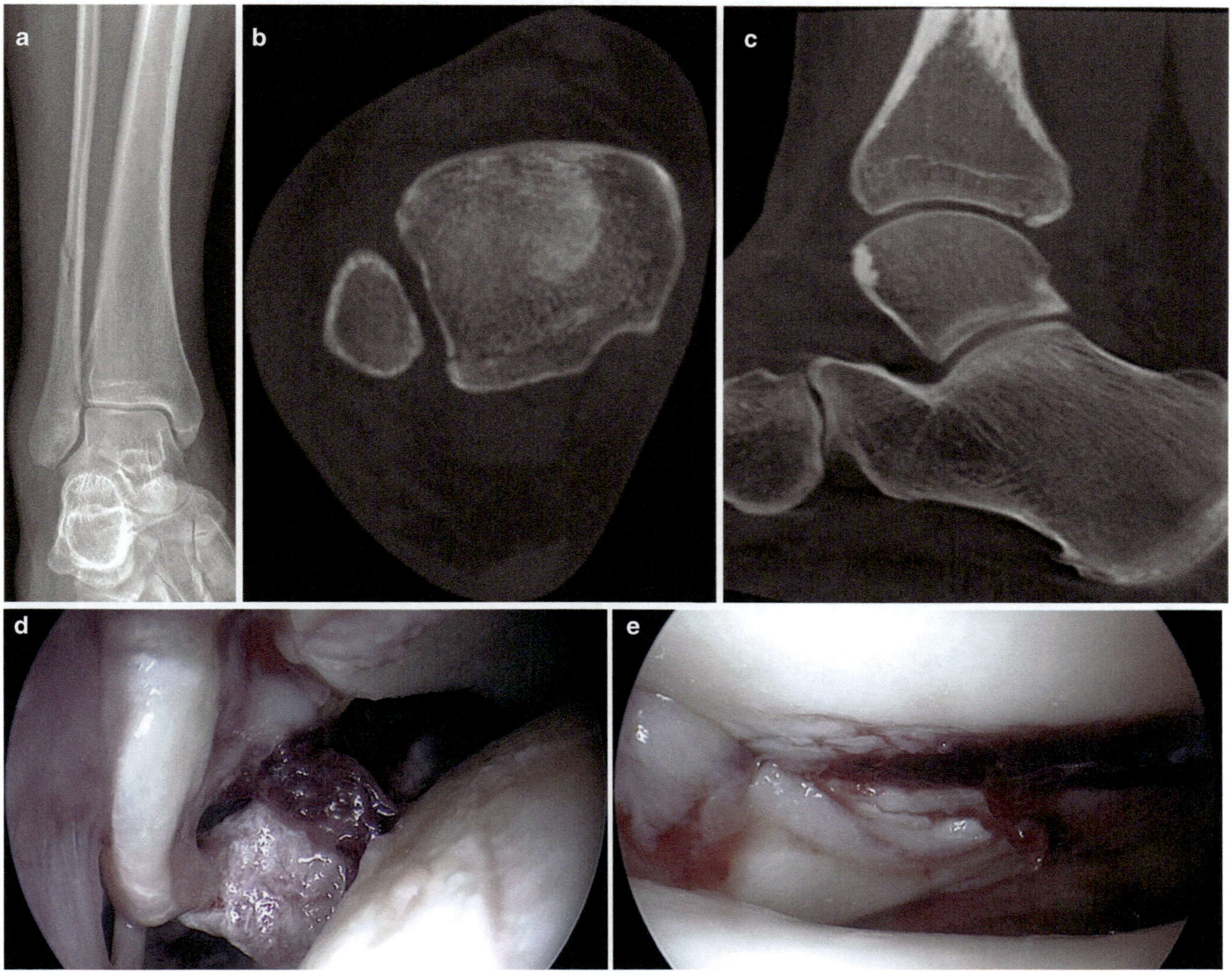

Fig. 4.20 This 59-year-old female patient sustained a pronation-external rotation trauma to her right ankle during a competition in orienteering. (**a**) The AP plain radiograph shows a minimally displaced Type Weber C-fracture without dislocation of the distal fibula. (**b**) The non-weight-bearing CT scan in the horizontal plane evidences a well-positioned fibula in the incisura and a non-dislocated avulsion fragment of posterior malleolus (Volkman). (**c**) The sagittal view confirms the Volkman fragment not being dislocated. (**d**) Arthroscopy, in contrast, evidences a complete distal rupture of the AITFL with the remaining stump with some gapping and posterior dislocation of the fibula. (**e**) The strong PITFL is intact, but there is a bony avulsion with minimal dislocation (Volkman fragment). In addition, a complete rupture of the superficial deltoid ligament was found (not shown). After plate fixation of the fibular fracture, the deltoid ligament was repaired. As the external rotation test still showed the same amount of widening of the tibiofibular clear space (TFCS), and the lateral hook test remained positive, a suture button was used to stabilize the syndesmosis. With this, the patient resumed the former level of sports and remained pain free

4.7.2 Chronic Injuries

In chronic injuries, arthroscopy permits to assess the position of fibula in the incisura and the stability of the ankle joint provided by the syndesmotic ligaments (Fig. 4.21). The incompetence of the syndesmotic ligaments is often detected when manually testing under arthroscopic visualization (Fig. 4.22). Such dynamic maneuvers during ankle arthroscopy may help to assess the stability of the syndesmosis in the coronal, sagittal, and transversal planes. Furthermore, they can also help in syndesmosis reduction [52]. The syndesmotic integrity can be assessed by inserting a 3-mm probe into the distal tibiofibular joint and turning it gently around its long axis in the syndesmosis [11, 78].

Sequential dissection of the ligaments has shown that the AITFL, IOL, and PITFL are needed to be injured to produce coronal plane syndesmotic instability [79]. Arthroscopic assessment of such instability should occur along the posterior margin of the incisura (Fig. 4.23). If instability exists posteriorly, similar findings found anteriorly suggest a concomitant deltoid injury [79].

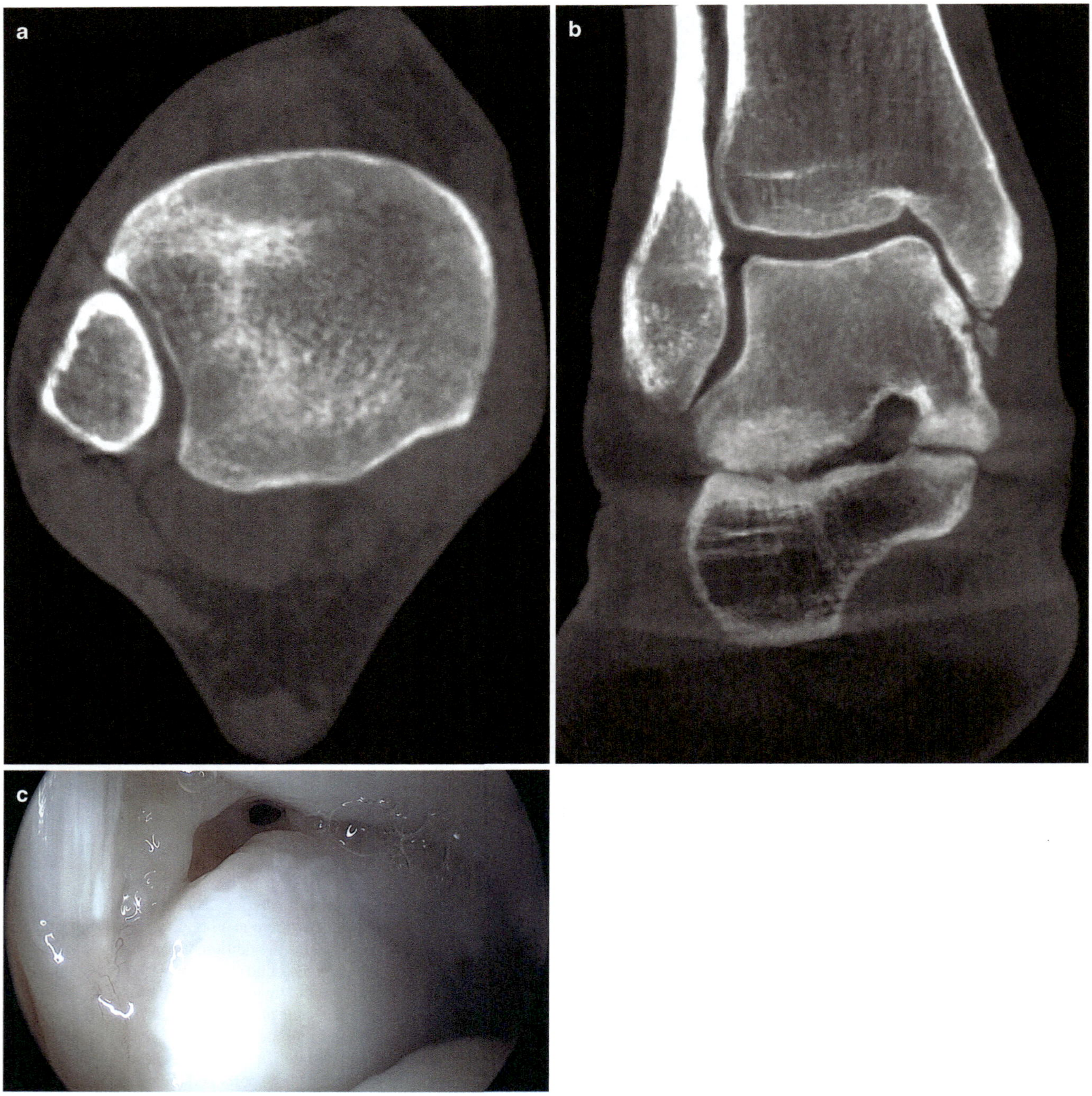

Fig. 4.21 This 47-year-old former female soccer player experienced progressive pain at the lateral ankle. She mentioned having sustained a mid-shaft fracture of the fibula after a direct trauma 8 years earlier that had been treated conservatively. (**a**) Weight-bearing CT scan shows the fibula slightly internally rotated and translated anteriorly in the incisura. (**b**) A distinct overlength of the fibula is seen in the coronal plane as is a slight varus talar tilt. (**c**) Arthroscopic assessment evidences significant lateral instability of the ankle with a rather thin AITFL that seems to be incompetent in its distal part. The fibula is translated slightly anterior and synovial tissue is seen in the lateral clear space until the posterior aspect of the incisura (asterisk). A substantial incompetence of the superficial deltoid ligament was also found (not shown). A correcting osteotomy of the fibula was performed, the ATFL and the CFL were reconstructed with the aid of a free plantaris tendon graft (see Fig. 4.29), and the deltoid ligament was reconstructed. With this, the patient resumed the former level of sports and remained pain free

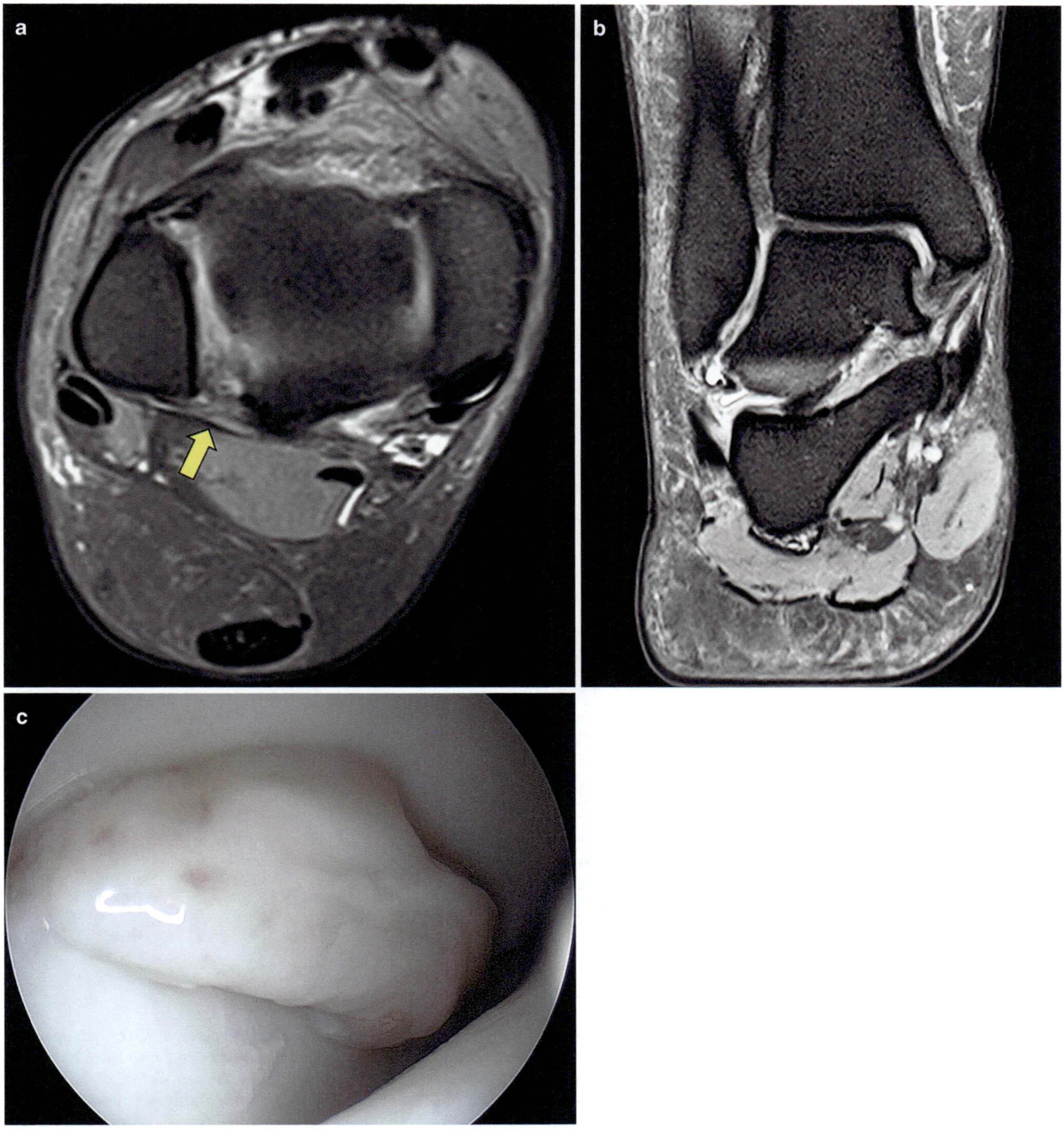

Fig. 4.22 This 25-year-old female nurse suffered from lateral ankle instability after a severe sprain on the stairs. After open revision of the peroneal tendons and repair of the ATFL 6 months earlier, she showed up with persistent lateral ankle pain and a feeling of instability that did not allow her to resume her professional activity. Clinical investigation revealed pain over the AITFL, a positive squeeze and external rotation stress tests. (**a**) MRI shows a partial lesion of the AITFL and widening of the lateral clear space especially in its posterior part (arrow). (**b**) In the coronal plane, a distinct widening of the lateral and medial clear space can be seen. Notice the substantial synovial tissue between the distal fibula and tibia. (**c**) Arthroscopic assessment evidences hypertrophic synovial tissue that plops into the joint when manually compressing the fibula against the tibia (squeeze test), while the tissue mass disappears when compression is removed; with this maneuver, the significant coronal plane instability of the syndesmosis can be verified. The ATFL and AITFL were reconstructed with the aid of a free plantaris tendon graft. The fixation of the graft to the anterior tubercle of tibia was done by a screw with a washer (see Fig. 4.29b)

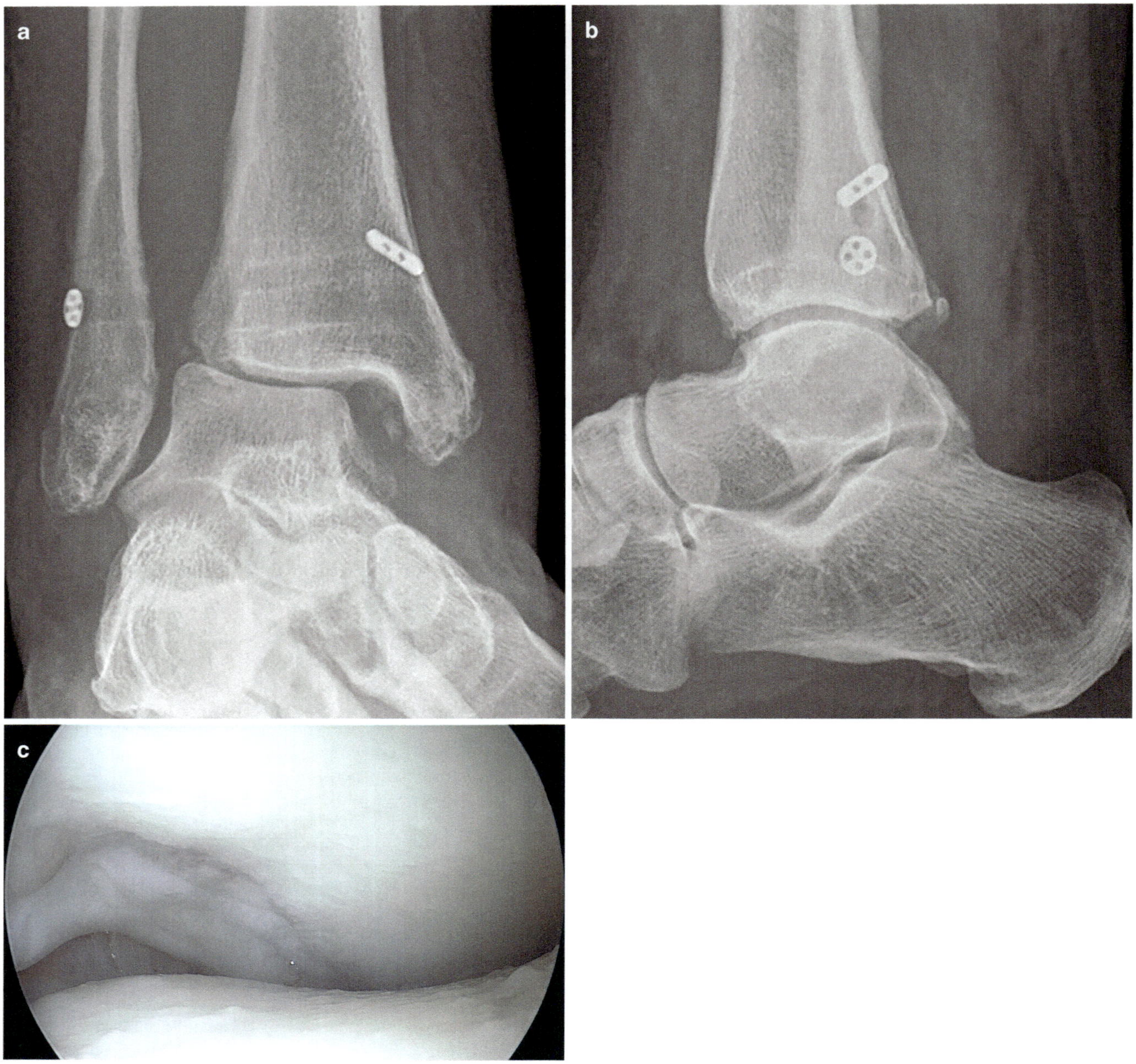

Fig. 4.23 This 48-year-old female farmer sustained a Maisonneuve type fracture 9 months earlier that was first treated by closed reduction of the distal fibula and fixation by two tricortical screws. When the screws were removed after 10 weeks, the syndesmosis was found to be unstable; therefore, a percutaneous fixation with a suture button was performed. Standard weight-bearing radiographs show the incompetent syndesmosis with significant gapping and a substantial widened medial clear space in the (**a**) AP view and (**b**) lateral view. (**c**) Intraoperative arthroscopy visualizes the scarred soft tissue in the widened lateral tibiofibular clear space. It also covers the articular surface of the fibula as a result of soft tissue interposition. Analogously, soft tissue interposition was found in the medial clear space (not shown). Treatment and evolution are shown in Fig. 4.30

Arthroscopic evaluation is furthermore helpful to detect syndesmotic ligament hypertrophy with resulting anterolateral impingement (Fig. 4.24) [80].

While using stress radiography could not distinguish between intact and single-ligament disruption and was unreliable in distinguishing between sequential transection models, arthroscopy significantly predicted isolated disruption of the AITFL or the deltoid ligaments [81]. Also, probing arthroscopically, allowed for differentiation between most patterns of ligament injuries, including sequential transections.

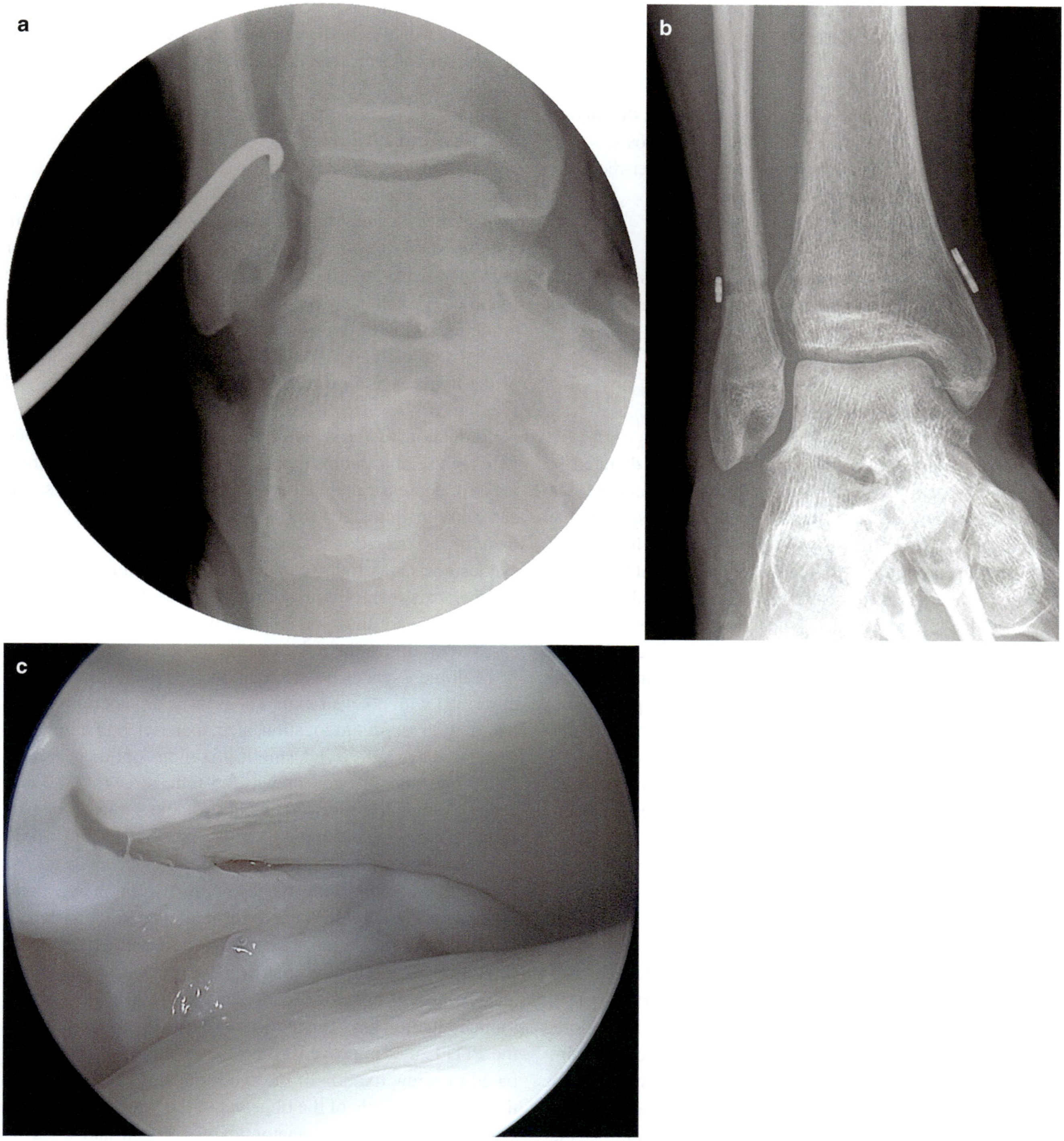

Fig. 4.24 This 26-year-old male soccer player sustained a high ankle sprain 2.5 years earlier that was surgically treated. (**a**) Intraoperative lateral hook test confirmed the instability of the syndesmosis. (**b**) Therefore, repair of the lateral ankle ligaments and the AITFL were performed. A suture button was used to protect the repaired AITFL. (**c**) 2.5 years later, the patient complains about persistent pain and some instability feeling in his lateral ankle not allowing him to resume full sports activity. Arthroscopic assessment shows scarred soft tissues in the lateral tibiofibular clear space with scar formation of the anterolateral capsular explaining anterior soft tissue impingement pain. After arthroscopic debridement (not shown), the patient regained full sports activity

4.8 Conservative Treatment and Rehabilitation

- Treatment of acute syndesmotic injuries is dictated by the stability of the deltoid and syndesmosis.
- Isolated syndesmotic injuries require longer recovery periods than lateral ankle sprains.

While acute syndesmotic injuries may be successfully treated with conservative measures, chronic injuries require, in most instances, surgical treatment.

4.8.1 Conservative Treatment

The treatment of acute syndesmotic injuries is dictated by the stability of the deltoid and syndesmosis. Patients who have been diagnosed with isolated syndesmotic sprains may be treated nonoperatively with good results [46, 82–85]. Published rehabilitation protocols include variable periods of immobilization and non-weight-bearing based on injury severity [46, 83, 85]. Isolated syndesmotic injuries have been noted to require longer recovery periods than lateral ankle sprains, 62 versus 15 days for return to sport in one study [84]. Despite the variability among the study participants with respect to the severity of isolated syndesmotic sprains, good results have been reported in numerous studies [83, 86]. Nonetheless, nonoperative management of isolated stable syndesmotic sprains is feasible, showing good results when patients are selected appropriately.

4.8.2 Rehabilitation

The rehabilitation process is implemented in three phases: acute (I), subacute (II), and integration to sport (III) [87]. The protocols for each phase of rehabilitation are tailored individually to achieve the goals of joint protection, minimization of inflammatory response, and pain control for the acute phase; restoration of mobility, strength, and gait for the subacute phase; and increased strength, neuromuscular control, and sports-specific tasks for the last phase.

4.9 Surgical Management

- Successful outcome requires anatomic reduction of the syndesmosis.
- The first and most critical step of syndesmotic reduction is anatomic reduction of the fibula including restoration of length, alignment, and rotation.
- Various fixation methods are available.

Reconstruction is recommended when syndesmotic rupture is identified in both acute and chronic settings to prevent progression of arthritis and disability.

4.9.1 Acute Injuries

Operative stabilization of the tibiofibular syndesmosis is indicated when syndesmotic instability is confirmed either in acute unstable isolated syndesmotic injuries (Fig. 4.25) or intraoperatively after definitive fixation of concomitant ankle fractures (Fig. 4.26) [88]. Successful outcome requires anatomic reduction of the syndesmosis [64]. The first and most critical step of syndesmotic reduction is anatomic reduction of the fibula including restoration of length, alignment, and rotation.

Reduction of the syndesmosis is commonly performed with the use of a clamp (Fig. 4.27); however, numerous studies have demonstrated that positioning of the clamp or screw can cause malreduction [89, 90]. In a cadaveric model, placement of the reduction clamp in a neutral position across the syndesmosis was found to have fewer malreductions of the syndesmosis than oblique placement [91]. Direct visualization of the syndesmosis is important and is advocated for all cases to minimize the risk of malreduction.

Multiple syndesmotic fixation methods have been described with no clear expert consensus or superior combination with respect to location, size, material, and number of cortices engaged. Syndesmotic fixation options include using one screw, two screws, 3.5-mm screw(s), 4.5-mm screw(s), metallic screw(s), bioabsorbable screw(s) or performing supra-syndesmotic fixation, trans-syndesmotic fixation, or suture button fixation.

Ankle fractures with syndesmotic disruption are commonly associated with a posterior malleolar fracture where the PITFL is intact and attached to the fractured fragment (Fig. 4.28) [92]. There is controversy regarding management and fixation of posterior malleolar fractures; however, anatomic reduction has been shown to re-establish the tension of the PITFL and improved syndesmotic stability when compared to screw fixation of the syndesmosis [92]. Fracture of the Chaput tubercle of the tibia and of the Wagstaffe tubercle of the fibula should be anatomically reduced and fixed by screws with or without support of plates.

4.9.2 Chronic Injuries

If chronic instability to the distal tibiofibular syndesmosis is verified, various reconstruction options are available. While debridement may be enough in some patients [4, 93, 94], others need additional stabilization using a positioning screw, suture button [22, 93, 95, 96], or even a more complex reconstruction such as an osteotomy, medialization and proximalization of the tibial insertion of the AITFL [97–99],

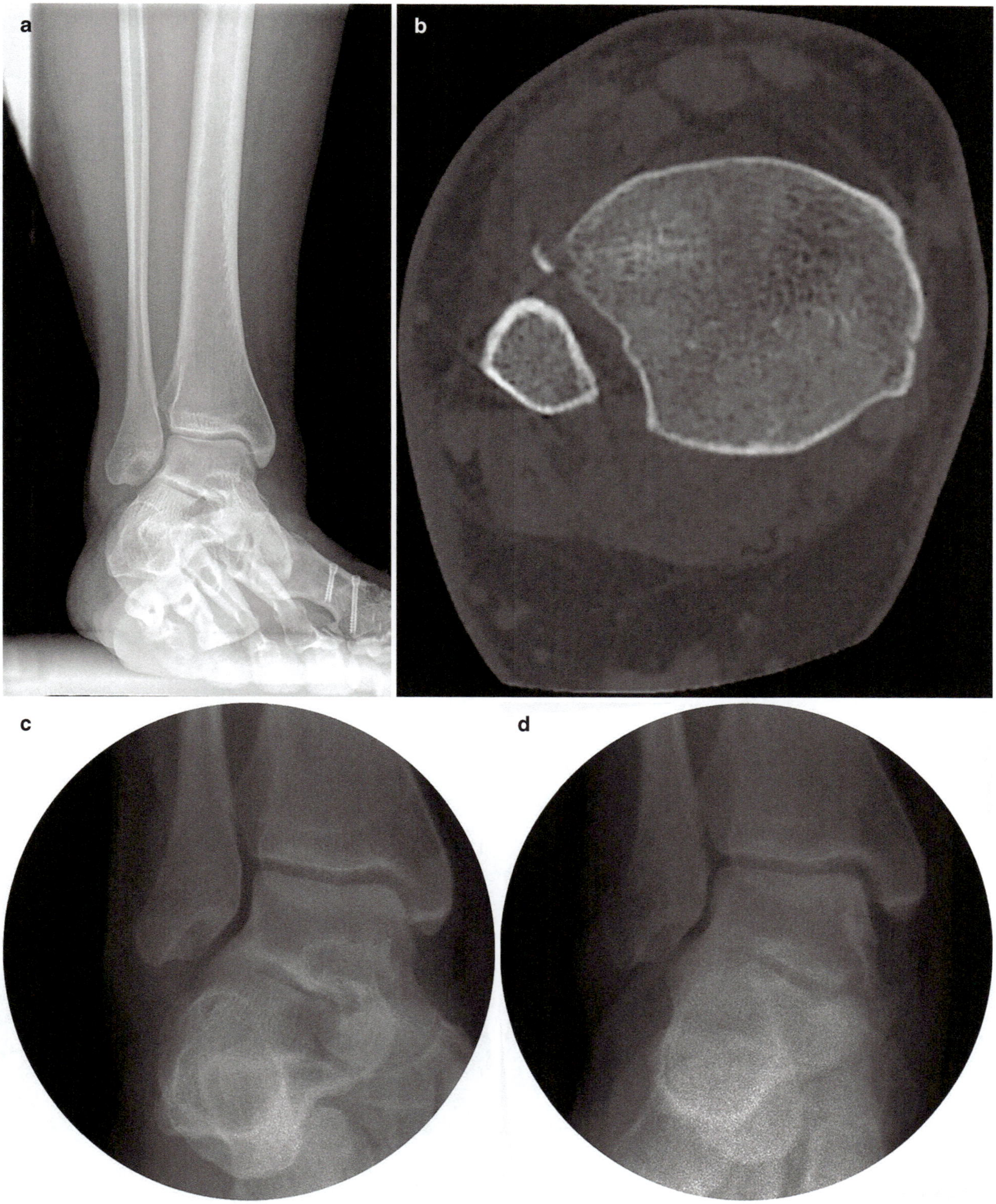

Fig. 4.25 *Surgical technique: Chronic lateral instability, partial rupture of the syndesmosis: ligament reconstruction and suture button.* This 28-year-old female high-level volleyball player was suffering from recurrent ankle sprains since a severe sprain 2 years earlier that was treated conservatively. Since then, she was doing sports only with wearing a protective ankle brace. Despite this, she sustained a further complex ankle sprain. Clinically, a hematoma and tenderness are found over the ATFL and AITFL. (**a**) The AP plain radiograph shows a congruent ankle mortise. (**b**) However, the CT scan evidences a bony avulsion of the AITFL at the tibial tubercle. As compared with intraoperative fluoroscopy without stress (**c**), external rotation stress shows distinct widening of the medial clear space and lateral tibiofibular clear space (**d**). (**e**) Arthroscopy confirms a partial tear of the AITFL, and it evidences a substantial instability of the fibula in the shallow incisura mainly in the sagittal plane. Beside this, a significant anterolateral rotational instability of the talus within the mortise is found. (**f**) Surgical exploration shows the incompetent ATFL and hematoma with partial rupture of the AITFL at the tibial tubercle. (**g**) The ATFL is reconstructed with the aid of a free plantaris tendon graft and the syndesmosis is stabilized with a suture button. (**h**) Fluoroscopic control of the suture button. (**i**) While applying external rotation stress, the syndesmosis is seen to be stable

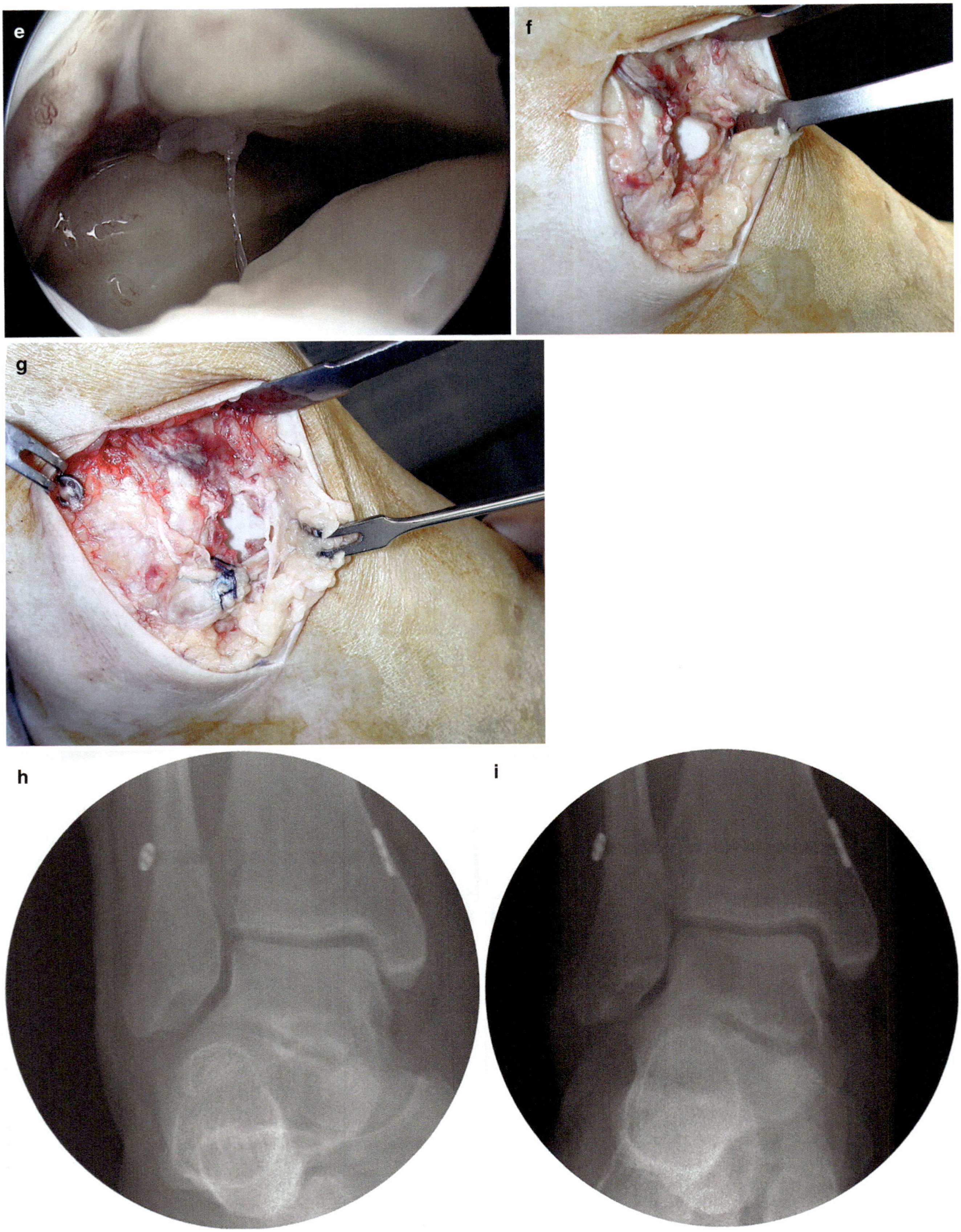

Fig. 4.25 (continued)

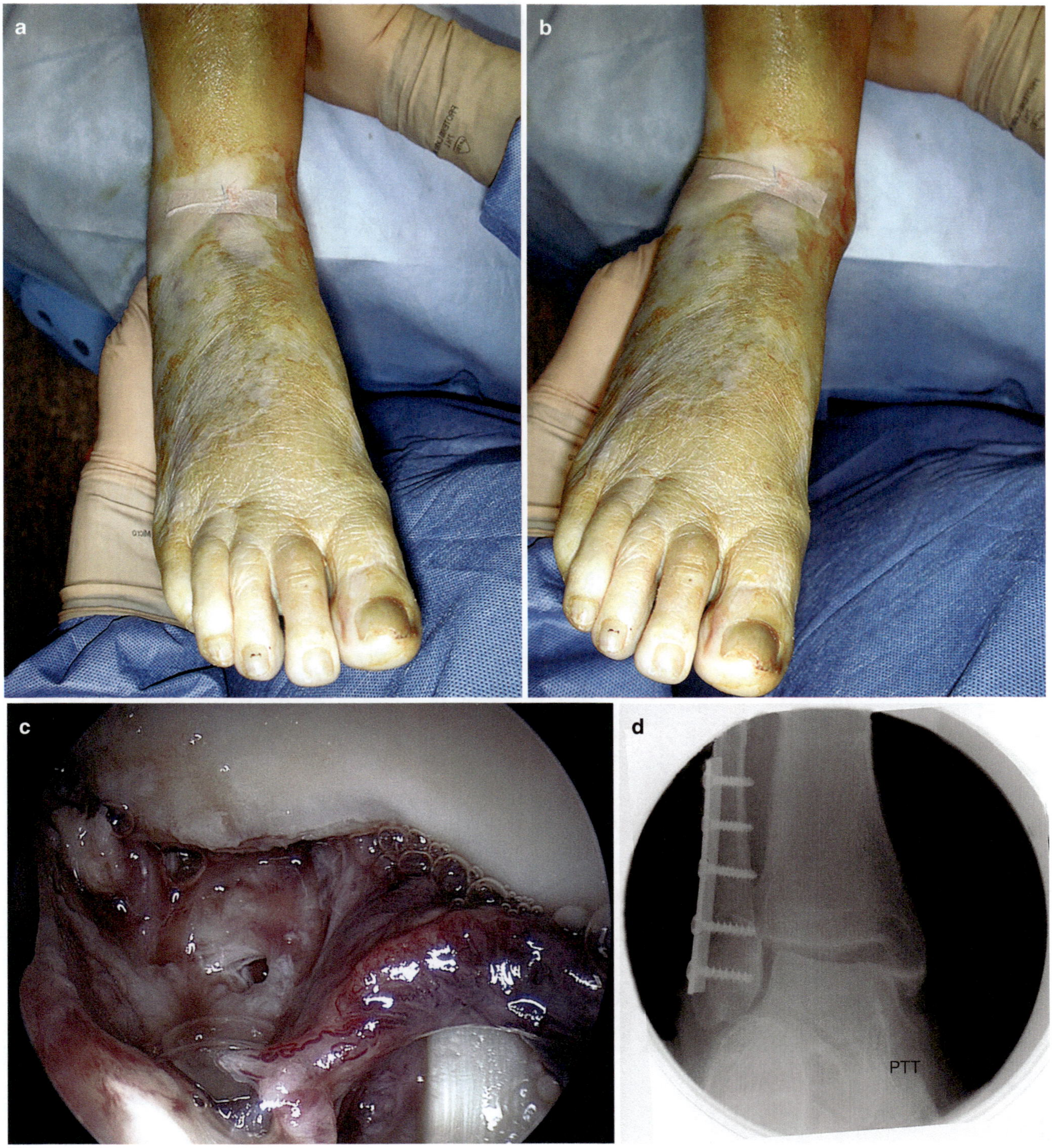

Fig. 4.26 *Surgical technique: Global instability after ankle fracture, deltoid ligament repair*. Sixty-one-year-old female patient after a complex injury to her right ankle (same patient as Fig. 4.27). (**a**) Supination and (**b**) pronation testing shows the complex lateral and medial instability. (**c**) Arthroscopy reveals a complete tear of the superficial deltoid also involving the deep portion substantially; thus, the posterior tibial tendon (PTT) is visible. (**d**) After plate fixation of the fibula, fluoroscopy shows persistent medial instability with a valgus tilt of the talus. (**e**) Surgical exploration of the medial ankle shows the extended rupture of the deltoid ligament. (**f**) First, the deep posterior deltoid is repaired. (**g**) Then, the anterior superficial deltoid ligament is repaired. (**h**) With this, the ankle has become stable, including the syndesmosis; thus, no further fixation of the syndesmosis is necessary. (**i**) Plain AP radiograph while weight-bearing after 5 years showing a stable ankle despite some valgus misalignment of the hindfoot. The patient is completely pain free and not limited in any activity

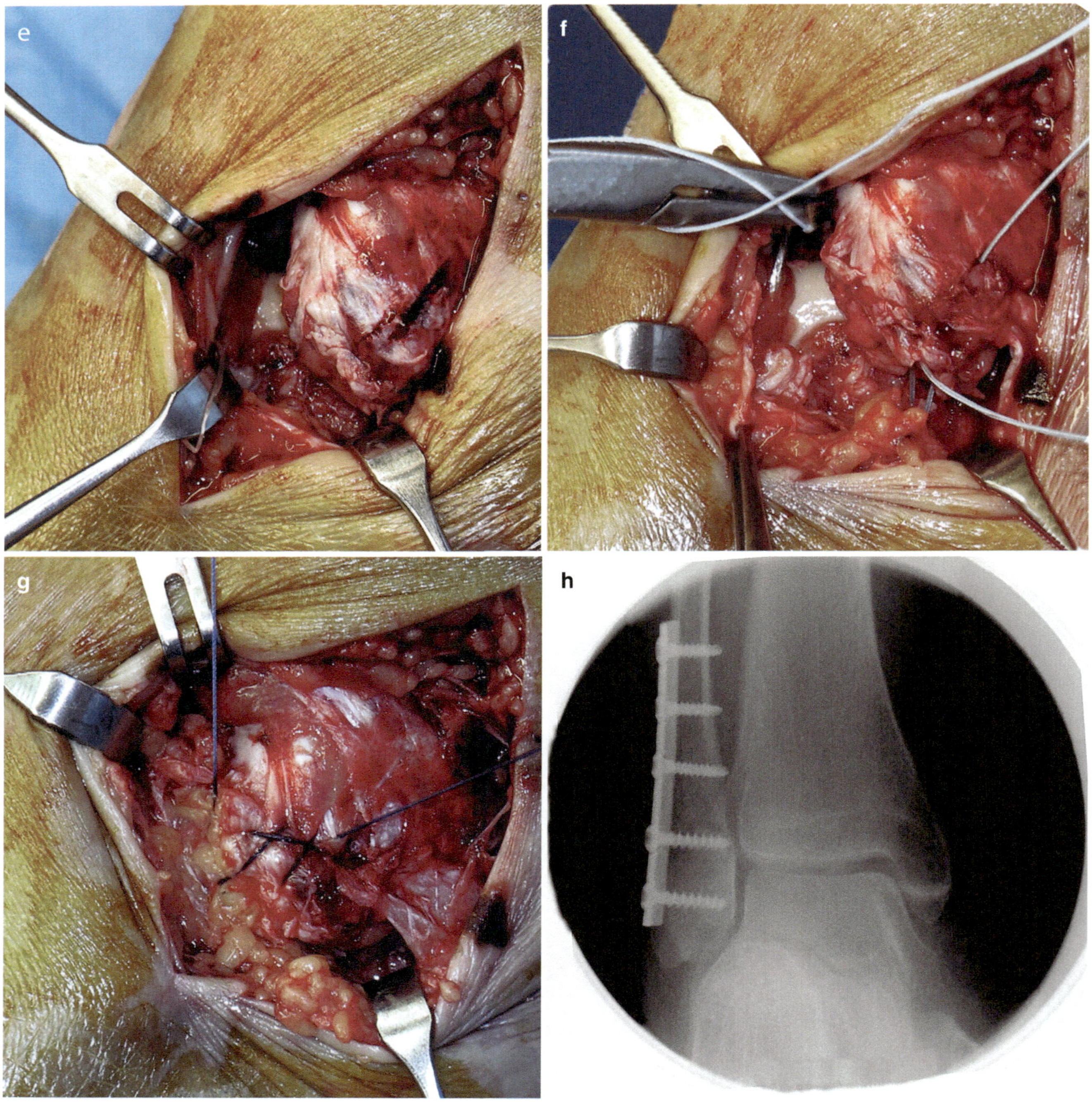

Fig. 4.26 (continued)

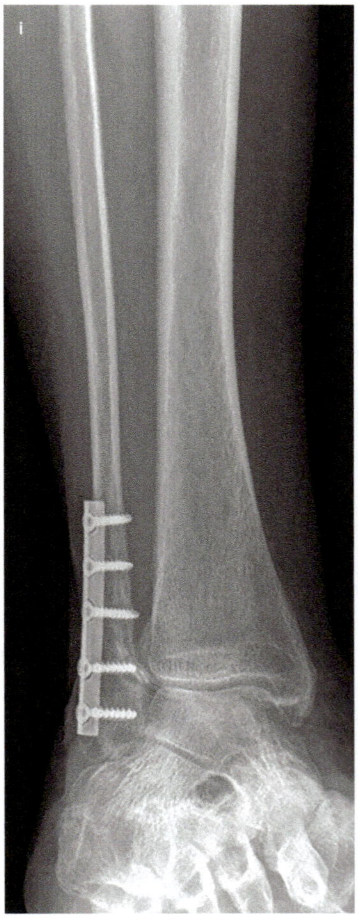

Fig. 4.26 (continued)

and/or a reconstruction of the AITFL with an autograft [4, 78]. Specific techniques for AITFL reconstruction were reported using the semitendinosus tendon [100], the gracilis tendon [101], the plantaris tendon [97], the split peroneus longus tendon [102], or hamstring tendon [103] (Fig. 4.29). In most instances, a positioning screw was recommended for temporary protection of the ligamentous reconstruction. In long-standing disorders, a tibiofibular fusion may be necessary (Fig. 4.30) [44, 104].

A correcting osteotomy of either the tibia or fibula, or of both is required in malunited ankle fractures, especially after a pronation-external rotation trauma, to balance the ankle joint (Fig. 4.31) [105]. With this, the scarred syndesmotic ligaments are tightened. Usually no additional stabilization of the syndesmosis is necessary to get a stable ankle mortise.

4.9.3 Postoperative Management

Postoperative care begins with immobilization of the ankle in a splint or boot, with no weight-bearing permitted for a period of 4–6 weeks. Range-of-motion exercises and resistance training should begin a few days after surgery, as tolerated by the patient. Progressive weight-bearing in a boot and strengthening exercises can subsequently be introduced after 4–6 weeks. Patients can return to competitive sports at 10–12 weeks, depending on injury severity.

4.10 Outcome

- Most reports focus on treatment of syndesmotic injuries associated with ankle fractures, showing overall satisfactory results after various treatment modalities.
- In posterior malleolar fractures where the posterior inferior tibiofibular ligament is usually intact, posterior malleolar fixation yields better stabilization of the syndesmosis, with restoration of 70% of normal syndesmotic stiffness compared with 40% after syndesmotic fixation alone.

Only a few reports are available on the outcome of surgically treated chronic syndesmotic injuries; most of them reported an increase of postoperative outcome scores [106–110]. More reports are available on the treatment of syndesmotic injuries associated with ankle fractures. These show overall satisfactory results after various treatment modalities [87]. A number of studies have found no major differences with regard to using 3.5- or 4.5-mm screws [111], tricortical and quadricortical screws [112, 113], trans-syndesmotic and supra-syndesmotic screws [114], stainless steel and titanium screws [112], or metal and bioabsorbable

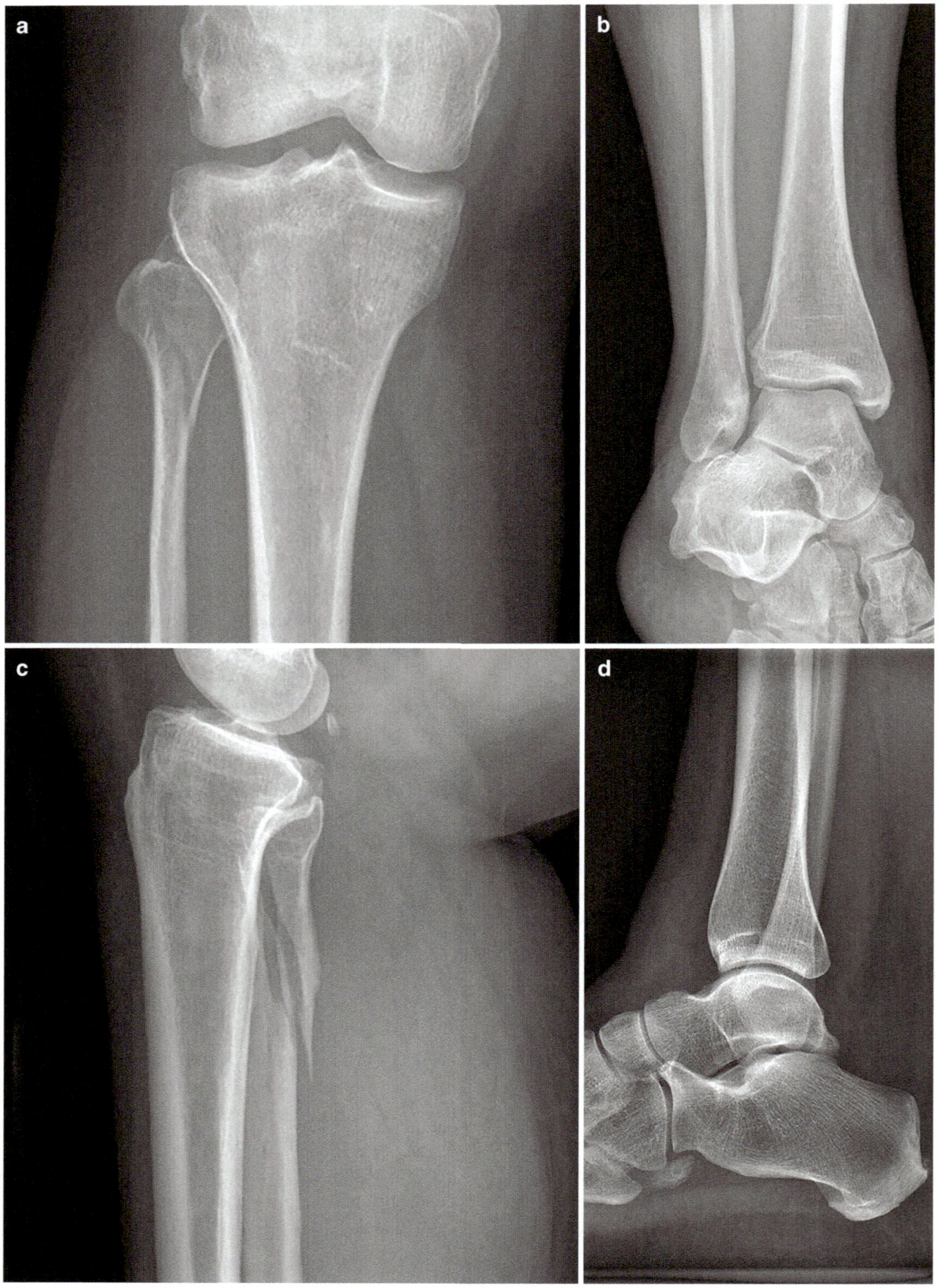

Fig. 4.27 *Surgical technique: Maisonneuve fracture, syndesmotic reconstruction with screws.* Thirty-one-year-old competitive mountain climber who sustained a complex external rotation trauma while wearing high-shaft shoes. (**a–d**) Plain non-weight-bearing radiographs showing a Maisonneuve type high tibial fracture with moderate gapping of the syndesmosis. (**e**) Arthroscopy shows the rupture of the AITFL. (**f**) The displaced fibula cannot be seen in the tibial incisura. The deltoid ligament shows a partial rupture (not shown). Intraoperative fluoroscopy (**g**) without and (**h**) with external rotation stress evidences moderate instability of the syndesmosis probably due to limited injury to the deltoid ligament. (**i**) The distal fibula is exposed and open reduction with the aid of a clamp is performed and (**j**) checked by fluoroscopy; thereafter, holes are drilled for the insertion of two 3.5-mm tricortical position screws. Notice the oblique anterolateral direction of the screw insertion that should account for approximately 30°. Fluoroscopic control shows correct position in the (**k**) coronal and (**l**) sagittal plane. (**m–o**) Screw position is postoperatively confirmed by CT scan. The position screws were removed after 8 weeks. (**p–r**) Weight-bearing CT scan 1 year after the surgery, showing persistent correct position of the fibula in all three planes. The patient is pain free and has resumed his former level of climbing sports

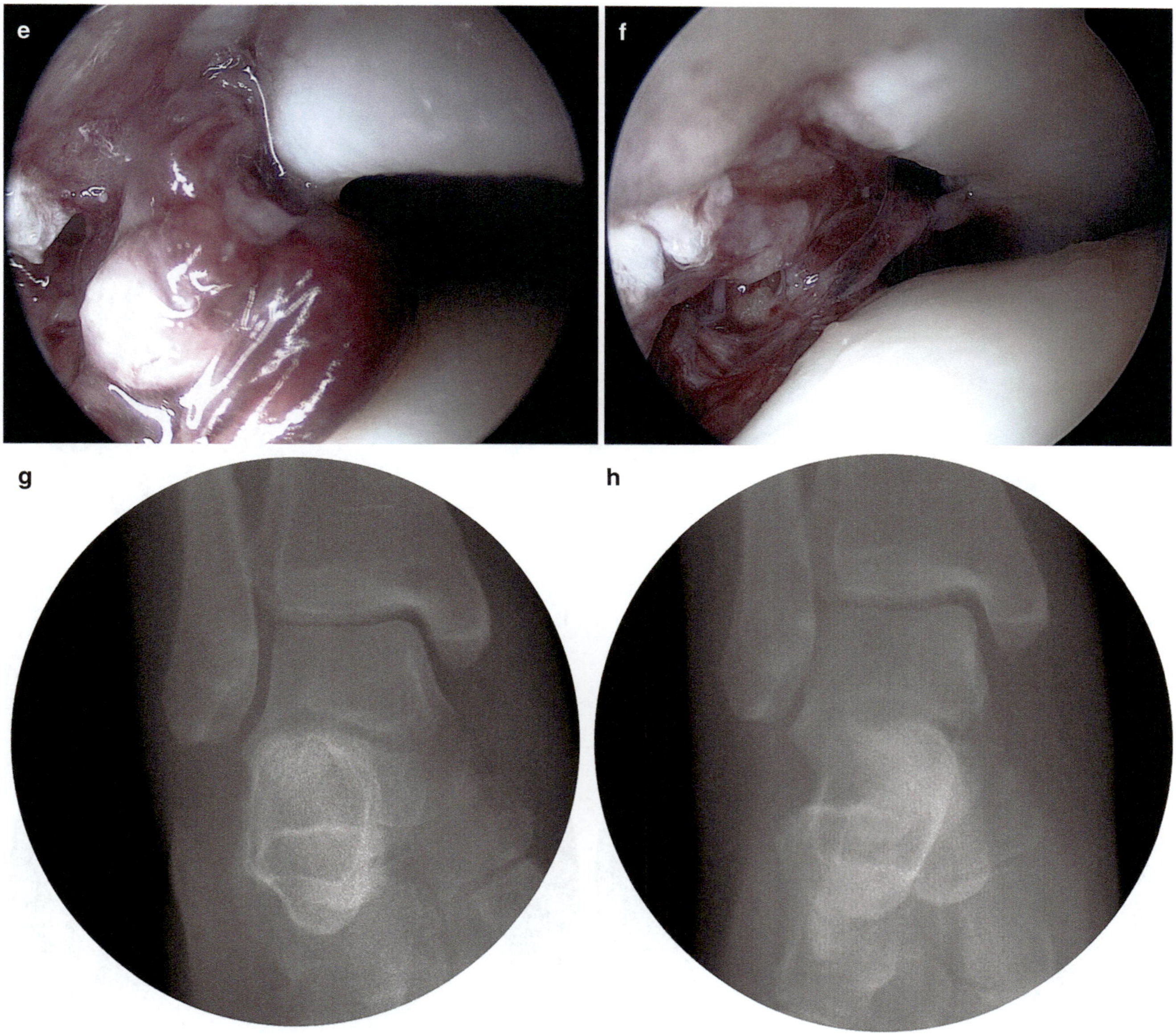

Fig. 4.27 (continued)

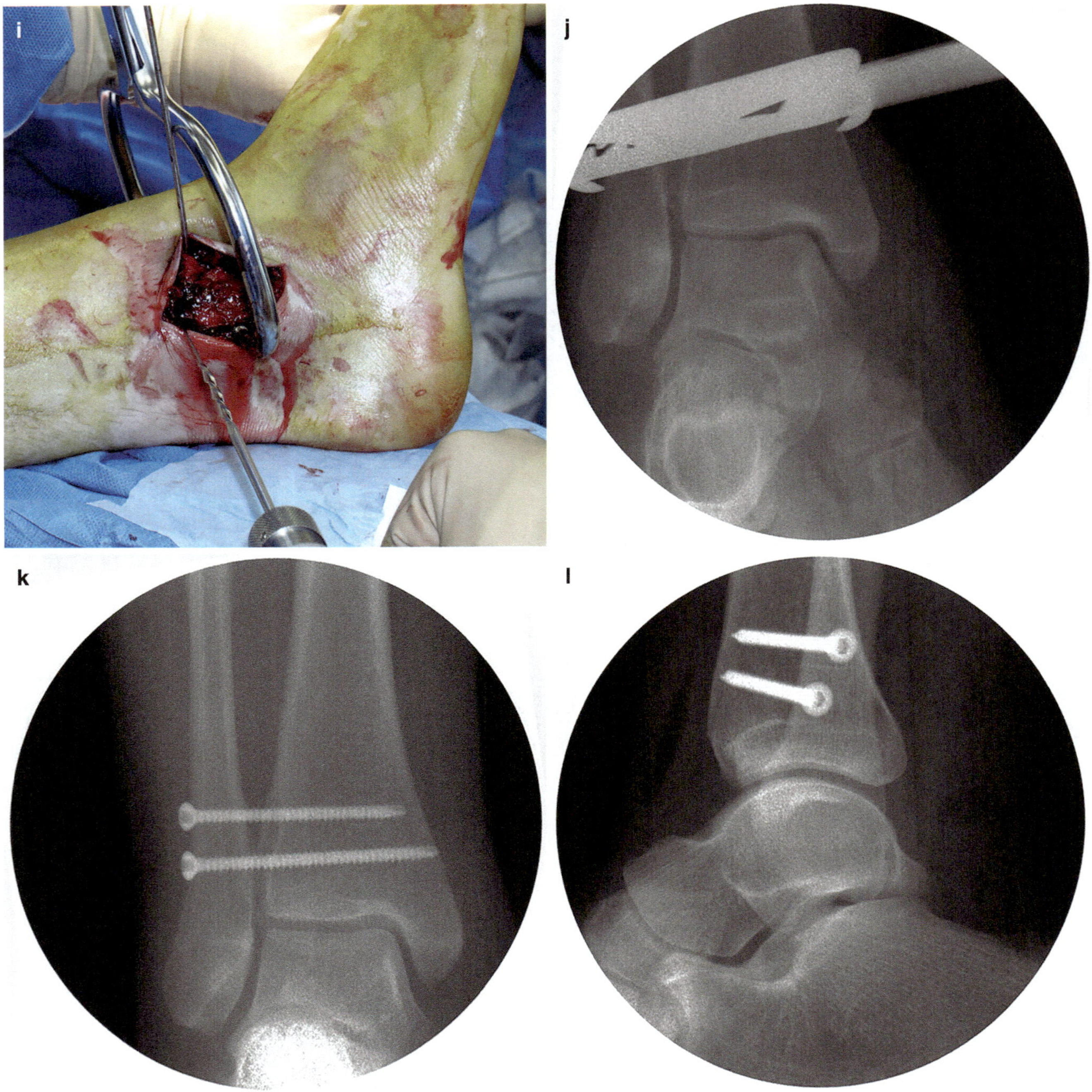

Fig. 4.27 (continued)

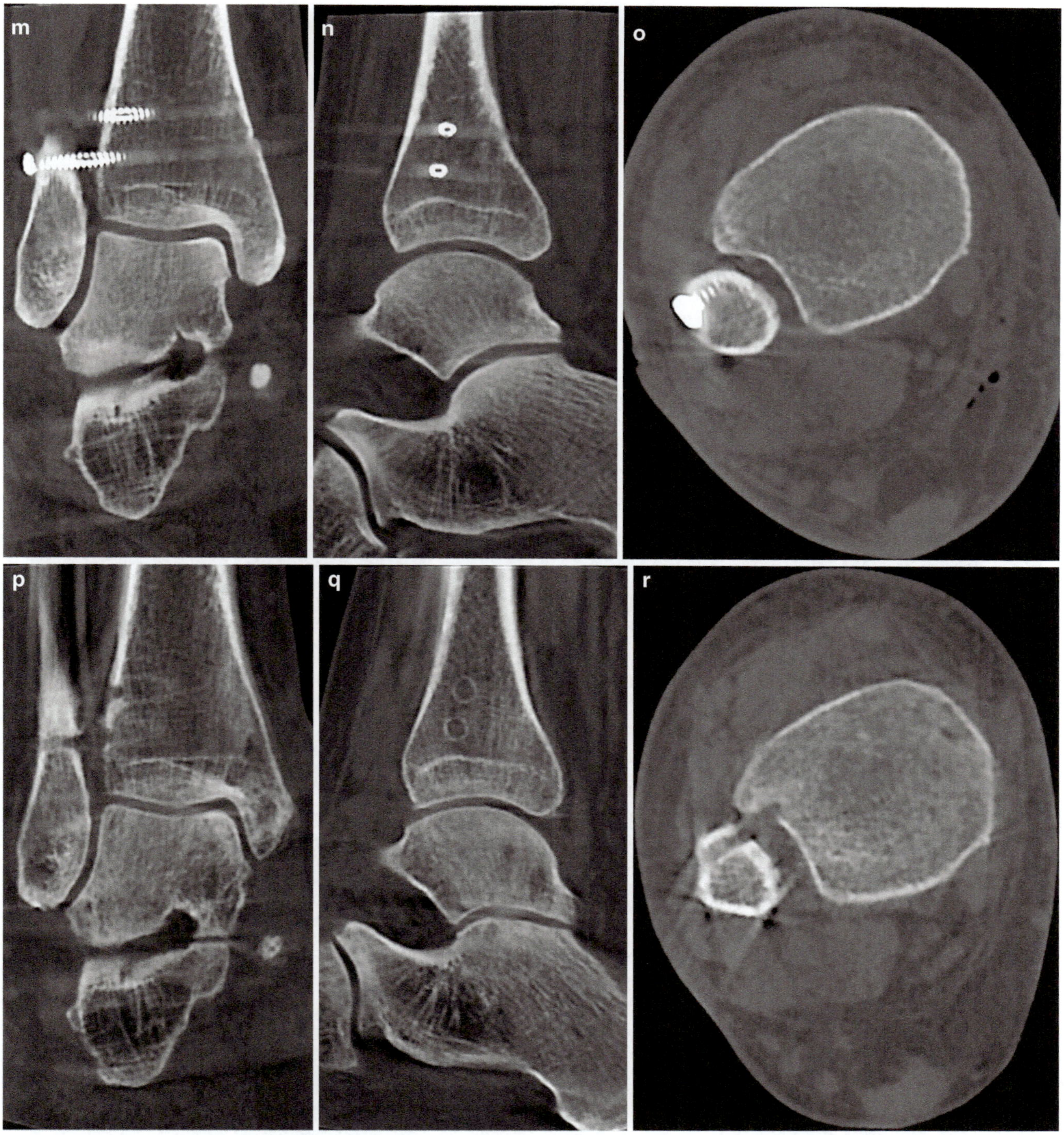

Fig. 4.27 (continued)

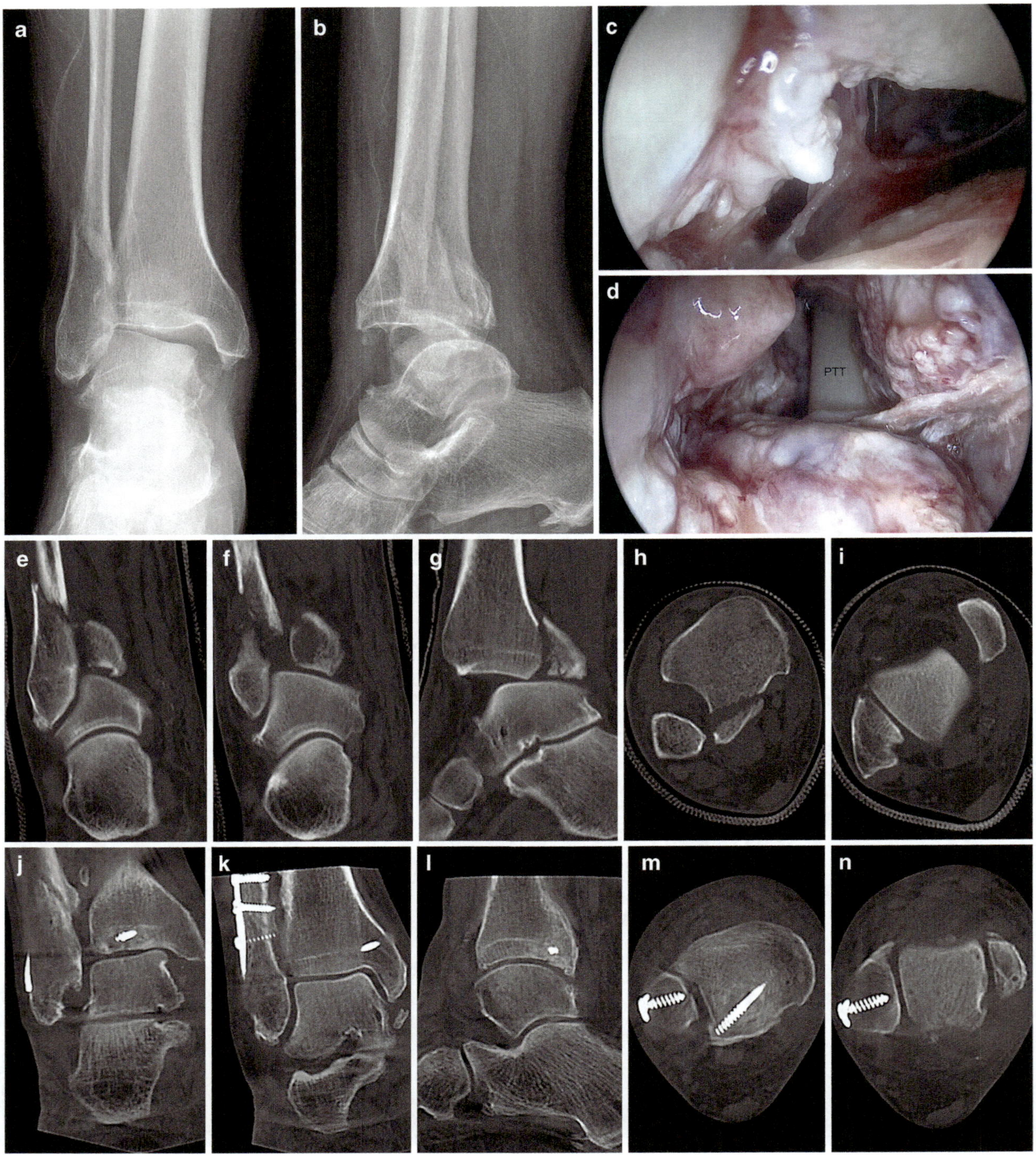

Fig. 4.28 *Surgical technique: Bony avulsion of the posterior syndesmosis (Volkman) and complete rupture of the deltoid: Reconstruction by fracture fixation and deltoid ligament repair.* Sixty-six-year-old Curling player who sustained a complex eversion-external rotation trauma while practicing competitive sports. (**a**) Plain AP radiograph shows a Weber Type C-fracture with lateral dislocation of the talus. (**b**) The lateral view evidences a fracture of the posterior malleolus (Volkman) with posterior dislocation of the talus. (**c**) Arthroscopy visualizes the ruptured AITFL and the empty incisura due to fibular dislocation. (**d**) On medial side, the deltoid ligament is seen completely torn, thus exposing the posterior tibial tendon (PTT). Preoperative CT scan: (**e**) The distal fibula is attached to posterolateral tibial fragment indicating an intact PITFL. (**f**) Whereas, the fibula is disconnected to anterior tibia indicating a torn AITFL. (**g**) The Volkman fragment is substantially dislocated. (**h**) In the coronal view, the regular connection between the fibula and Volkman fragment is confirmed. (**i**) Further distally, the talus is seen to follow the fibula, while the medial clear space is widely open subsequent to deltoid ligament rupture. Weight-bearing CT scans 6 months after internal fixation of the fibula and Volkman fragment as well as deltoid ligament reconstruction: (**j**) Coronal plane view showing a regular position of the posterior tibiofibular joint and Volkman fragment after fibula and posterior tibial fixation. (**k**) The anterior fibula is also anatomically reduced. (**l**) The posterior malleolar (Volkman) fragment is integrated in an anatomic position. (**m**, **n**) This is also seen in the horizontal view. Plain radiographs 1 year after surgery showing the restored and stable ankle in both the (**o**) coronal and (**p**) sagittal planes. The ankle congruity is restored with an anatomically positioned talus. Notice that no additional syndesmotic fixation was necessary after having fixed the Volkman fragment

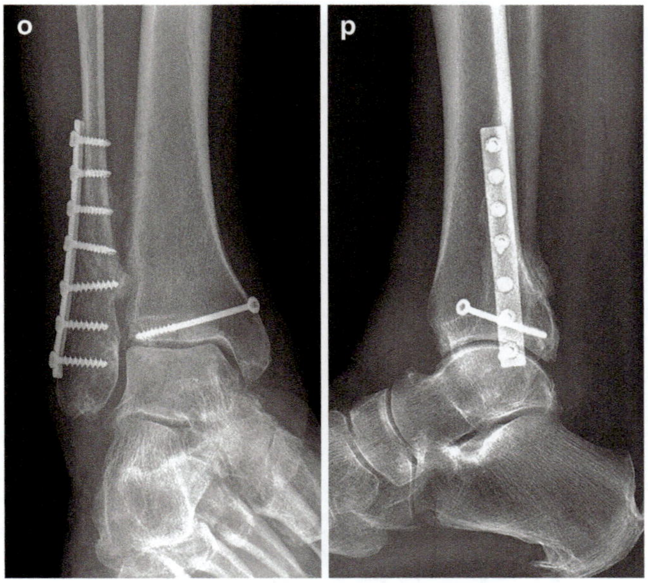

Fig. 4.28 (continued)

screws [115–120]. A slightly better functional outcome was reported with the use of suture buttons [121]. The malreduction rate in syndesmotic injuries treated with screws when compared to suture buttons was higher [122]. In posterior malleolar fractures where the posterior inferior tibiofibular ligament is usually intact, posterior malleolar fixation yielded better stabilization of the syndesmosis, with restoration of 70% of normal syndesmotic stiffness after posterior malleolar fixation compared with 40% after syndesmotic fixation alone [92]. Posterior malleolar fixation may also improve the accuracy of ankle fracture reduction, resulting in improved fibular reduction in terms of rotation, length, and translation.

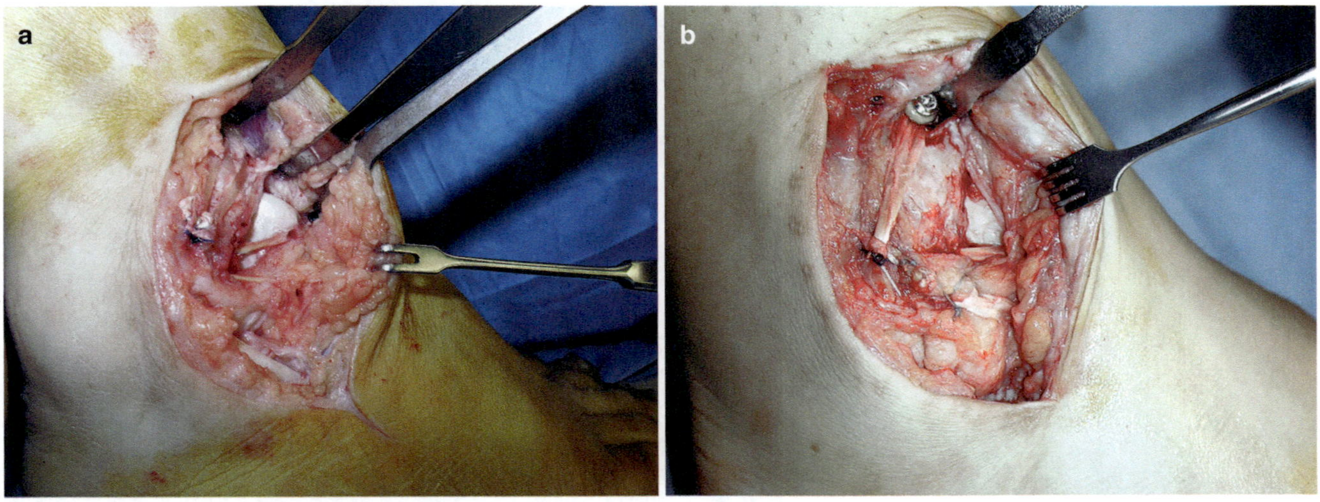

Fig. 4.29 *Surgical technique: Chronic unstable syndesmosis reconstructed with a free plantaris tendon graft.* (**a**) In this 47-year-old female patient (same patient as Fig. 4.21), the ATFL and the AITFL are reconstructed by a free plantaris tendon graft. First, the bony tunnels are made in the distal fibula and the talar neck (technique see Fig. 2.35); then, two tunnels are made in the anterior tubercle of tibia. This allows to reroute the plantaris tendon graft first from the distal fibula to the talar neck and back to the fibula, from there to the anterior tubercle and back again to the fibula. While the foot is held in a neutral foot position, the graft is tightened and then secured by some sutures. (**b**) In this 25-year-old female patient (same patient as Fig. 4.22), a screw with a washer is used to fix the plantaris tendon graft to the anterior tubercle of the tibia after having formed a loop

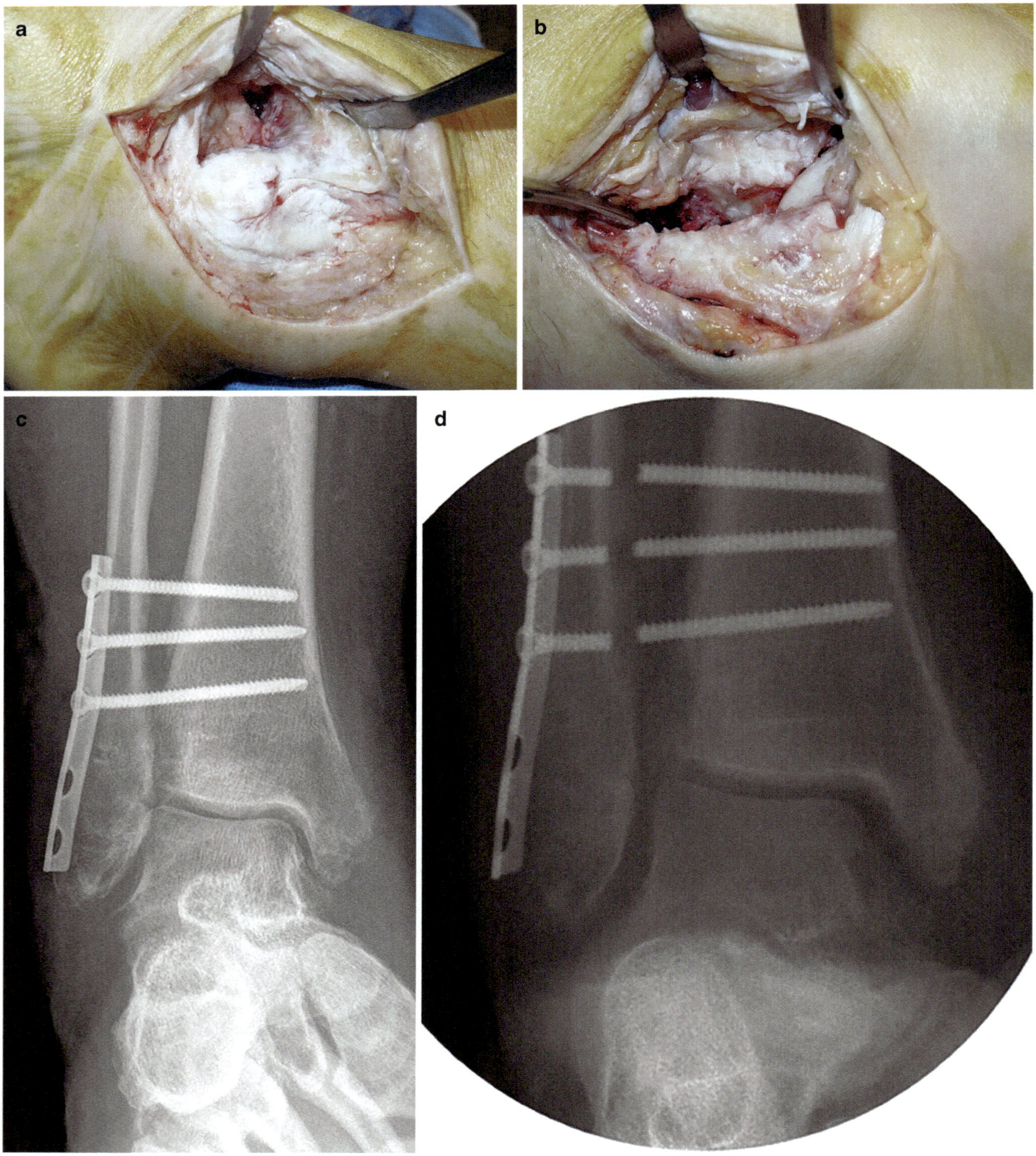

Fig. 4.30 *Surgical technique: Chronic unstable syndesmosis reconstructed with a tibiofibular fusion*. Forty-eight-year-old patient with a persistent incompetent syndesmosis after a Maisonneuve type fracture treated by a suture button (same patient as Fig. 4.23). (**a**) Surgical exposure of the medial ankle shows the incompetent deltoid ligament and the wide medial clear space which is first cleaned. (**b**) Surgical exposure of the lateral ankle shows the wide lateral tibiofibular clear space which is cleaned and then debrided to the subchondral bone. (**c**) After anatomic reduction of the fibula, three screws are used over a third tubular plate to get maximal compression to the interposed allograft. (**d**) After 16 weeks, the screws are broken as a result of a not fused and still unstable syndesmosis. (**e**) A revision fusion is performed with a more extended allograft and a longer plate with which the fusion is able to heal within 4 months

e

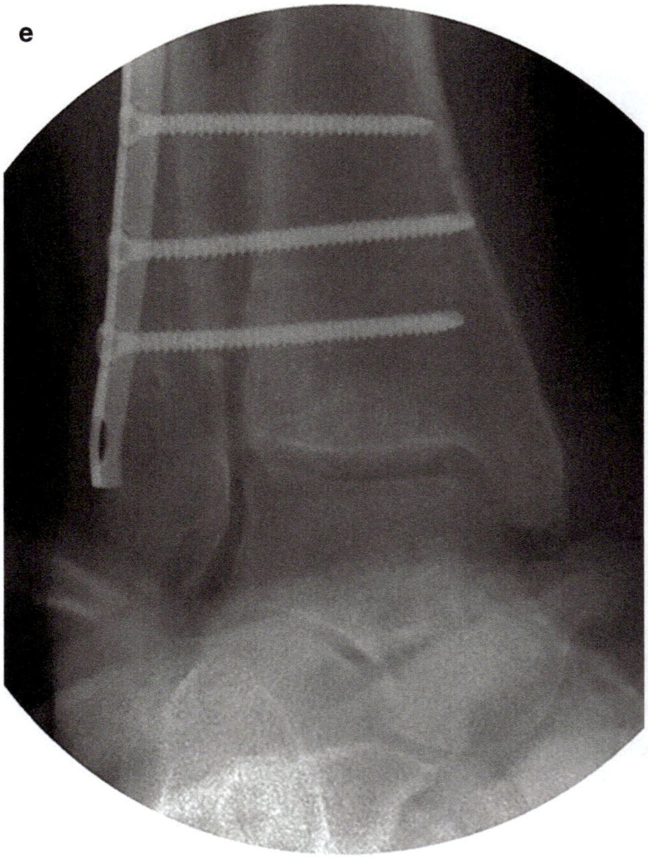

Fig. 4.30 (continued)

4.11 Complications

- Malreduction of syndesmosis is common and results in chronic pain and instability.
- Loss of the lateral buttress allows the talus to shift towards lateral with a subsequent increase of ankle peak load that might result in osteoarthritis.

Malreduction of the syndesmosis is common with reported rates of malreduction in approximately 25–50% of the cases [57, 123]. A malreduction of the syndesmosis of just 1.5 mm can portend poor clinical results [89, 124].

Hardware-related complications associated with suture button fixation are similar to those of screw fixation and include soft tissue irritation (2%), discomfort (2%), infection (2%), and no reported cases of breakage or loosening in the included studies [125]. Unique complications associated with suture button fixation include tendon entrapment from the medial button [126]. Additional but rare complications associated with suture button fixation but also present with screw fixation include distal tibia fracture (Fig. 4.32) [127, 128].

Fixation of the syndesmosis results in the loss of physiological motion at tibiofibular joint and resultant alteration in normal biomechanics [129]. The limitation in motion leads

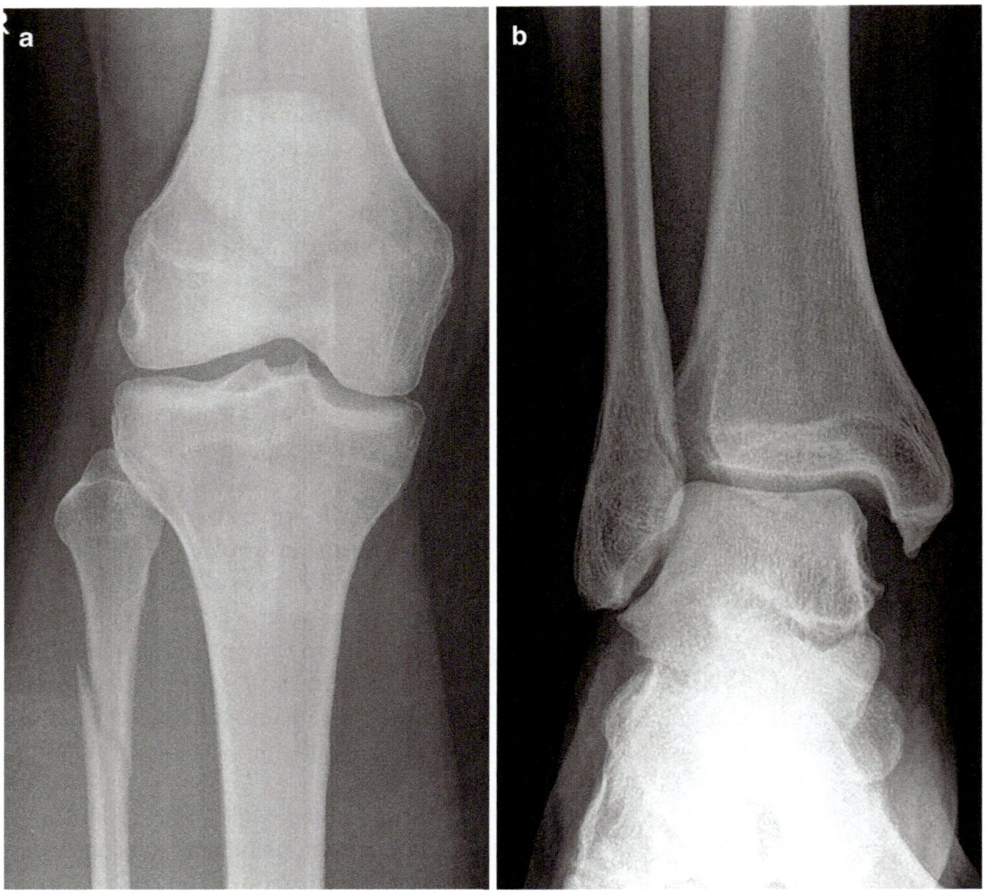

Fig. 4.31 *Surgical technique: Chronic unstable syndesmosis in a non-balanced ankle treated with distal tibial and fibular correcting osteotomies*. This 39-year-old competitive motorcycle driver sustained a Maisonneuve type fracture of his right ankle. (**a**, **b**) Plain AP radiographs show the high tibial fracture and the widened syndesmosis as well as medial clear space of the ankle, with lateralization of talus that follows the fibula. (**c**, **d**) In the lateral views, the spiral fracture of proximal fibula is seen and a tiny bony avulsion at the posterior tibia as well. In the emergency setting, the fracture was reduced with a clamp and two percutaneously inserted position screws. (**e**) The AP view under fluoroscopy shows a well-reduced ankle with one screw at the proximal end of the incisura, and a second screw more proximal. (**f**) The position of fibula looks correct in the sagittal plane as well. Notice the tricortical screw fixation with rather short screws, thus providing minimal resistance against rotational forces of the fibula. Furthermore, there exists a screw hole below the upper screw, indicating that the surgeon failed first. No treatment was done for the deltoid ligament. (**g**) Postoperatively the fibula looks a bit externally rotated with a slightly widened lateral tibiofibular clear space. (**h**) In the lateral view, the ankle looks well reduced. The screws were removed after 10 weeks. (**i**) Three months later, the patient showed up with chronic pain over his distal fibula and in the sinus tarsi. Furthermore, he was experiencing a feeling of ankle instability when walking. In the AP view, a callus is seen in the area of the upper screw hole as a result of a fatigue fracture associated with a widening of the lateral tibiofibular clear space. The lateral tibiotalar joint space has become distinctly narrower, however with the talus showing a regular medial clear space. (**j**) On the lateral view, a talocalcaneal overlap of >50% (yellow arrow) and a sinus tarsi impingement (red arrow) as a result of a valgus malalignment of the heel is seen. This can also be seen on the hindfoot alignment view (**k**). Therefore, correcting osteotomies are indicated to balance the ankle and unload the syndesmosis. (**l**) After exposure of the distal tibia through a short medial approach, the closing wedge osteotomy is marked by two K-wires to guide the saw plate. Two incomplete cuts are performed to preserve the lateral cortex. (**m**) Then a wedge is removed, and the osteotomy is closed over a plate fixed first to the distal fragment and then to the proximal tibia, thereby the talus is seen to follow the medial malleolus. While the medial clear space is closed, the talofibular joint is open and the fibula is too short. Therefore, an oblique fibular osteotomy is performed. (**n**) The fibula is lengthened until the appropriate position is achieved, and then fixed by a plate. The ankle is now well balanced with high congruency of all compartments and a well-repositioned fibula with a regular lateral tibiofibular clear space, and it is also well balanced in the sagittal plane (**o**). The syndesmosis is stable as tested by the lateral hook test (not shown). Apparently, the scarred syndesmosis was tightened by the lengthening of the distal fibula, stabilizing it. (**p**–**r**) One year postoperatively, plain radiographs under weight-bearing show a well-balanced ankle. The implants were removed 2 months later. (**s**–**u**) 10 years after surgery, the patient is pain free without any limitations in his daily life and activities. The plane radiographs evidence some degenerative changes, but with preserved joint congruity and articular space

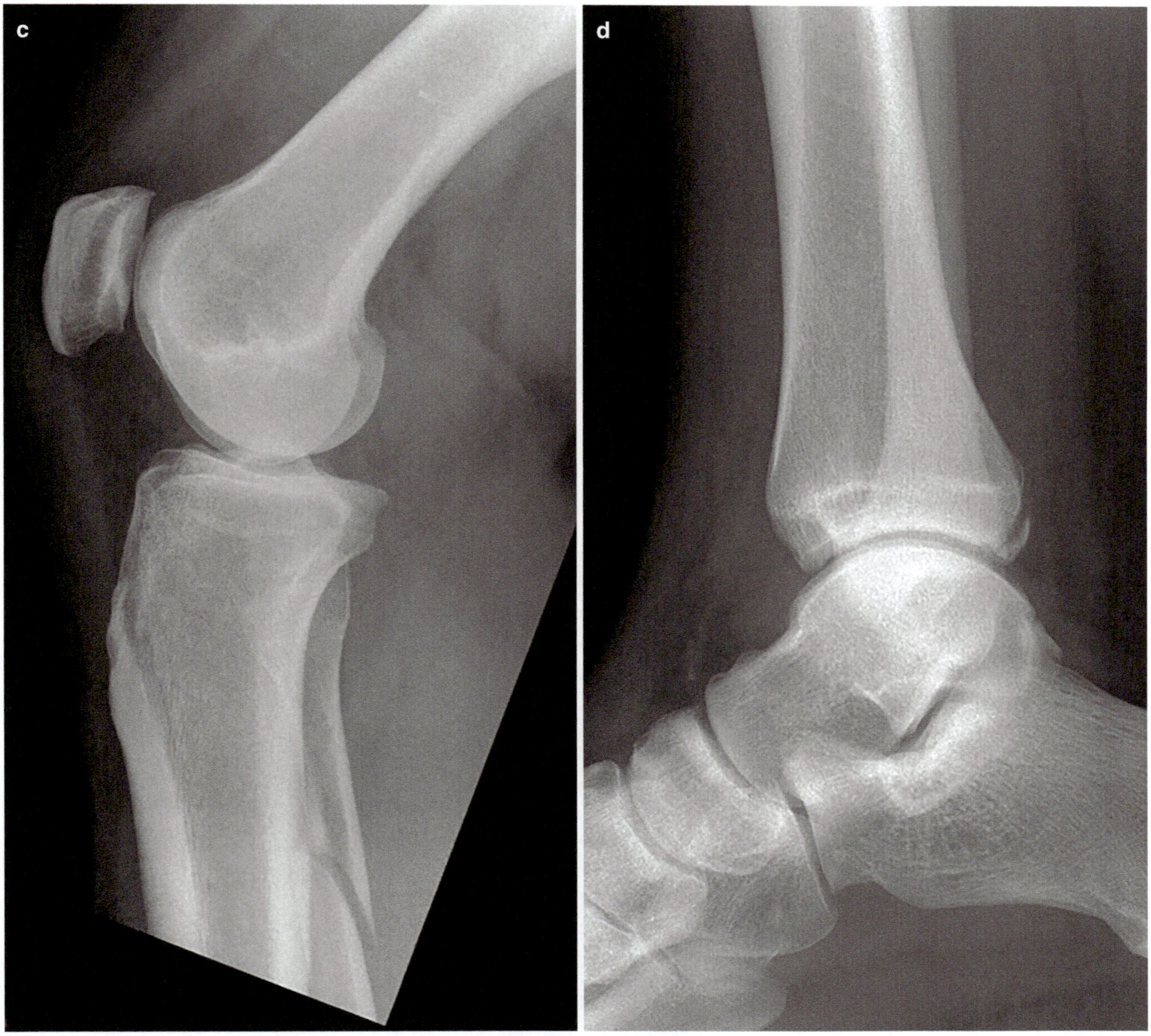

Fig. 4.31 (continued)

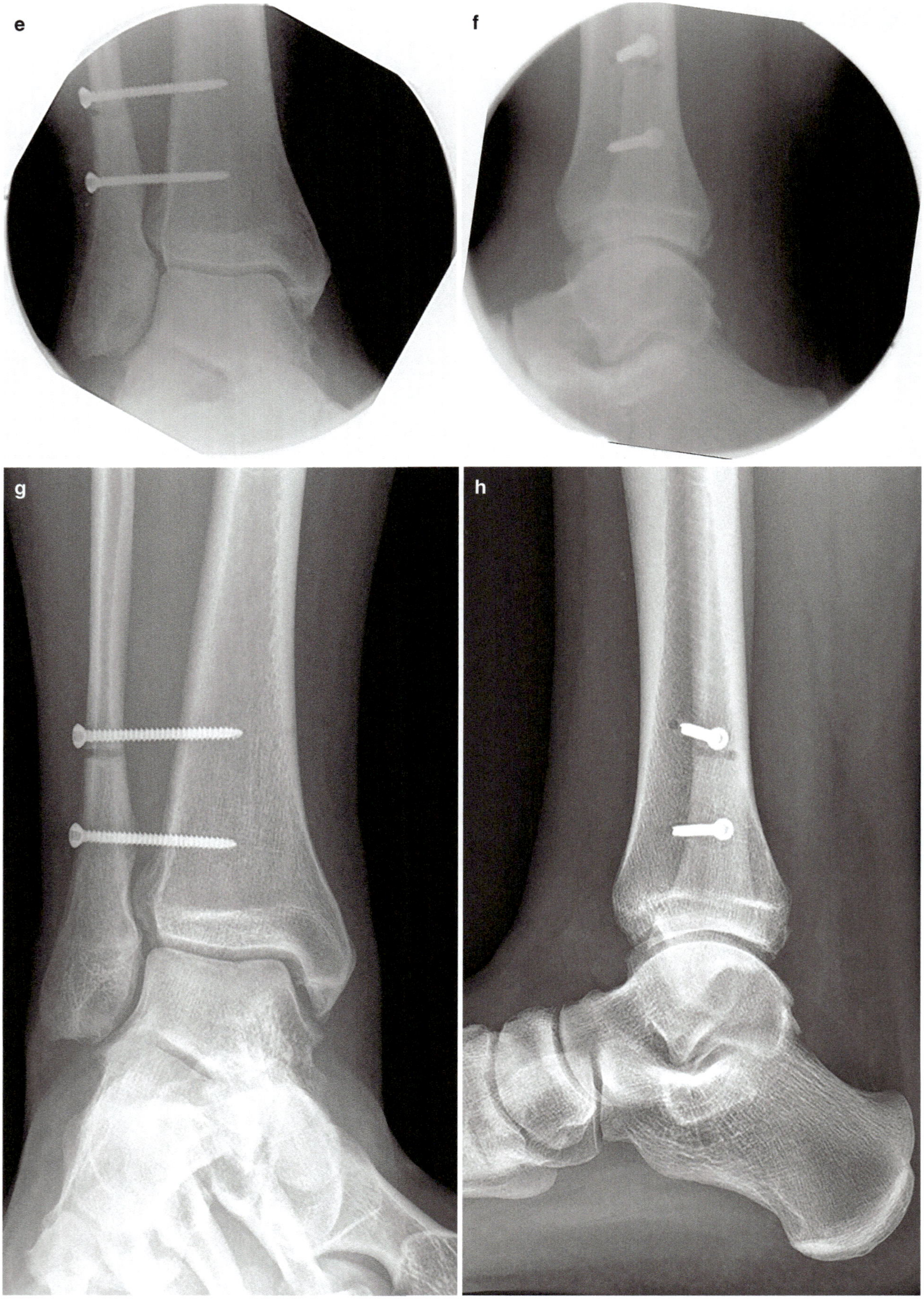

Fig. 4.31 (continued)

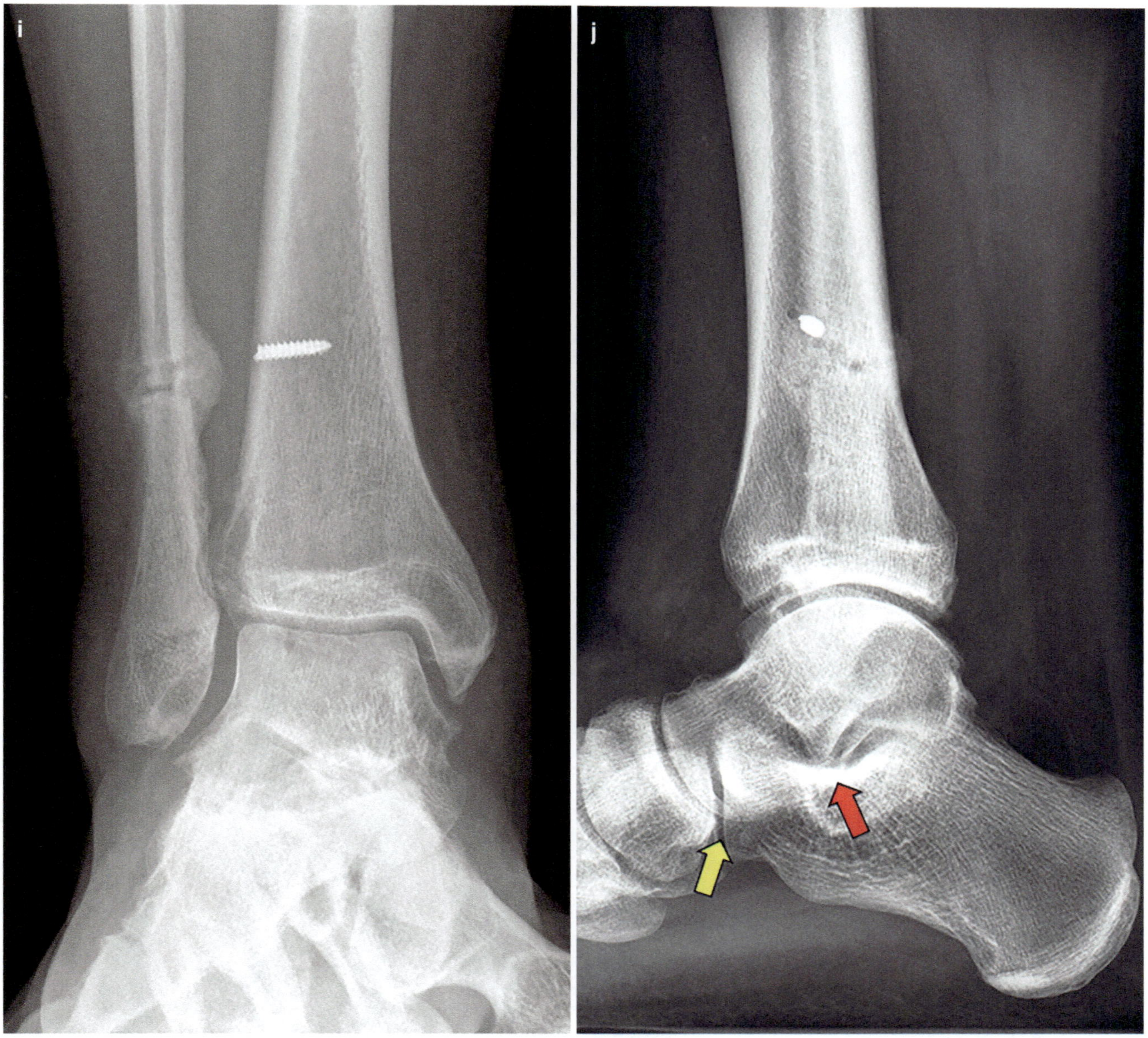

Fig. 4.31 (continued)

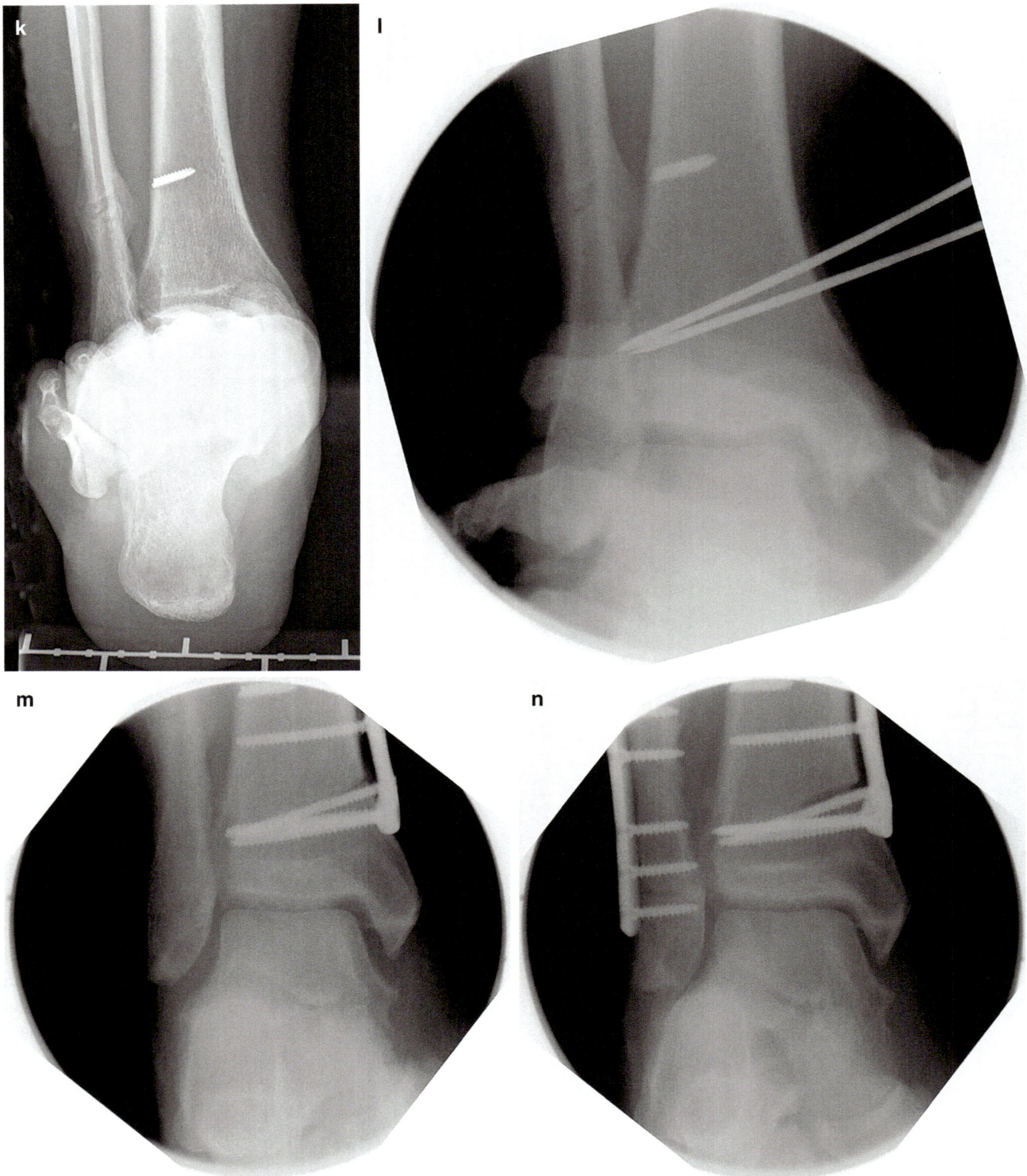

Fig. 4.31 (continued)

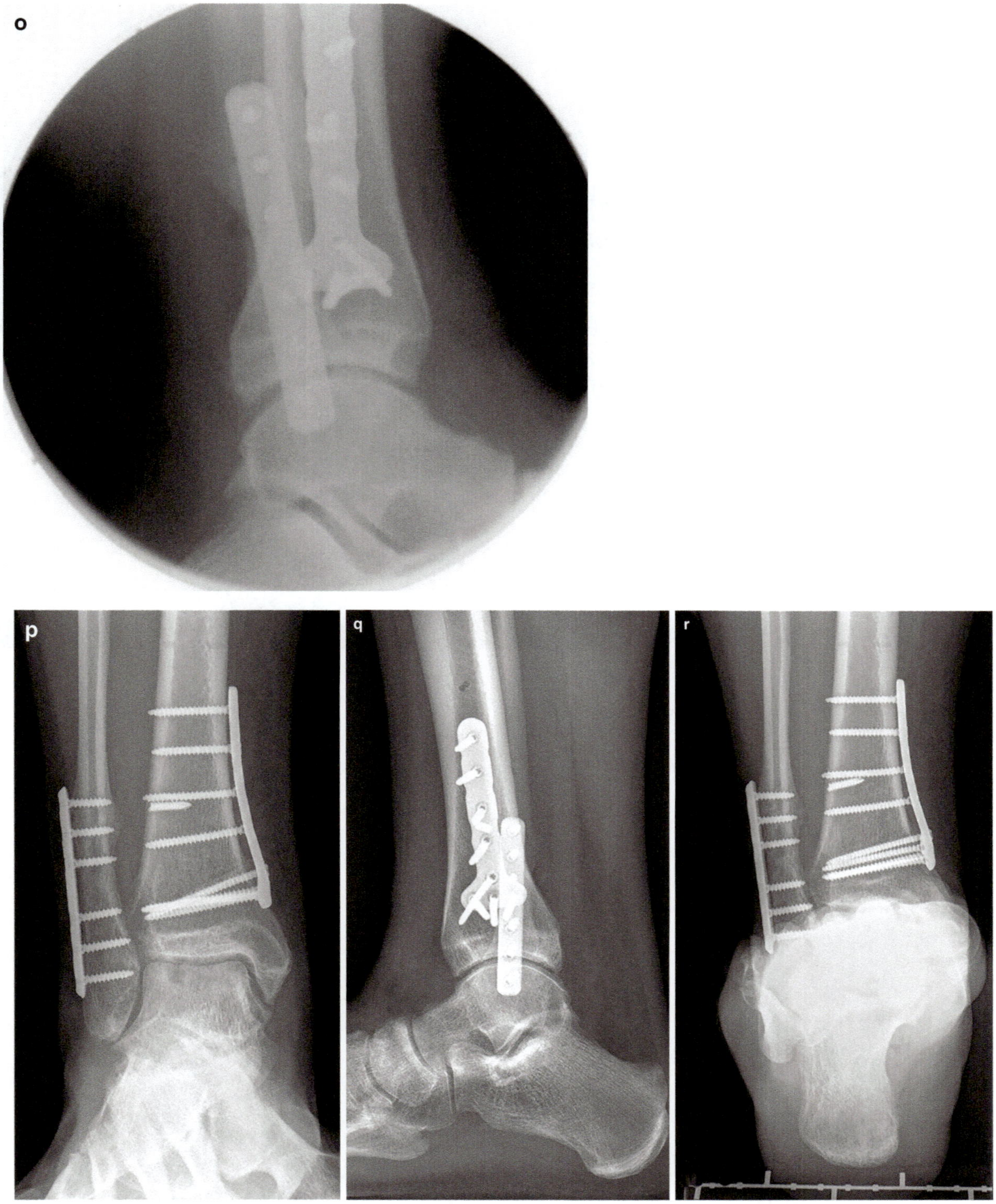

Fig. 4.31 (continued)

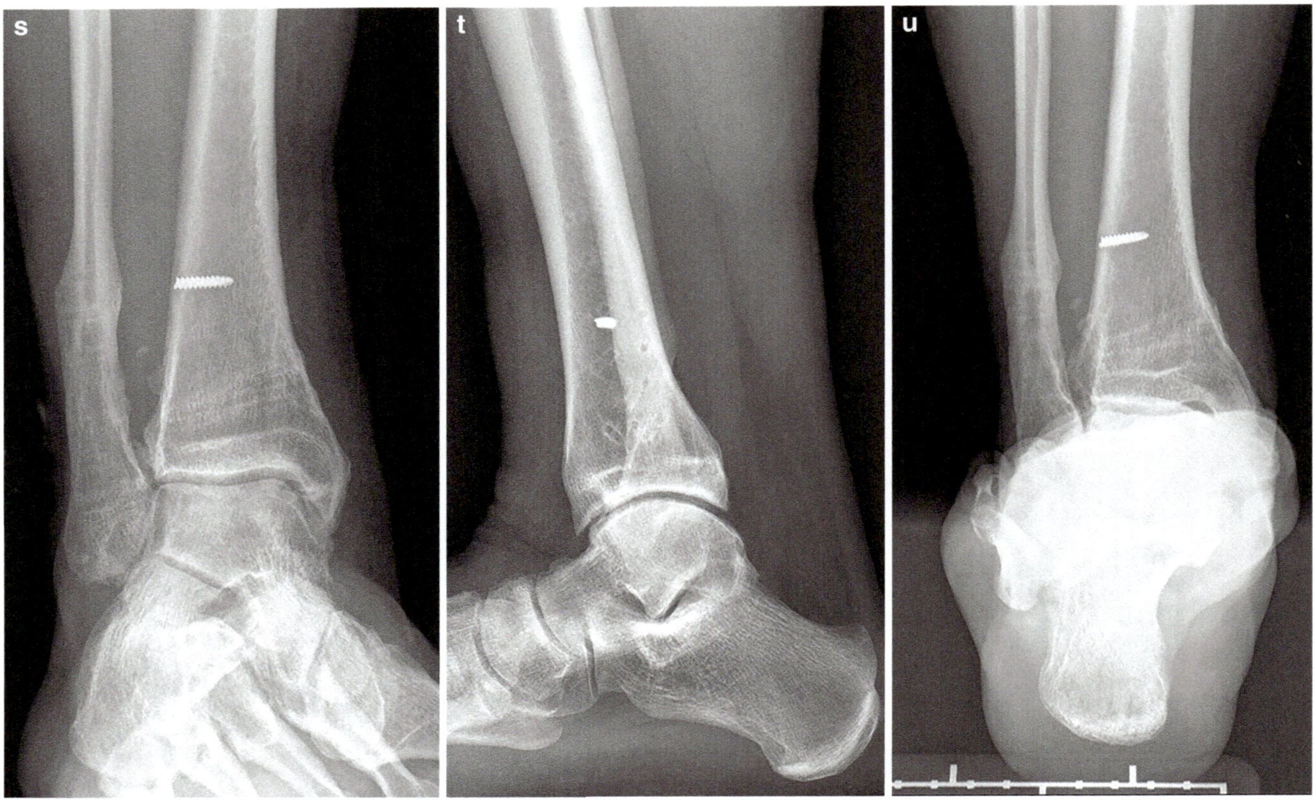

Fig. 4.31 (continued)

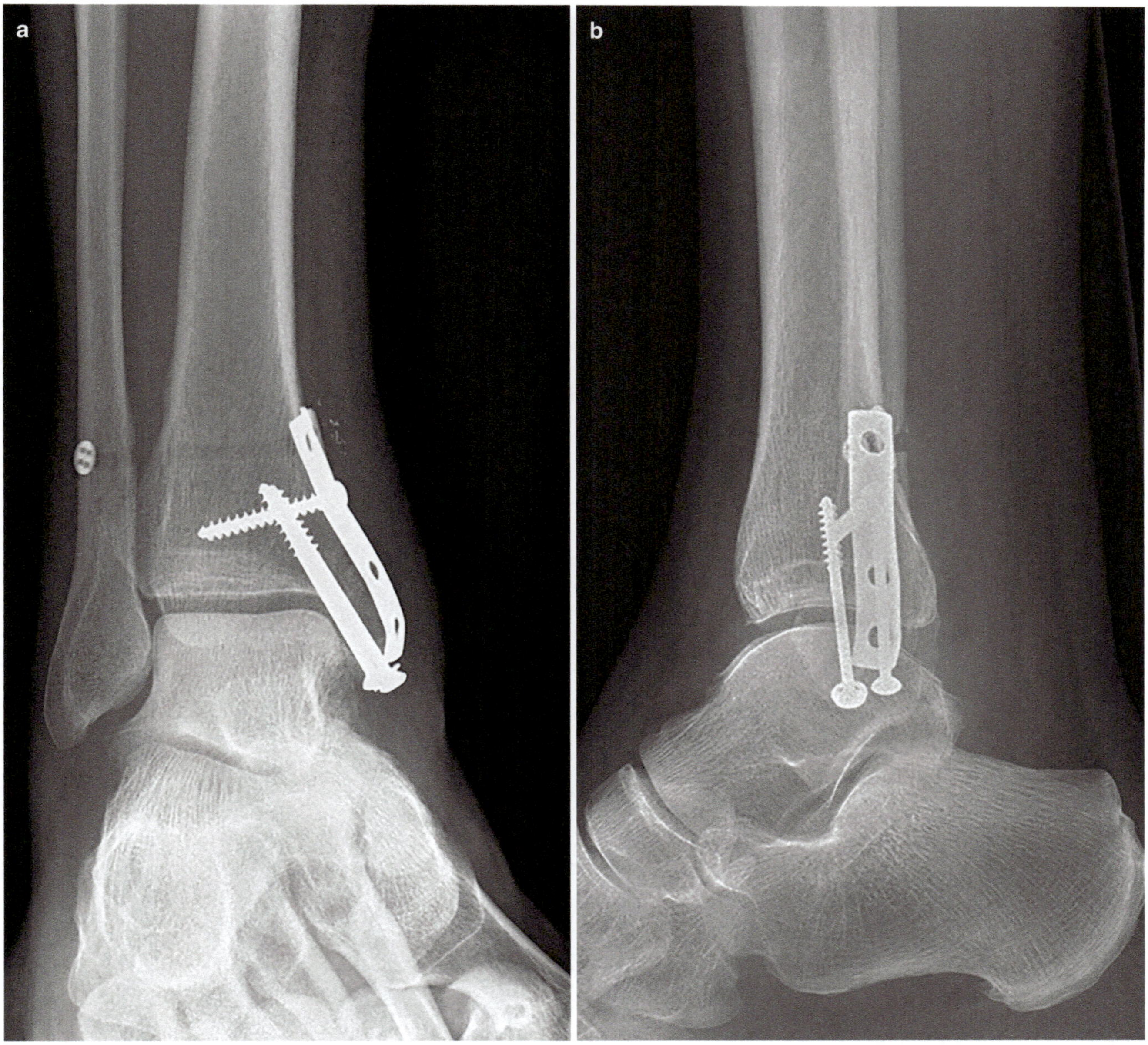

Fig. 4.32 This 49-year-old male patient sustained a Maisonneuve type injury with a non-displaced high fibular fracture and a fracture of the medial malleolus while hiking. (**a**) Postoperative plain radiograph at 6 weeks after fixation of the medial malleolus by a plate and two compression screws as well as syndesmosis stabilization using a suture button. (**b**) The lateral view shows the posterior position of the plate of which the proximal hole was used to fix the suture button. With this, drilling was made along the posterior cortex of fibula. (**c**) Five weeks later, the patient felt acute pain while walking, without a trauma. Plain radiographs show the stress fracture along the drill canal of the suture button and the distal tibia tilted into varus and retrocurvatum position. (**c**) AP view; (**d**) lateral view

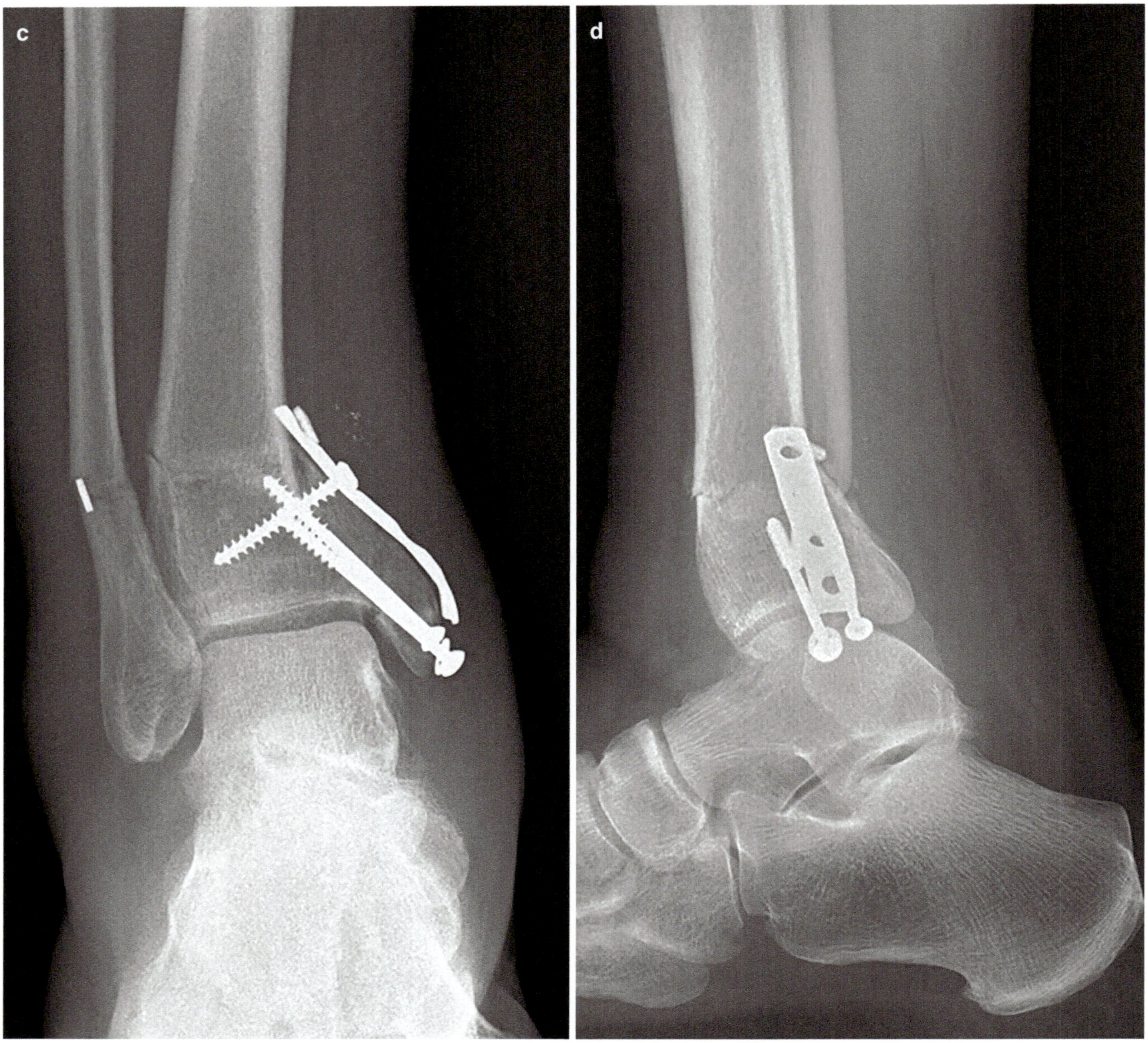

Fig. 4.32 (continued)

to increased stress placed across the syndesmotic screws, leading to high screw failure rates [130]. Currently there is no clear evidence supporting routine syndesmotic screw removal or retention [131].

Additional reported complications of syndesmotic injuries are the development of heterotopic ossifications and more rarely tibiofibular synostosis with questionable functional consequences [86].

4.12 Conclusions

- Initial diagnosis of a syndesmotic injury is crucial.
- Appropriate treatment of syndesmotic injuries is crucial for the outcome.

Injuries to the syndesmosis are relatively common in certain athletic populations. Although many of these injuries can be treated nonsurgically, it is important to differentiate between stable and unstable injuries. Recent literature has improved our understanding of the sequence, severity, and significance of ligament disruption associated with injury to the syndesmosis, which has aided clinicians in determining treatment decisions and prognosis. Trans-syndesmotic screw fixation remains a common and effective fixation method for syndesmotic injuries. No consensus exists regarding screw size, screw quantity, number of cortices, postoperative care, and the necessity of implant removal. In clinical and biomechanical studies, the suture button has shown promising results as an alternative method for managing syndesmotic injuries. The key advantages of suture buttons include more physiological motion, a significantly lower incidence of malreduction, and no need for routine implant removal.

References

1. Hopkinson WJ, St Pierre P, Ryan JB, Wheeler JH. Syndesmosis sprains of the ankle. Foot Ankle. 1990;10(6):325–30.
2. Markolf KL, Jackson S, McAllister DR. Force and displacement measurements of the distal fibula during simulated ankle loading tests for high ankle sprains. Foot Ankle Int. 2012;33(09):779–86.
3. Yuen CP, Lui TH. Distal tibiofibular syndesmosis: anatomy, biomechanics, injury and management. Open Orthop J. 2017;11:670–7.
4. Ogilvie-Harris DJ, Reed SC. Disruption of the ankle syndesmosis: diagnosis and treatment by arthroscopic surgery. Arthroscopy. 1994;10(5):561–8.
5. Xenos JS, Hopkinson WJ, Mulligan ME, Olson EJ, Popovic NA. The tibiofibular syndesmosis. Evaluation of the ligamentous structures, methods of fixation, and radiographic assessment. J Bone Joint Surg Am. 1995;77(6):847–56.
6. Harris J, Fallat L. Effects of isolated Weber B fibular fractures on the tibiotalar contact area. J Foot Ankle Surg. 2004;43(1):3–9.
7. Ramsey PL, Hamilton W. Changes in tibiotalar area of contact caused by lateral talar shift. J Bone Joint Surg Am. 1976;58(3):356–7.
8. Mavi A, Yildirim H, Gunes H, Pestamalci T, Gumusburun E. The fibular incisura of the tibia with recurrent sprained ankle on magnetic resonance imaging. Saudi Med J. 2002;23(7):845–9.
9. Ebraheim NA, Lu J, Yang H, Rollins J. The fibular incisure of the tibia on CT scan: a cadaver study. Foot Ankle Int. 1998;19(5):318–21.
10. Kelikian H, Kelikian S. Disorders of the ankle. Philadelphia, PA: W.B. Saunders Co; 1985. p. 4–8.
11. Bartonicek J. Anatomy of the tibiofibular syndesmosis and its clinical relevance. Surg Radiol Anat. 2003;25(5–6):379–86.
12. Kim S, Huh YM, Song HT, Lee SA, Lee JW, Lee JE, et al. Chronic tibiofibular syndesmosis injury of ankle: evaluation with contrast-enhanced fat-suppressed 3D fast spoiled gradient-recalled acquisition in the steady state MR imaging. Radiology. 2007;242(1):225–35.
13. van Moppes FI, Meijer F, van den Hoogenband CR. Arthrographic differential diagnosis between ruptures of the anterior talofibular ligament, the joint capsule and the anterior tibiofibular ligament. Rofo. 1980;133(5):534–9.
14. Bassett FH III, Gates HS III, Billys JB, Morris HB, Nikolaou PK. Talar impingement by the anteroinferior tibiofibular ligament. A cause of chronic pain in the ankle after inversion sprain. J Bone Joint Surg Am. 1990;72(1):55–9.
15. Nikolopoulos CE, Tsirikos AI, Sourmelis S, Papachristou G. The accessory anteroinferior tibiofibular ligament as a cause of talar impingement: a cadaveric study. Am J Sports Med. 2004;32(2):389–95.
16. Subhas N, Vinson EN, Cothran RL, Santangelo JR, Nunley JA II, Helms CA. MRI appearance of surgically proven abnormal accessory anterior-inferior tibiofibular ligament (Bassett's ligament). Skelet Radiol. 2008;37(1):27–33.
17. Ebraheim NA, Taser F, Shafiq Q, Yeasting RA. Anatomical evaluation and clinical importance of the tibiofibular syndesmosis ligaments. Surg Radiol Anat. 2006;28(2):142–9.
18. Van de Perre S, Vanhoenacker FM, De Vuyst D, Parizel R. Imaging anatomy of the ankle. JBR-BTR. 2004;87(6):310–4.
19. Golano P, Mariani PP, Rodriguez-Niedenfuhr M, Mariani PF, Ruano-Gil D. Arthroscopic anatomy of the posterior ankle ligaments. Arthroscopy. 2002;18(4):353–8.
20. Oh CS, Won HS, Hur MS, Chung IH, Kim S, Suh JS, et al. Anatomic variations and MRI of the intermalleolar ligament. AJR Am J Roentgenol. 2006;186(4):943–7.
21. Rosenberg ZS, Cheung YY, Beltran J, Sheskier S, Leong M, Jahss M. Posterior intermalleolar ligament of the ankle: normal anatomy and MR imaging features. AJR Am J Roentgenol. 1995;165(2):387–90.
22. Ogilvie-Harris DJ, Reed SC, Hedman TP. Disruption of the ankle syndesmosis: biomechanical study of the ligamentous restraints. Arthroscopy. 1994;10(5):558–60.
23. Hu WK, Chen DW, Li B, Yang YF, Yu GR. Motion of the distal tibiofibular syndesmosis under different loading patterns: a biomechanical study. J Orthop Surg (Hong Kong). 2019;27(2):2309499019842879.
24. Peter RE, Harrington RM, Henley MB, Tencer AF. Biomechanical effects of internal fixation of the distal tibiofibular syndesmotic joint: comparison of two fixation techniques. J Orthop Trauma. 1994;8(3):215–9.
25. Vukicevic S, Stern-Padovan R, Vukicevic D, Keros P. Holographic investigations of the human tibiofibular interosseous membrane. Clin Orthop Relat Res. 1980;151:210–4.
26. Hunt KJ, Goeb Y, Behn AW, Criswell B, Chou L. Ankle joint contact loads and displacement with progressive syndesmotic injury. Foot Ankle Int. 2015;36(9):1095–103.
27. Kumar A, Charlebois SJ, Cain EL, Smith RA, Daniels AU, Crates JM. Effect of fibular plate fixation on rotational stability of simulated distal tibial fractures treated with intramedullary nailing. J Bone Joint Surg Am. 2003;85(4):604–8.
28. Sproule JA, Khalid M, O'Sullivan M, McCabe JP. Outcome after surgery for Maisonneuve fracture of the fibula. Injury. 2004;35(8):791–8.
29. Stufkens SA, van den Bekerom MP, Doornberg JN, van Dijk CN, Kloen P. Evidence-based treatment of maisonneuve fractures. J Foot Ankle Surg. 2011;50(1):62–7.
30. Lloyd J, Elsayed S, Hariharan K, Tanaka H. Revisiting the concept of talar shift in ankle fractures. Foot Ankle Int. 2006;27(10):793–6.
31. Thordarson DB, Motamed S, Hedman T, Ebramzadeh E, Bakshian S. The effect of fibular malreduction on contact pressures in an ankle fracture malunion model. J Bone Joint Surg Am. 1997;79(12):1809–15.
32. Sarsam IM, Hughes SP. The role of the anterior tibio-fibular ligament in talar rotation: an anatomical study. Injury. 1988;19(2):62–4.

33. Mait AR, Forman JL, Nie B, Donlon JP, Mane A, Forghani AR, et al. Propagation of syndesmotic injuries during forced external rotation in flexed cadaveric ankles. Orthop J Sports Med. 2018;6(6):2325967118781333.
34. Rosati E, Medina MA. The role of the tibiofibular interosseous membrane in the repair of fractures of the tibia and fibula. Ital J Orthop Traumatol. 1987;13(4):521–5.
35. Xu D, Wang Y, Jiang C, Fu M, Li S, Qian L, et al. Strain distribution in the anterior inferior tibiofibular ligament, posterior inferior tibiofibular ligament, and interosseous membrane using digital image correlation. Foot Ankle Int. 2018;39(5):618–28.
36. Manyi W, Guowei R, Shengsong Y, Chunyan J. A sample of Chinese literature MRI diagnosis of interosseous membrane injury in Maisonneuve fractures of the fibula. Injury. 2000;31(Suppl 3):C107–10.
37. Scranton PE. Isolated syndesmotic injuries: diastasis of the ankle in the athlete. Tech Foot Ankle Surg. 2002;1(2):88–93.
38. Boytim MJ, Fischer DA, Neumann L. Syndesmotic ankle sprains. Am J Sports Med. 1991;19(3):294–8.
39. Inman VT. The joints of the ankle. Baltimore, MD: Williams & Wilkins; 1976.
40. Riegels-Nielsen P, Christensen J, Greiff J. The stability of the tibio-fibular syndesmosis following rigid internal fixation for type C malleolar fractures: an experimental and clinical study. Injury. 1983;14(4):357–60.
41. Hintermann B, Regazzoni P, Lampert C, Stutz G, Gachter A. Arthroscopic findings in acute fractures of the ankle. J Bone Joint Surg Br. 2000;82(3):345–51.
42. Ramasamy P, Ward A. Distal tibiofibular joint dislocation with an intact fibula: a classification system. Injury. 2003;34(11):862–5.
43. Fincher AL. Early recognition of syndesmotic ankle sprains. Int J Athl Ther Train. 1999;4(2):42–3.
44. Katznelson A, Lin E, Militiano J. Ruptures of the ligaments about the tibio-fibular syndesmosis. Injury. 1983;15(3):170–2.
45. Menelaus MB. Injuries of the anterior inferior tibio-fibular ligament. Aust N Z J Surg. 1961;30:279–87.
46. Brosky T, Nyland J, Nitz A, Caborn DN. The ankle ligaments: consideration of syndesmotic injury and implications for rehabilitation. J Orthop Sports Phys Ther. 1995;21(4):197–205.
47. Michelson JD, Waldman B. An axially loaded model of the ankle after pronation external rotation injury. Clin Orthop Relat Res. 1996;328:285–93.
48. Sman AD, Hiller CE, Refshauge KM. Diagnostic accuracy of clinical tests for diagnosis of ankle syndesmosis injury: a systematic review. Br J Sports Med. 2013;47(10):620–8.
49. Teitz CC, Harrington RM. A biochemical analysis of the squeeze test for sprains of the syndesmotic ligaments of the ankle. Foot Ankle Int. 1998;19(7):489–92.
50. Lin CF, Gross ML, Weinhold P. Ankle syndesmosis injuries: anatomy, biomechanics, mechanism of injury, and clinical guidelines for diagnosis and intervention. J Orthop Sports Phys Ther. 2006;36(6):372–84.
51. Bauer AB, Wilsona EM, Chiodo MG. Injuries of the distal lower extremits syndesmosis. Curr Orthop Pract. 2009;20(2):111–6.
52. Lui TH, Ip K, Chow HT. Comparison of radiologic and arthroscopic diagnoses of distal tibiofibular syndesmosis disruption in acute ankle fracture. Arthroscopy. 2005;21(11):1370.
53. Ebraheim NA, Elgafy H, Padanilam T. Syndesmotic disruption in low fibular fractures associated with deltoid ligament injury. Clin Orthop Relat Res. 2003;409:260–7.
54. Harper MC, Keller TS. A radiographic evaluation of the tibiofibular syndesmosis. Foot Ankle. 1989;10(3):156–60.
55. Weber BG. Injuries of the ankle. Bern: Hans Huber; 1972.
56. Beumer A, van Hemert WL, Niesing R, Entius CA, Ginai AZ, Mulder PG, et al. Radiographic measurement of the distal tibiofibular syndesmosis has limited use. Clin Orthop Relat Res. 2004;423:227–34.
57. Gardner MJ, Demetrakopoulos D, Briggs SM, Helfet DL, Lorich DG. Malreduction of the tibiofibular syndesmosis in ankle fractures. Foot Ankle Int. 2006;27(10):788–92.
58. Nielson JH, Gardner MJ, Peterson MG, Sallis JG, Potter HG, Helfet DL, et al. Radiographic measurements do not predict syndesmotic injury in ankle fractures: an MRI study. Clin Orthop Relat Res. 2005;436:216–21.
59. Pakarinen HJ, Flinkkila TE, Ohtonen PP, Hyvonen PH, Lakovaara MT, Leppilahti JI, et al. Syndesmotic fixation in supination-external rotation ankle fractures: a prospective randomized study. Foot Ankle Int. 2011;32(12):1103–9.
60. Stoffel K, Wysocki D, Baddour E, Nicholls R, Yates P. Comparison of two intraoperative assessment methods for injuries to the ankle syndesmosis. A cadaveric study. J Bone Joint Surg Am. 2009;91(11):2646–52.
61. Jiang KN, Schulz BM, Tsui YL, Gardner TR, Greisberg JK. Comparison of radiographic stress tests for syndesmotic instability of supination-external rotation ankle fractures: a cadaveric study. J Orthop Trauma. 2014;28(6):e123–7.
62. Ebraheim NA, Lu J, Yang H, Mekhail AO, Yeasting RA. Radiographic and CT evaluation of tibiofibular syndesmotic diastasis: a cadaver study. Foot Ankle Int. 1997;18(11):693–8.
63. Ahn TK, Choi SM, Kim JY, Lee WC. Isolated syndesmosis diastasis: computed tomography scan assessment with arthroscopic correlation. Arthroscopy. 2017;33(4):828–34.
64. Krahenbuhl N, Weinberg MW, Davidson NP, Mills MK, Hintermann B, Saltzman CL, et al. Imaging in syndesmotic injury: a systematic literature review. Skelet Radiol. 2018;47(5):631–48.
65. Krähenbühl N, Bailey TL, Weinberg MW, Davidson NP, Hintermann B, Presson AP, et al. Is load application necessary when using computed tomography scans to diagnose syndesmotic injuries? A cadaver study. Foot Ankle Surg. 2019;26(2):198–204.
66. Malhotra K, Welck M, Cullen N, Singh D, Goldberg AJ. The effects of weight bearing on the distal tibiofibular syndesmosis: a study comparing weight bearing-CT with conventional CT. Foot Ankle Surg. 2019;25(4):511–6.
67. Osgood GM, Shakoor D, Orapin J, Qin J, Khodarahmi I, Thawait GK, et al. Reliability of distal tibio-fibular syndesmotic instability measurements using weightbearing and non-weightbearing cone-beam CT. Foot Ankle Surg. 2019;25(6):771–81.
68. Richter M, Seidl B, Zech S, Hahn S. PedCAT for 3D-imaging in standing position allows for more accurate bone position (angle) measurement than radiographs or CT. Foot Ankle Surg. 2014;20(3):201–7.
69. Krahenbuhl N, Bailey TL, Weinberg MW, Davidson NP, Hintermann B, Presson AP, et al. Impact of torque on assessment of syndesmotic injuries using weightbearing computed tomography scans. Foot Ankle Int. 2019;40(6):710–9.
70. Oae K, Takao M, Naito K, Uchio Y, Kono T, Ishida J, et al. Injury of the tibiofibular syndesmosis: value of MR imaging for diagnosis. Radiology. 2003;227(1):155–61.
71. Takao M, Ochi M, Oae K, Naito K, Uchio Y. Diagnosis of a tear of the tibiofibular syndesmosis. The role of arthroscopy of the ankle. J Bone Joint Surg Br. 2003;85(3):324–9.
72. Warner SJ, Garner MR, Schottel PC, Hinds RM, Loftus ML, Lorich DG. Analysis of PITFL injuries in rotationally unstable ankle fractures. Foot Ankle Int. 2015;36(4):377–82.
73. Chun KY, Choi YS, Lee SH, Kim JS, Young KW, Jeong MS, et al. Deltoid ligament and tibiofibular syndesmosis injury in chronic

lateral ankle instability: magnetic resonance imaging evaluation at 3T and comparison with arthroscopy. Korean J Radiol. 2015;16(5):1096–103.
74. Chan KB, Lui TH. Role of ankle arthroscopy in management of acute ankle fracture. Arthroscopy. 2016;32(11):2373–80.
75. Lucas DE, Watson BC, Simpson GA, Berlet GC, Hyer CF. Arthroscopic evaluation of syndesmotic instability and malreduction. Foot Ankle Spec. 2016;9(6):500–5.
76. Takao M, Ochi M, Naito K, Iwata A, Kawasaki K, Tobita M, et al. Arthroscopic diagnosis of tibiofibular syndesmosis disruption. Arthroscopy. 2001;17(8):836–43.
77. Watson BC, Lucas DE, Simpson GA, Berlet GC, Hyer CF. Arthroscopic evaluation of syndesmotic instability in a cadaveric model. Foot Ankle Int. 2015;36(11):1362–8.
78. Beumer A, Heijboer RP, Fontijne WP, Swierstra BA. Late reconstruction of the anterior distal tibiofibular syndesmosis: good outcome in 9 patients. Acta Orthop Scand. 2000;71(5):519–21.
79. Massri-Pugin J, Lubberts B, Vopat BG, Wolf JC, DiGiovanni CW, Guss D. Role of the deltoid ligament in syndesmotic instability. Foot Ankle Int. 2018;39(5):598–603.
80. Harper MC. Delayed reduction and stabilization of the tibiofibular syndesmosis. Foot Ankle Int. 2001;22(1):15–8.
81. Feller R, Borenstein T, Fantry AJ, Kellum RB, Machan JT, Nickisch F, et al. Arthroscopic quantification of syndesmotic instability in a cadaveric model. Arthroscopy. 2017;33(2):436–44.
82. Dattani R, Patnaik S, Kantak A, Srikanth B, Selvan TP. Injuries to the tibiofibular syndesmosis. J Bone Joint Surg Br. 2008;90(4):405–10.
83. Nussbaum ED, Hosea TM, Sieler SD, Incremona BR, Kessler DE. Prospective evaluation of syndesmotic ankle sprains without diastasis. Am J Sports Med. 2001;29(1):31–5.
84. Sman AD, Hiller CE, Rae K, Linklater J, Black DA, Refshauge KM. Prognosis of ankle syndesmosis injury. Med Sci Sports Exerc. 2014;46(4):671–7.
85. Williams GN, Jones MH, Amendola A. Syndesmotic ankle sprains in athletes. Am J Sports Med. 2007;35(7):1197–207.
86. Taylor DC, Englehardt DL, Bassett FH III. Syndesmosis sprains of the ankle. The influence of heterotopic ossification. Am J Sports Med. 1992;20(2):146–50.
87. Hunt KJ, Phisitkul P, Pirolo J, Amendola A. High ankle sprains and syndesmotic injuries in athletes. J Am Acad Orthop Surg. 2015;23(11):661–73.
88. Fort NM, Aiyer AA, Kaplan JR, Smyth NA, Kadakia AR. Management of acute injuries of the tibiofibular syndesmosis. Eur J Orthop Surg Traumatol. 2017;27(4):449–59.
89. Hamoui M, Ali M, Lovas F, Bonnel F. Troubles de rotation de la malléole fibulaire après ostéosynthèse des fractures de cheville (évaluation radiologique standard et scanographique, à propos de 20 cas). Med Chir Pied. 2008;24:155–66.
90. Miller AN, Barei DP, Iaquinto JM, Ledoux WR, Beingessner DM. Iatrogenic syndesmosis malreduction via clamp and screw placement. J Orthop Trauma. 2013;27(2):100–6.
91. Phisitkul P, Ebinger T, Goetz J, Vaseenon T, Marsh JL. Forceps reduction of the syndesmosis in rotational ankle fractures: a cadaveric study. J Bone Joint Surg Am. 2012;94(24):2256–61.
92. Gardner MJ, Brodsky A, Briggs SM, Nielson JH, Lorich DG. Fixation of posterior malleolar fractures provides greater syndesmotic stability. Clin Orthop Relat Res. 2006;447:165–71.
93. Han SH, Lee JW, Kim S, Suh JS, Choi YR. Chronic tibiofibular syndesmosis injury: the diagnostic efficiency of magnetic resonance imaging and comparative analysis of operative treatment. Foot Ankle Int. 2007;28(3):336–42.
94. Ogilvie-Harris DJ, Gilbart MK, Chorney K. Chronic pain following ankle sprains in athletes: the role of arthroscopic surgery. Arthroscopy. 1997;13(5):564–74.
95. Ryan PM, Rodriguez RM. Outcomes and return to activity after operative repair of chronic latent syndesmotic instability. Foot Ankle Int. 2016;37(2):192–7.
96. Schuberth JM, Jennings MM, Lau AC. Arthroscopy-assisted repair of latent syndesmotic instability of the ankle. Arthroscopy. 2008;24(8):868–74.
97. Colcuc C, Fischer S, Colcuc S, Busse D, Bliemel C, Neun O, et al. Treatment strategies for partial chronic instability of the distal syndesmosis: an arthroscopic grading scale and operative staging concept. Arch Orthop Trauma Surg. 2016;136(2):157–63.
98. Jain SK, Kearns SR. Ligamentous advancement for the treatment of subacute syndesmotic injuries. Report of a new technique in 5 cases. Foot Ankle Surg. 2014;20(4):281–4.
99. Wagener ML, Beumer A, Swierstra BA. Chronic instability of the anterior tibiofibular syndesmosis of the ankle. Arthroscopic findings and results of anatomical reconstruction. BMC Musculoskelet Disord. 2011;12:212.
100. Zamzami MM, Zamzam MM. Chronic isolated distal tibiofibular syndesmotic disruption: diagnosis and management. Foot Ankle Surg. 2009;15(1):14–9.
101. Yasui Y, Takao M, Miyamoto W, Innami K, Matsushita T. Anatomical reconstruction of the anterior inferior tibiofibular ligament for chronic disruption of the distal tibiofibular syndesmosis. Knee Surg Sports Traumatol Arthrosc. 2011;19(4):691–5.
102. Grass R, Rammelt S, Biewener A, Zwipp H. Peroneus longus ligamentoplasty for chronic instability of the distal tibiofibular syndesmosis. Foot Ankle Int. 2003;24(5):392–7.
103. Morris MW, Rice P, Schneider TE. Distal tibiofibular syndesmosis reconstruction using a free hamstring autograft. Foot Ankle Int. 2009;30(6):506–11.
104. Olson KM, Dairyko GH Jr, Toolan BC. Salvage of chronic instability of the syndesmosis with distal tibiofibular arthrodesis: functional and radiographic results. J Bone Joint Surg Am. 2011;93(1):66–72.
105. Hintermann B, Barg A, Knupp M. Corrective supramalleolar osteotomy for malunited pronation-external rotation fractures of the ankle. J Bone Joint Surg Br. 2011;93(10):1367–72.
106. Espinosa N, Smerek JP, Myerson MS. Acute and chronic syndesmosis injuries: pathomechanisms, diagnosis and management. Foot Ankle Clin. 2006;11(3):639–57.
107. Miyamoto W, Takao M. Management of chronic disruption of the distal tibiofibular syndesmosis. World J Orthop. 2011;2(1):1–6.
108. Rammelt S, Zwipp H, Grass R. Injuries to the distal tibiofibular syndesmosis: an evidence-based approach to acute and chronic lesions. Foot Ankle Clin. 2008;13(4):611–33, vii–viii.
109. van den Bekerom MP, de Leeuw PA, van Dijk CN. Delayed operative treatment of syndesmotic instability. Current concepts review. Injury. 2009;40(11):1137–42.
110. Wolf BR. Syndesmosis injuries in the athlete: when and how to operate. Curr Opin Orthop. 2002;13(2):151–4.
111. Rao SE, Muzammil S, Khan AH. Syndesmosis fixation in bimalleolar Weber C ankle fractures; comparison of 3.5 and 4.5-mm screws. Prof Med J. 2008;15:49–53.
112. Beumer A, Campo MM, Niesing R, Day J, Kleinrensink GJ, Swierstra BA. Screw fixation of the syndesmosis: a cadaver model comparing stainless steel and titanium screws and three and four cortical fixation. Injury. 2005;36(1):60–4.
113. Moore JA Jr, Shank JR, Morgan SJ, Smith WR. Syndesmosis fixation: a comparison of three and four cortices of screw fixation without hardware removal. Foot Ankle Int. 2006;27(8):567–72.
114. Kukreti S, Faraj A, Miles JN. Does position of syndesmotic screw affect functional and radiological outcome in ankle fractures? Injury. 2005;36(9):1121–4.

115. Ahmad J, Raikin SM, Pour AE, Haytmanek C. Bioabsorbable screw fixation of the syndesmosis in unstable ankle injuries. Foot Ankle Int. 2009;30(2):99–105.
116. Hovis WD, Kaiser BW, Watson JT, Bucholz RW. Treatment of syndesmotic disruptions of the ankle with bioabsorbable screw fixation. J Bone Joint Surg Am. 2002;84(1):26–31.
117. Kaukonen JP, Lamberg T, Korkala O, Pajarinen J. Fixation of syndesmotic ruptures in 38 patients with a malleolar fracture: a randomized study comparing a metallic and a bioabsorbable screw. J Orthop Trauma. 2005;19(6):392–5.
118. Sinisaari IP, Luthje PM, Mikkonen RH. Ruptured tibio-fibular syndesmosis: comparison study of metallic to bioabsorbable fixation. Foot Ankle Int. 2002;23(8):744–8.
119. Sun H, Luo CF, Zhong B, Shi HP, Zhang CQ, Zeng BF. A prospective, randomised trial comparing the use of absorbable and metallic screws in the fixation of distal tibiofibular syndesmosis injuries: mid-term follow-up. Bone Joint J. 2014;96-B(4):548–54.
120. Thordarson DB, Samuelson M, Shepherd LE, Merkle PF, Lee J. Bioabsorbable versus stainless steel screw fixation of the syndesmosis in pronation-lateral rotation ankle fractures: a prospective randomized trial. Foot Ankle Int. 2001;22(4):335–8.
121. Schepers T. Acute distal tibiofibular syndesmosis injury: a systematic review of suture-button versus syndesmotic screw repair. Int Orthop. 2012;36(6):1199–206.
122. Naqvi GA, Cunningham P, Lynch B, Galvin R, Awan N. Fixation of ankle syndesmotic injuries: comparison of tightrope fixation and syndesmotic screw fixation for accuracy of syndesmotic reduction. Am J Sports Med. 2012;40(12):2828–35.
123. Franke J, von Recum J, Suda AJ, Grutzner PA, Wendl K. Intraoperative three-dimensional imaging in the treatment of acute unstable syndesmotic injuries. J Bone Joint Surg Am. 2012;94(15):1386–90.
124. Sagi HC, Shah AR, Sanders RW. The functional consequence of syndesmotic joint malreduction at a minimum 2-year follow-up. J Orthop Trauma. 2012;26(7):439–43.
125. Inge SY, Pull Ter Gunne AF, Aarts CAM, Bemelman M. A systematic review on dynamic versus static distal tibiofibular fixation. Injury. 2016;47(12):2627–34.
126. Welck MJ, Ray P. Tibialis anterior tendon entrapment after ankle tightrope insertion for acute syndesmosis injury. Foot Ankle Spec. 2013;6(3):242–6.
127. Citak M, Backhaus M, Muhr G, Kalicke T. Distal tibial fracture post syndesmotic screw removal: an adverse complication. Arch Orthop Trauma Surg. 2011;131(10):1405–8.
128. Hohman DW, Affonso J, Marzo JM, Ritter CA. Pathologic tibia/fibula fracture through a suture button screw tract: case report. Am J Sports Med. 2011;39(3):645–8.
129. Huber T, Schmoelz W, Bolderl A. Motion of the fibula relative to the tibia and its alterations with syndesmosis screws: a cadaver study. Foot Ankle Surg. 2012;18(3):203–9.
130. Hamid N, Loeffler BJ, Braddy W, Kellam JF, Cohen BE, Bosse MJ. Outcome after fixation of ankle fractures with an injury to the syndesmosis: the effect of the syndesmosis screw. J Bone Joint Surg Br. 2009;91(8):1069–73.
131. Dingemans SA, Rammelt S, White TO, Goslings JC, Schepers T. Should syndesmotic screws be removed after surgical fixation of unstable ankle fractures? A systematic review. Bone Joint J. 2016;98-B(11):1497–504.

5 Medial Ankle Instability (Including Spring Ligament)

The deltoid ligament is a complex structure that spans from the medial malleolus to the navicular, talus, and calcaneus. Its superficial components are also connected to the plantar calcaneonavicular ligaments (spring ligament). It is primarily responsible for stabilizing the medial side of the ankle. It limits anterior, posterior, and lateral translation of the talus and restrains talar abduction [1–4]. The superficial and deep components hereby have different functions, the superficial deltoid resists eversion of the hindfoot, and the deep deltoid is the primary restraint to external rotation of the talus [2].

Injuries to the deltoid ligament complex often occur in combination with injuries to other structures of the foot, such as ankle fractures, syndesmosis injuries, or lateral ligament injuries [5, 6]. Among all ankle sprains in an athletic patient cohort, isolated deltoid ligament injuries were found in 5–15% of the cases [7, 8]. Generally, however, it has been suggested that the medial ankle ligaments are injured more often than believed [9–11]. Typically, injuries to the medial ankle ligaments occur during running downstairs, landing on uneven surfaces and dancing while the body simultaneously rotates in the opposite direction. A key feature of the patients' history is whether or not they have sustained a pronation (eversion) trauma, e.g., an outward rotation of the foot during simultaneous inward rotation of the tibia. Excessive lateral rotation of the foot may injure the tibiofibular and interosseous ligaments at the syndesmosis, as has been discussed in Chap. 3. Additionally, the anterior fibers of the deltoid ligament may also be affected by these extreme rotation injuries. In practice, however, it is not so easy to identify which structures could be affected according to the injury mechanism. Patients often remember suffering an acute ankle sprain or even multiple ankle sprains; however, they are not able to clearly describe the injury mechanism. Complete deltoid ligament ruptures are sometimes seen in association with lateral malleolar fractures [12–15] or bimalleolar fractures [16, 17].

Chronic deltoid ligament insufficiency can be found in patients with concomitant conditions including posterior tibial tendon disorder, trauma and sports related deltoid disruptions, valgus talar tilting with previous triple arthrodesis or total ankle arthroplasty.

One concern may be whether posterior tibial tendon (PTT) dysfunction and medial ankle instability are distinct conditions. Although possible, it is not clear yet if, or to which extent, medial ankle instability may cause secondary PTT dysfunction over time, as the tendon may become elongated and/or ruptured [18–21].

5.1 Anatomy of the Deltoid-Spring Ligament Complex

- Though it is generally agreed that the deltoid ligament has superficial and deep components, there are many different interpretations of the individual bands that constitute these two components
- The superficial deltoid forms a functional unit with the spring ligament complex to support and stabilize the talar head

In the literature, various anatomic descriptions of the medial collateral (deltoid) ligaments exist (Fig. 5.1a); however, it is generally agreed that it has superficial and deep components (Fig. 5.1b) [1, 3, 22–28]. Beyond this basic classification, there are however many different interpretations of the individual bands that constitute these two components. Sarrafian [26] described 13 different interpretations (proposed between 1822 and 1979); more have been suggested since [22, 27, 29]. In an osteoligamentous preparation of 60 ankles from 39 cadavers, the tibiospring (TSL) and tibiocalcaneal (TCL) ligaments were found in 100% of the specimens, while the prevalence rates of other components lay within the range of 63.3–96.7% [28]. The tibionavicular

B. Hintermann, R. Ruiz, *Foot and Ankle Instability*, https://doi.org/10.1007/978-3-030-62926-7_5

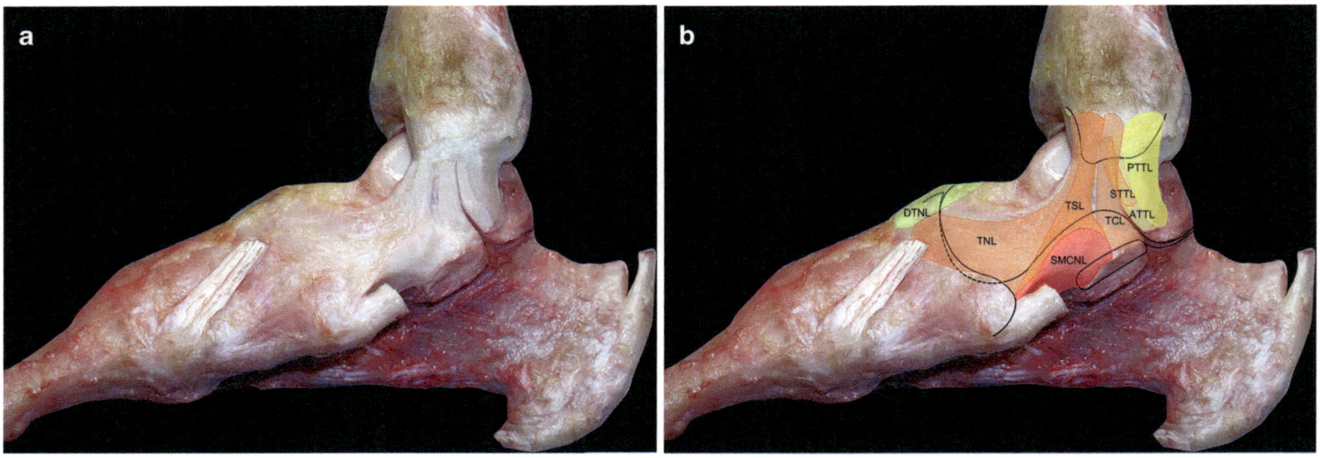

Fig. 5.1 Medial view of the foot and ankle. (**a**) The deltoid ligament spans from the medial malleolus to the navicular, talus, and calcaneus. It cannot be functionally separated from the plantar calcaneonavicular ligaments (Spring ligament). (**b**) The tibionavicular (TNL), tibiospring (TSL), tibiocalcaneal (TCL), and superficial posterior tibiotalar (STTL) ligaments form the superficial deltoid, whereas the deep anterior tibiotalar (ATTL) and the deep posterior tibiotalar (PTTL) ligaments form the deep deltoid. The tibiospring ligament (TSL) has a broad connection to the superomedial part of the spring ligament (SMCNL), building up a sling around the talar head. The tibionavicular ligament (TNL) is a thickening of the dorsomedial capsular of the talonavicular joint, as is the dorsal talonavicular ligament (DTNL) on the dorsolateral aspect of the joint

(TNL) and deep posterior tibiotalar ligaments (PTTL) were the thinnest and thickest, respectively, while the other ligaments had similar thicknesses. The possible absence of a component, particularly of the superficial layer, might compromise joint stability in acute ankle injuries [30].

As the tibioligamentous portion of the superficial deltoid has a broad insertion on the spring ligament (Fig. 5.1), this ligament complex may interplay with the deltoid ligament in terms of stabilizing the medial ankle joint and thus is functionally not separable from it.

5.1.1 Superficial Components of the Deltoid Ligament

The superficial deltoid ligament includes the tibionavicular (TNL), the tibiospring (TSL), the tibiocalcaneal (TCL), and the superficial posterior tibiotalar (STTL) ligaments (Fig. 5.1) [22, 23, 26, 28, 29].

5.1.1.1 The Tibionavicular Ligament

The tibionavicular ligament (TNL) forms the most anterior part of the deltoid ligament, originating from the anterior border of the anterior colliculus and inserting onto the dorsomedial aspect of the navicular bone; occasionally, its fibers extend onto the spring ligament (Fig. 5.1) [22, 23]. In up to 60% of the specimens, the TNL could not be identified as a separate ligament [22, 23, 26, 28, 29].

5.1.1.2 The Tibiospring Ligament

The tibiospring ligament (TSL) is the most superficial ligament, extending distally and almost perpendicularly from its origin on the medial malleolus, to form the most superficial attachment to the superior border of the plantar calcaneonavicular ligament (spring ligament) (Fig. 5.1) [1, 22, 23, 26, 28, 29].

5.1.1.3 The Tibiocalcaneal Ligament

The tibiocalcaneal Ligament (TCL) originates from the medial surface of the anterior colliculus and inserts onto the medial border of the sustentaculum tali (Fig. 5.1) [22, 23, 26, 28, 29], with a few fibers occasionally attaching to the spring ligament [26]. There is general agreement that the TCL is the strongest superficial component of the medial collateral ligament complex [25, 26, 28, 29].

5.1.1.4 The Superficial Posterior Tibiotalar Ligament

The superficial posterior tibiotalar ligament (STTL) originates from the intercollicular groove (medial surface of the posterior colliculus and the posterior part of the anterior colliculus) to attach to both the medial talar tubercle and the sustentaculum tali (Fig. 5.1) [25, 26, 28, 29].

5.1.2 Deep Components of the Deltoid Ligament

The deep deltoid ligament includes the deep anterior tibiotalar (ATTL) and the deep posterior tibiotalar (PTTL) ligaments (Fig. 5.1). Several authors [22, 23, 25, 26, 28, 29] have reported the presence of two deep tibiotalar ligaments (anterior and posterior), whereas others [27] have observed only a single deep ligament.

5.1.2.1 The Deep Posterior Tibiotalar Ligament

The deep posterior tibiotalar ligament (PTTL) originates from the intercollicular groove and inserts onto the medial surface of the talus under the tail of the articular facet. It may reach as far back as the posteromedial talar tubercle (Fig. 5.1) [26]. The PTTL is the only deep ligament that is observed consistently [22, 28, 29].

5.1.2.2 The Deep Anterior Tibiotalar Ligament

The deep anterior tibiotalar ligament (ATTL) originates on the anterior colliculus as well as the medial malleolus and inserts onto the medial surface of the talus, just distal to the anterior part of the medial articular facet (Fig. 5.1) [26, 29]. The ATTL has been described to be variable in size, sometimes being hardly discernible and sometimes completely absent [25, 28].

5.1.3 The Spring Ligament Complex

There is much confusion in the literature as to which anatomic structure is the true "spring ligament" (Figs. 5.2, and 5.3). Some investigators believe that this complex is formed by two major components [26, 31–35]: the superomedial calcaneonavicular ligament (SMNCL) and the inferior calcaneonavicular ligament (ICNL). Davis et al. [31], in a dissection study of 38 fresh-frozen feet, analyzed the anatomy of the spring ligament in more detail. They consistently observed a stronger and larger medial portion, the SMNCL, and a smaller lateral portion, the ICNL. While the SMCNL was found to have histologic properties that suggest significant load bearing, the histology of the ICNL suggested a pure tensile load function. The deltoid ligament and the PT

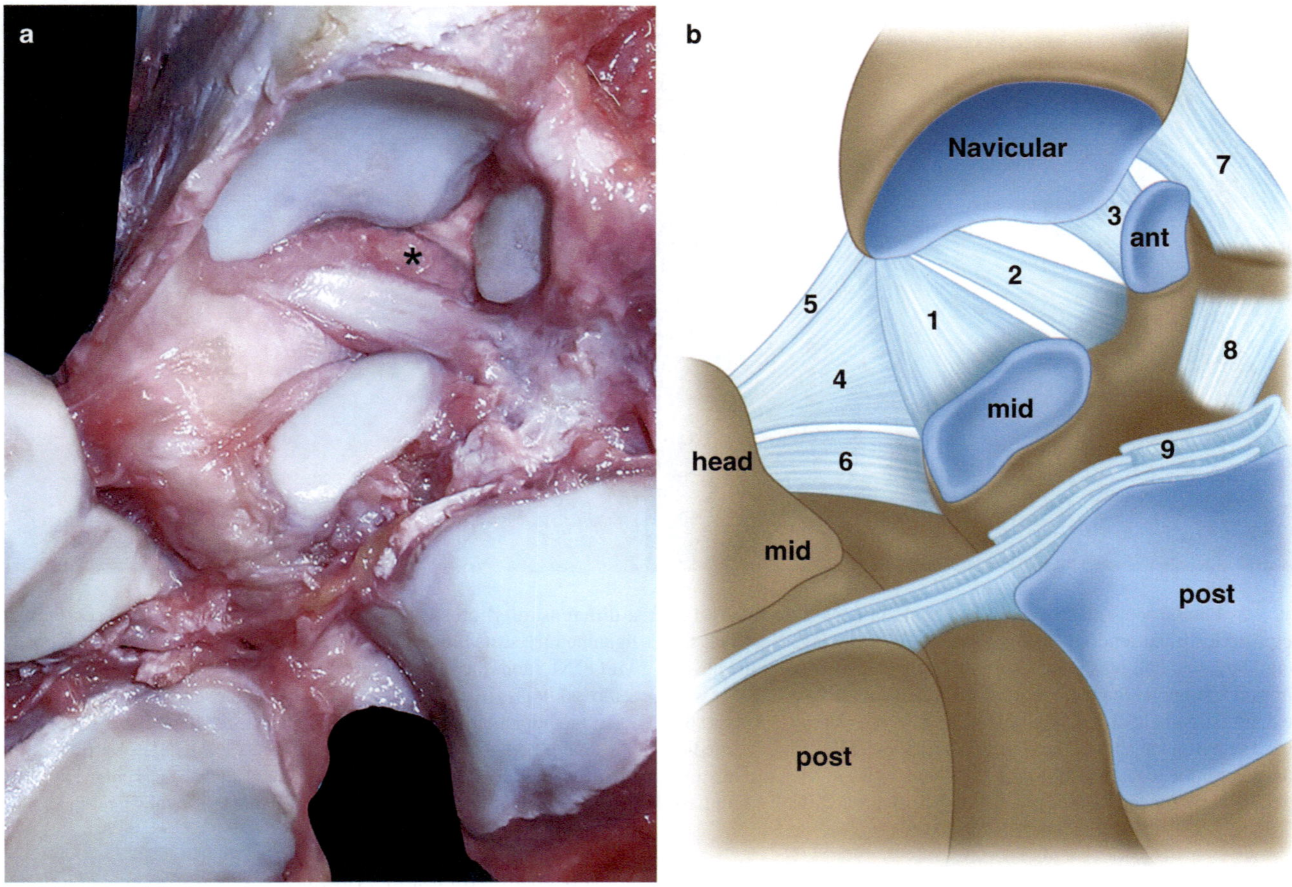

Fig. 5.2 Spring ligament complex, dorsal view after removal of the talus, exposing the acetabulum pedis. (**a**) Photograph, (**b**) Drawing. The spring ligament complex provides an articular surface for the talar head. Note the fibrocartilage that articulates with inferior and medial aspects of the talar head. The superomedial calcaneonavicular ligament (SMCNL, 1) has a broad attachment on the anteromedial margin of the middle facet of the sustentaculum tali, coursing anteriorly, upward and medially to the superomedial aspect of the navicular. With its triangular shape, it shares a broad insertion area with the tibiospring ligament (TSL, 4). Its smooth dorsal surface is covered with fibrocartilage and articulates with the medioplantar talar head. The medioplantar oblique calcaneonavicular ligament (MPOCNL; 2), which is composed of two bundles, arises from the coronoid fossa and courses obliquely in an anteromedial direction to attach onto or just below the navicular tuberosity. The inferior calcaneonavicular ligament (ICNL, 3) also arises from the coronoid fossa to the navicular beak, being clearly separated from the MPOCNL by fat tissue (Asterisk). 1 = superomedial calcaneonavicular ligament, 2 = medioplantar oblique calcaneonavicular ligament, 3 = inferior calcaneonavicular ligament, 4 = tibiospring ligament, 5 = tibionavicular ligament, 6 = tibiocalcaneal ligament, 7 = lateral calcaneonavicular ligament, 8 = cervical ligament, 9 = talocalcaneal interosseous ligament, ant = anterior calcaneal facet, mid = middle calcaneal facet, post = posterior calcaneal facet

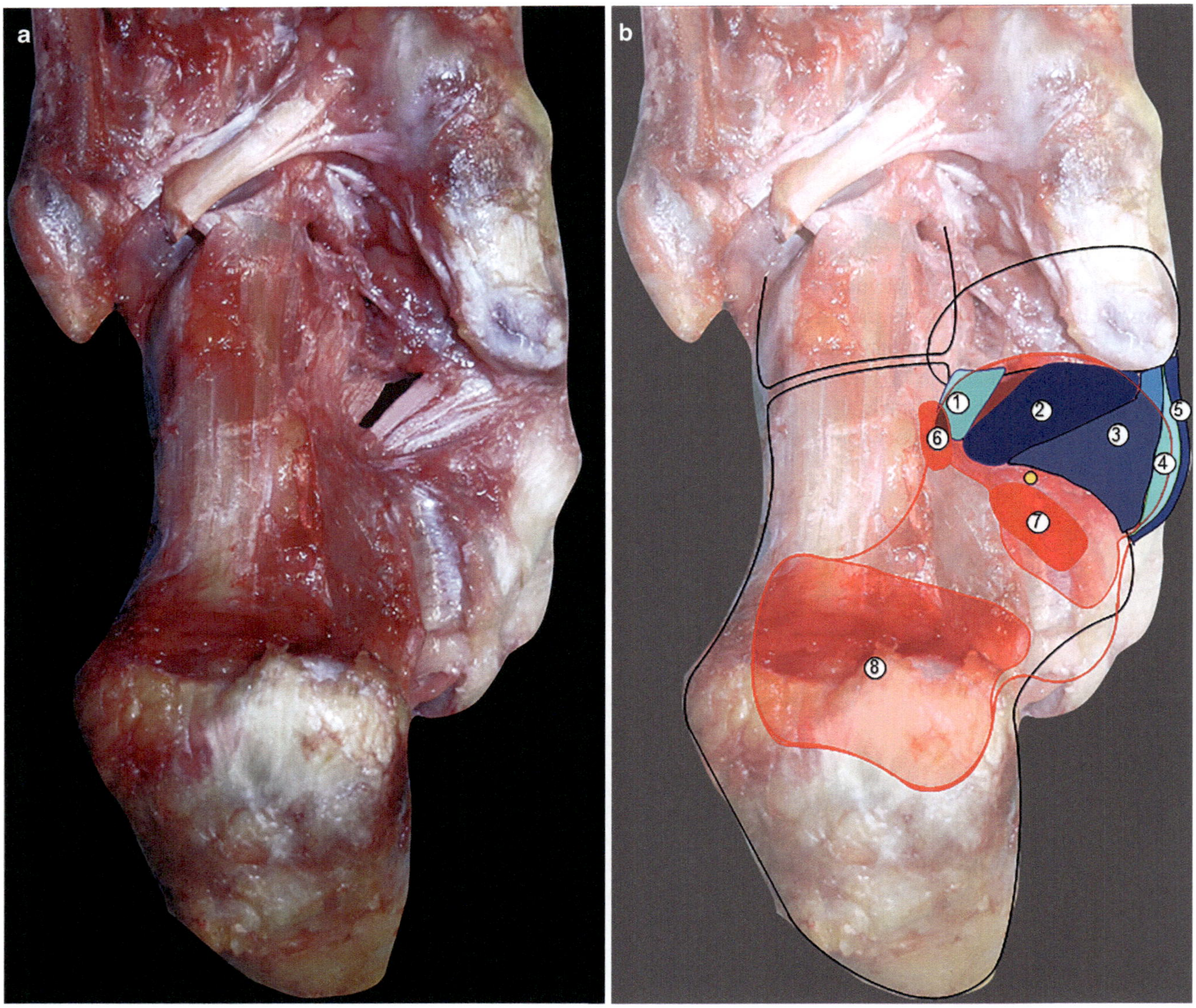

Fig. 5.3 Plantar view of the spring ligament complex after removal of the posterior tibial tendon. (**a**) Photograph, (**b**) Drawing. Note that the spring ligament complex connects the anterior calcaneus with the navicular, and it supports the major part of the talar head. It forms a sling with the deltoid ligament around the talar head, thus providing stability to the talus against plantarflexion and internal rotation. Fibers of the medioplantar oblique calcaneonavicular ligament (MPOCNL) are distinct from the superomedial calcaneonavicular ligament (SMCNL) and have a different insertion site on the navicular tuberosity. Between the two ligamentous structures, some fat can be found. The fat between the MPOCNL and the inferior calcaneonavicular ligament (ICNL) was removed in this image. 1 = inferior calcaneonavicular ligament (ICNL), 2 = medioplantar oblique calcaneonavicular ligament (MPOCNL), 3 = superomedial calcaneonavicular ligament (SMCNL), 4 = tibiospring ligament (TSL), 5 = talonavicular ligament (TNL), 6 = anterior calcaneal facet, 7 = middle calcaneal facet, 8 = posterior calcaneal facet

tendon had direct attachments to the SMCNL in all specimens. An articular facet composed of fibrocartilage was found in each SMCNL specimen.

More recently, Taniguchi and coworkers [35] reported a third component lying beneath the cartilaginous surface of the complex that is known as the medioplantar oblique calcaneonavicular ligament (MPOCNL); this finding has been further supported by other dissections and MRI studies [32, 33, 36]. Golano and coworkers [37] have described this ligament as being the medial fascicle of the ICNL, whereas they named the "true" ICNL as the lateral fascicle of the ICNL.

The spring ligament complex receives its blood supply from penetrating branches of the medial plantar artery and the calcaneal artery [31]. Indirect contributions arise at the sites of its ligamentous attachments to the navicular and sustentaculum tali. The central third of the spring ligament complex is largely avascular.

5.1.3.1 The Superomedial Calcaneonavicular Ligament

The superomedial calcaneonavicular ligament (SMCNL) originates from the superomedial aspect of the sustentacu-

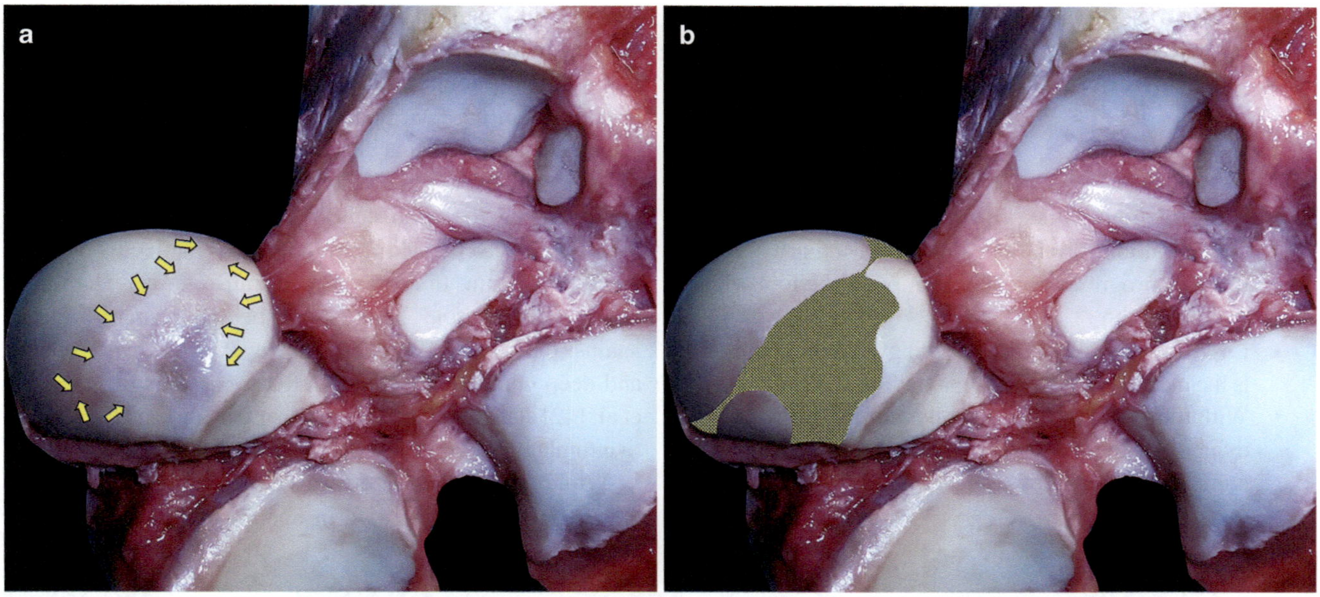

Fig. 5.4 Inferior view of the talar head and dorsal view of the acetabulum pedis. (**a**) The footprints of the spring ligament complex on the inferior articular surface of the talar head can be well seen, in particular in the area of the medioplantar oblique calcaneonavicular ligament (arrows). Note the poor quality of the cartilage in this area, which is thinner and uneven. (**b**) The footprints correspond well with the map of the spring ligament complex

lum tali and the anterior edge of the anterior facet of the calcaneus (Figs. 5.2, and 5.3) [26]. The triangular-shaped ligament fans out, concave laterally, to insert broadly on the edge of the navicular facet. In the contact area with the talar head, the SMCNL is covered by a poorly demarcated plate of fibrocartilaginous tissue, providing a smooth transitional surface for talar head articulation (Fig. 5.4) [31]. The central region of the articular surface of the ligament is thicker than the medial margin bordering the medioplantar oblique calcaneonavicular ligament [35]. The SMCNL is intimate with the posterior tibial tendon. The superficial fibers of the SMCNL are flattened by the posterior tibial tendon, which lies on its medial surface, and attach to the tendinous sheath thereof. The transitional zone between the SMCNL and the tibiospring ligament (TSL), a division of the superficial deltoid ligament, can be consistently seen [36].

5.1.3.2 The Medioplantar Oblique Calcaneonavicular Ligament

The medioplantar oblique calcaneonavicular ligament (MPOCNL) attaches between the anterior and middle facets of the calcaneus (coronoid fossa), in the sustentaculum tali, just inferior and slightly posterior to the attachment of the inferior calcaneonavicular ligament (ICNL). The fibers of the MPOCNL course obliquely in an anteromedial direction to attach to or just below the navicular tuberosity [26, 31]. While there is fatty tissue between its lateral border and the ICNL, its medial border is closely related to and sometimes inseparable from the SMCNL. The MPOCNL has a consistent striated and heterogeneous appearance with one to three bundles and can be clearly visualized on removal of the talus and the fibrocartilage that covers the spring ligament complex. It is the thinnest portion of the spring ligament complex [32, 35, 36].

In contrast to Sarrafian [26] who described this ligament as representing the ICNL and being the true spring ligament, Davis et al. [31] questioned, as others [38], the term spring ligament, as "the two structures (SMCN and ICN ligaments) appear grossly and histologically more like a sling than a spring" [31]. According to Gray [39], there is no real evidence that the spring ligament is particularly resilient, and Hardy [38] reported that the plantar calcaneonavicular ligament is a purely collagenous ligament and does not possess elastic properties.

The interlaced fibers of the two ligaments form a gentle concavity around the talar head [31]. Thereby the SMCNL, MPOCNL, and the superficial deltoid (TSL and TNL) create a complex of ligaments that support the talar head and stabilize the talocalcaneonavicular joint. A relationship between laxity of this ligament complex and medial ankle instability has been suggested [10].

5.1.3.3 The Inferior Calcaneonavicular Ligament

The inferior calcaneonavicular ligament (ICNL), which constitutes the lateral part of the spring ligament fibrocartilage complex, is a strip-like bundle of wide and short fibers that originate in the notch between the anterior and middle facets of the calcaneus and terminate on the navicular beak.

The ICNL is completely separated from the MPOCNL by fatty tissue and is the thickest component of the spring ligament complex [32, 33, 35, 36].

5.2 Biomechanics of Medial Ankle Instability (Including Spring Ligament)

- As the deltoid is the primary restraint against talar abduction and pronation, loss of its integrity may result in progressive destabilization of the foot with overpronation
- Loss of support of the deltoid-spring ligament complex is the main underlying cause of flatfoot deformity
- With their tendons, the deep flexor muscles act as a dynamic support of the deltoid-spring ligament complex

The deltoid ligament and the spring ligament complex work as one functional unit, each playing its specific role.

Close [40] found the deltoid ligament to be a strong restraint, limiting talar abduction. With all lateral structures removed, he found that the intact deltoid ligament allows only 2 mm of spreading between the talus and medial malleolus. When the deep deltoid ligament was released, the talus could be separated from the medial malleolus by a distance of 3.7 mm. In contrast to Rasmussen [41], Harper [3] claimed the deltoid ligament to be the primary restrain against pronation of the talus, however, with the superficial and deep components equally effective in this regard. Nigg et al. [42] stated that the deltoid ligament appears to be sensitive to plantarflexion, external rotation, and pronation.

While early studies described the posterior fibers of the deltoid ligament as being tight in dorsiflexion and the anterior

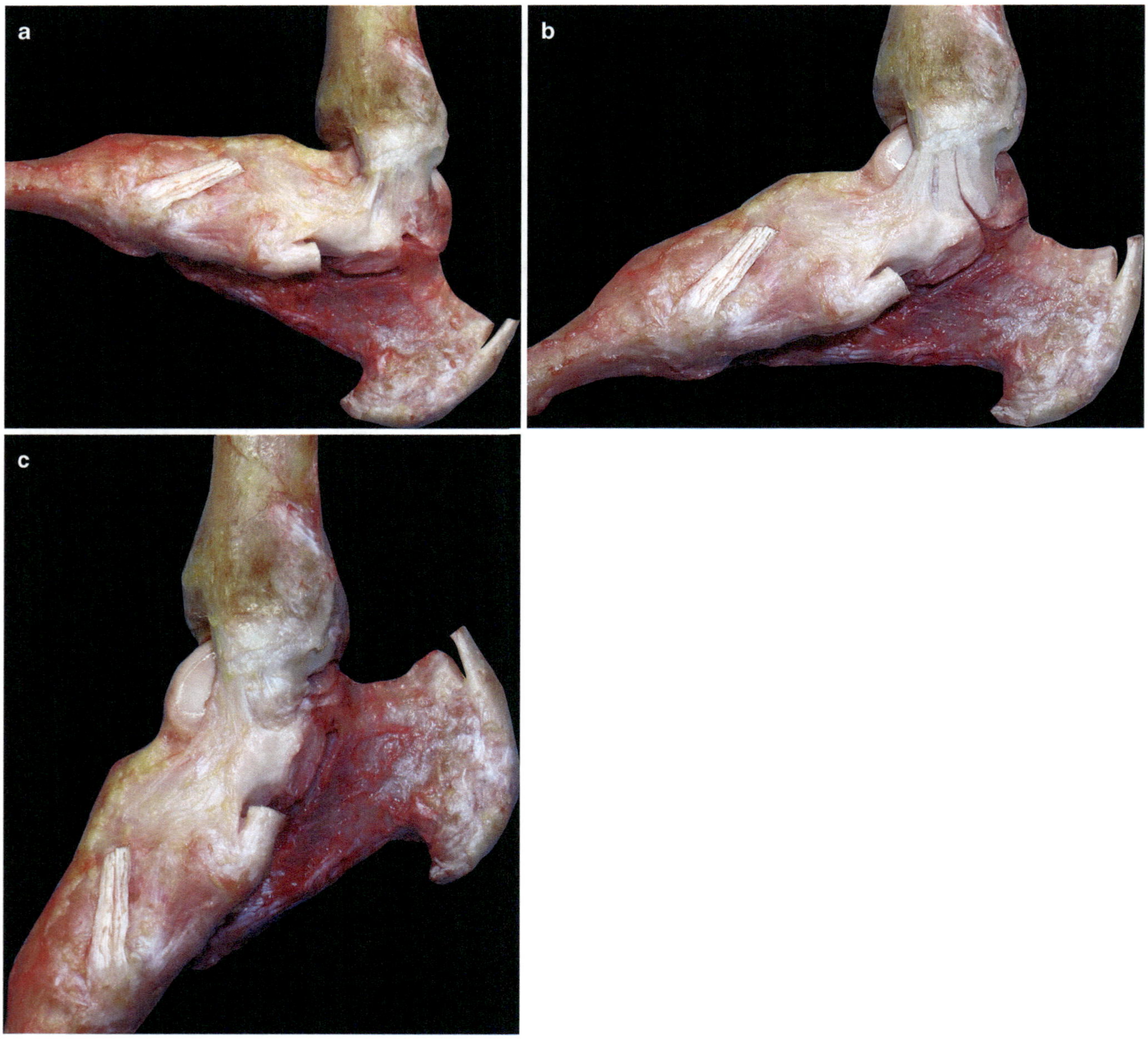

Fig. 5.5 Medial view of the foot and ankle showing the position of the deltoid ligament. (**a**) dorsiflexion, (**b**) neutral position, (**c**) plantarflexion. Note the changes of position and tension of the different portions of the deltoid ligament during the range of sagittal plane motion

fibers in plantarflexion [43], other studies reported movements that show a more isometric pattern of elongation of the TCL compared with both the TNL and STTL (Fig. 5.5) [44–46].

Hintermann et al. [47] and Sommer et al. [48], studied in vitro, the role of the ankle ligaments in the coupling mechanism between the foot and the leg, especially in transferring movement between calcaneal eversion/inversion and tibial rotation. While sectioning of the lateral ligaments did not significantly affect the tibial rotation and foot eversion-inversion for a given dorsi-plantarflexion, deltoid ligament resection highly changed the movement transfer, especially during plantarflexion. Apparently, the coupling mechanism of the ankle joint complex does markedly depend on the integrity of the deltoid ligament.

Earll et al. [2] found that the TCL sectioning produced the greatest changes in both the contact area (decreased up to 43%) and peak pressure (increased up to 30%). Siegler et al. [27] reported the increasing order of ultimate load to be TCL, TNL, and STTL. These observations emphasize the role of the TCL in guiding ankle rotations on the medial side, similar to the calcaneofibular (CFL) ligament on the lateral side.

The static soft tissue restraints of the medial longitudinal arch include the spring ligament complex, superficial deltoid ligament, medial talonavicular joint capsule, plantar fascia, and the talocalcaneal ligament. Several ligaments were found to have pathological changes in patients with adult acquired flatfoot deformities; however, the spring ligament complex and talocalcaneal interosseous ligament were most frequently implicated [19]. All patients with posterior tibial tendon insufficiency demonstrated some degree of spring ligament complex attenuation on MRI and 74% were diagnosed with a spring ligament tear. Although posterior tibial tendon dysfunction is the most common cause of flatfoot deformity, traumatic rupture of the spring ligament complex without posterior tibial tendon dysfunction has also been reported to result in flatfoot deformity [49–51].

5.3 Conclusions and Clinical Implications

- Besides maintaining medial ankle stability, the superficial portion of the medial ankle ligaments play a significant role in maintaining rotational ankle stability
- Besides maintaining medial ankle stability in the coronal plane, the deep portion of the deltoid ligament plays a significant role in maintaining rotational medial ankle stability
- Besides preventing foot pronation, the deltoid-spring ligament complex plays a crucial role in the maintenance of the plantar arch

Obviously, besides maintaining medial ankle stability, the superficial portion of the medial ankle ligaments play a significant role in maintaining rotational ankle stability. It has been shown that the loss of the TNL and TSL leads to a measurable increase in eversion/pronation without any tilting of the talus or gapping of the subtalar joint [41, 42, 52]. It has also been shown that the loss of the TNL and the TSL allows an increase in internal rotation of the leg [53]. In fact, the loss of the TNL and TSL restraint unlocks the subtalar joint, allowing further eversion/pronation. It is this increase in eversion/pronation and probably also some laxity of the anterior talofibular (ATFL) ligament that may lead to symptomatic instability. Keeping this in mind, no tilting is necessary at either ankle or subtalar levels to experience functional instability. The question however remains, to which extent this pronation movement is physiological. Boss et al. [22] and Hintermann et al. [10] described the interval as a conjunction of a tiny layer of connective fibers between the TCL and TSL. It has been suggested that these two ligaments get separated distinctly until the connecting fibers within the interval become tightened, thereby working as dynamic restraints against pronation force (Fig. 5.6). A lesion along this interval was found in 37 of 52 patients (71%) who experienced symptomatic medial ankle instability [10].

The deep portion of the deltoid ligament (ATTL and PTTL) plays a significant role in maintaining rotational medial ankle stability. It has been shown that loss of the ATTL and PTTL leads to a measurable increase of talus tilting while the foot is loaded [40]. With this, the talus progressively disconnects from the tibia and furthermore, the pivoting of the talus along the medial malleolus will be lost. This leads to a lateral shift of the center of rotation and thus a lateral shift of the articular load. These changes of biomechanics are detrimental for the integrity of the ankle joint complex and will result in progressive deformation and destabilization of the hindfoot, leading to overload of the lateral tibiotalar joint [2]. This process may become particularly critical with the loss of the PT function and subsequent chronic overload as well as degenerative disease of its tendon.

A crucial role in the stabilization mechanism of the talocalcaneonavicular (peritalar) joint may be attributed to the spring ligament. Furthermore, the SMCNL, MPOCNL, and ICNL create, in conjunction with the superficial deltoid (TSL and TNL), a complex of ligaments which support the talar head and thereby stabilize the medial ankle and peritalar joints. Moreover, recent studies have shown that besides preventing the foot pronation, the deltoid-spring ligament complex plays a crucial role in the plantar arch maintenance [54, 55]. While the posterior tibial tendon dynamically supports this ligament function (Fig. 5.7), it only plays a secondary role in the plantar arch maintenance, thus not being able to protect the foot against progressive flatfoot development once the ligamentous structures have failed [19, 56].

The PT muscle is the most powerful subtalar invertor, it has the longest moment arm and the largest physiologic cross-sec-

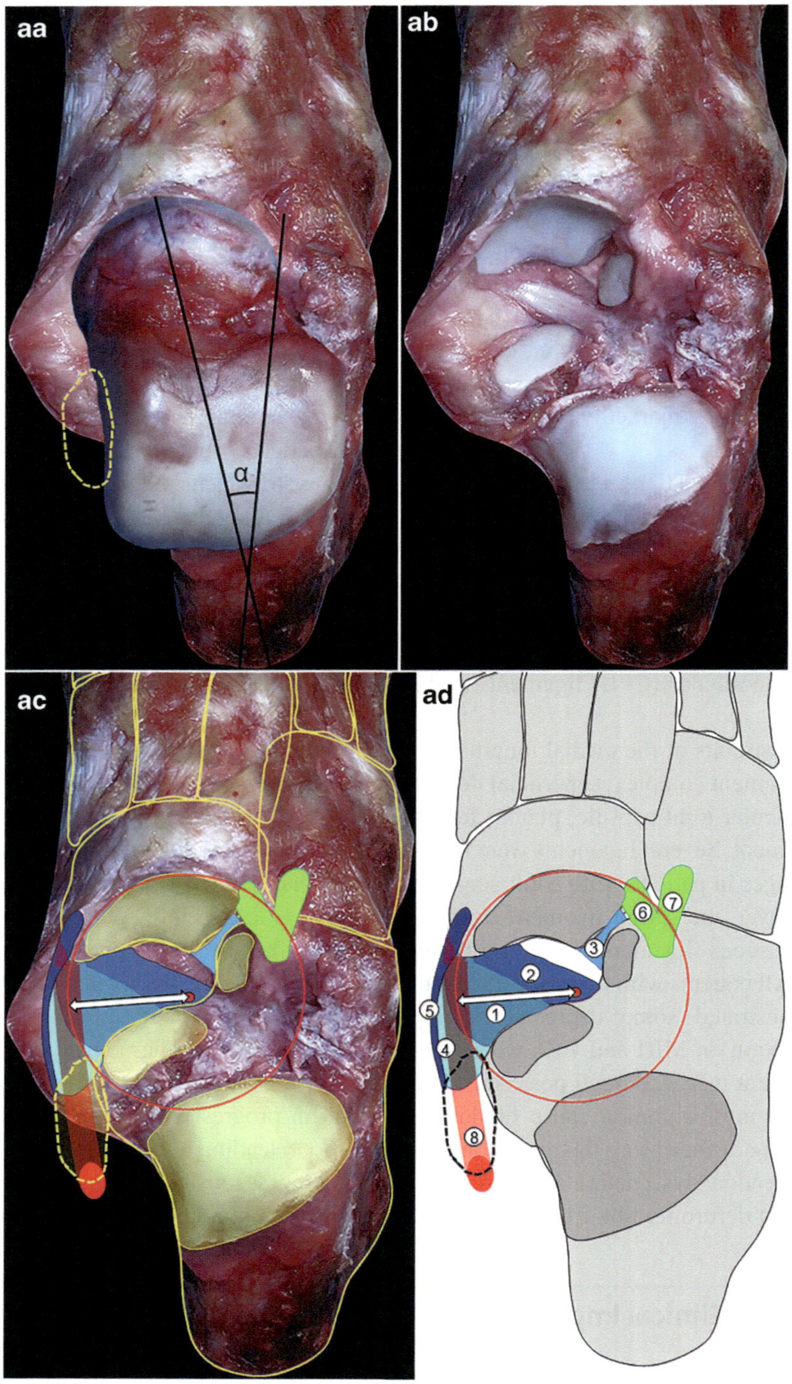

Fig. 5.6 Dorsal view of the coxa pedis showing the calcaneonavicular (spring) ligament complex in the various foot positions. (**A**) Neutral foot position: (**aa**) The talus is sitting on top of the calcaneus with a talocalcaneal angle α of 22°. The dotted yellow line shows the position of the medial malleolus. (**ab**) Situs of the facets of the calcaneus and the articular surface of the navicular after removal of the talus. (**ac**) The spring ligament forms, in conjunction with parts of the superficial deltoid and bifurcate ligament, a strong ligamentous construct which supports and surrounds the talar head, thus providing support and stability. Note the missing bony support of the talar head on the medial side, where the spring and tibiospring ligaments (TSL) provide the support and stabilization. As the tibiocalcaneal ligament (TCL) is in loose contact with the TSL through the interval, the TCL does not provide restrain against abduction of the forefoot, e.g., external rotation of the talonavicular (TN) joint about its own rotational axis. The posterior tibial (PT) tendon runs beneath the superomedial calcaneonavicular ligament (SMCNL) and TSL, thus having a leverage to the axis of rotation of the TN joint, which corresponds to the size of the radius of the circle given by the TN joint. (**ad**) Drawing, as (**ac**). (**B**) Foot in pronation: (**ba**) The talocalcaneal angle α has increased to 32°. (**bb**) The acetabulum pedis has opened medially. (**bc**) The line of action of the PT tendon has moved laterally, thus its leverage to the center of rotation of the TN joint has decreased substantially. (**bd**) Drawing, as (**bc**). (**C**) Foot in supination: (**ca**) the talocalcaneal angle α has decreased to 10°. (**cb**) The medial side of the acetabulum pedis has closed, e.g., the distance between the anterior facet of the calcaneus and the tuberosity of the navicular has decreased. (**cc**) The direction of the medioplantar oblique calcaneonavicular ligament (MPOCNL), the SMCNL, and TSL has changed, as the navicular tuberosity has approached the medial malleolus. Note the line of action of the PT tendon with an increased leverage about the axis of rotation of TN joint when compared to the foot in pronation. (**cd**) Drawing, as (**cc**). 1 = superomedial calcaneonavicular ligament (SMCNL), 2 = medioplantar oblique calcaneonavicular ligament (MPOCNL), 3 = inferior calcaneonavicular ligament (ICNL), 4 = tibiospring ligament (TSL), 5 = tibionavicular ligament (TNL), 6 lateral calcaneonavicular ligament (LCNL), 7 = medial calcaneocuboid ligament (MCCL), 8 = posterior tibial (PT) tendon

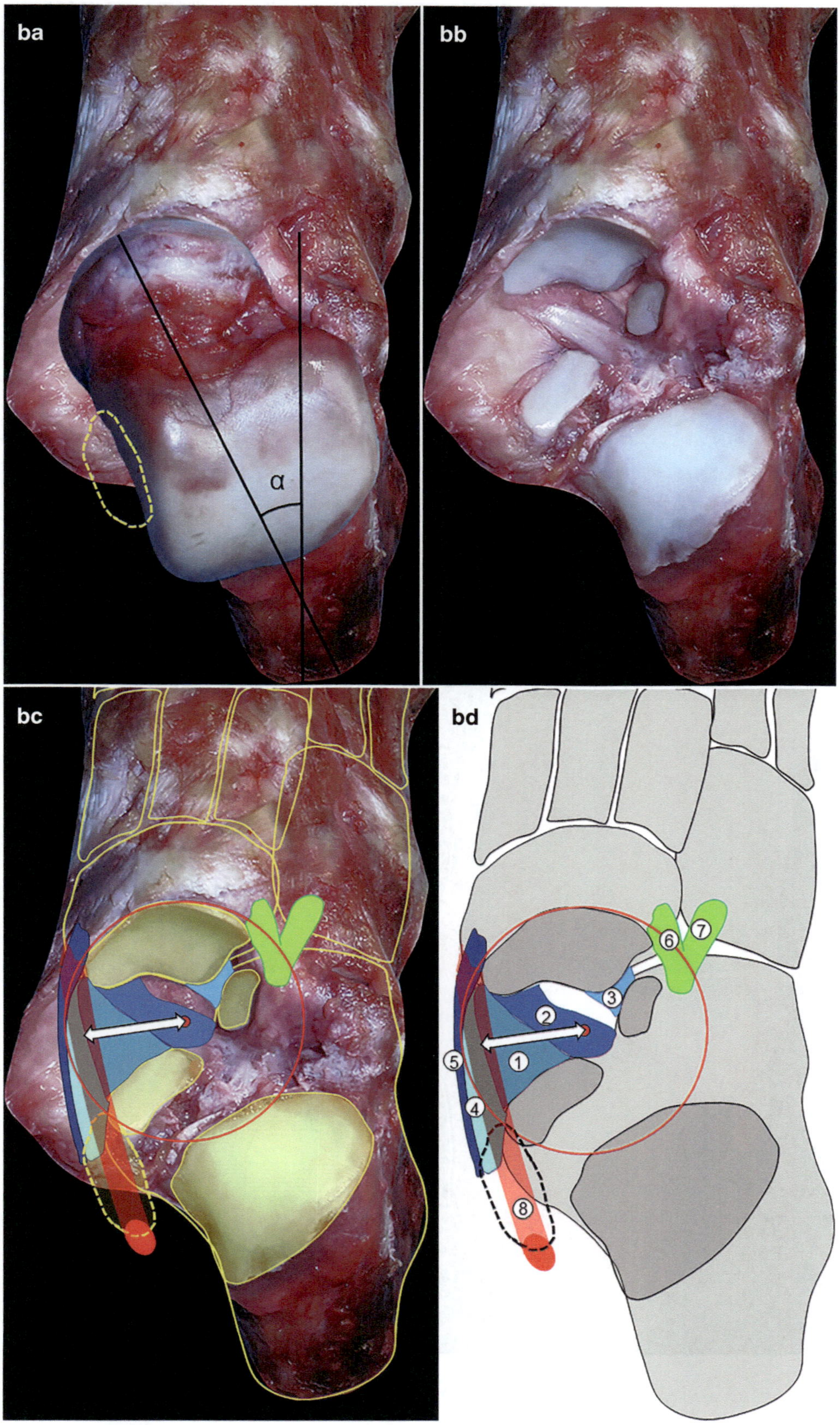

Fig. 5.6 (continued)

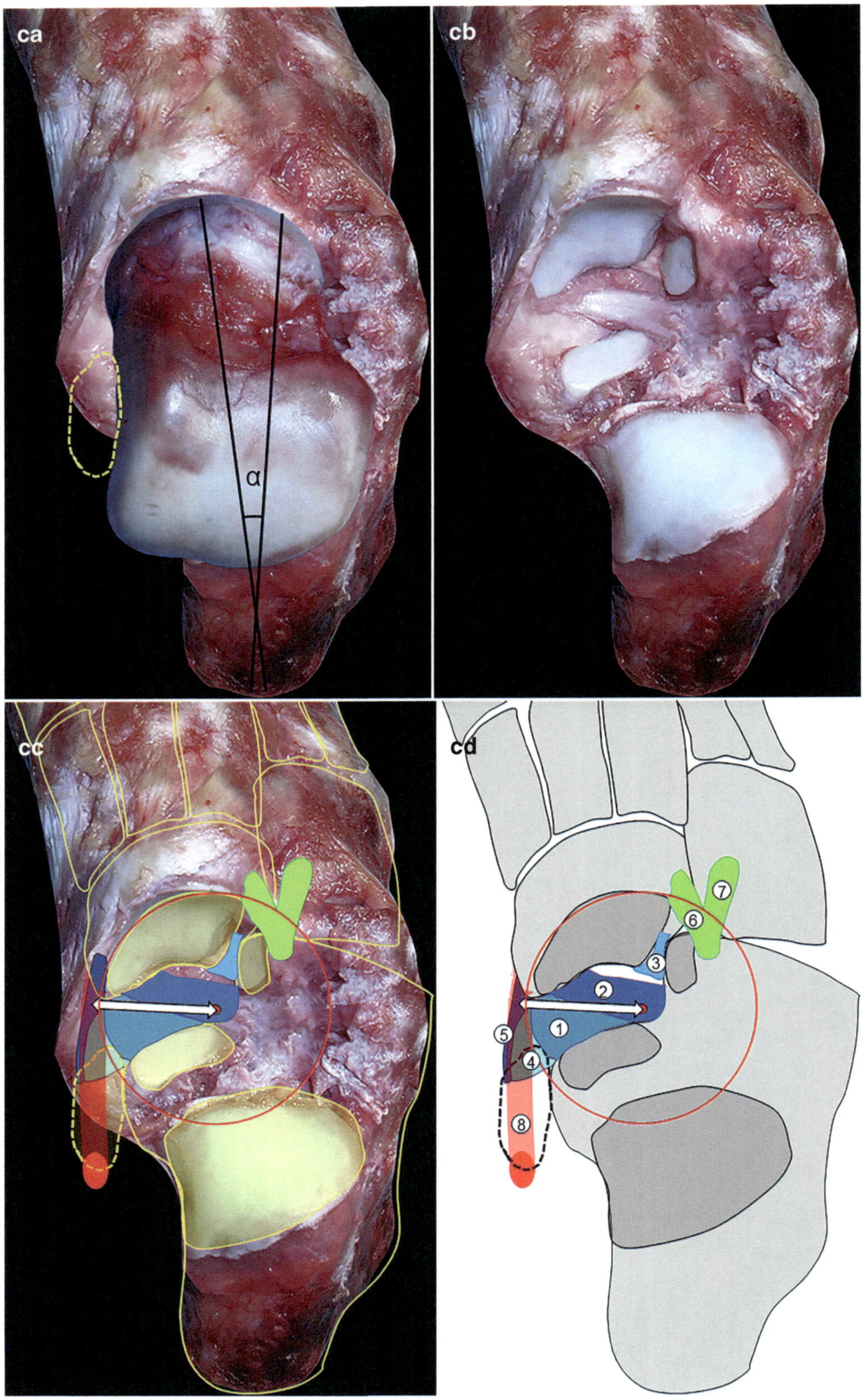

Fig. 5.6 (continued)

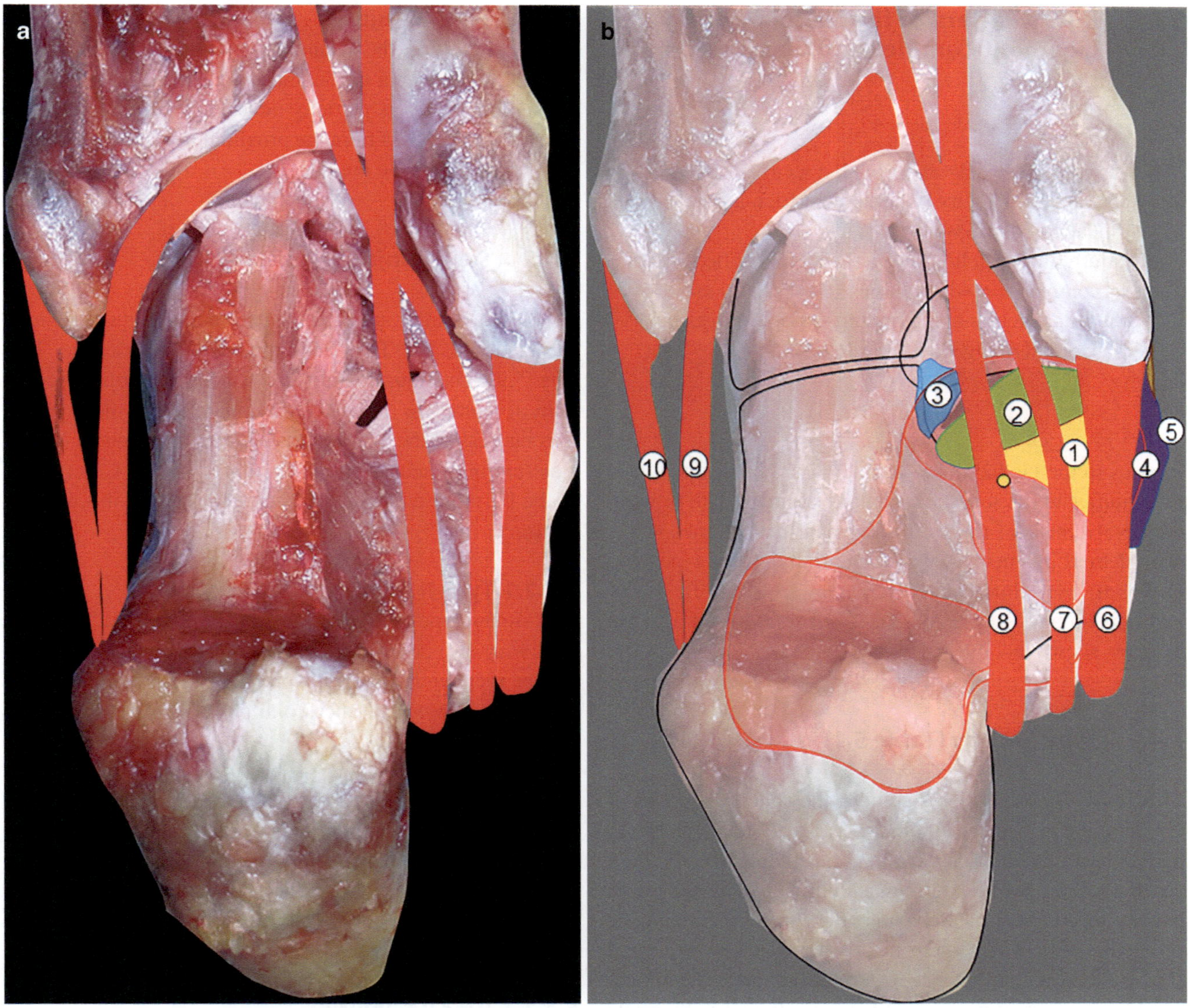

Fig. 5.7 Plantar view (same specimen as Fig. 5.6). (**a**) The posterior tibial (PT, 6), flexor digitorum longus (FDL, 7), and flexor hallucis longus (FHL, 8) tendons run beneath the spring ligament complex, thus being active stabilizers and supporting this ligament complex. On the lateral side, they are opposed to the peroneus brevis (PB, 10) and peroneus longus (PL, 9) tendons. (**b**) The PT muscle has the longest lever to the center of rotation of the talonavicular joint (yellow circle). 1 = superomedial calcaneonavicular ligament (SMCNL), 2 = medioplantar oblique calcaneonavicular ligament (MPOCNL), 3 = inferior calcaneonavicular ligament (ICNL), 4 = tibiospring ligament (TSL), 5 = tibionavicular ligament (TNL)

tion [57, 58]. During gait, when the foot is on firm ground, the PT tendon will not be able to produce plantar flexion, internal rotation nor inversion of the foot; however, it will instead push the medial malleolus forward, providing an external rotation moment on the leg. This external rotation of the leg is transmitted to the talus, moving its head laterally. The navicular follows the talar head, so the medial column is placed over the lateral column. By this active mechanism, the foot converts into a rigid structure for propulsion, a stiff lever to allow for the Achilles-calcaneus plantar system to push-off. Failure to achieve external rotation of the leg during the stance phase will fail to externally rotate the talus, thus first, the medial column will suffer medial plantar tensile stress for which it is not prepared to cope with, and second, the force provided by the Achilles tendon will not act on the metatarsophalangeal break line but on the midtarsal joint, contributing to the pronatory deforming forces.

5.4 Injury Pattern of the Deltoid-Spring Ligament Complex and Classification

- Injuries to the deltoid-spring ligament includes various types of injury patterns for which a new classification is proposed
- Injuries to the deltoid ligament complex often occur in combination with injuries to other structures of the foot, such as ankle fractures, syndesmosis injuries, or lateral ligament injuries

Injuries to the medial ankle ligaments can be differentiated into injuries to the superficial deltoid ligament with or without involvement of the spring ligament and injuries to the deep deltoid ligament. A classification into three types was proposed by Hintermann et al. in 2003 [10]. Later, Hintermann and Ruiz (FAC 2021, *in press*) added a fourth Type, as shown in Table 5.1.

5.4.1 Type I-Injury (Table 5.1)

This most common injury includes the superficial layer of the deltoid ligament at its tibial periosteal attachment with partial discontinuity, delamination or a complete tear with or without lesion of the flexor retinaculum. Typically, the lesion is seen to continue caudally into the interval between the TSL and TCL. These were mostly found to be separated (Fig. 5.8). As a consequence, external rotation at the talonavicular joint increases and the tibia tends to internally rotate when the foot is loaded. Often, PT muscle activation is able to compensate for this deformity.

5.4.1.1 Type I A-Injury

This injury type includes the TNL and TSL. Typically, a delamination of the deep ligament portion at the tibial insertion is found, while the superficial fibers may remain intact. In most instances, the tear extends distally, resulting in a partial tear of the interval.

5.4.1.2 Type I B-Injury

In this injury type, the tear extends further to the TCL, which is also partially detached from its tibial insertion, showing a partial delamination. The anterior colliculus of the medial malleolus is free from ligaments, leaving just a tiny superficial layer of the TNL and TSL left at the proximal insertion site. In contrast to Type I A-injuries, the remaining ligaments are typically thickened and show transmural scar formation. In most instances, the tear extends into the interval.

5.4.1.3 Type I C-Injury

In this injury type, the delamination of the TCL involves the whole insertion area at the anterior colliculus, leaving just the superficial layers partially intact. The TNL and TSL are completely detached from the proximal insertion site and the tear also involves the interval.

5.4.2 Type II-Injury (Table 5.1)

This less common injury is located mainly within the midsubstance of the TSL and may also include the TNL (Fig. 5.9). The injury pattern can vary from partial discontinuity to complete rupture. As a consequence, the ligamentous buttress of the talar head is lost when the foot is loaded, resulting in pronation and abduction of the foot. Activation of the PT muscle may partially compensate for this deforming force.

5.4.2.1 Type II A-Injury

This injury type consists of a partial tear of the TSL. The TNL may also be involved. The resulting incompetence can best be seen while the foot is pronated and/or the forefoot is abducted. In most instances, the posterior part of the TSL remains intact.

5.4.2.2 Type II B-Injury

The TSL shows a complete tear that allows direct visualization of the talar neck and sometimes even the proximal articular surface of the medial talar head. The resulting defect is typically small and can be closed while the foot is held in supinated and adducted position.

5.4.2.3 Type II C-Injury

The tear also involves part of the TCL, resulting in a major defect that cannot be closed by holding the foot in a supinated and adducted position.

5.4.3 Type III-Injury (Table 5.1)

The injury is located distally at the insertion to the navicular and involves mainly the distal part of the TNL, TSL, SMCNL, and MPOCNL (Fig. 5.10a). The rupture may continue along the navicular with avulsion of the PT tendon at its insertion to the tuberosity of the navicular bone (Fig. 5.10b). This configuration is often seen in the presence of an accessory external tibial bone that is detached along its connection to the navicular bone (Fig. 5.11). As a consequence, the support of the talar head is lost when the foot is loaded, which results in plantarflexion of the talus and abduction as well as pronation of the foot, whereas activation of PT muscle, depending on its involvement in the injury, may be able to resist partially against the

Table 5.1 Classification of injury patterns to the deltoid-spring ligament complex

Type I-Lesion

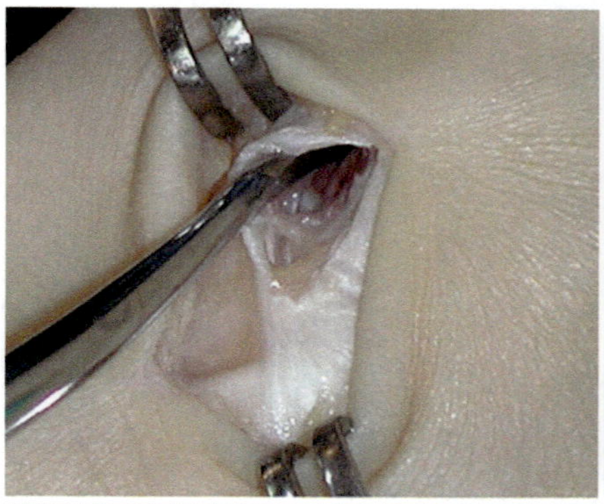	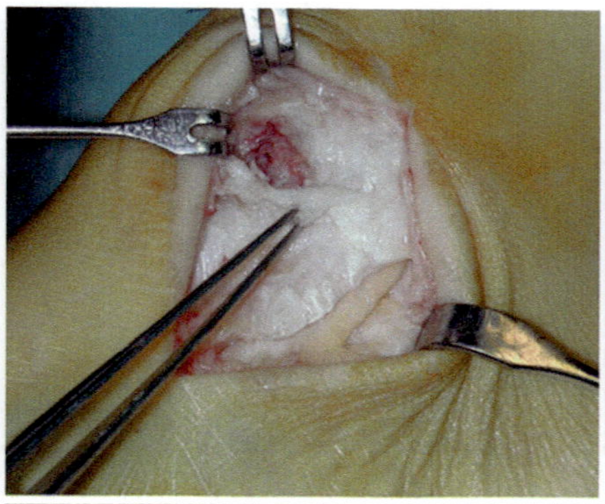	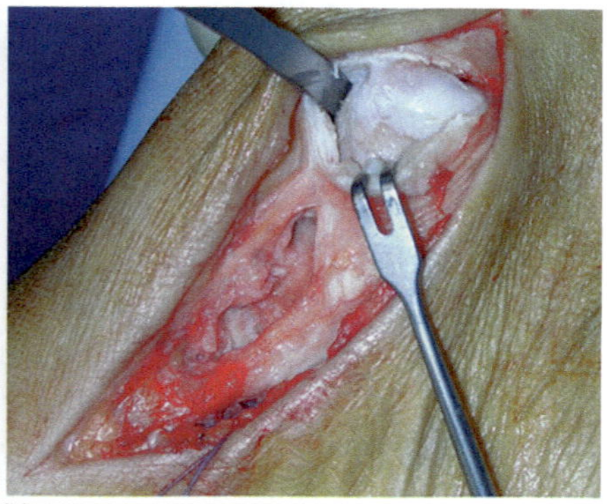
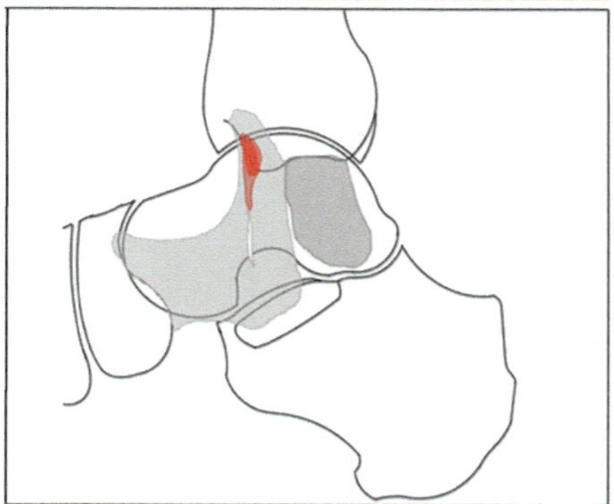	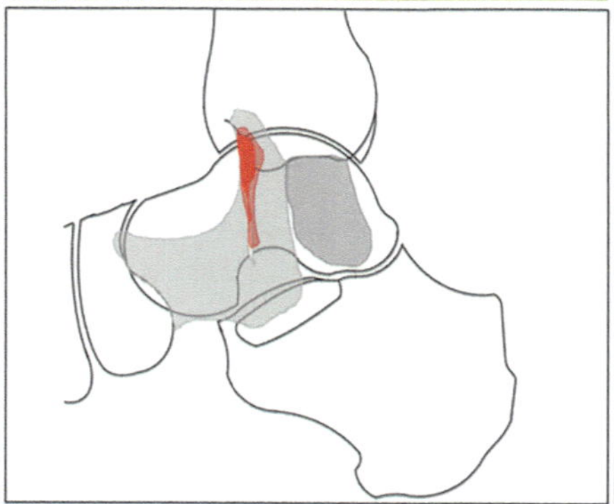	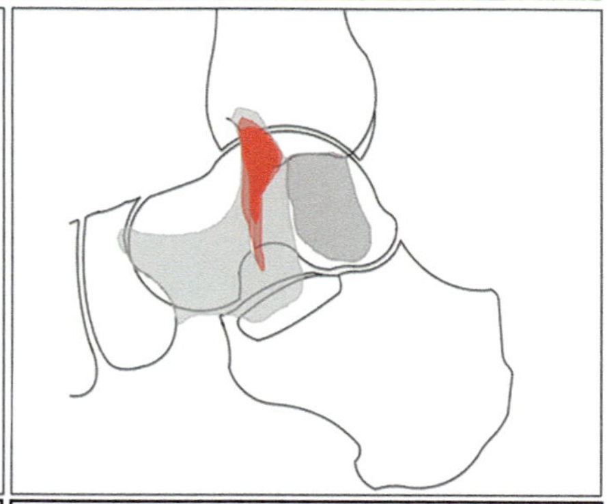
Delamination of TNL and TSL from proximal insertion, partial tear of interval	Avulsion of TNL, TSL and partial TCL from proximal insertion, (partial) tear of interval	Avulsion of TNL, TSL and TCL from proximal insertion, tear of interval

Type II-Lesion

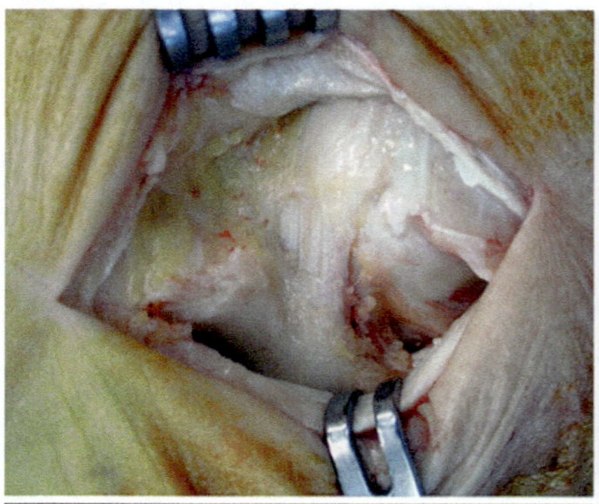	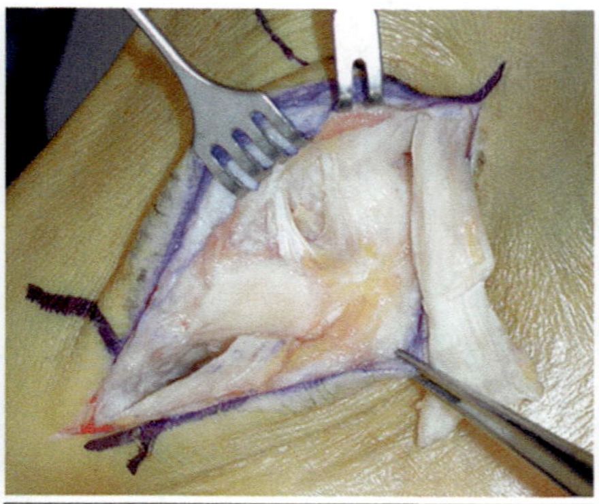	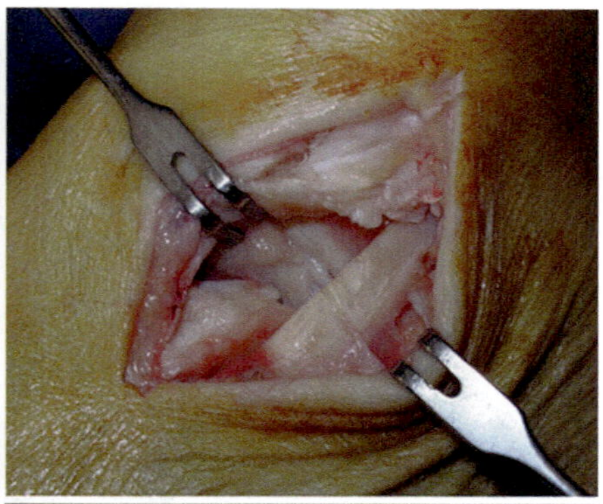
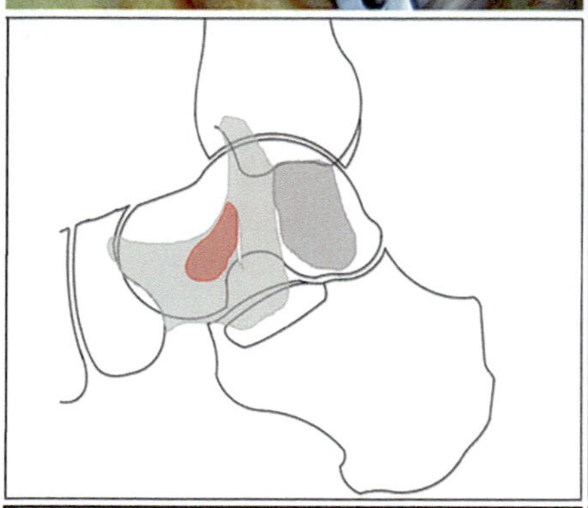	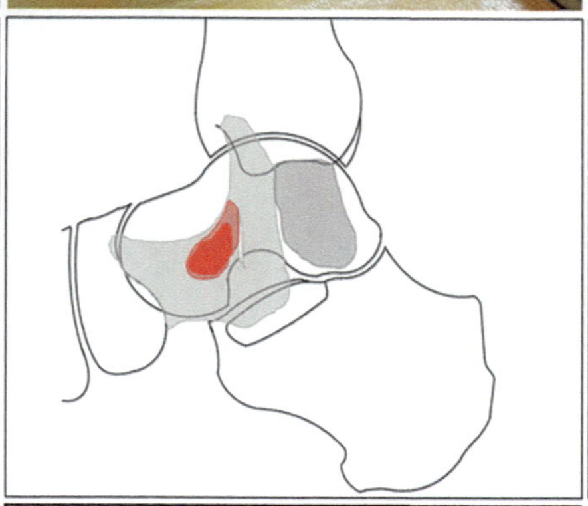	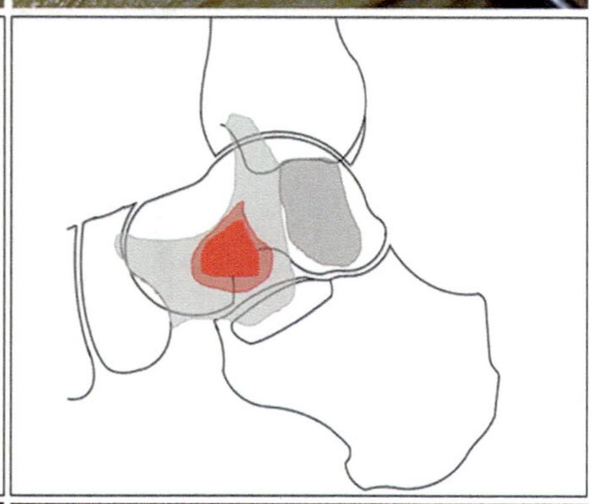
Partial tear of TNL and TSL, resulting in partial discontinuity	Complete tear of TSL that can be closed while the foot is supinated/adducted	Complete tear of TSL that cannot be closed while the foot is supinated/adducted

Table. 5.1 (continued)

Type III-Lesion

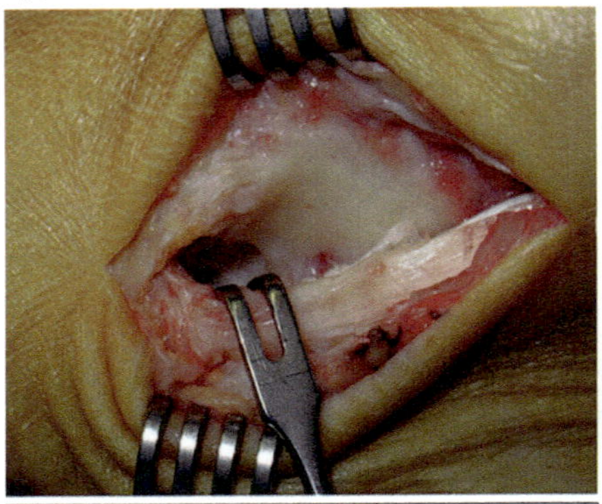	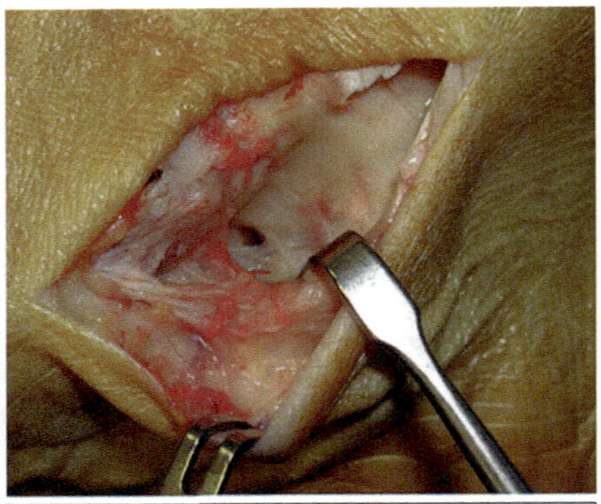	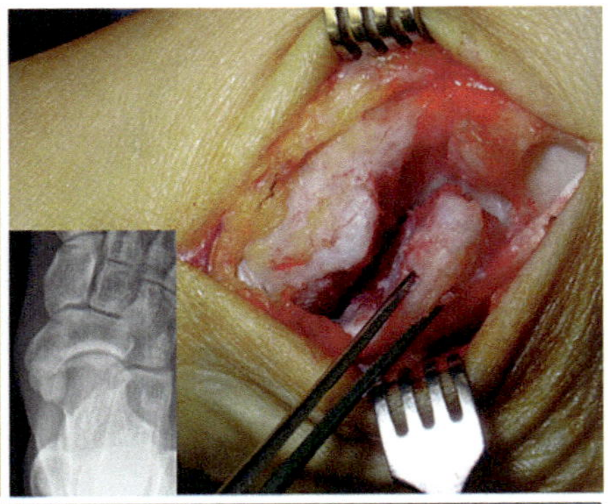
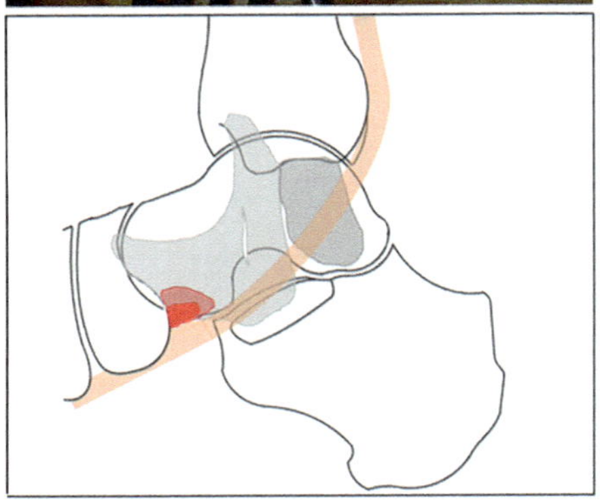	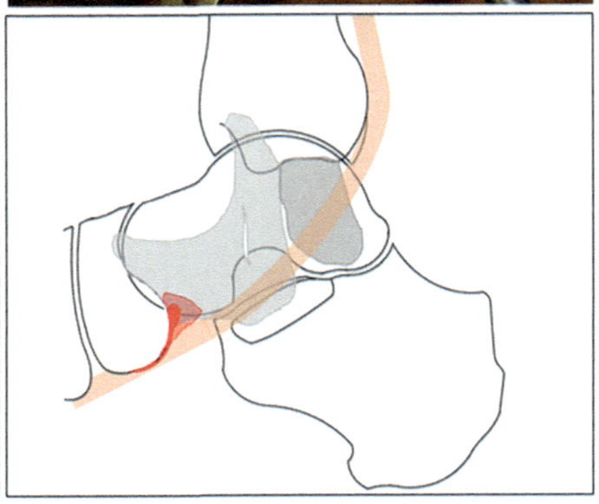	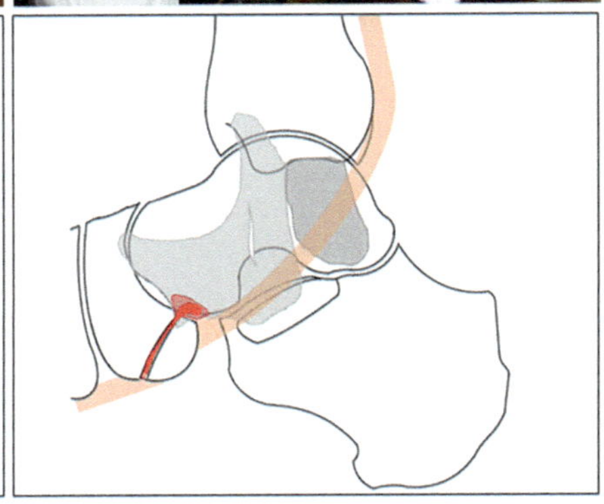
Isolated avulsion of MPOCNL and SMCNL from navicular, PT tendon intact	(Partial) avulsion of MPOCNL and SMCNL from navicular, avulsion of PT tendon from navicular	Bony avulsion of PT tendon, partial tear of SMCNL and MPOCNL from navicular

Type IV-Lesion

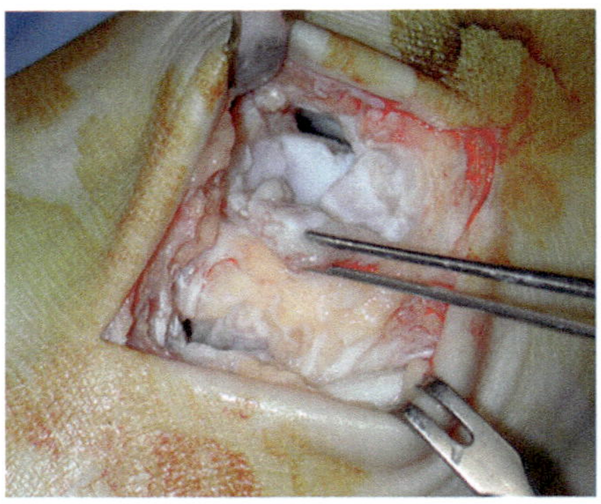	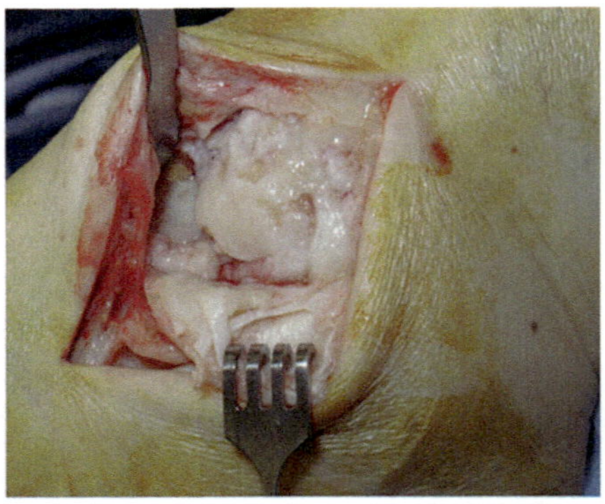	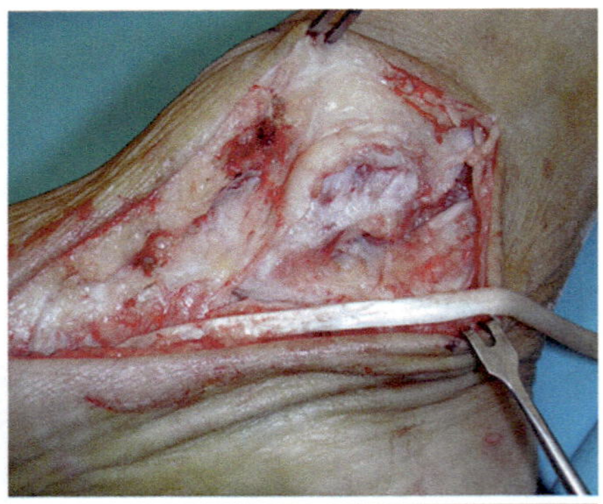
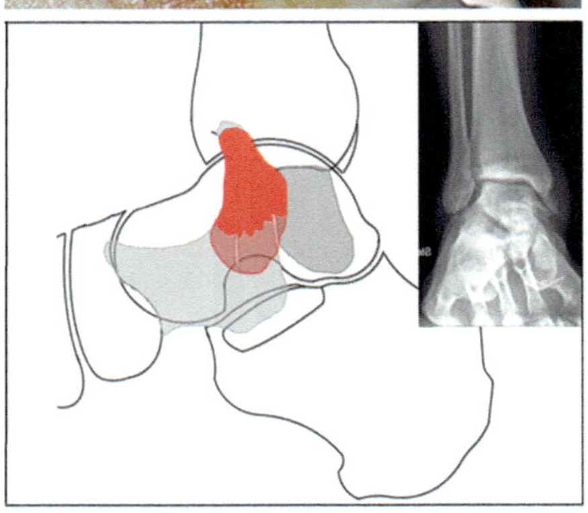	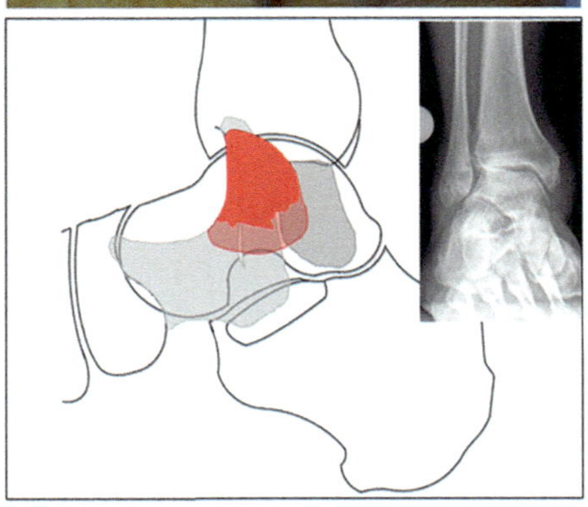	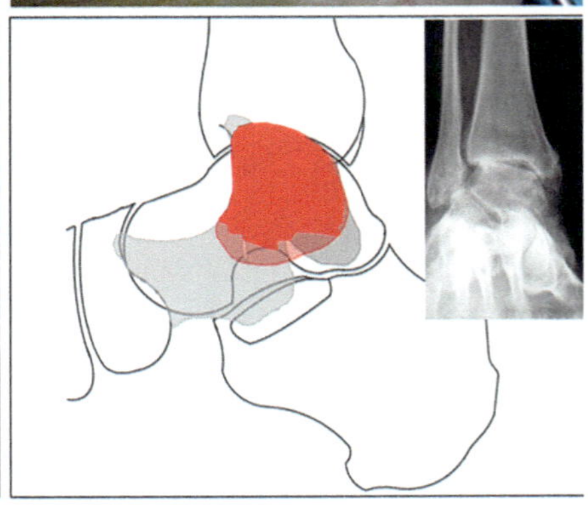
Avulsion of TNL, TSL, TCL and STTL, partial tear of ATTL; Talar tilt < 5°	Avulsion of TNL, TSL, TCL, STTL, and ATTL, partial tear of PTTL; Talar tilt < 10°	Tear of whole deltoid (TNL, TSL, TCL, STTL, ATTL and PTTL); Talar tilt > 10°

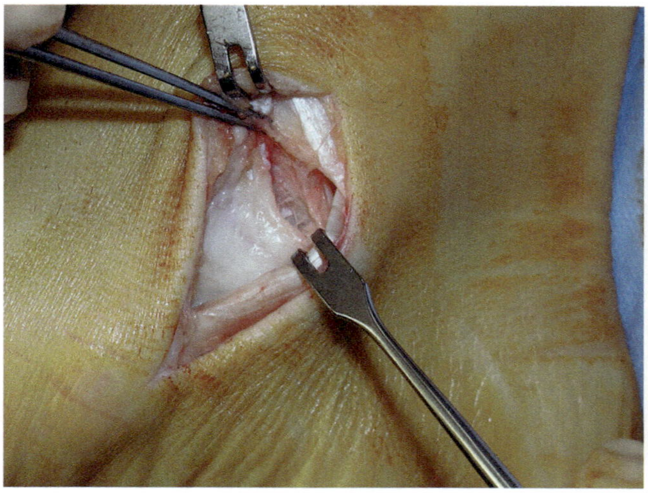

Fig. 5.8 The type I-injury includes the superficial layer of the deltoid ligament at its tibial periosteal attachment with partial discontinuity, delamination or a complete tear, typically extending caudally into the interval between the TSL and TCL. As a consequence, when the foot is loaded, the interval will be distracted, thus enabling the foot to externally rotate at the talonavicular joint, whereas the tibia tends to internally rotate. Because the PT tendon runs perpendicularly to the lesion, PT muscle activation is able to actively resist against this instability and imminent deformity, respectively

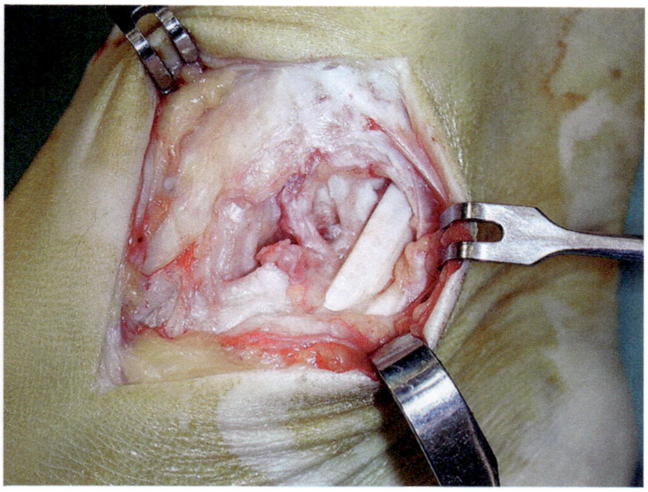

Fig. 5.9 The Type II-injury includes mainly the mid-substance of the TSL and may also include the TNL. The injury pattern can vary from partial discontinuity to complete rupture. As a consequence, when the foot is loaded, the ligamentous buttress of the talar head becomes incompetent, resulting in pronation and abduction of the foot. Because the TP tendon runs obliquely to the lesion, PT muscle activation may only partially compensate for this deforming force

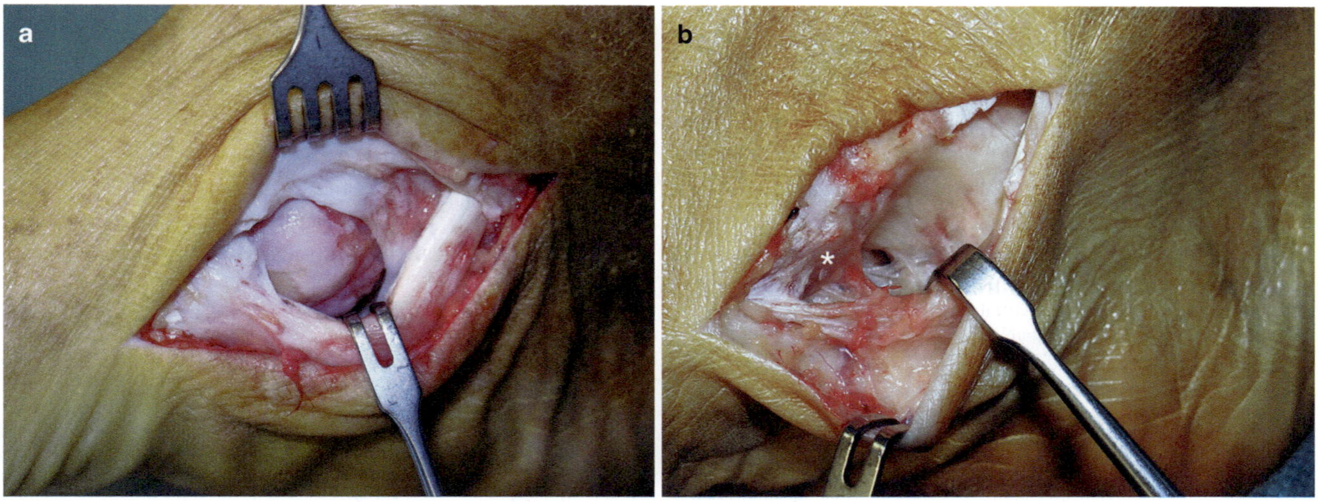

Fig. 5.10 The Type III-injury is located distally at the insertion to the navicular and involves mainly the distal part of the TNL, TSL, SMCNL, and MPOCNL (**a**). The rupture may continue along the navicular (Asterisk) with avulsion of the PT tendon at its insertion to the tuberosity of the navicular bone (**b**). As a consequence, when the foot is loaded, the ligamentous support of the talar head is lost, which results in plantarflexion of the talus and abduction as well as pronation of the foot, whereas activation of PT muscle may or may not be able to resist against the deforming forces, depending on its involvement in the injury

deforming forces. No talar tilt can be seen radiographically in the AP view under weight-bearing and/or valgus stress view.

5.4.3.1 Type III A-Injury

In this injury type, an avulsion of the ICNL and SMCNL from the navicular can be seen, while the PT tendon is not affected. The defect can best be seen intraoperatively, while the foot is slightly supinated, and the PT tendon is kept away with a hook.

5.4.3.2 Type III B-Injury

In this injury type, the PT tendon is also affected. Typically, an avulsion of the tendon can be seen at its main insertion site at the tuberosity of the navicular, while its connection to the plantar ligamentous network remains intact. The ICNL

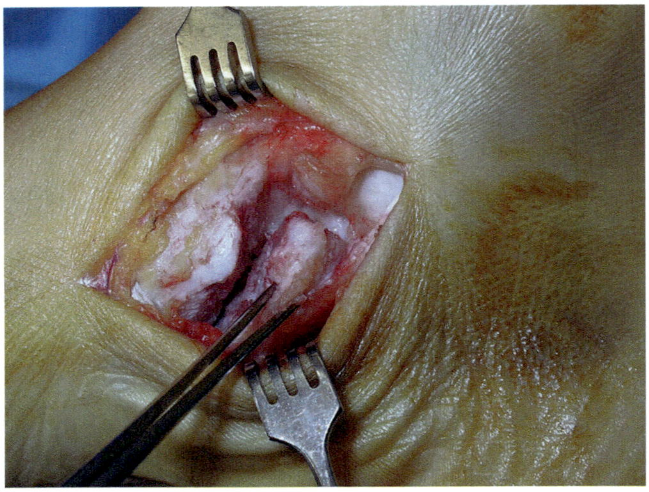

Fig. 5.11 A special configuration among the Type III-injury is an avulsion of the PT tendon in the presence of an accessory external tibial bone that has become disconnected from the navicular bone subsequent to a pronation-abduction trauma to the foot. In rare cases, an acute avulsion fracture from the navicular can be found. In most instances, this lesion is associated to a limited tear of TNL, TSL, SMNCL, and MPOCNL along their distal insertion to the navicular

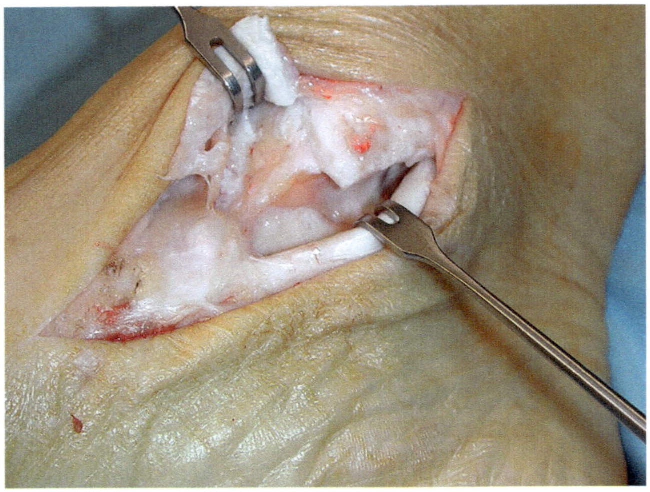

Fig. 5.12 The Type IV-injury includes the deep deltoid, mainly the ATTL and PTTL; in most instances, the TCL is also involved, but in general not the TSL and TNL, which remain intact as is also the case for the spring ligament. As a consequence, when the foot is loaded, the talus tilts into valgus, which gradually results in valgus deformity of the hindfoot and supination deformity of the forefoot that cannot be compensated by activating the PT muscle. Typically, a talar tilt can be seen radiographically in the AP view under weight-bearing and/or valgus stress view, meaning that the destabilization process also involves the tibiotalar (ankle) joint

and SMCNL may also evidence an avulsion; if present, it is usually rather small.

5.4.3.3 Type III C-Injury

In contrast to Type III B-injuries, there is a bony avulsion of the PT tendon from the navicular. In most instances, this injury type can be seen with the presence of an external tibial bone that has become disconnected from the navicular bone subsequent to a pronation-abduction trauma to the foot. In rare cases, an acute avulsion fracture from the navicular can be found.

5.4.4 Type IV-Injury (Table 5.1)

Injuries to the deep medial ankle ligaments (Fig. 5.12) can occur at the proximal insertion to the medial malleolus, in the mid-substance of the ligaments or at the distal insertion to the talus. While the injury is typically found for ATTL at its proximal tibial insertion, involving also the superficial layers of the deltoid, injuries to the PTTL are mostly seen near its medial talar insertion [59]. The ICNL and SMCNL (spring ligament), in contrast, are usually not affected. As a consequence, the talus tilts into valgus when the foot is loaded, which gradually results in valgus deformity of the hindfoot and supination deformity of the forefoot that cannot be compensated by activating the PT muscle. Typically, a talar tilt can be seen radiographically in the AP view under weight-bearing and/or valgus stress view, meaning that the destabilization process has also involved the tibiotalar (ankle) joint.

5.4.4.1 Type IV A-Injury

This type of injury results mainly in a tear of the proximal area of the TNL, TSL, TCL, and STTL, partially involving the ATTL as well. The resulting valgus tilt is <5°.

5.4.4.2 Type IV B-Injury

In this type of injury, the tear extends further posteriorly, involving the ATTL and partially also the PTTL. The resulting valgus tilt may increase up to 10°.

5.4.4.3 Type IV C-Injury

The whole deltoid ligament is disrupted with a valgus destabilization that exceeds 10° of valgus tilt when the foot is loaded.

5.5 Injury Mechanism

- Injuries to the superficial deltoid ligament occur during running down the stairs, landing on uneven surfaces and dancing while the body simultaneously rotates in the opposite direction

- Injuries to the deep deltoid ligament are mostly seen after a direct eversion trauma
- Injuries to the spring ligament most likely result from a direct or indirect trauma that enforces the foot into pronation and abduction, sometimes including an injury to the PT tendon at its insertion

A key feature of the patients' history is whether they have sustained an eversion trauma, i.e., an outward rotation of the foot during simultaneous inward rotation of the tibia.

5.5.1 Injuries to the Superficial Deltoid Ligament

Typically, injuries to the superficial deltoid ligament occur during running down the stairs, landing on uneven surfaces and dancing while the body simultaneously rotates in the opposite direction. Medial instability should be suspected on the basis of patients reporting a "giving way" feeling, especially towards medial when walking on even ground, downhill, or downstairs. Patients also report sensing pain at the anteromedial aspect of the ankle and sometimes pain around the lateral ankle, especially during dorsiflexion of the foot [10, 11, 60]. Chronic injury may result from overload in patients with an acquired flatfoot deformity [20, 61, 62].

5.5.2 Injuries to the Deep Deltoid Ligament

Injuries to the deep deltoid ligament, in contrast, are mostly seen after a direct eversion trauma, as sustained in contact sports when the foot is enforced in acute eversion by a load applied from lateral to the foot on the ground, e.g., when the foot cannot escape.

5.5.3 Injuries to the Spring Ligament

Little is known about the injury mechanism to the spring ligament [63]. A direct or indirect trauma that enforces the foot into pronation and abduction may most likely result in an injury to the spring ligament that may include an injury to the PT tendon at its insertion. It has been suggested that the presence of an accessory bone (external tibial bone) may expose the SMNCL to injuries because of its fibrous connection to the navicular that may become incompetent after a pronation trauma (Hintermann & Ruiz, *in press*). Chronic injury may result from overload in acquired flatfoot deformity [20, 62].

5.6 Clinical Findings

- In an acute injury, local pain and swelling may be the main clinical findings
- In a chronic injury, an asymmetrical planus and pronation deformity of the affected foot is the main clinical finding to indicate medial ankle instability
- Compensatory over function of the deep flexors, such as plantar flexion of the great toe, may also indicate loss of medial ankle stability

With the patient bearing weight, asymmetrical planus and pronation deformity of the affected foot to indicate medial ankle instability can be seen (Fig. 5.13a, b) [10, 60]. Typically, the excessive valgus of the hindfoot and pronation of the foot disappear while the patient is asked to correct the hindfoot pronation and thereby to activate the PT muscle (Fig. 5.13c). Analogously, the excessive valgus of the hindfoot and pronation of the foot disappear while the patient is asked to go in tiptoe position (Fig. 5.13d). With this, a primary PT tendon dysfunction is excluded. If hindfoot valgus is not fully corrected, it can either be due to a PT tendon dysfunction or an incompetent deep deltoid (Fig. 5.14). In the case of an injury to the spring ligament including an avulsion of PT tendon, the patient is no longer able to stabilize the medial ankle (Fig. 5.15).

Pain on palpation along the anterior medial gutter was described to be the hallmark of medial ankle instability, being present in all observed patients [10]. While pain along the PT tendon may be present, its inversion force is typically not compromised.

When the deep deltoid is involved, valgus misalignment of the heel can be found when compared to the contralateral, non-affected, side. All variations of associated flatfoot deformities can be seen when the PT tendon has subsequently become insufficient. In particular, the forefoot gradually experiences a supination deformity. The patient typically presents with a dorsal pseudexostosis of the first metatarsal head due to an elevated (dorsiflexed) position of the first metatarsal that may be misinterpreted as a hallux rigidus (Fig. 5.16a). When the patient is asked to activate the PT muscle for correcting the pronation position, the great toe is seen to go into plantarflexion as the patient uses the flexor hallucis longus as a medial ankle stabilizer (Fig. 5.16b). In an advanced stage, when walking barefoot, the patient may even use the plantarflexed great toe to stabilize the foot (Fig. 5.17). Clinical stress investigation is most reliable when the patient is seated on the table with hanging feet. While the heel is taken with one hand and the tibia with the other hand, a valgus tilt stress is applied to the

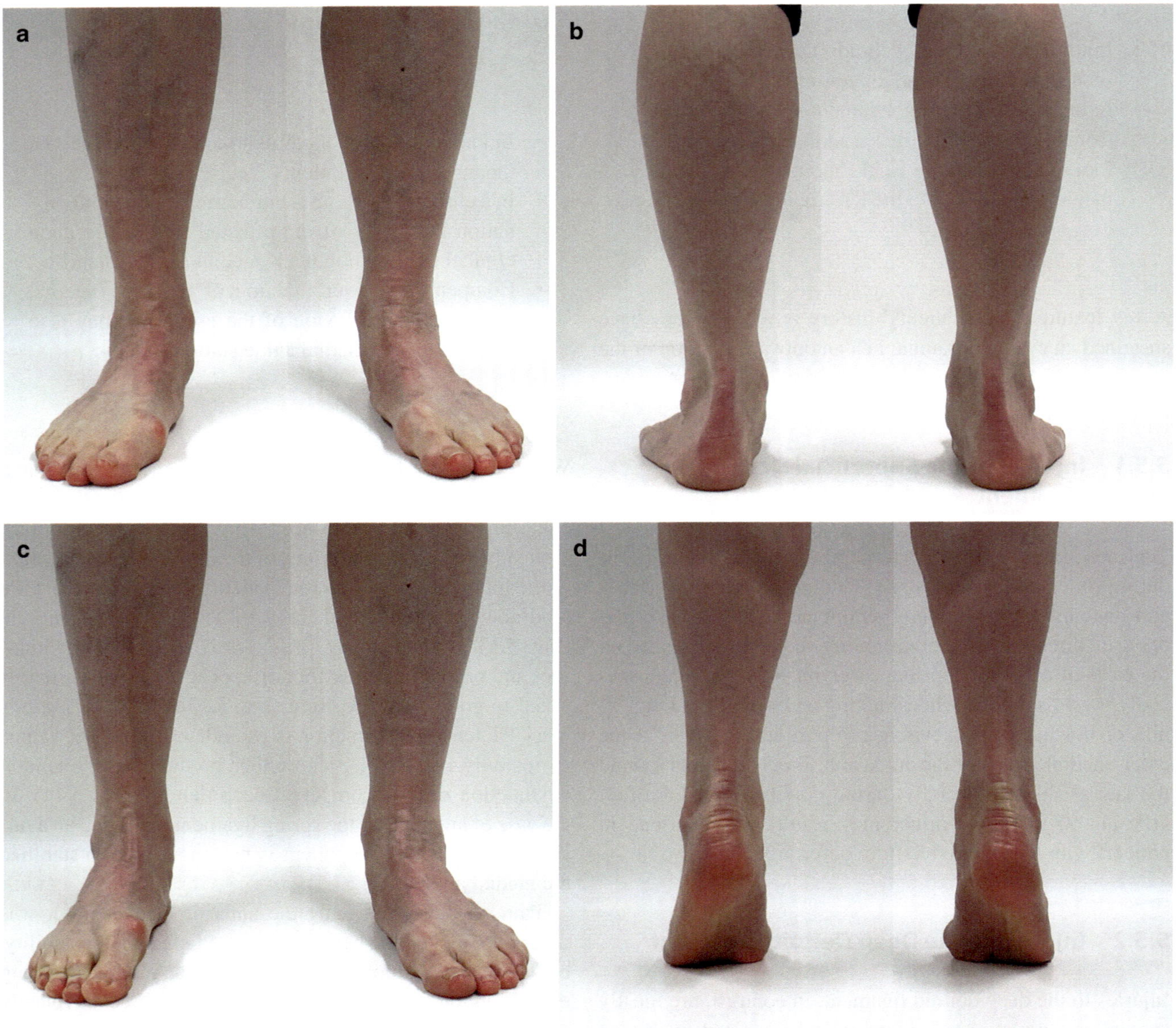

Fig. 5.13 Medial ankle instability in a 46-year-old male patient who sustained a pronation trauma of his right foot 16 months ago. Under conservative treatment, the patient has persistent pain on the medial ankle and progressively also along the PT tendon. Pain is also indicated on the dorsal aspect of the first MTP joint. (**a**) Frontal view, relaxed position. Bilateral flatfoot with increased prominence of the medial malleolus and a valgus and pronatus position of the great toe of the right foot, with a pseudexostosis on the medial and dorsal aspect of the MTP I-head. (**b**) Posterior view, relaxed position. Bilateral flattening of the arch and abduction of the forefoot, with increased prominence of the medial malleolus. (**c**) Anterior view. When the patient is asked to correct the position of his affected right foot by activating the PT muscle, the medial prominence is seen to disappear as the arch is restored. Note the activation of the anterior tibial muscle and the raising of the first metatarsal, associated with a flexion contracture position of the toes. The pseudexostosis becomes more evident on the dorsal aspect of the first metatarsal head. (**d**) Posterior view. In tiptoe position, the hindfoot is seen corrected symmetrically and the medial prominence has completely disappeared

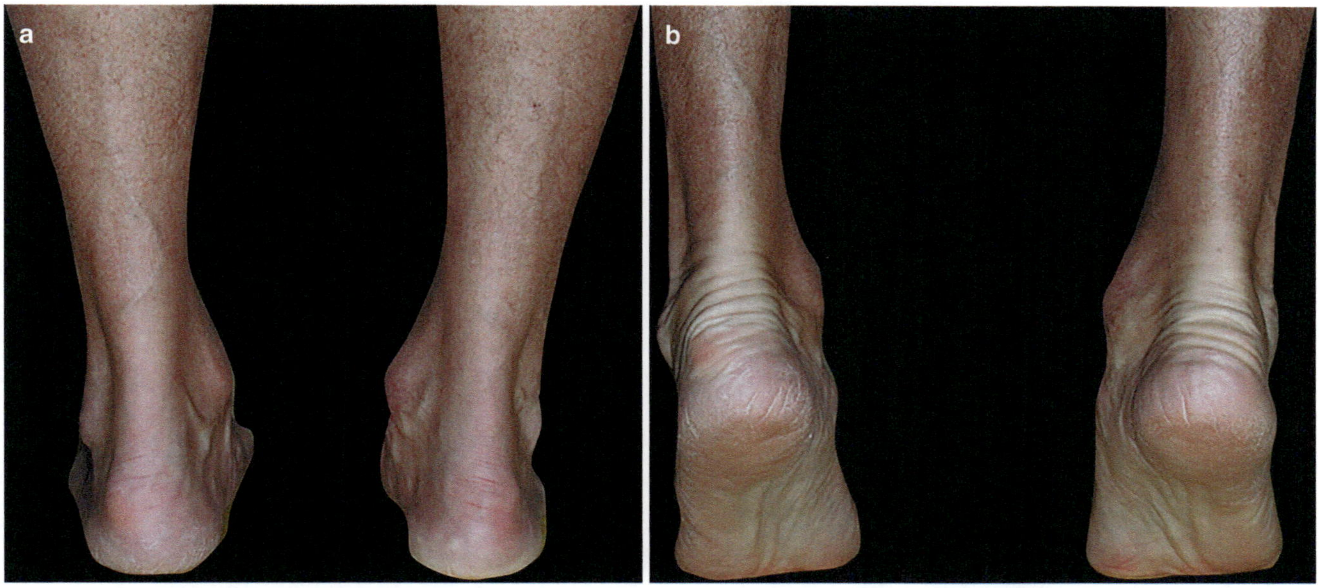

Fig. 5.14 This 58-year-old male patient with painful medial ankle instability took part in ultra-marathons until 14 months ago, when he sustained a pronation trauma of his right ankle while downhill running. He sensed progressive pain along the PT tendon. The clinical picture in (**a**) relaxed position. The right affected foot shows a substantial prominence of the medial malleolus due to an internally rotated position of the leg. Furthermore, there exists a distinct valgus misalignment of the hindfoot. (**b**) In tiptoe position, the medial prominence is seen to disappear only partially and some valgus misalignment of the hindfoot persists

heel, and the result compared with the contralateral side. Then, while holding the foot in slight plantarflexion and abduction, an anterior drawer stress is applied and again compared to the contralateral side (Fig. 5.18).

5.7 Imaging

- Standard weight-bearing radiographs serve to identify structural changes of the foot and ankle and additionally, to exclude bony pathologies
- CT scan is indicated in the case of coalitions and suspected bony avulsions
- MRI, though not necessary on a regular basis, can be helpful to assess deltoid ligament injuries regarding their location and extent

Standard weight-bearing radiographs are taken to assess structural changes of the foot and ankle and additionally to exclude bony pathologies (Fig. 5.19). To assess the deformity, it is mandatory to ask the patient to stay in a relaxed position; when asking the patient to correct the deformity, obtained radiographs will serve to determine to which extent the deformity is correctable (Fig. 5.20). If a talocalcaneal coalition is suspected or an avulsion fracture is seen that involves the articular surfaces, computed tomography (CT) should be performed (Fig. 5.21). MRI, though not necessary on a regular basis, can be helpful to assess deltoid ligament injuries regarding their location and extent (Fig. 5.22) [59, 64–67]. When the medial clear space is enlarged, but less than 5 mm, an MRI analysis has been recommended because of its increased accuracy and decreased false positive rate for surgery [68]. Comparing MRI and surgical findings for superficial deltoid ligament tears has shown a sensitivity of 83.3% (45/54) and specificity of 93.9% (31/33) and for deep deltoid ligament tears a sensitivity of 96.3% (26/27) and specificity of 97.9% (46/47) [69]. Sonography can also be helpful in detecting an acute injury to the deltoid (Fig. 5.23).

5.8 Arthroscopy

- Arthroscopy has evolved to being a helpful preoperative diagnostic tool
- Arthroscopy can show the extent and location of the deltoid injury and the resulting amount of instability

Ankle arthroscopy was found to be a helpful diagnostic tool to confirm clinically suspected instability of the medial and lateral ankle, and to detect additional structural changes such

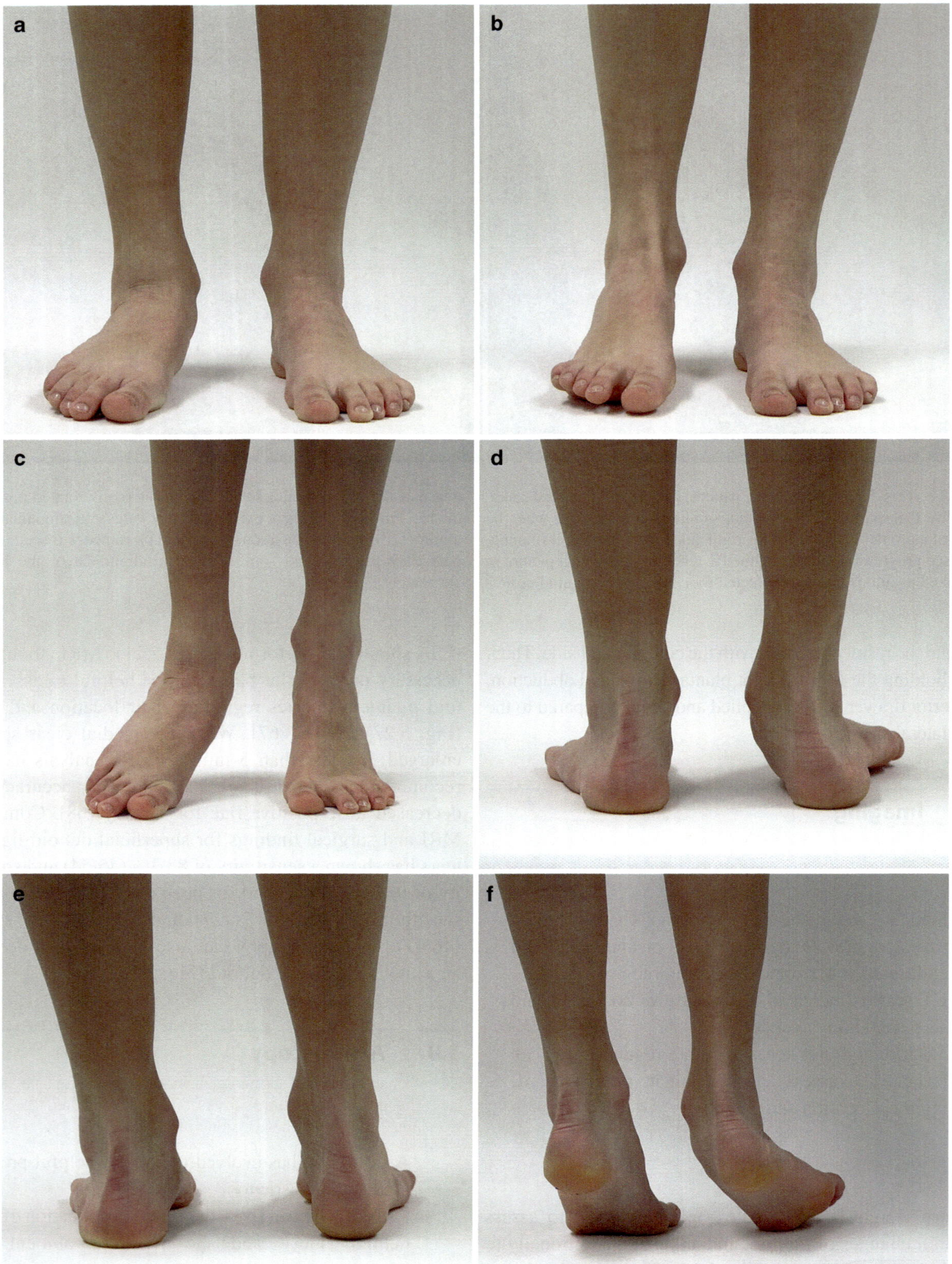

Fig. 5.15 This 16-year-old volleyball player sustained an acute eversion-pronation trauma of her right foot 14 months earlier and is complaining about persistent medial instability. She can hardly control her right foot when walking, especially when she is getting tired. (**a**) Frontal view, relaxed position. The foot is everted, with little abduction of the forefoot. (**b**) Frontal plane. In an attempt to correct the position of her affected foot, she is using mainly the anterior tibial muscle; however, she fails to do so unless she unloads the hindfoot. (**c**) Frontal plane. She is also not able to stabilize the foot when going into tiptoe position. (**d**) Posterior view, relaxed position. The foot is seen everted, with some little forefoot abduction. Notice the impressive prominence of the medial malleolus due to an internally rotated position of the leg. (**e**) Posterior view. When asked to correct the foot deformity, the deformity is seen to be almost completely corrected as the patient unloads her heel. Notice the calf atrophy as a consequence of reduced use. (**f**) Posterior view. While trying to go into tiptoe position, the eversion-pronation deformity is seen not to be corrected, resulting in a touch-down of the medial forefoot only

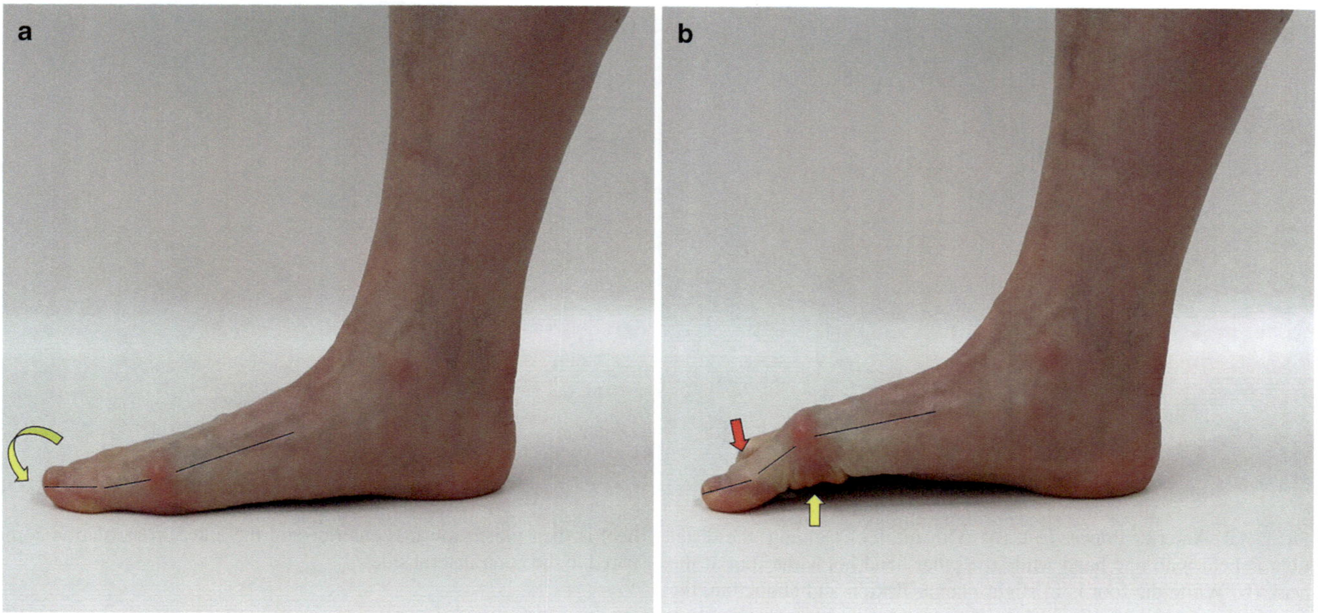

Fig. 5.16 Medial view of the foot in the same patient as Fig. 5.13. (**a**) Relaxed position. The arch is flattened and the great toe evidences some pronation which gives the impression of a pseudexostosis over the medial aspect of the first metatarsal head. (**b**) When the patient is asked to correct his foot position by activating the PT muscle, the first metatarsal is seen to raise up (yellow arrow), whereas the great toe shows a plantarflexion contracture with subsequent hyperextension in the IP-joint of the great toe (red arrow). The pronation of the great toe has disappeared and the pseudexostosis is now seen more on the dorsal aspect of the first metatarsal head

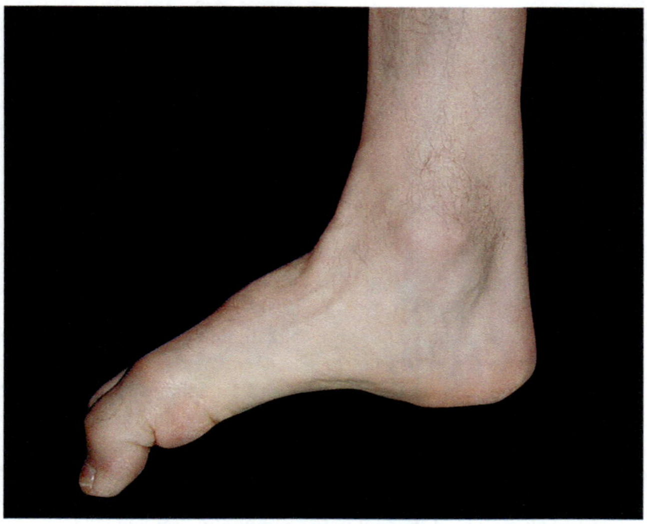

Fig. 5.17 Medial view of the foot in a 58-year-old male patient who has been suffering from medial ankle instability for 34 months. When asked to walk barefoot, he uses plantarflexion of the great toe including the end phalanx to increase the power of the flexor hallucis longus muscle to stabilize the medial arch

as cartilage lesions [60, 70, 71]. In contrast to the lateral side, the instability pattern on the medial side of the ankle is associated with an increased anterior shift of the talus associated to a distinctly increased opening of the medial tibiotalar joint when pull is applied to the slightly plantarflexed foot.

5.8.1 Acute Injury

In an acute injury to deltoid ligament, arthroscopy can show the extent and location of the deltoid injury and the resulting amount of instability (Table 5.2; Figs. 5.24, 5.25, and 5.26).

5.8.2 Chronic Injury

In a chronic injury to the deltoid ligament, arthroscopy can show the extent and location of the deltoid injury and the resulting amount of instability (Table 5.3; Figs. 5.27, 5.28, 5.29, and 5.30).

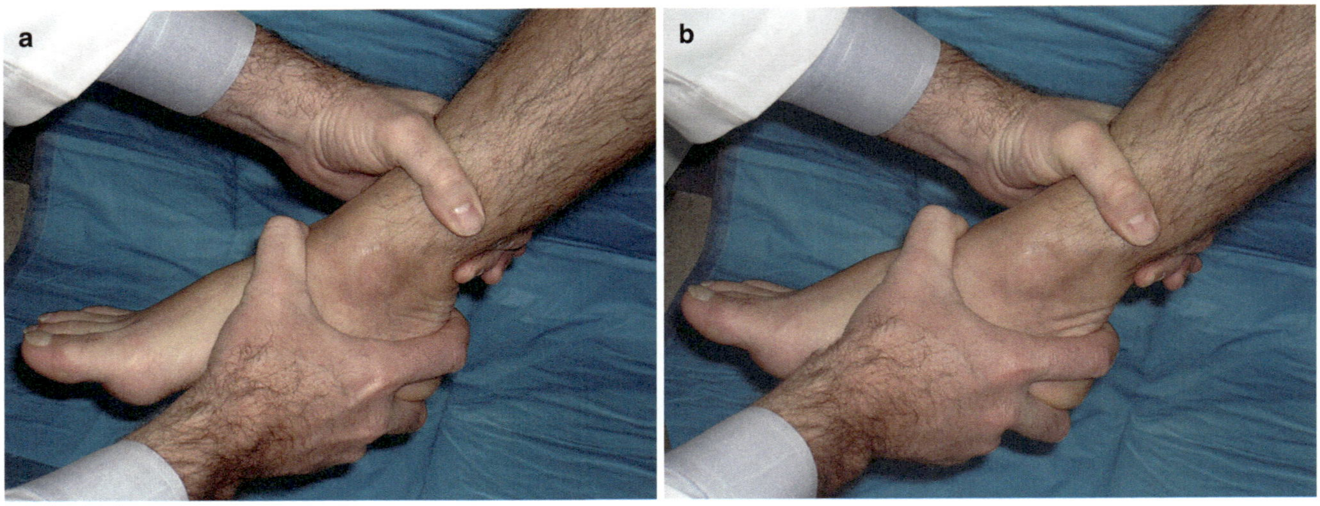

Fig. 5.18 Anterior drawer test. (**a**) With the foot hanging, the distal tibia is held with one hand while the other hand holds the foot at the heel. (**b**) While the foot is in slight plantar flexion and abduction, the heel is then pulled towards anterior and the anterior translation compared to the contralateral side

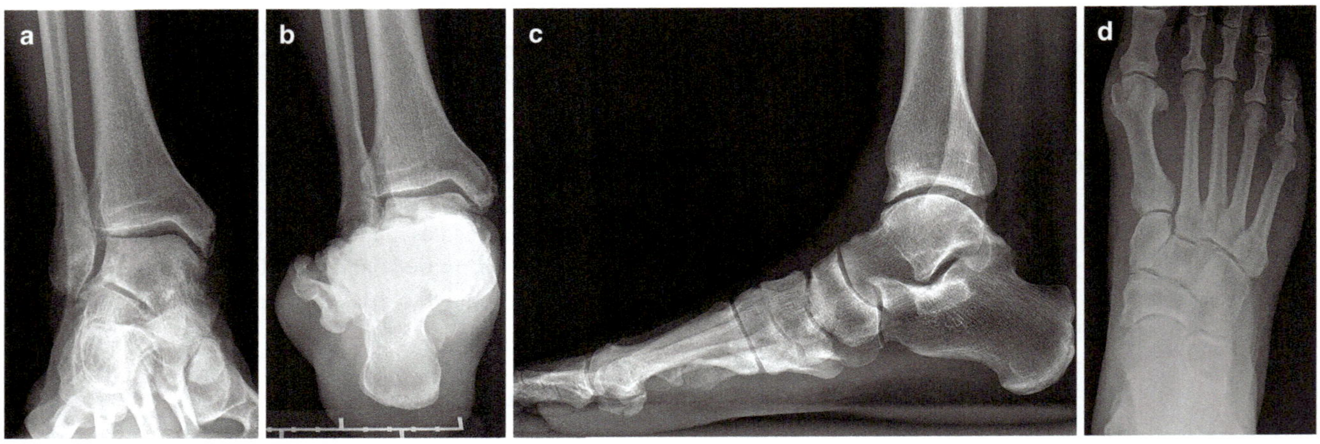

Fig. 5.19 This 51-year-old former ice hockey player sustained a severe pronation trauma 3 years earlier and is complaining about progressive pain on the anterior aspect of the medial malleolus as well as on the lateral aspect of the ankle. Standard radiographs under weightbearing were taken. (**a**) The AP view of the ankle shows a gapping of the medial tibiotalar joint with a talar tilt of 8°. Note the higher bone density on the lateral tibiotalar joint with increased trabecular formation subsequent to the lateralized force transmission, whereas the medial tibiotalar joint shows a rarefication of bony trabeculae. (**b**) The hindfoot alignment view shows an increased gapping, a talar tilt in the anterior tibiotalar joint, and a valgus malalignment of the heel with an increased valgus moment arm. (**c**) The lateral view of the foot shows osteophyte formation on the anterior border of the tibia and a slight closure of the sinus tarsi without bony impingement. This osteophyte has become a main stabilizer of the ankle against anterior extrusion of the talus; therefore, resection of this osteophyte would destabilize the ankle and shouldn't be considered. (**d**) The DP view of the foot shows preserved alignment of the foot with a minimally pronounced uncoverage of talar head

a

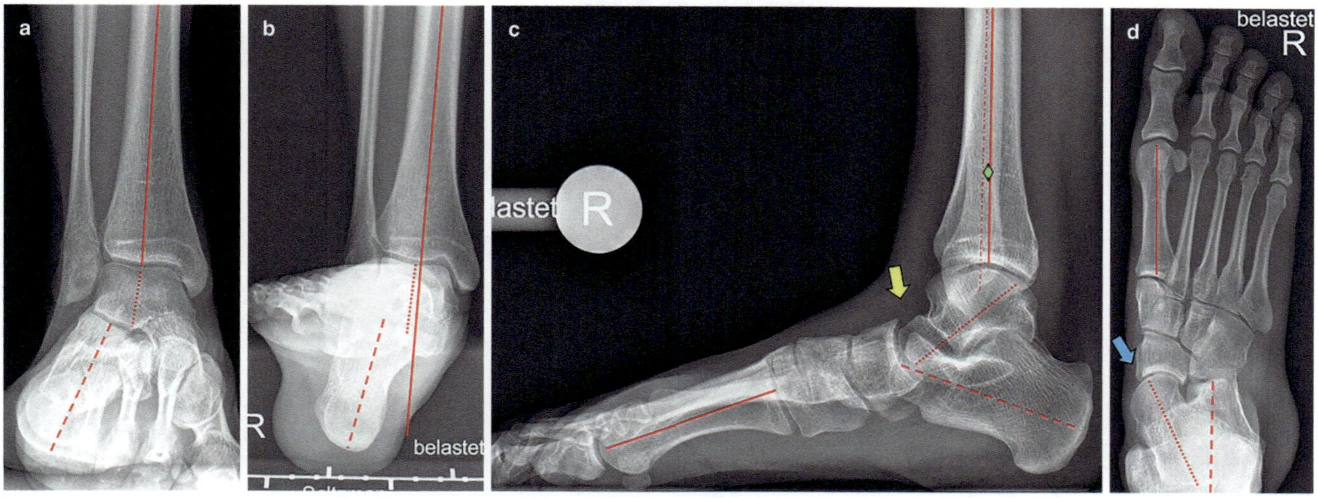

b

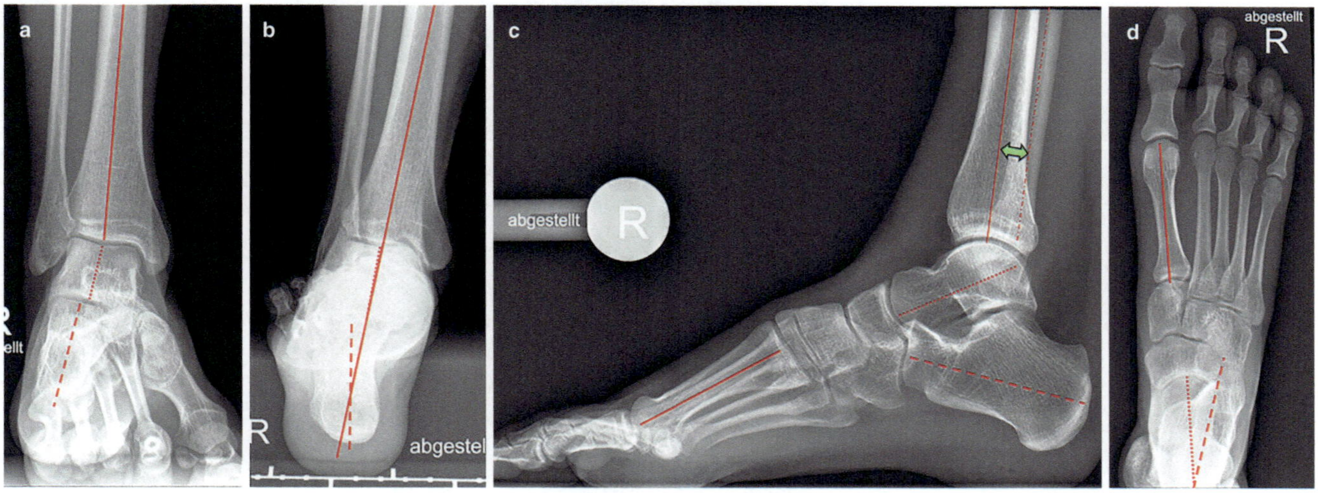

Fig. 5.20 Standard radiographs in the same patient as Fig. 5.15. (**a**) The radiographs were first taken with the foot loaded while the patient is asked to stay in relaxed position; (**b**) thereafter, the patient is asked to correct the deformity. Notice the changes occurring in all planes, with collapse of the arch, increased talocalcaneal angles, hindfoot valgus, uncoverage of talar head (blue arrow), sag at talonavicular joint (yellow arrow), and internal rotation of tibia (green arrow). **a**) AP view, **b**) alignment view, **c**) lateral view, and **d**) DP view

In an early stage of chronic medial ankle instability (Fig. 5.27, Grade 1), a synovialitis spot can be seen at the anteromedial corner of the ankle which often interposes into the joint space, whereas in a more chronic stage, osteophyte formation can be found at this location, often also involving the anterior aspect of the medial malleolus. Due to this increased shifting movement of the talus towards anterior, out of ankle mortise, a contrecoup lesion to the cartilage of the medial aspect of the talus can consistently be found [60]. Another typical finding is the bald anterior aspect of the medial malleolus, where a periosteum scar can be seen at the original insertion site of the TNL and TSL, whereas these ligaments are retracted. When applying valgus stress to the ankle, some opening of the medial clear space but no opening of the medial tibiotalar joint can be seen, as long as the deep layers of the deltoid ligament (ATTL and PTTL) are competent.

In Grade 2 instability (Fig. 5.28), when applying valgus stress to the ankle, in contrast, the medial clear space is typically seen to open substantially until the deep fibers of the ligament are tensioned, whereas the superficial deltoid remains incompetent. Some opening of the medial

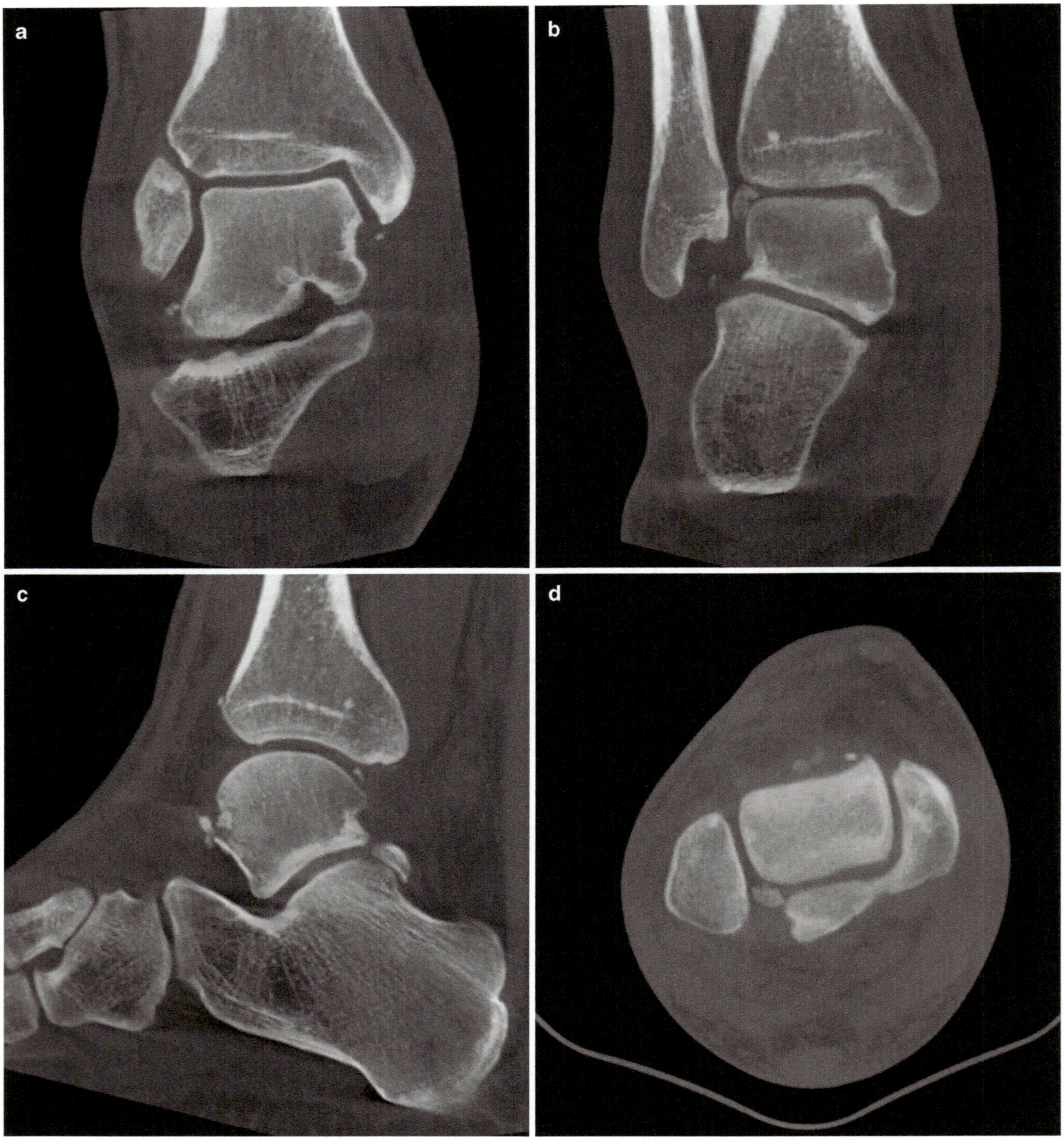

Fig. 5.21 This 26-year-old handball player sustained an acute eversion trauma when his opponent hit his lower leg from lateral while the foot was loaded. These weight-bearing CT scans were taken 9 days after injury. (**a**, **b**) Coronal views showing a congruent tibiotalar joint with bony fragments in the sinus tarsi and beneath the tip of medial malleolus. Furthermore, a bigger fragment can be seen in the lateral gutter. (**c**) Lateral view of the foot showing a fragmentation at the lateral talar neck and a further fragment in the posterior tibiotalar joint. (**d**) Horizontal view showing the intraarticular fragment in the dorsal aspect of the tibiofibular joint

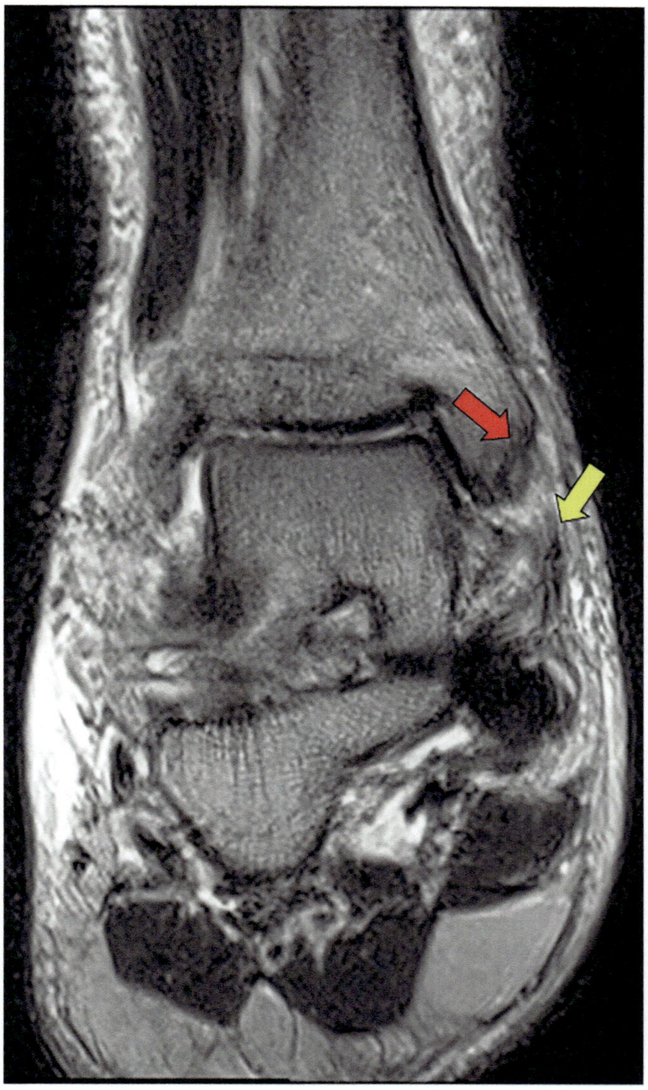

Fig. 5.22 A coronal view in an MRI of a 24-year-old footballer after a severe eversion trauma showing a complete rupture of the deltoid along the medial malleolus (red arrow). The tear is proximal in the depicted superficial deltoid (yellow arrow)

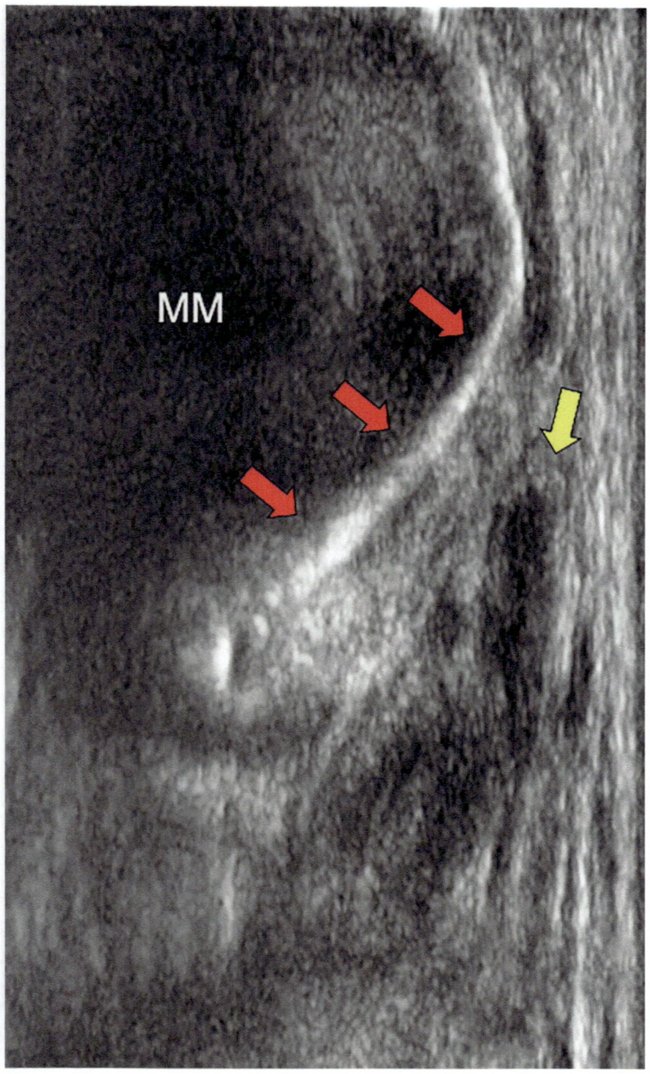

Fig. 5.23 Sonography in the same patient as Fig. 5.21, shows the tear along the bony insertion (red arrows), extending proximally subperiosteally, with complete detachment of the deltoid (yellow arrow)

Table 5.2 Arthroscopic findings in acute medial ankle instability

	Arthroscopic findings	Stress X-ray	Figure
Grade 1	Only the superficial deltoid is involved; its continuity is preserved while the hematoma beneath the synovia is seen	TT – MCS +	5.24
Grade 2	The deep deltoid is also involved, but its continuity is still preserved	TT + MCS ++	5.25
Grade 3	The superficial and deep deltoid are torn, typically allowing to see the PT and FDL tendons	TT +++ MCS +	5.26

TT talar tilt, *MCS* medial clear space, *PT* posterior tibial, *FDL* flexor digitorum longus

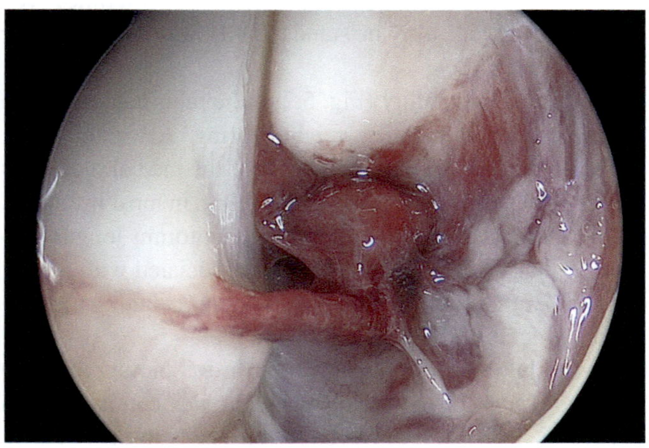

Fig. 5.24 Arthroscopic findings in acute injuries to the deltoid ligament, Grade 1: Only the superficial deltoid is involved; its continuity is typically preserved while the hematoma beneath the synovia is seen

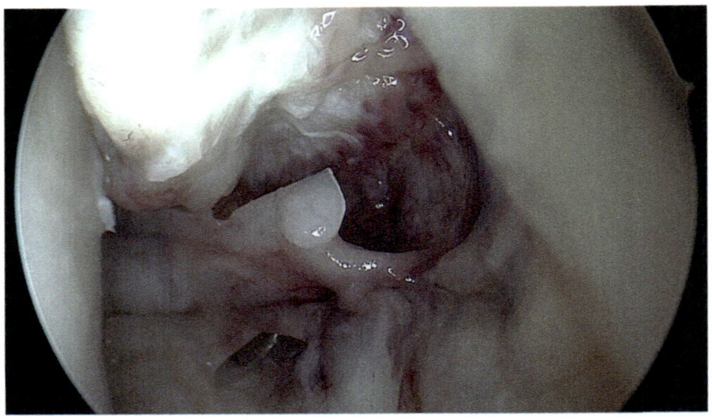

Fig. 5.25 Arthroscopic findings in acute injuries to the deltoid ligament, Grade 2: The deep deltoid is also involved, but its continuity is still preserved, thus no or very little medial talar tilt can be seen when applying valgus stress to the hindfoot

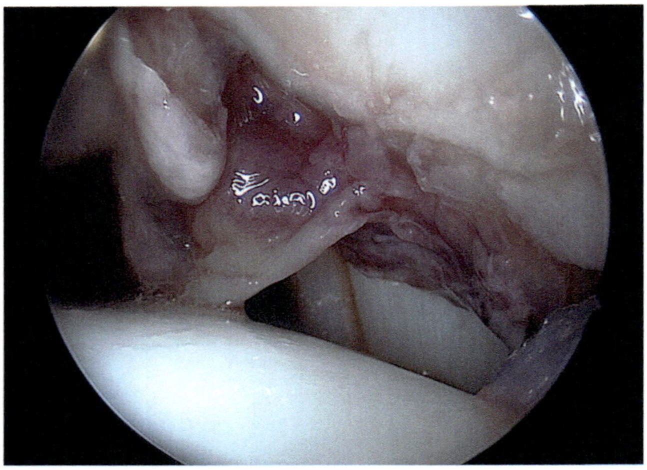

Fig. 5.26 Arthroscopic findings in acute injuries to the deltoid ligament, Grade 3: The superficial and deep deltoid are torn, typically allowing to see the posterior tibial and flexor digitorum longus tendons

clear space and distinct opening of the medial tibiotalar joint can be verified under fluoroscopy and sometimes seen to a lesser extent also in standard AP radiographs under weight-bearing.

In Grade 3 instability (Fig. 5.29), the talus has tilted into valgus as seen in the weight-bearing AP radiograph. Arthroscopically, the inferior aspect of the medial malleolus can be seen free from ligaments, allowing, in most instances, to see the posterior tibial and flexor digitorum longus tendons. Often, the Grade 3 injuries are associated with a bony avulsion of the anterior colliculus, seldom including the posterior colliculus (Fig. 5.30).

Recently, the feasibility of an arthroscopic approach to the whole span of the spring ligament was confirmed in a cadaveric study [72]; however, it still needs to be validated for its benefit in clinical use.

Table 5.3 Arthroscopic findings in chronic medial ankle instability

	Arthroscopic Findings	Stress X-ray	Figure
Grade 1	– Synovialitis spot at anteromedial corner of tibiotalar joint – Osteophyte formation at anterior edge of medial malleolus – Bald anterior aspect of medial malleolus – Superficial cartilage lesion at medial aspect of talus	TT – MCS +	5.27
Grade 2	– The deep deltoid is also involved, but its continuity is still preserved – Bald anterior aspect of medial malleolus extending to the tip with missing superficial deltoid – Superficial cartilage lesion at medial aspect of talus	TT + MCS ++	5.28
Grade 3A	– The deep deltoid is torn, typically allowing to see the PT and FDL tendons – Bald medial malleolus – Deep cartilage lesion at medial aspect of talus	TT +++ MCS ++	5.29
Grade 3B	– Avulsion of deltoid with a bony fragment, typically allowing to see the PT and FDL tendons – Deep cartilage lesion at medial aspect of talus	TT +++ MCS +	5.30

TT talar tilt, *MCS* medial clear space, *PT* posterior tibial, *FDL* flexor digitorum longus

5.9 Conservative Treatment and Rehabilitation

- Usually, an acute isolated injury to the deltoid ligament can be conservatively managed
- In young patients and athletes, early surgical intervention results in a better functional outcome and earlier return to sports

An acute isolated injury to the deltoid ligament should be conservatively managed for 3–6 months unless there is an associated pathologic condition that necessitates earlier surgical intervention. The aim of treatment is to stabilize the ankle, align it well and rehabilitate for asymptomatic function. There is evidence, however, that in young patients and athletes, early surgical intervention results in a better functional outcome and much earlier return to sports, thus suggesting not to delay surgical treatment [6, 10, 11, 73, 74]. A reason for conservative treatment by some surgeons may be the anatomical difficulties in separating and defining the

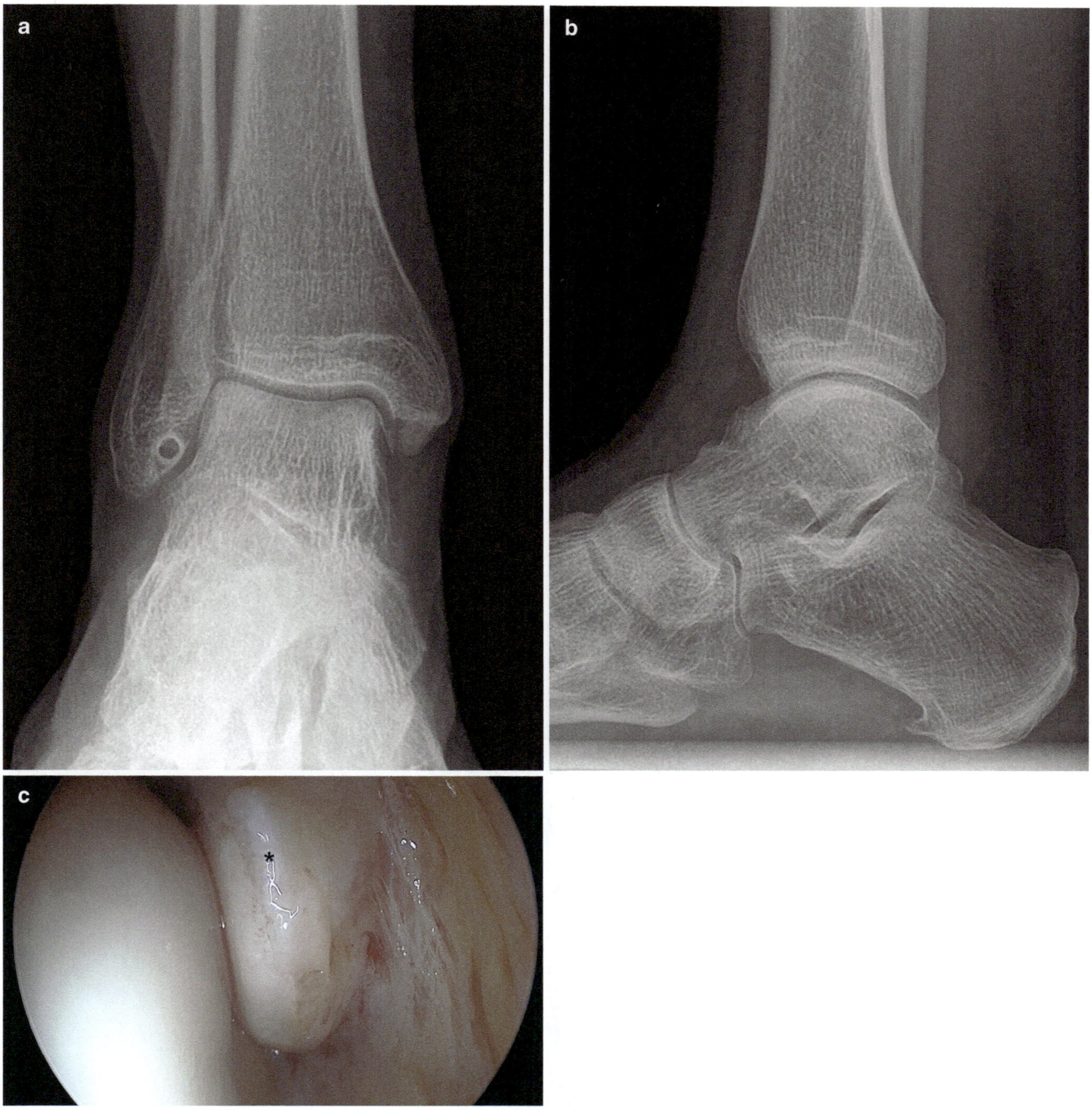

Fig. 5.27 Arthroscopic findings in chronic injuries to the deltoid ligament, Grade 1. This 32-year-old female patient underwent non-anatomic reconstruction of the lateral ankle ligament with the use of a tendon allograft 7 years ago. (**a**) The AP standard radiograph shows an overload of the lateral tibiotalar joint with increased trabecular formation and some impaction of the lateral tibial plafond as a result of the tight fibulotalar joint. (**b**) The lateral radiograph of the ankle. (**c**) Arthroscopy shows a bald talus with a retracted and scarred superficial deltoid. The deep layers of the deltoid are intact, checked by valgus stress application (not shown). Note the osteophyte formation (Asterisk) on the anterior aspect of the malleolus caused by the antero-posterior shifting movement of the medial malleolus subsequent to the tight lateral compartment. Furthermore, some superficial damage to the cartilage on the medial aspect of the talus is visible as a result of the shifting movement

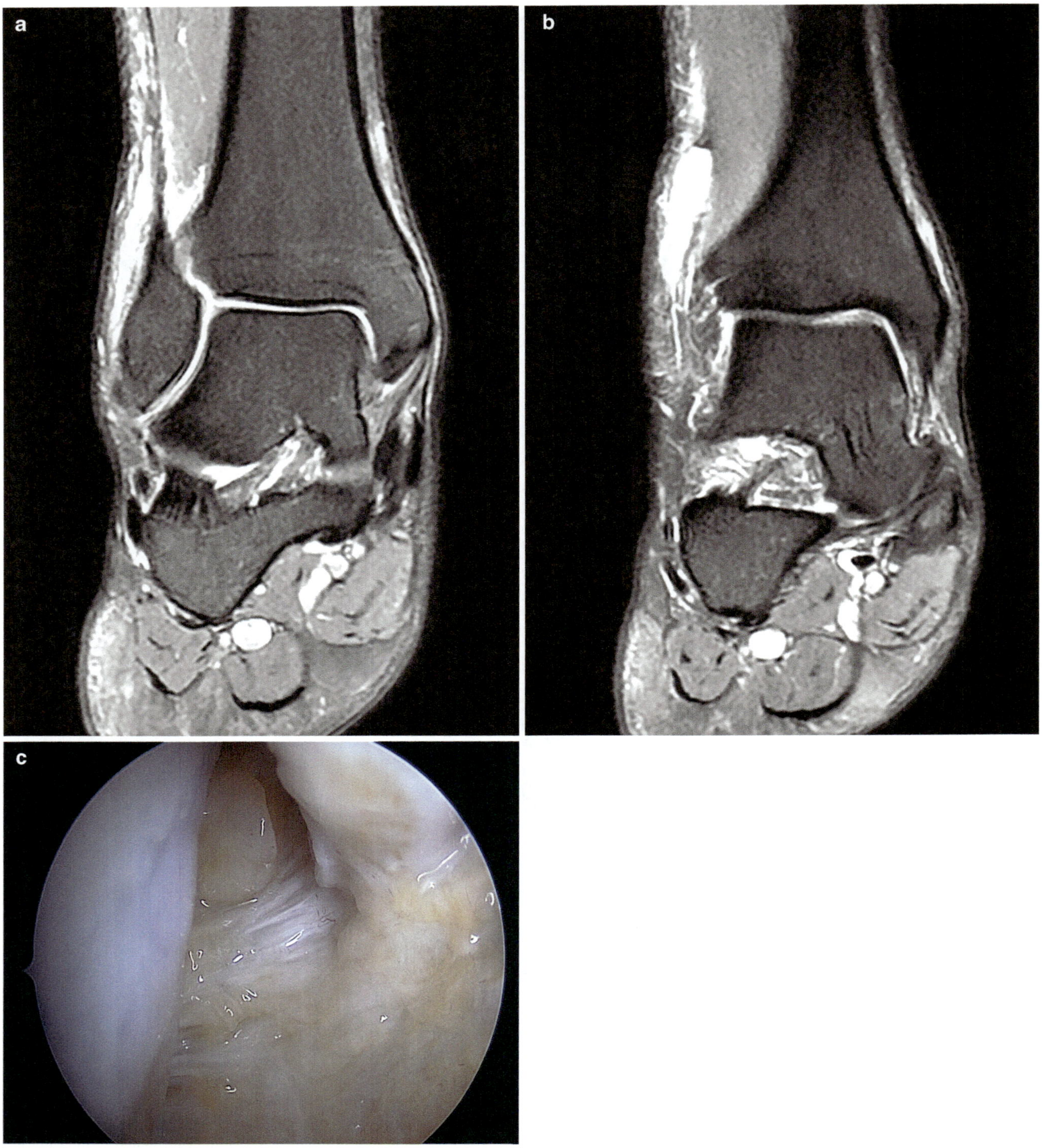

Fig. 5.28 Arthroscopic findings in chronic injuries to the deltoid ligament, Grade 2. This 42-year-old former volleyball player with a globally unstable ankle experienced recurrent ankle sprains since a severe sprain 13 years ago. (**a**) MRI shows substantial damage to the lateral ankle ligaments with potential incompetence of the syndesmotic ligaments as well. The deltoid shows an extended avulsion of the superficial layers from the medial malleolus. The deep layers also evidence some scarring. (**b**) A cut more anteriorly shows the thinned superficial deltoid (tibiospring and tibionavicular ligaments) with extended scarring. (**c**) Arthroscopically, the medial malleolus is found to be bald distally to the tip with a periosteum scar at the avulsion site of the superficial deltoid. When applying valgus stress, the medial tibiotalar joint is typically seen to open until the deep fibers of the ligament are tensioned, this shows that the continuity of the deltoid is still preserved

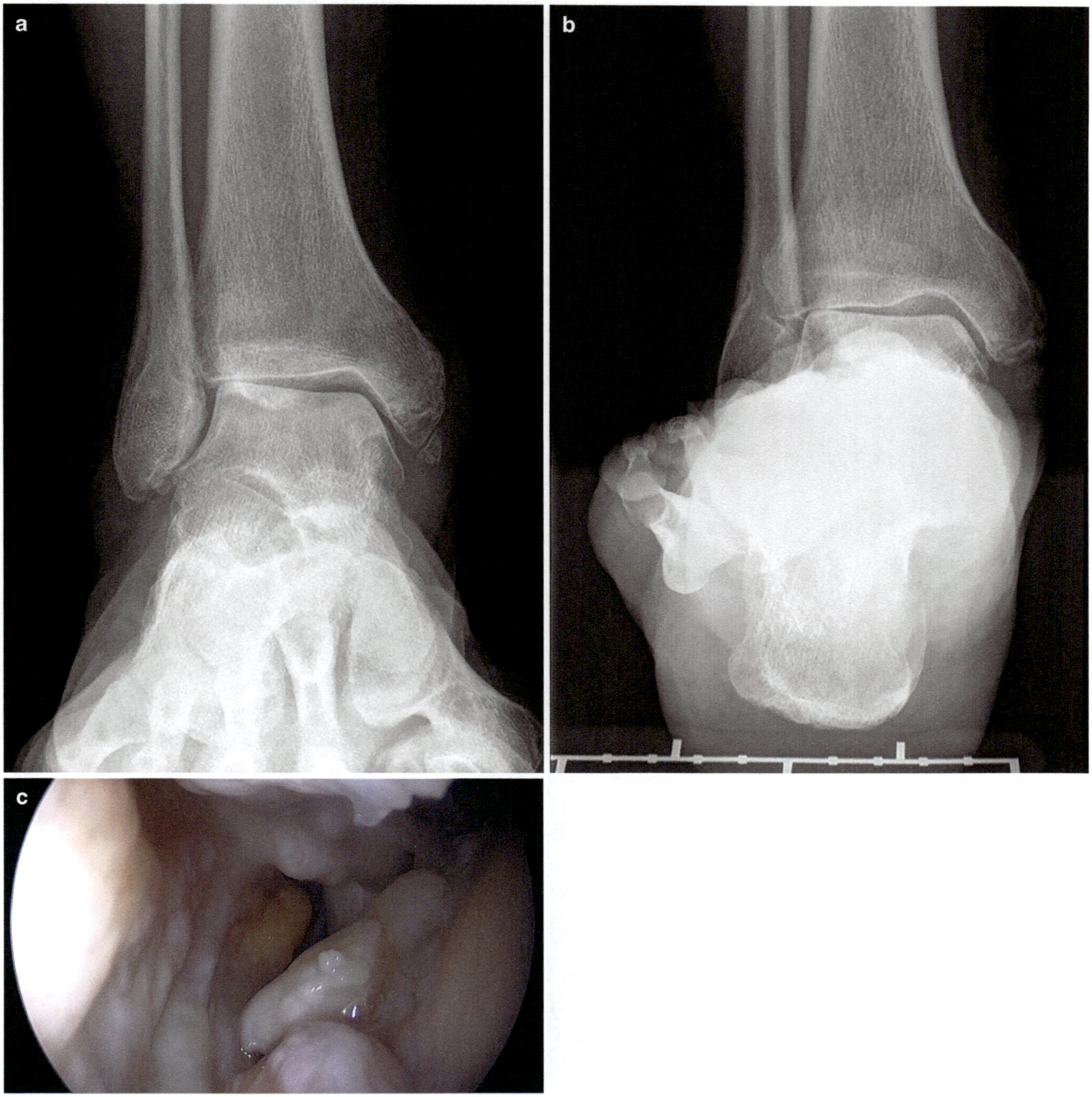

Fig. 5.29 Arthroscopic findings in chronic injuries to the deltoid ligament, Grade 3-A. A 54-year-old former soccer player complained about increasing pain in his lateral ankle after having sustained multiple severe ankle sprains. He also felt like experiencing lateral ankle instability. (**a**) The AP standard radiograph under weight-bearing shows a medial talar tilt with narrowing of the lateral tibiotalar joint and an increased density of the subchondral bone in this area. Furthermore, a small bony fragment is visible that has not been displaced from the medial malleolus while the talus has tilted into valgus. (**b**) The medial gapping of the tibiotalar joint space can also be seen in the hindfoot alignment view. Note the impaction of the medial tibial plafond at its anterior aspect, a typical finding in patients with severe rotational ankle instability that initially started with an instability of the lateral ankle. (**c**) Arthroscopically, the medial malleolus is found completely free from ligaments, allowing to see the posterior tibial tendon. Severe cartilage lesions on the medial aspect of the talus are also found

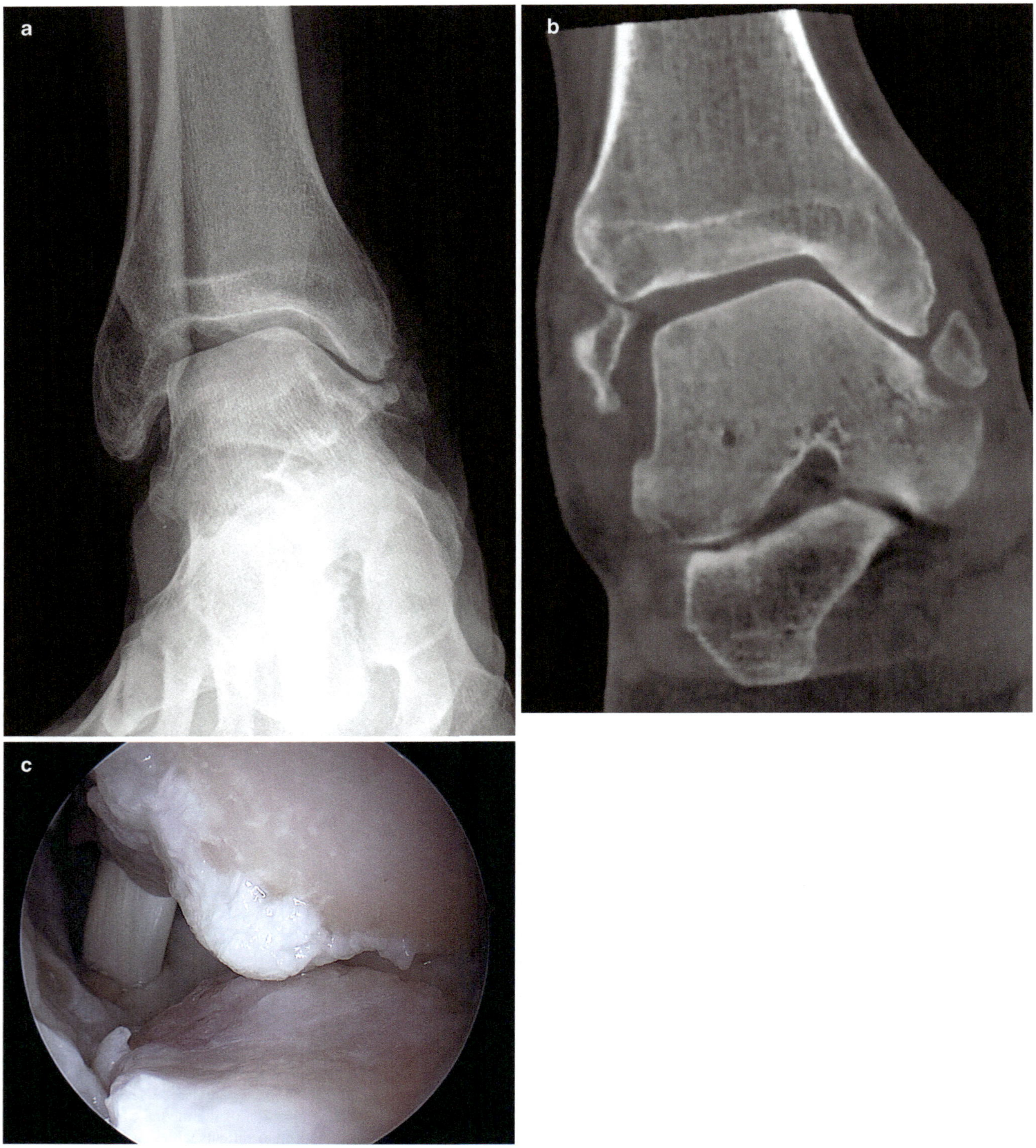

Fig. 5.30 Arthroscopic findings in chronic injuries to the deltoid ligament, Grade 3-B. A 44-year-old former basketball player sustained multiple severe ankle sprains. Besides experiencing a feeling of instability, she senses medial ankle pain due to a varus malaligned ankle. (**a**) The standard AP radiograph under weight-bearing shows the varus configuration of the distal tibia and the varus tilt of the talus within the ankle mortise, with a compensatory valgus tilt of the subtalar joint. Note the bony fragment beneath the tip of medial malleolus. (**b**) The weight-bearing CT scan shows the size and extent of the bony fragment as well as the gapping of the lateral tibiotalar and talofibular joints. (**c**) Arthroscopically, the big bony fragment extending to the posterior aspect of the medial malleolus can be seen, with disruption of the sheath of the posterior tibial tendon. Severe cartilage lesions are present. The deltoid ligament is mainly preserved (not shown), indicating that the fracture occurred during a severe ankle sprain or as consequence of chronic stress

individual components of the deltoid, as well as the variability of their presence, which may lead to hesitance in proceeding with surgical management.

5.9.1 Type I and Type II-Injuries

The majority of the Type I and Type II-injuries can be treated conservatively without surgery. This is especially true for an intra-substance tear of the ligament, with no evidence of PT tendon pathology. Besides prescription of anti-inflammatory medication in the acute phase and a brace and/or orthotics in the form of a medial foot arch support, temporary restriction from physical activities is advised.

5.9.2 Type III-Injuries

In more serious type III sprains or in patients who are unable to bear weight, a cast may be used. Like lateral sprains, a cast immobilization of 2–3 weeks is typically recommended, followed by longer functional rehabilitation with an emphasis on proprioceptive training. The use of a boot for up to 6 weeks is reasonable, as this prevents valgus tilt as well as anterior and lateral translation of the talus and thus removes any strain that may be placed through the deltoid. Additionally, it allows the patient to perform dorsiflexion and plantar flexion exercises that would normally be restricted by a cast. This prevents capsular scarring of the ankle joint, potentially facilitating an earlier return to sports.

5.9.3 Type IV-Injuries

After an acute Type IV injury, surgical management is advised. For a chronic injury, if PT tendon function is preserved, a conservative treatment may be considered and the same measures as for Type III-injuries are used.

5.10 Surgical Management of Medial Ankle Instability

- Reconstruction of all affected structures is mandatory to restore the stability of the medial ankle joint complex
- In complete tears of the deep deltoid with a talar tilt >5°, surgical reconstruction might be critical
- In long-standing deformities, additional osteotomies may be indicated to balance and stabilize the ankle joint complex
- Additional soft tissue procedures may be necessary in the case of posterior tibial dysfunction

The main strategy is to reconstruct all affected structures to restore the stability of the medial ankle joint complex (Table 5.1). In the case of an extended injury with a long-standing instability, especially in Type IV-injuries, the

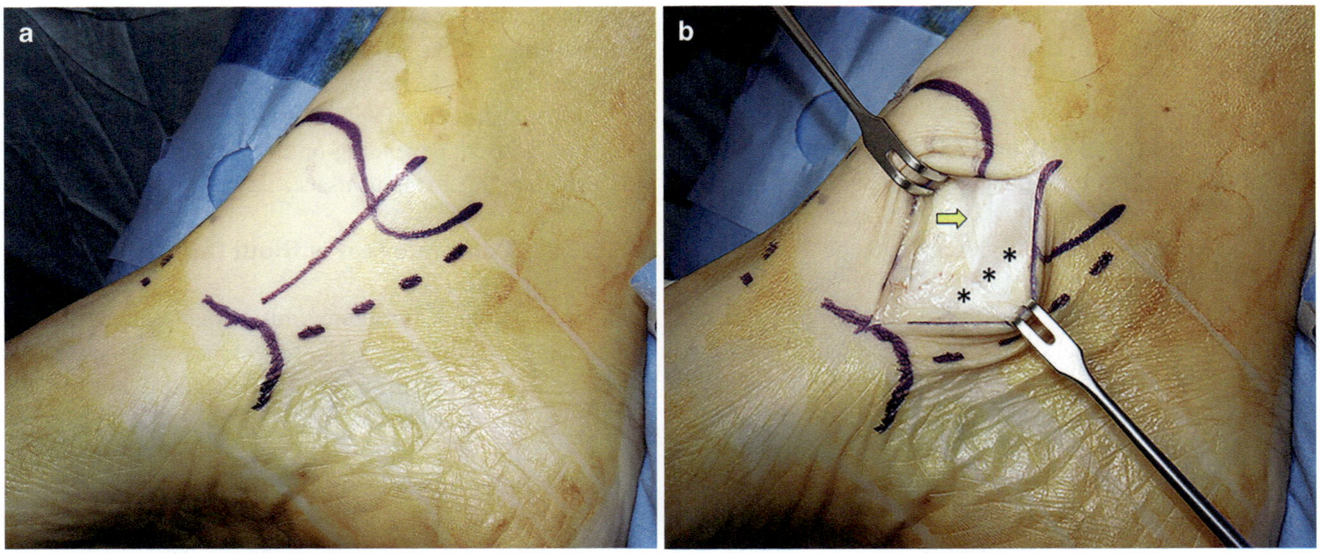

Fig. 5.31 *Surgical Technique: Surgical approach to the superficial deltoid.* (**a**) A gently curved incision is made along a line starting 2 cm cranial to the tip of the medial malleolus, going towards the medial aspect of the navicular bone, approximately 1 cm anterior to the PT tendon (dotted line), to expose the retinaculum that covers the deltoid ligament. The length of the incision depends on the extent of the injury. (**b**) If an injury to the spring ligament and/or distal PT tendon is suspected, the sheath of the PT tendon is dissected along its anterior insertion to the retinaculum (3 asterisks). Note the interval between the TCL and the TSL (arrow)

question is whether a primary reconstruction is feasible or whether the use of an autograft or allograft is necessary [75–83]. Correcting osteotomies to support the reconstructed soft tissue structures may also be considered [6, 10].

Surgical exposure starts with a gently curved incision along a line starting 2 cm cranially to the tip of the medial malleolus, going towards the medial aspect of the navicular bone (Fig. 5.31). Its length depends on the location and extension of the ligament lesion. After dissection of the extensor retinaculum, the anterior aspect of the deltoid ligament is exposed. Then, a longitudinal incision of the tendon sheath allows to explore the PT tendon and to identify the spring ligament. The TNL and TSL are then explored. While the foot is moved into pronation/abduction, the site of injury can be detected.

5.10.1 Proximal Tear of Deltoid Ligament (Type I-Injury)

In a Type I-injury, the ligamentous incompetence will be found mainly along the interval and the proximal insertion of the superficial layers of the deltoid.

In the case of an *acute injury* (Fig. 5.32a), a hematoma will be found. The fascia may be found mostly intact (Fig. 5.32b) and the extent as well as severity of the lesion can only be seen after further dissection (Fig. 5.32c). Transosseous sutures or a suture anchor are used for reattachment of the torn superficial deltoid ligament (Fig. 5.32d, e).

In a chronic setting, the superficial ligament can be found disconnected from the medial malleolus even when thickened. The rupture along the interval between the TSL and TCL may be visible or, if incomplete, be detected by manual testing.

5.10.1.1 Injury to TNL and TSL (Type I A)

A short longitudinal incision along the interval between the TSL and TCL, where usually a small fibrous septum without adherent connective fibers is present, is made to expose the anterior aspect of the medial malleolus. Typically, the deep part of the TCL is found to be disconnected from the medial malleolus, whereas the superficial part remains connected (Fig. 5.33a). After having roughened the anterior colliculus of the medial malleolus, an anchor is placed to aid refixation of the TNL and TSL, to reattach the deep part of the TCL to the medial malleolus (Fig. 5.33b, c), and to further close the interval (Fig. 5.33d–g). Additional size 0 resorbable sutures are used to enhance reattachment of the TNL and TSL at their proximal insertion and to close the tendon sheath (Fig. 5.33h).

5.10.1.2 Injury to the TNL, TSL and a Partial Injury to the TCT (Type I B)

After debridement of the insertion area at the medial malleolus, the ligament is meticulously debrided from the scar tissue (Fig. 5.34). One to two bony anchors are used to reattach the ligaments and additional sutures are used to firmly close the interval.

5.10.1.3 Injury to the TNL, TSL, and TCT (Type I C)

The surgical reconstruction starts similar to the one for a Type II B-injury (Fig. 5.35). In most instances, 2–3 bony anchors will be necessary to firmly reattach the ligaments. Additional sutures are used to reconstruct the midpart of the TSL and the interval. In cases where there is a bony avulsion of the proximal deltoid, the bony surfaces can be debrided and then fixed back to the medial malleolus with the use of screws or plates (Fig. 5.36).

5.10.2 Intermediate Tear of Deltoid Ligament (Type II-Injury)

A Type II-injury is characterized by a mid-substance tear involving parts (Fig. 5.37a) or all layers (Fig. 5.37b, c) of the superficial ligaments; in the case of a complete tear, the talar neck or proximal medial aspect of the talar head is exposed. Pronation of the foot and/or abduction of the forefoot permits better assessment of the severity and extent of the tear.

5.10.2.1 Incomplete Tear (Type II A)

If there is a partial rupture (Fig. 5.38), with the deep layers intact, a primary reconstruction by zigzag suturing, as is done in dynamic reconstruction, is usually enough for firm reconstruction. If the rupture involves all layers of the TSL, multiple non-resorbable sutures may be required to get a strong reconstruction (Fig. 5.39). Sometimes an anchor needs to be used, depending on the location and quality of the remaining ligamentous tissue.

5.10.2.2 Complete Tear without Defect (Type II B)

If there is a complete rupture with a small defect, a direct repair can be made (Fig. 5.40). Sometimes an anchor needs to be used, depending on the location and quality of the remaining ligamentous tissue.

5.10.2.3 Complete Tear with Defect (Type II C)

If there is a transmural lesion with a major defect (Fig. 5.41), the scarred borders of the ligament are debrided first. An anchor is placed on the anterior colliculus of the medial malleolus and the ruptured area of the TSL is grabbed by a zig-

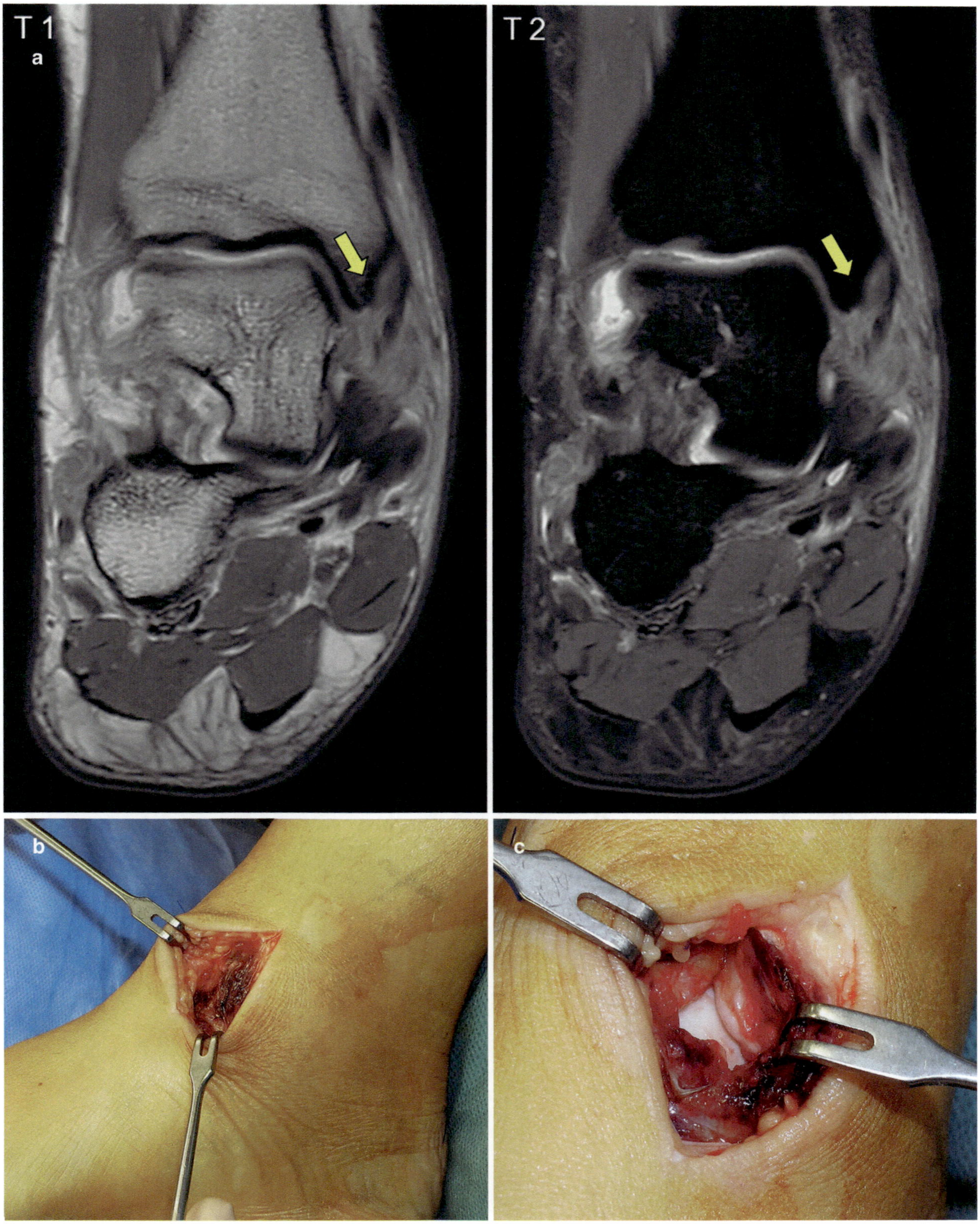

Fig. 5.32 *Surgical Technique: Repair of an acute proximal injury to the superficial deltoid (Injury Type I).* Acute severe pronation trauma of the right ankle in a 26-year-old female high-level floor ball player with a history of conservatively treated recurrent sprains. Currently presenting with a hematoma on the medial and lateral aspect of the ankle with tenderness. Preoperative arthroscopy revealed a Grade 2-injury with involvement of the superficial and also partially the deep deltoid ligament (Fig. 5.25). (**a**) MRI showing the avulsion of the superficial deltoid along the medial malleolus (arrow). (**b**) After incision of the skin, an extended hematoma is found while the fascia is mostly intact. (**c**) The extent of the lesion can be seen after further dissection of the fascia at the injury site. Note that the injury extends to the outer side of the medial malleolus, with avulsion of the ligament from the medial malleolus. (**d**) A suture button is placed on the anterior aspect of the medial malleolus, just above its tip, allowing to reattach the ligament (**e**). Additional sutures are used to repair the ligament. This patient returned to competitive sports 3 months later and she played the world championships 2 weeks after that

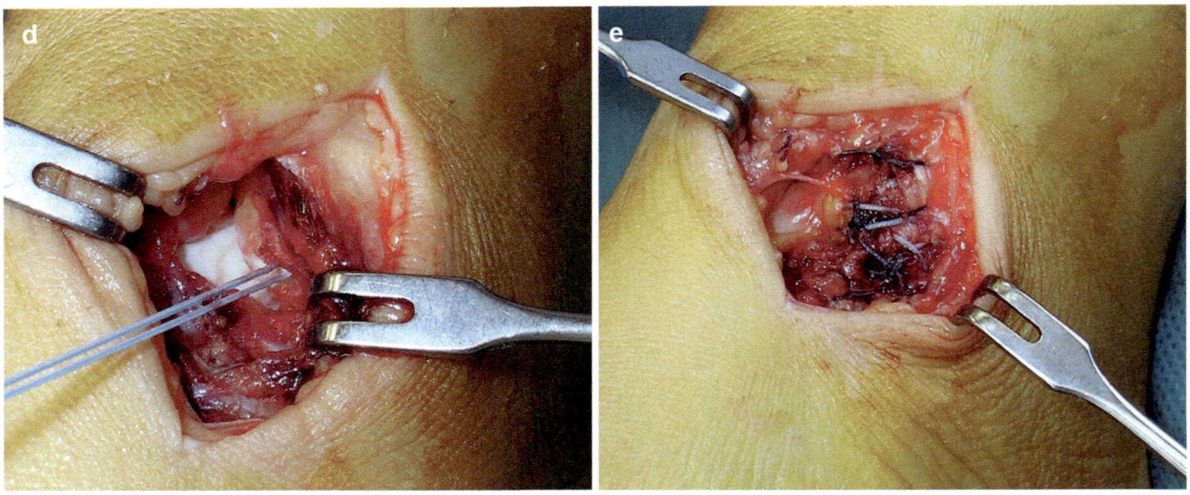

Fig. 5.32 (continued)

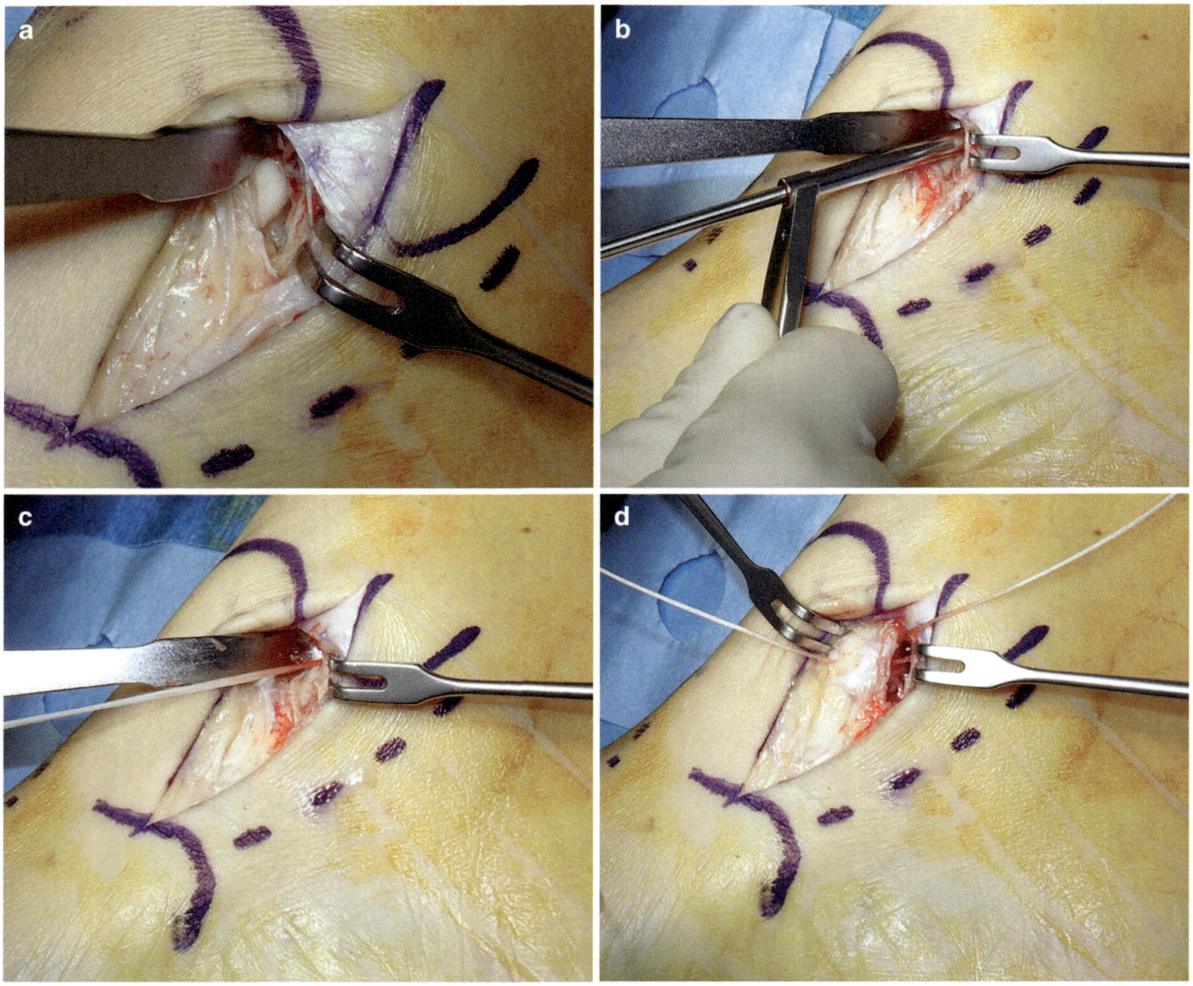

Fig. 5.33 *Surgical Technique: Repair of a chronic proximal injury to the superficial deltoid (Injury Type I A)*. A 36-year-old female triathlon athlete sustained a pronation trauma 18 months ago and is currently suffering from medial ankle pain on her right foot which hinders her from running on uneven ground and taking right turns. Furthermore, a feeling of instability is present, especially when tired. (**a**) The tiny retinaculum is dissected along the interval between the TSL and TCL to expose the anterior aspect of the medial malleolus. Typically, the deep part of the TCL is found to be disconnected from the medial malleolus, whereas the superficial part remains connected. (**b**) After having roughened the bony surface, a drill hole is made on the anterior aspect of the anterior colliculus. (**c**) A suture anchor is inserted. (**d**) First, the TSL is taken by the suture. (**e**) Then, the suture is turned posteriorwards to grab the TCL. (**f**) One to two further turns are done, followed by the second suture. (**f**) While the suture is tightened, the interval closes. (**g**) The knot is aimed to be placed anterior to the medial malleolus to not cause any irritation when wearing shoes. (**h**) Finally, the sheath of the PT tendon is closed with interrupted sutures

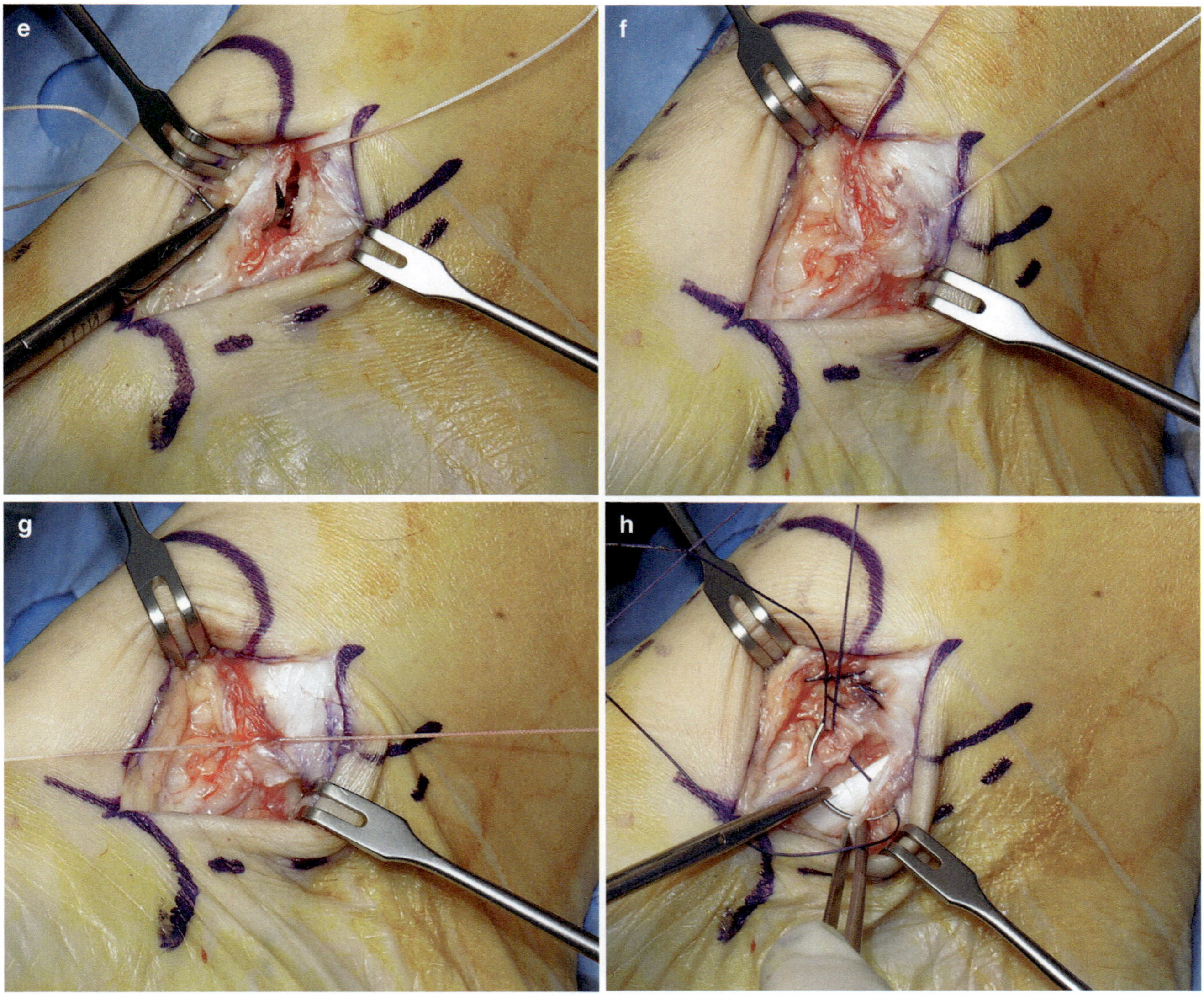

Fig. 5.33 (continued)

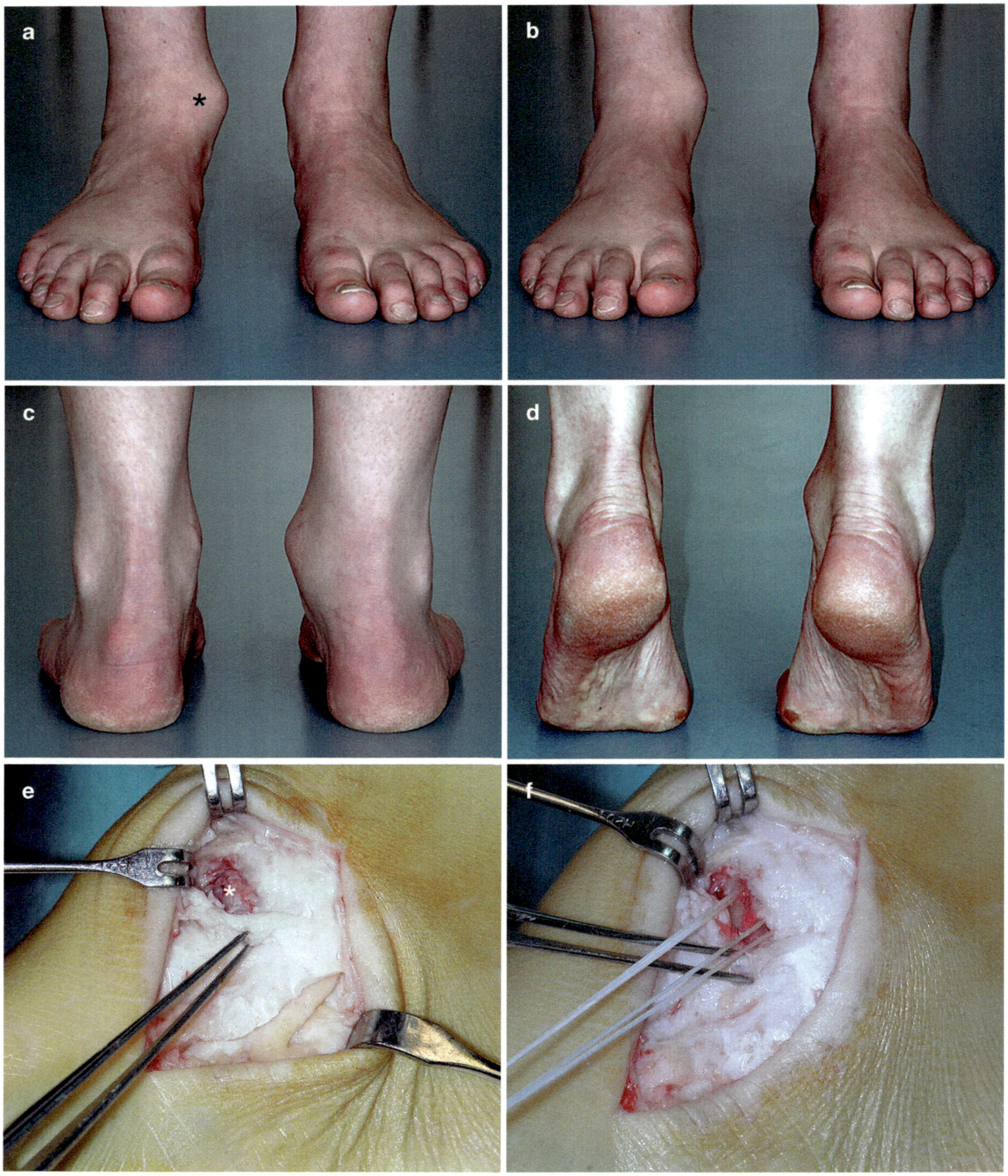

Fig. 5.34 *Surgical Technique: Repair of a chronic proximal injury to the superficial deltoid (Injury Type I B).* This 24-year-old sports student sustained a pronation trauma 15 months ago when landing after a jump from the high bar. Initially, there was a big hematoma on the anterior aspect of her right ankle. Despite protecting the ankle with tape bandages for sports exercises and performing intensive physiotherapy, the symptoms increased enforcing her to think about dropping out of university. Clinical investigation: (**a**) When standing relaxed, the medial prominence of her right ankle is seen markedly due to the internal rotation of the tibia. Pain on palpation is found at the anteromedial corner of the tibiotalar joint (asterisk) and along the PT tendon. (**b**) When asking the patient to correct the pronation deformity by activating the PT muscle, the tibia is seen to externally rotate, thereby the medial prominence is decreased, however still markedly bigger than the unaffected contralateral side. (**c**) Analogously, the heel is seen in valgus when relaxed. Note that there is no forefoot abduction. (**d**) The heel misalignment is seen to completely disappear when the patient is asked to go in tiptoe position, indicating a normal PT function. (**e**) Surgical exploration evidences an avulsion of the TNL and TSL from the anterior colliculus with some extension into the TCL. The scarred ligament is typically thickened at the injury site (asterisk = Tip of medial malleolus [anterior colliculus]). (**f**) The anterior aspect of the medial malleolus is roughened, and two suture anchors are inserted to serve for tight reattachment of the torn ligaments. (**g–j**) Clinical appearance 16 years after surgical reconstruction showing symmetrical function of both ankles. After the surgical reconstruction, the patient was able to continue her studies in sports and has been working as a sports teacher, without any limitations, for the past 15 years

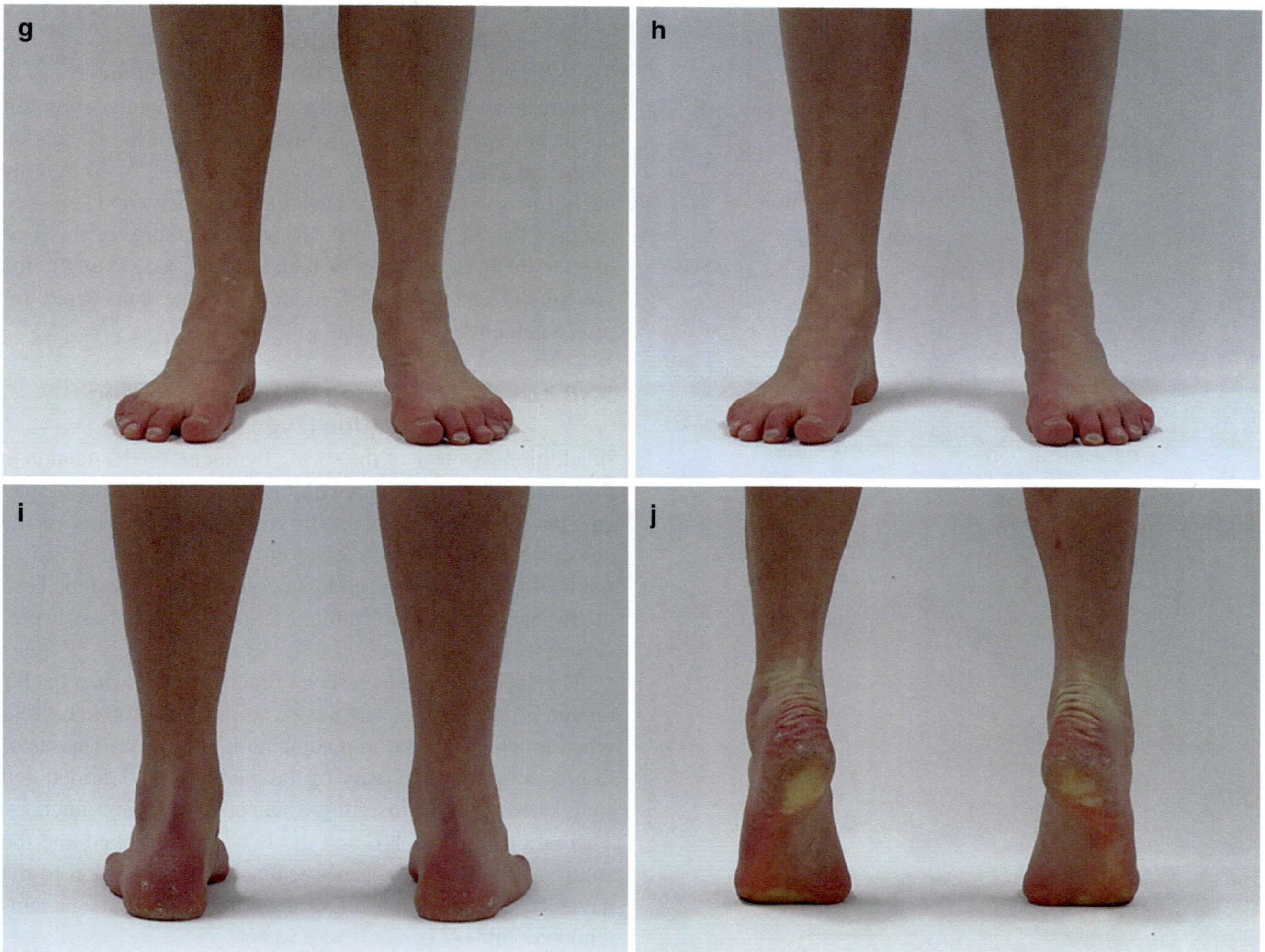

Fig. 5.34 (continued)

zag suture for dynamic reconstruction. If the defect cannot be properly closed, two flaps are prepared, of which one remains attached distally and the other one proximally. An anchor is used at the anterior colliculus of the medial malleolus and another one on the tubercle of the navicular bone to provide separate fixation of each flap. A zigzag suture technique is used to preserve elasticity of the reconstructed ligament and, most importantly, an overlap of the sutures is strictly avoided to not get a tenodese effect between the medial malleolus and navicular. Thereafter, additional size 0 resorbable sutures are used to enhance the stability of the reconstructed ligament. Alternatively, an augmentation with an autograft or internal brace can be considered to enhance the strength of the reconstructed ligament.

5.10.3 Spring Ligament Tear (Type III-Injury)

The Type III-lesion involves the calcaneonavicular (spring) ligament complex (Fig. 5.42a) and often also includes an avulsion injury of the PT tendon at the navicular tuberosity (Fig. 5.42b). Often the ligament complex is disconnected from the navicular bone, with some remaining tissue however, covering the lesion (Fig. 5.42c).

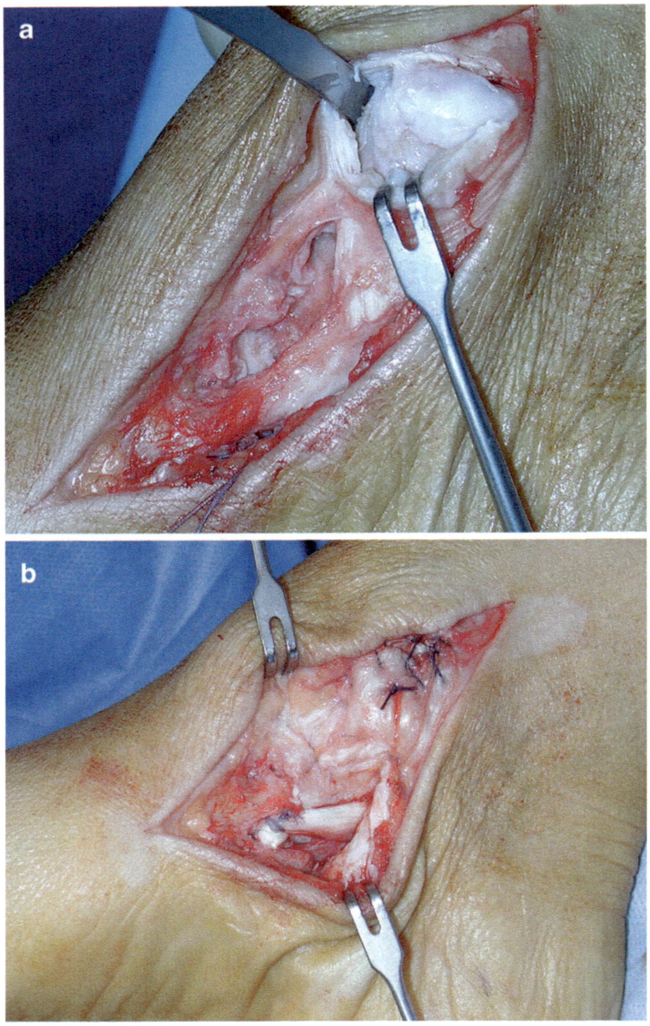

Fig. 5.35 *Surgical Technique: Repair of a chronic proximal injury to the superficial deltoid (Injury Type I C).* This 54-year-old female trail runner sustained a new severe sprain of her right hindfoot after experiencing recurrent sprains previously. Besides sensing pain on palpation and during loading around the medial malleolus, she also senses lateral ankle pain due to an impingement and peroneal tendon dislocation. (**a**) Surgical exploration evidences a complete avulsion of the superficial deltoid involving also the main part of the TCL. The insertion area of the TNL, TSL, and TCL is typically bald, with a pseudo-articulation surface due to the motion of the loaded ligaments while moving the foot. (**b**) After having roughened the insertion area, the torn ligaments are reattached by two bony anchors with sutures extended to the intermediate portion of the TSL followed by multiple sutures to obtain a strong ligament reconstruction. An FDL transfer was also done (technique see Fig. 5.57)

5.10.3.1 Tear of Spring Ligament with Intact PT Tendon (Type III A)

The SMCNL and ICNL are detached from the insertion on the navicular, sometimes with a small ligament portion left on the navicular, whereas the insertion area of the PT tendon on the navicular tuberosity remains intact (Fig. 5.43). A bony anchor is inserted into the navicular tuberosity and serves to reattach the SMCNL and ICNL. As the quality of the ligament at its distal end may be bad, a side-to-side suture to the very distal end of the PT tendon may be considered for reinforcement.

5.10.3.2 Tear of Spring Ligament Involving the PT Tendon (Type III B)

In addition to a tear of the spring ligament, the PT tendon is disconnected from the navicular tuberosity; however, it may still have an attachment to the distal plantar aspect of the navicular bone (Fig. 5.44). Additionally, the connection of the PT tendon through the ligamentous network to the base of the metatarsal bones and sustentaculum tali is still preserved (Fig. 5.45).

This lesion can be best seen intraoperatively when the PT tendon is pulled away with a hook towards medioplantar, and when moving the foot into supination/adduction. The insertion area on the tuberosity of the navicular is debrided and roughened before inserting one or two bony anchors. Thereafter, the SMCNL and the ICNL are grabbed and the suture is continued to firmly reattach the PT tendon to the navicular tuberosity to get a strong refixation of the ligament-tendon complex.

5.10.3.3 Bony Avulsion of PT Tendon with Spring Ligament Tear (Type III C)

In these injuries there is a bony avulsion of the PT tendon from the navicular bone, either as an acute fracture (Fig. 5.46) or a disconnection of an accessory external tibial bone (Fig. 5.47), typically associated with a partial rupture of the SMCNL along its insertion on the medioplantar aspect of the navicular.

In the case of an acute avulsion of the PT tendon, the fragment is usually too small for screw fixation (Fig. 5.48). After sharp resection of the fragment, refixation of the PT tendon is achieved by one or two bony anchors.

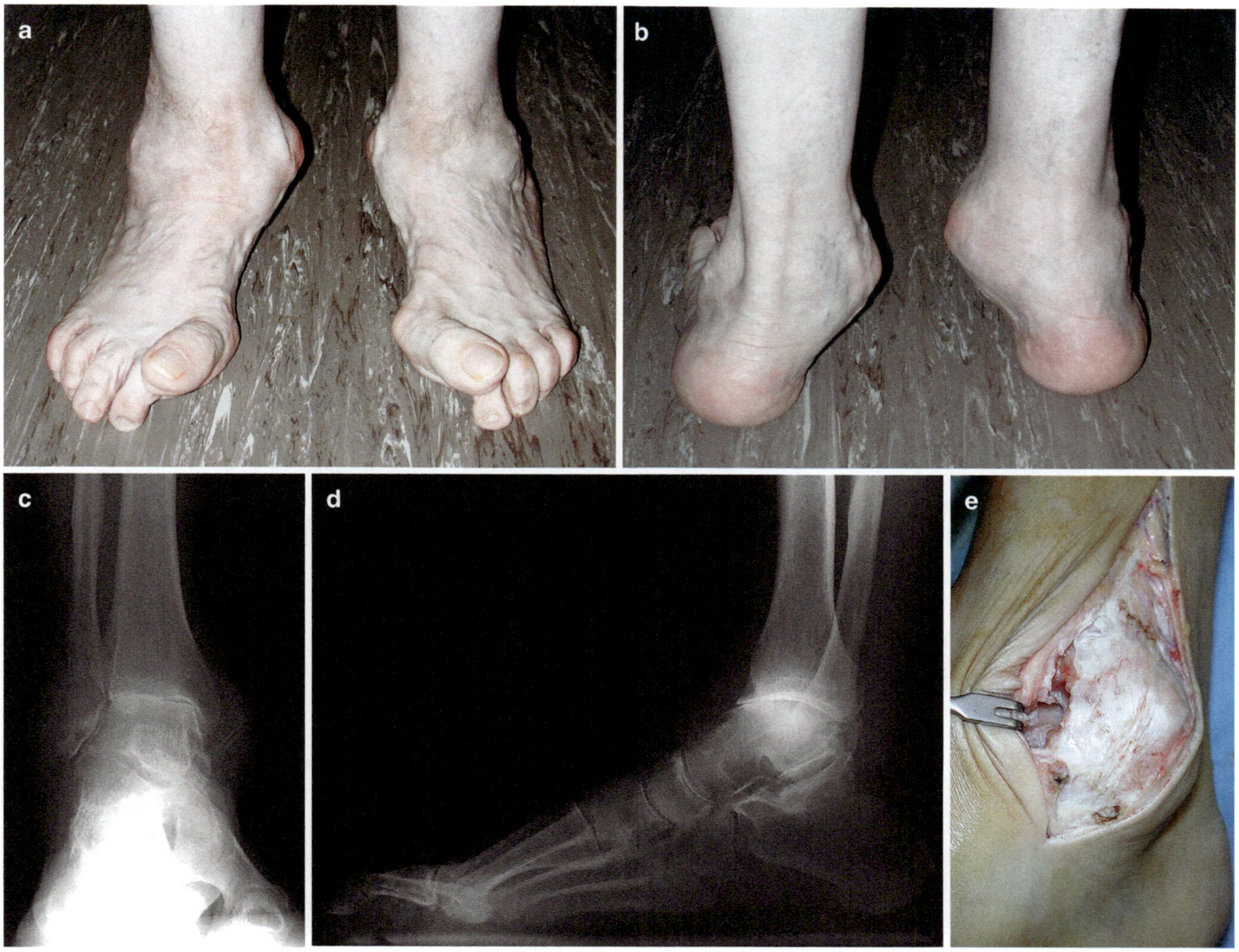

Fig. 5.36 *Surgical Technique: Repair of a chronic proximal injury to the superficial deltoid with bony avulsion (Injury Type I C).* This 52-year-old former national soccer goalkeeper sustained multiple ankle sprains during his carrier which were never appropriately treated and currently experiences progressive pain mainly on his right ankle that hinders him from walking for more than 10 min. (**a**) Clinical anterior view assessment shows the medial prominence of the ankle and the loss of the medial arch support. Impressively, there is a cock-up deformity of the great toe that has obviously lost its supporting function, whereas the lesser toes are still used for stabilization of the hindfoot through the flexor digitorum longus activation. (**b**) Posterior view showing the medial prominence of the ankle due to the internally rotated leg and the valgus malalignment of the heel, while the forefoot is in regular position. (**c**) AP standard radiographs under weight-bearing showing a slight valgus tilt with wear of the lateral tibiotalar joint and very little valgus malalignment. (**d**) The lateral view shows anterior extrusion of the talus with wear of the anterior tibiotalar joint. (**e**) Surgical exposure of the medial ankle shows the deltoid ligament scarred and elongated. (**f**) Further dissection evidences the naked medial malleolus covered by a smooth surface from the articulation with the bony avulsion of the deltoid. (**g**) The bony surfaces of both the malleolar and avulsion side are roughened. (**h**) Screw fixation of a compression plate and transosseous sutures are used for firm reattachment of the ligaments while the foot is held in a neutral position. (**i**) Exposure of the lateral ankle ligaments shows a similar injury pattern with complete avulsion. (**j**) The lateral ankle ligaments are reattached in a similar way. After an initial favorable evolution with return to a normal daily life, ankle osteoarthritis progressed, making total ankle replacement necessary 12 years later

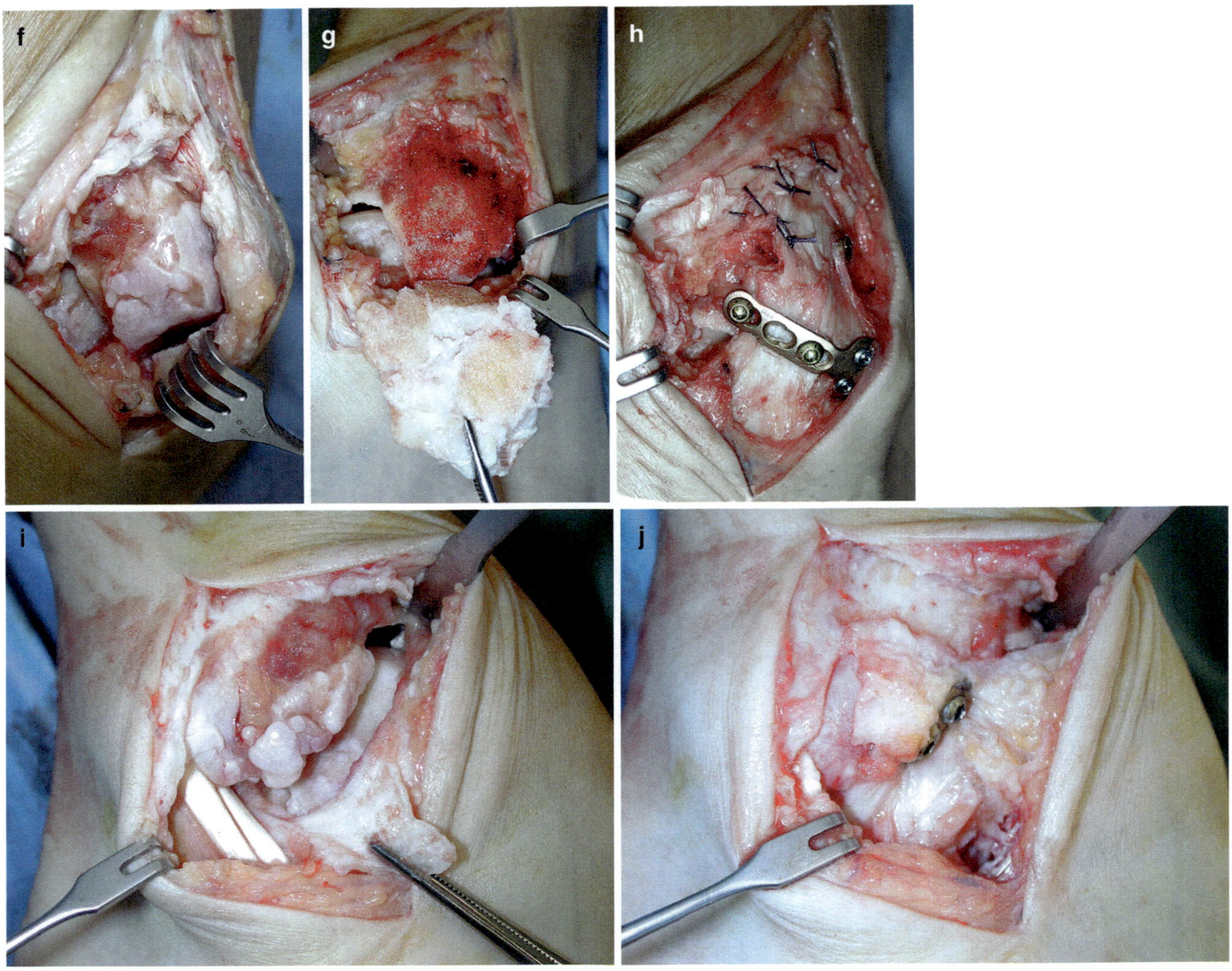

Fig. 5.36 (continued)

In the case of an accessory external tibial bone, it is separated from the navicular by dissecting the pseudarthrosis with a knife (Fig. 5.47). If the accessory bone is big enough for reattachment, e.g., approximately 5 mm of diameter, a bone cut is performed along the medial border of the navicular and thereafter on the accessory bone. While the foot is held in supination and adduction, and the PT tendon is pulled distally, the accessory bone is reduced against the navicular and thereafter fixed by one or two 3-mm screws. Additional transosseous sutures are used to enhance the fixation of the bone and the PT tendon to the dorsal aspect of the navicular. If the accessory bone is too small for refixation, it is excised, and the PT tendon is reattached with a bony anchor and transosseous sutures. Additional non-resorbable sutures are used to reattach the spring ligament and, if incompetent, the TNL and TSL ligaments are additionally reattached at their insertion site on the navicular.

5.10.4 Deep Deltoid Ligament Tear (Type IV-Injury)

Though it is still controversially discussed whether primary repair of the deltoid ligament is necessary after an acute injury with valgus instability of the ankle in the coronal plane, there is evidence that surgical repair may yield better results than non-surgical treatment [12, 13, 15, 84–86]. While the superficial deltoid ligament is ruptured along its insertion area on the medial malleolus, the deep deltoid ligament (ATTL and PTTL) is typically ruptured distally at its insertion onto the talus (Fig. 5.49). Both parts of the deltoid ligament are repaired by using bony anchors or transosseous sutures to reattach the stumps onto the bone at their insertion site. Additional sutures may be used to reattach the torn fibers.

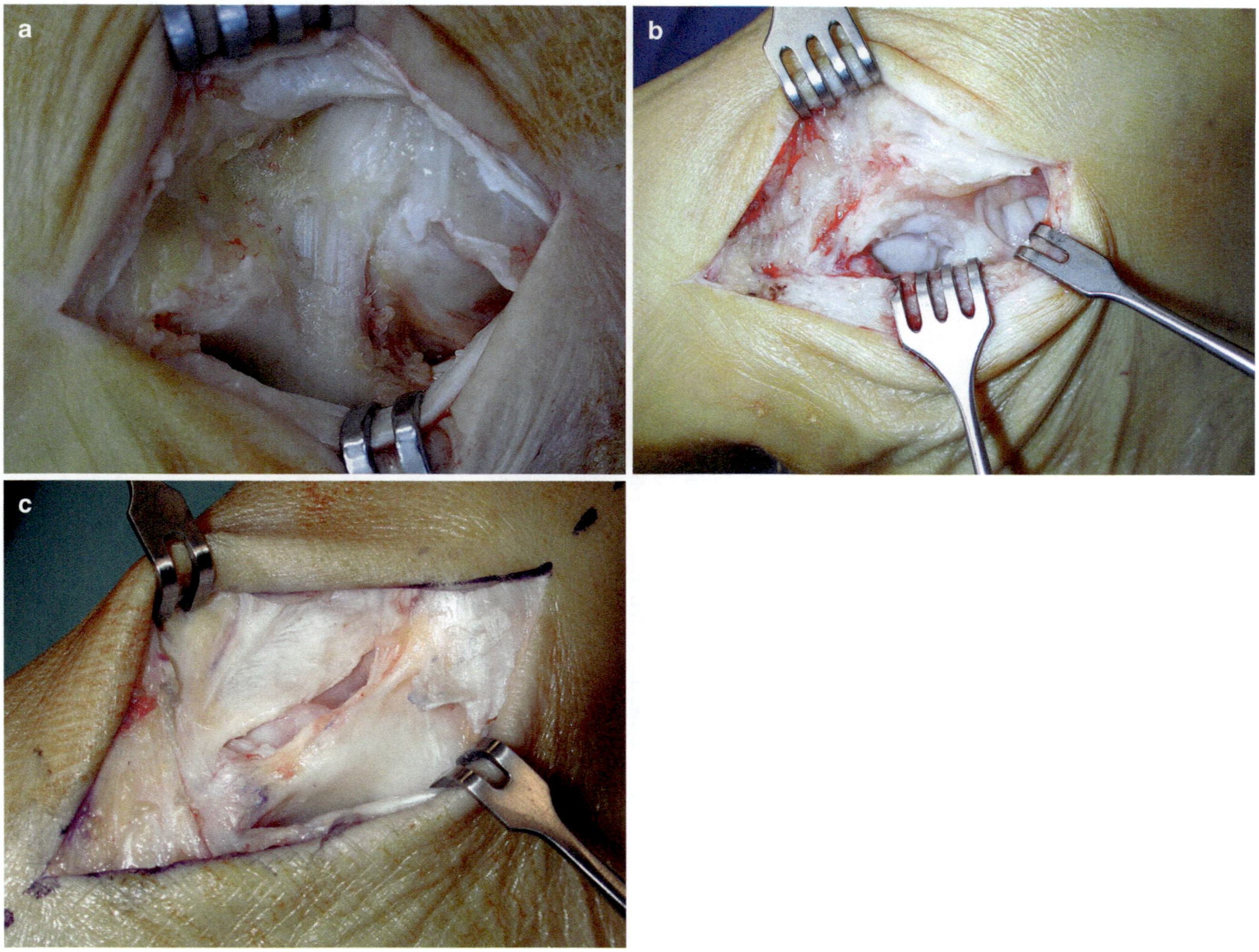

Fig. 5.37 *Surgical Technique: Exposure of a mid-substance tear of the superficial deltoid (Injury Type II).* A Type II-injury is characterized by a mid-substance tear of the superficial deltoid. (**a**) Partial rupture not involving all layers, thus the talar head cannot be seen. (**b**) Complete tear after a pronation trauma 8 weeks ago. (**c**) Complete long-standing tear with scarred and thickened borders showing the talar head. Pronation of the foot and/or abduction of the forefoot permits better assessment of the severity and extent of the tear

Chronic injuries with progressive valgus destabilization of the ankle are challenging to treat as they are, in most instances, associated with peritalar instability (Fig. 5.50) or peritalar subluxation (Fig. 5.51).

5.10.4.1 Incomplete Tear of the Deep Deltoid with a Talar Tilt <5° (Type IV A)

Though primary reconstruction of the deltoid ligament by its advancement and reattachment to the medial malleolus usually provides acceptable results intraoperatively (Fig. 5.52), in most instances, they are not able to resist the physiological force over time and thus fail. Augmentation with a free plantaris tendon graft (Fig. 5.53) and/or internal brace (Fig. 5.54) were found to be more effective in providing stability in the long run.

5.10.4.2 Subtotal Tear of the Deep Deltoid with a Talar Tilt <10° (Type IV B)

Several techniques using autograft or allograft tendons, or internal brace (Fig. 5.54) for reconstruction, have been proposed with acceptable intraoperative results. However, long-term data, especially showing whether they can resist against the applied physiological forces over time or whether they restrict motion [75–83], is still outstanding. The main surgical reconstruction challenges lie in the placement of the tunnels for the graft and the course of the reconstructed ligament. Quantitative analysis using available imaging modalities, to describe the anatomical origins and insertions of the individual superficial and deep deltoid constituents, may facilitate the development of the novel anatomical reconstruction possibilities and allow surgeons to plan the locations of the

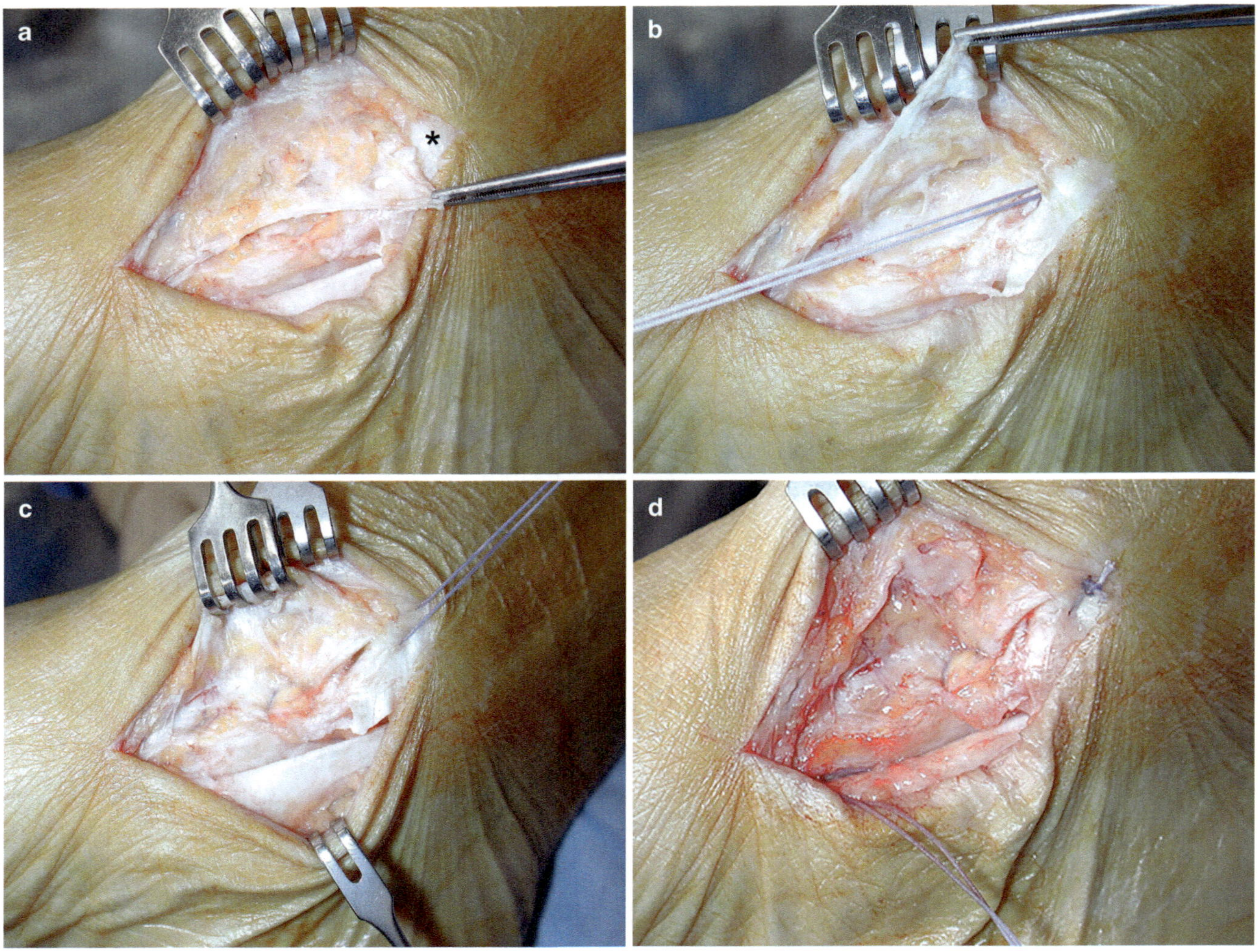

Fig. 5.38 *Surgical Technique: Repair of an incomplete mid-substance tear of the superficial deltoid (Injury Type II A).* This 44-year-old female runner sustained a pronation trauma while running in the snow 3 months ago. Since the patient had persistent pain and a feeling of instability with subsequent overload of the PT tendon despite shoe modifications, surgical repair was initiated. (**a**) After having opened the sheath of the PT tendon, the tinned extensor retinaculum is dissected from the deltoid (asterisk = tip of medial malleolus). (**b**) The retinaculum flap is kept away to expose the deltoid. Abduction-adduction movement of the foot may show the incompetent and partially torn deltoid. A bony anchor is inserted on the anterior aspect of the anterior colliculus. (**c**) A zigzag suture is performed for dynamic repair of the ligament and then tightened. (**d**) After having checked whether some pronation/abduction movement of the foot is still possible, a knot is made. This patient returned to full sports activity 4 months later

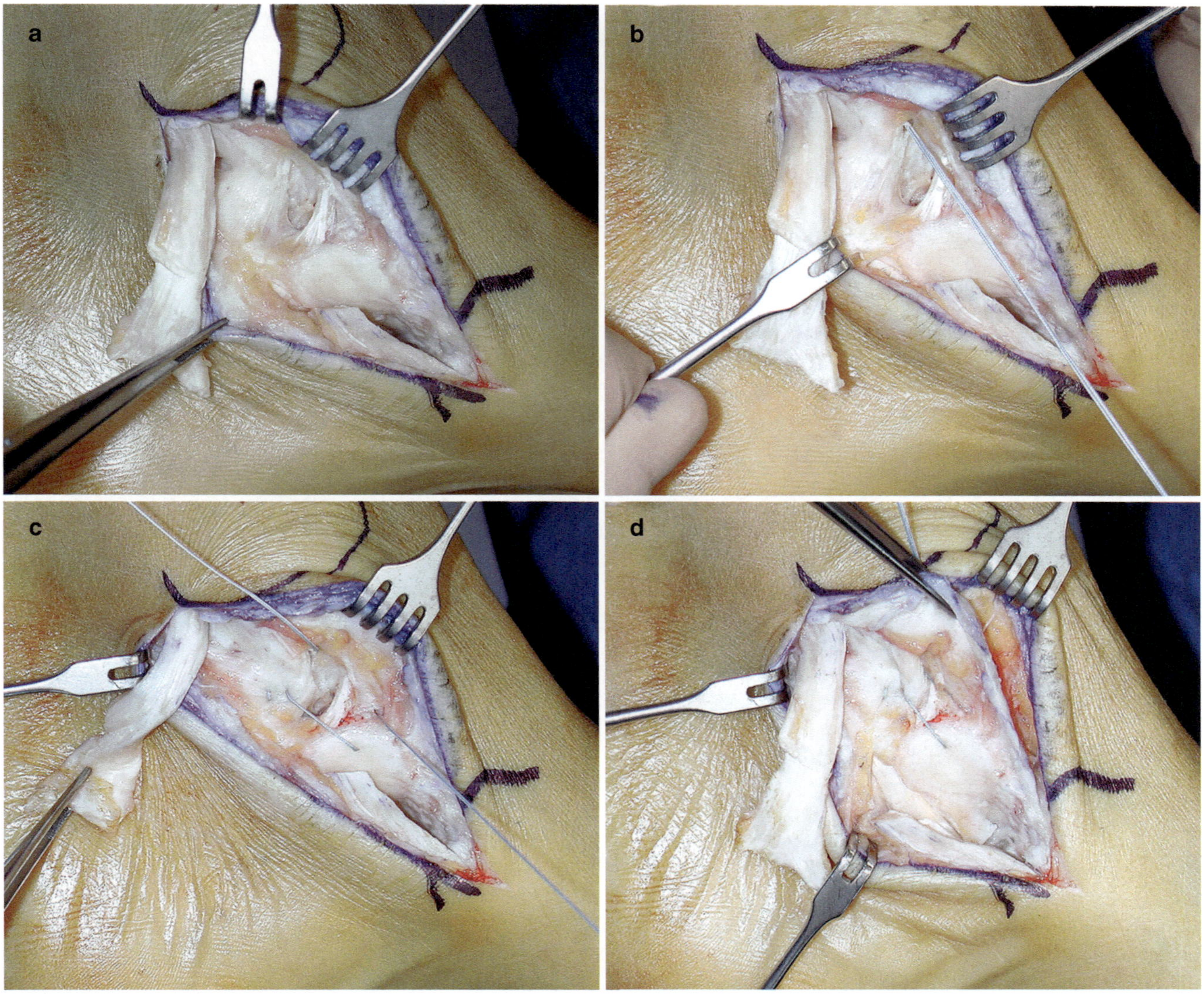

Fig. 5.39 *Surgical Technique: Repair of a small transmural midsubstance tear of the superficial deltoid (Injury Type II A).* This 53-year-old female patient experienced a pronation/abduction trauma of her foot while playing badminton 11 months ago and senses an onset of pain along the PT tendon when trying to practice any physical activity. She also notices having a medial instability of her foot that has become more difficult to actively control over time. (**a**) Surgical exposure evidenced an elongated PT tendon and a rather small and transmural rupture of the tibiospring ligament. The PT tendon is dissected by a Z-shaped cut close to its distal insertion (not shown). (**b**) A bony anchor is inserted on the anterior aspect of the medial malleolus. (**c**) Multiple sutures are done to close the defect. (**d**) The suture is finished while holding the foot in a slight supinated position. Thereafter, the PT tendon is reconstructed by shortening it 1 cm (surgical technique see Fig. 5.58)

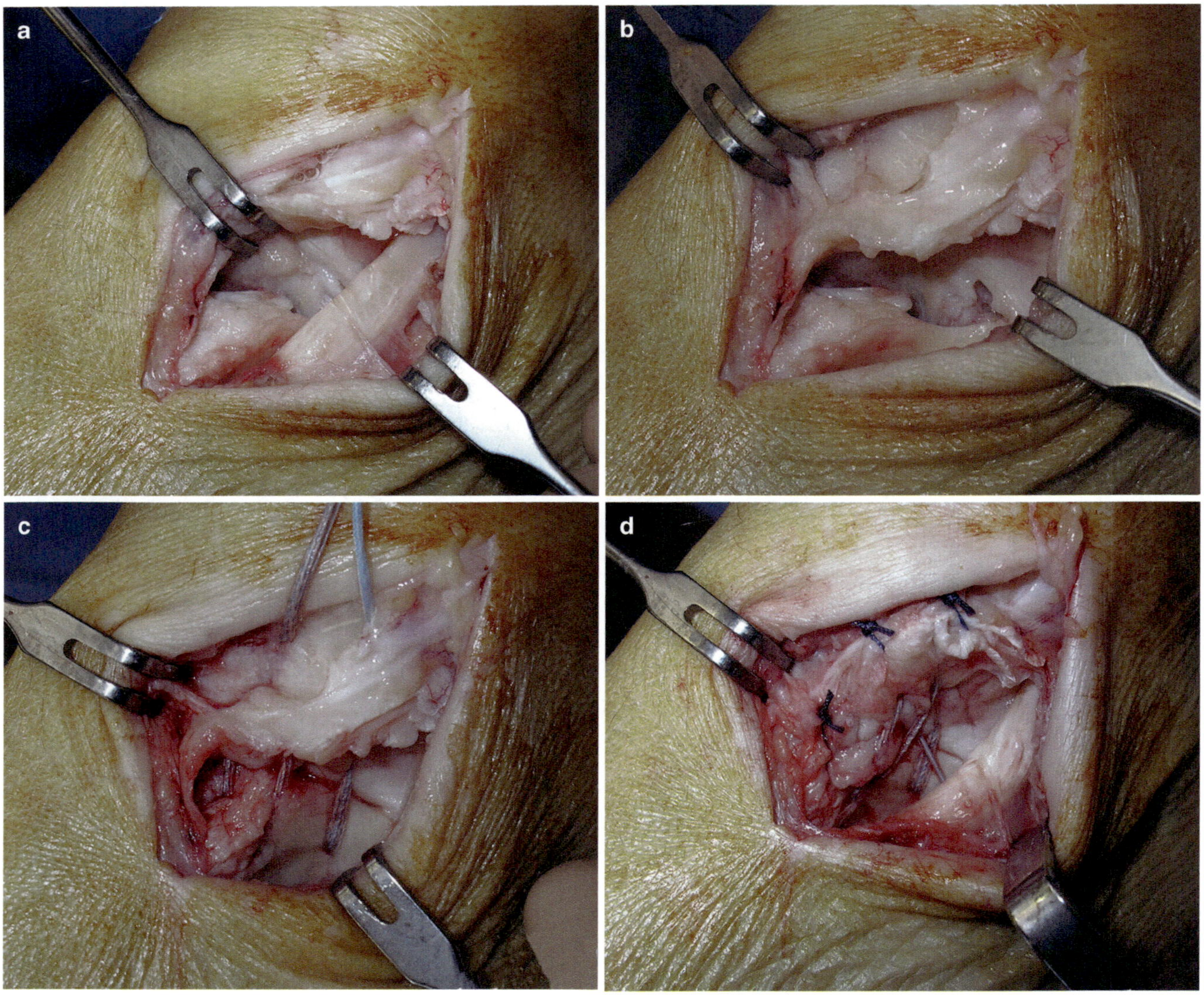

Fig. 5.40 *Surgical Technique: Repair of a complete mid-substance tear of the superficial deltoid (Injury Type II B).* This 38-year-old soccer player sustained a complex pronation-abduction trauma of his right foot 6 weeks ago which does not allow him to return to sports activities. He is complaining about experiencing pain on the medial aspect of his foot and he is uncapable of kicking a ball with his inner foot. (**a**) Surgical exploration shows the complete rupture that is mainly covered by the PT tendon.) (**b**) While the PT tendon is kept away, the extent of the tear is visible. (**c**) Multiple non-resorbable sutures are used to close the defect. (**d**) Additional resorbable sutures are used to finalize the reconstruction. This patient returned to playing soccer 4½ months later

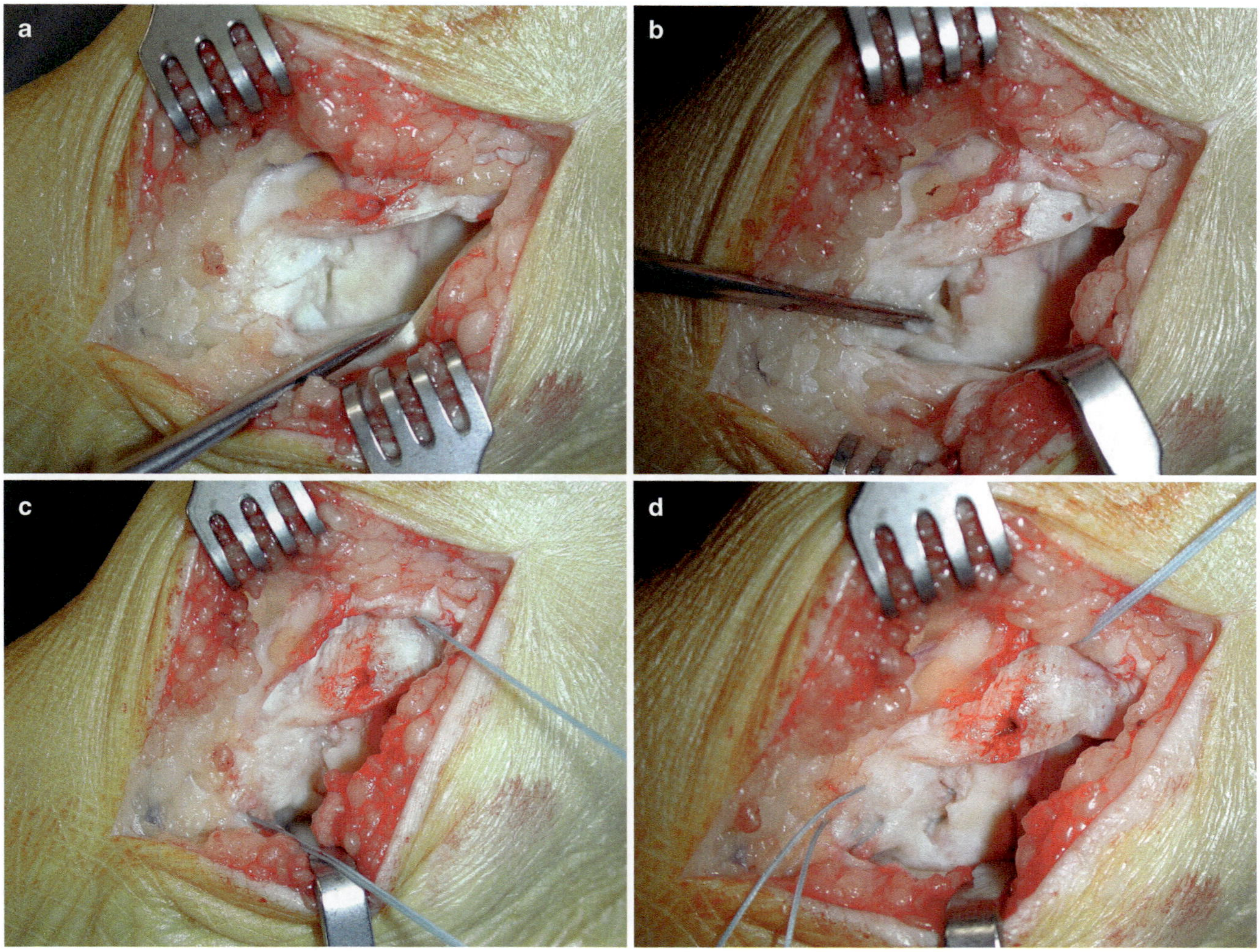

Fig. 5.41 *Surgical Technique: Repair of an extended complete mid-substance tear of the superficial deltoid (Injury Type II C).* This 58-year-old very active female patient suffering from bilateral overpronation since her childhood observed an increase of the deformity after having twisted her ankle 15 months earlier while slippering on ice. Additionally, she reported sensing retromalleolar pain. (**a**) Surgical exposure shows an extended transmural tear of the tibiospring ligament. (**b**) The tear extends into the superomedial calcaneonavicular ligament. (**c**) A bony anchor is inserted on the medial malleolus and another one to the tuberosity of the navicular. (**d**) Both sutures are used to grab the remaining ligament tissue. (**e**) The distal suture is continued to close the distal aspect of the tear. (**f**) The proximal suture is continued to close the proximal aspect of the tear, paying attention not to across the loop of the distal suture. (**g**) When tightening both sutures the tear is seen to close while a strong ligament construct is created. (**h**) After having checked that some abduction/pronation movement of the foot is preserved, a knot is made

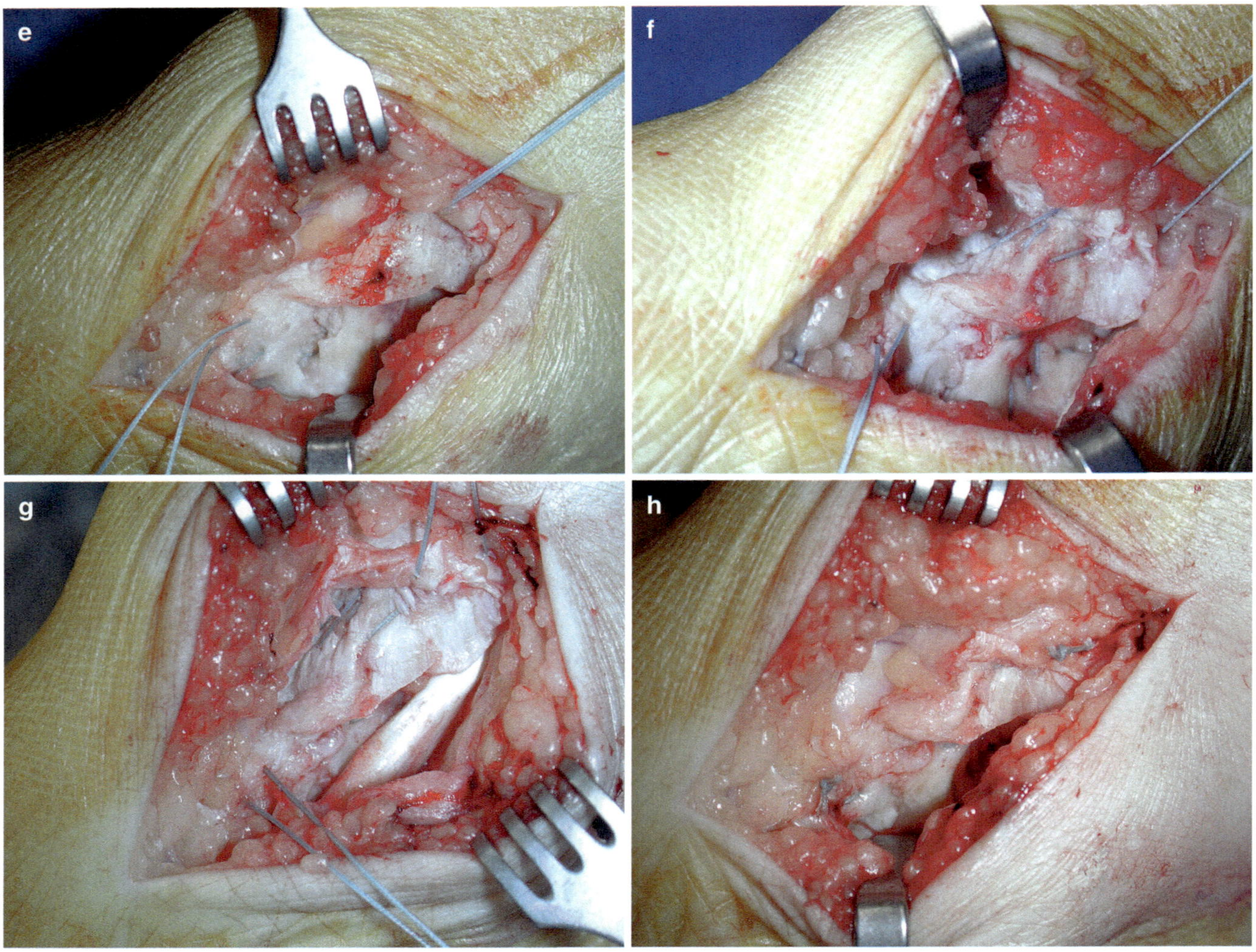

Fig. 5.41 (continued)

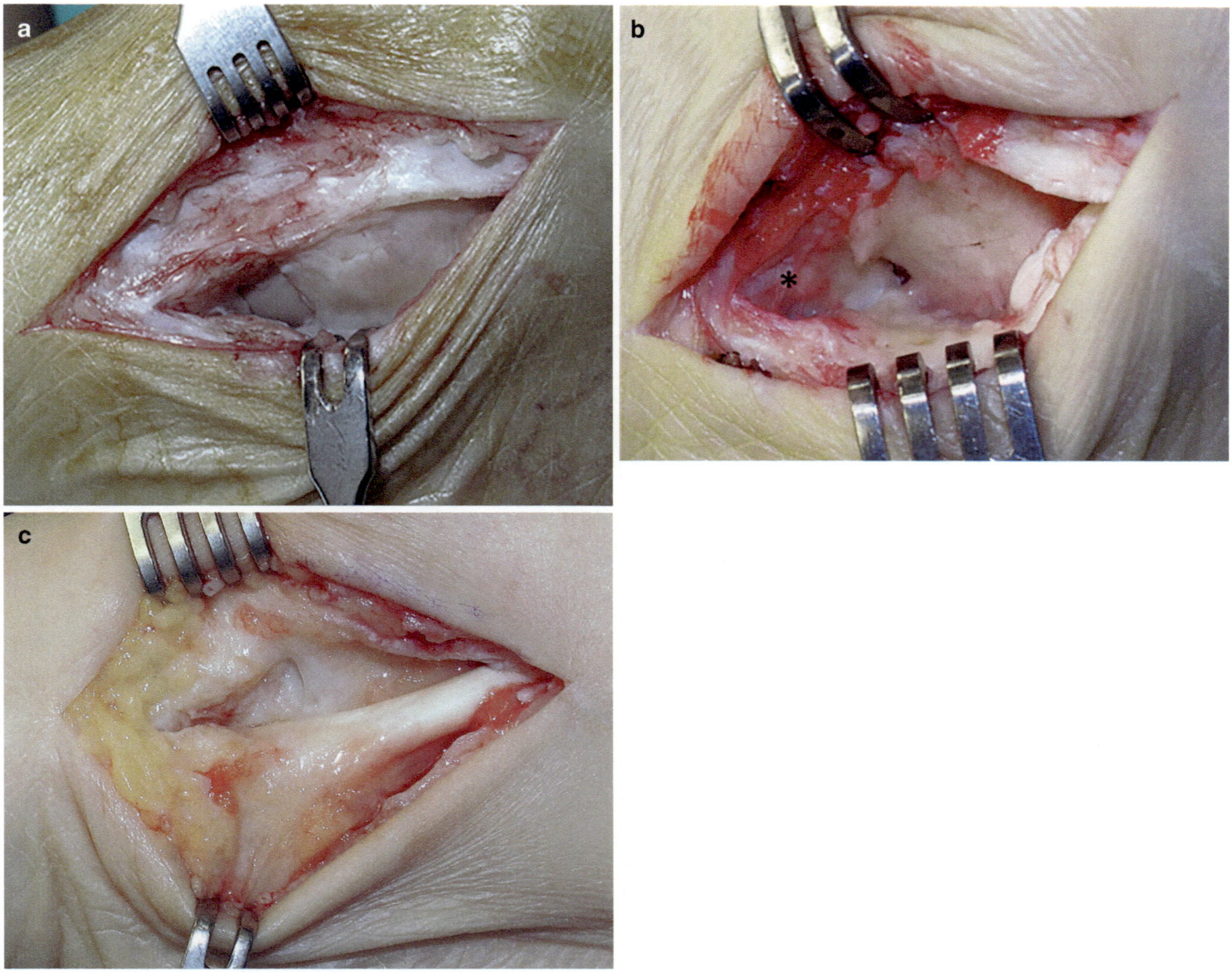

Fig. 5.42 *Surgical Technique: Exposure of a spring ligament tear (Injury Type III).* A Type III-lesion involves the calcaneonavicular (spring) ligament complex. (**a**) Isolated tear of the spring ligament. (**b**) Rather small tear of the spring ligament associated with an avulsion of the PT tendon from the tuberosity of the navicular (asterisk). (**c**) Some remaining tissue hides the avulsion of the PT tendon

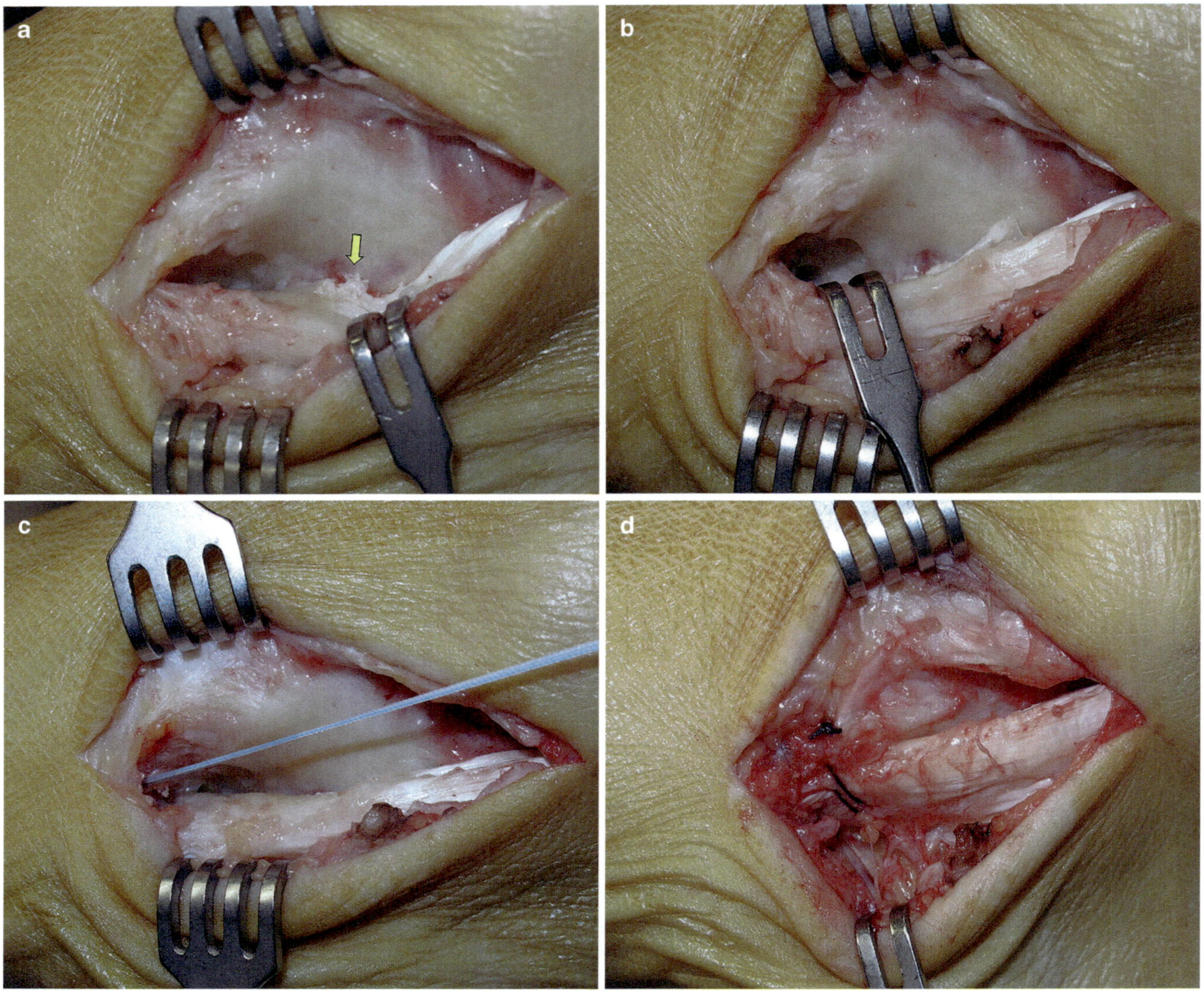

Fig. 5.43 *Surgical Technique: Repair of an isolated tear of the spring ligament (Injury Type III A).* This 39-year-old male mountain biker sustained a pronation trauma of his foot when toppling down a slope. Initially, he ignored the pain and swelling on the medial aspect of the foot and showed up 3 months later only when pain along the PT tendon occurred. (**a**) After having dissected the distal sheath of the PT tendon and evacuating some fluid, the PT tendon is found with some microruptures (arrow). Notice also the inflammatory response of the tendon sheath and the isolated rupture of the SMCNL and MPOCNL. (**b**) The lesion to the spring ligament can be better seen when the PT tendon is pulled away, a maneuver that also permits to ensure the integrity of its insertion to the navicular tuberosity. (**c**) A suture anchor is inserted to the navicular tuberosity and serves to reattach the spring ligament. (**d**) Due to the bad quality of the ligament on its distal part, a side-to-side suture to the very distal end of the PT tendon is used to reinforce the reconstruction

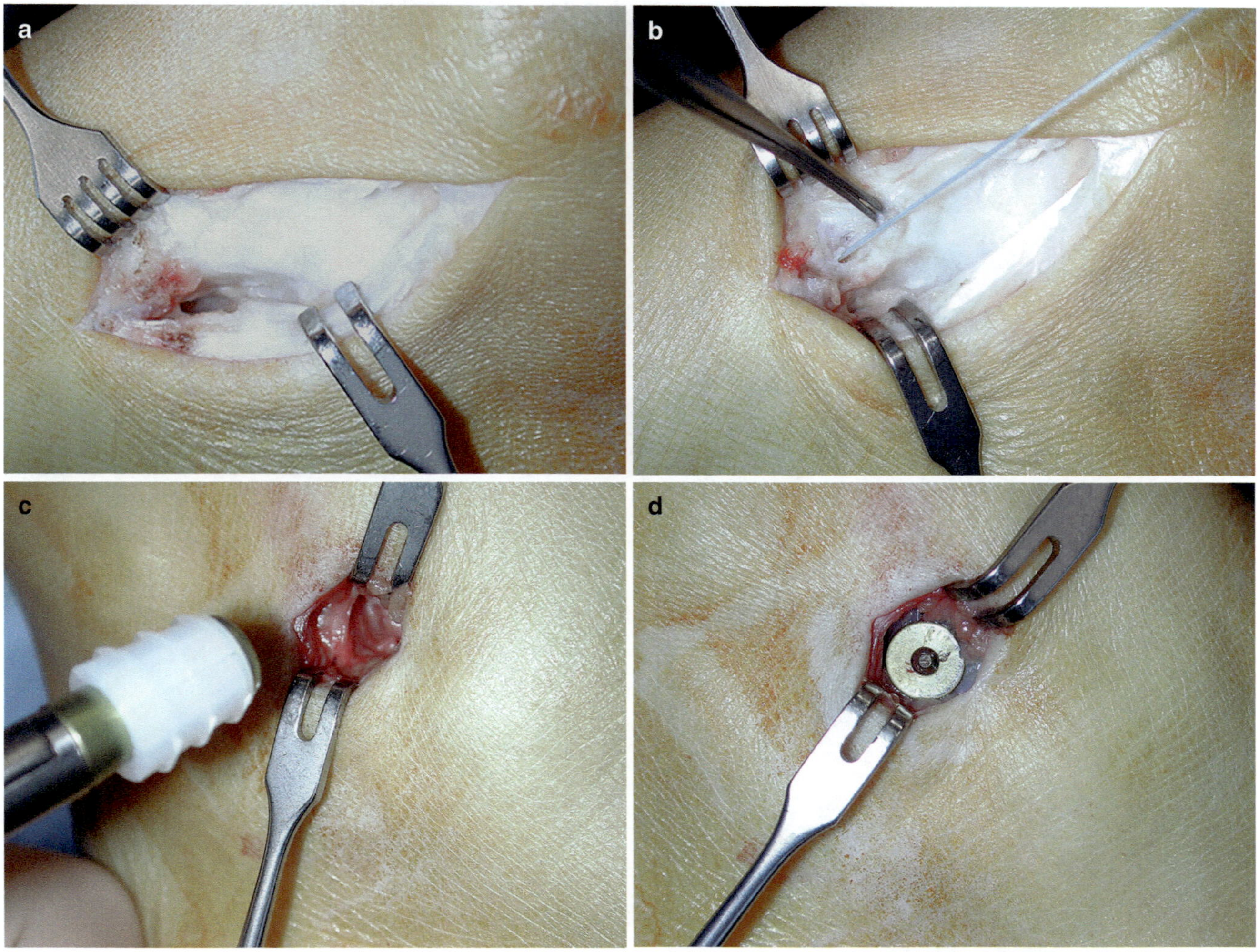

Fig. 5.44 *Surgical Technique: Repair of a tear of the spring ligament associated with an avulsion of the PT tendon with arthroreisis (Injury Type III B)*. Same patient as Fig. 5.15. (**a**) Surgical exploration shows an avulsion of PT tendon from navicular with incomplete tear of spring ligament (SMCNL). (**b**) A suture anchor is used for reattachment of PT tendon and repair of spring ligament. (**c**) In this young patient, an arthroreisis was done to protect the soft tissue reconstruction. The sinus tarsi is exposed through a small incision and the device is inserted. (**d**) Photograph showing the device inserted into the sinus tarsi. Radiographs 6 weeks after surgery showing the device in correct position; (**e**) lateral view, (**f**) DP view. The arthroreisis was removed 3 years later. Radiographs 1 year later show an unchanged foot configuration, indicating regained stability of the foot; (**g**) lateral view, (**h**) DP view. (**i–l**) Clinically, the foot shows a symmetric function to the contralateral unaffected foot. Notice the symmetric muscular configuration as a proof of fully regained function

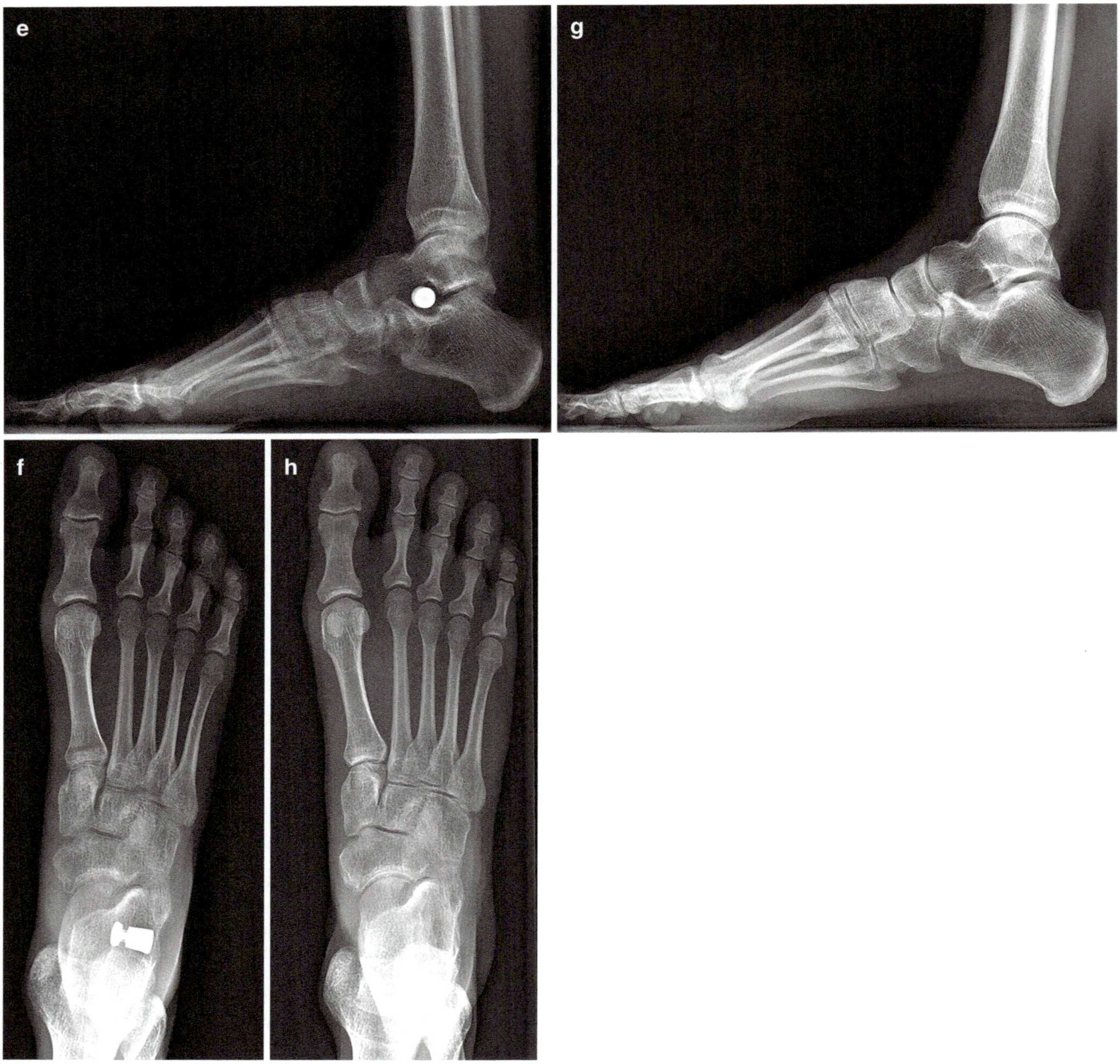

Fig. 5.44 (continued)

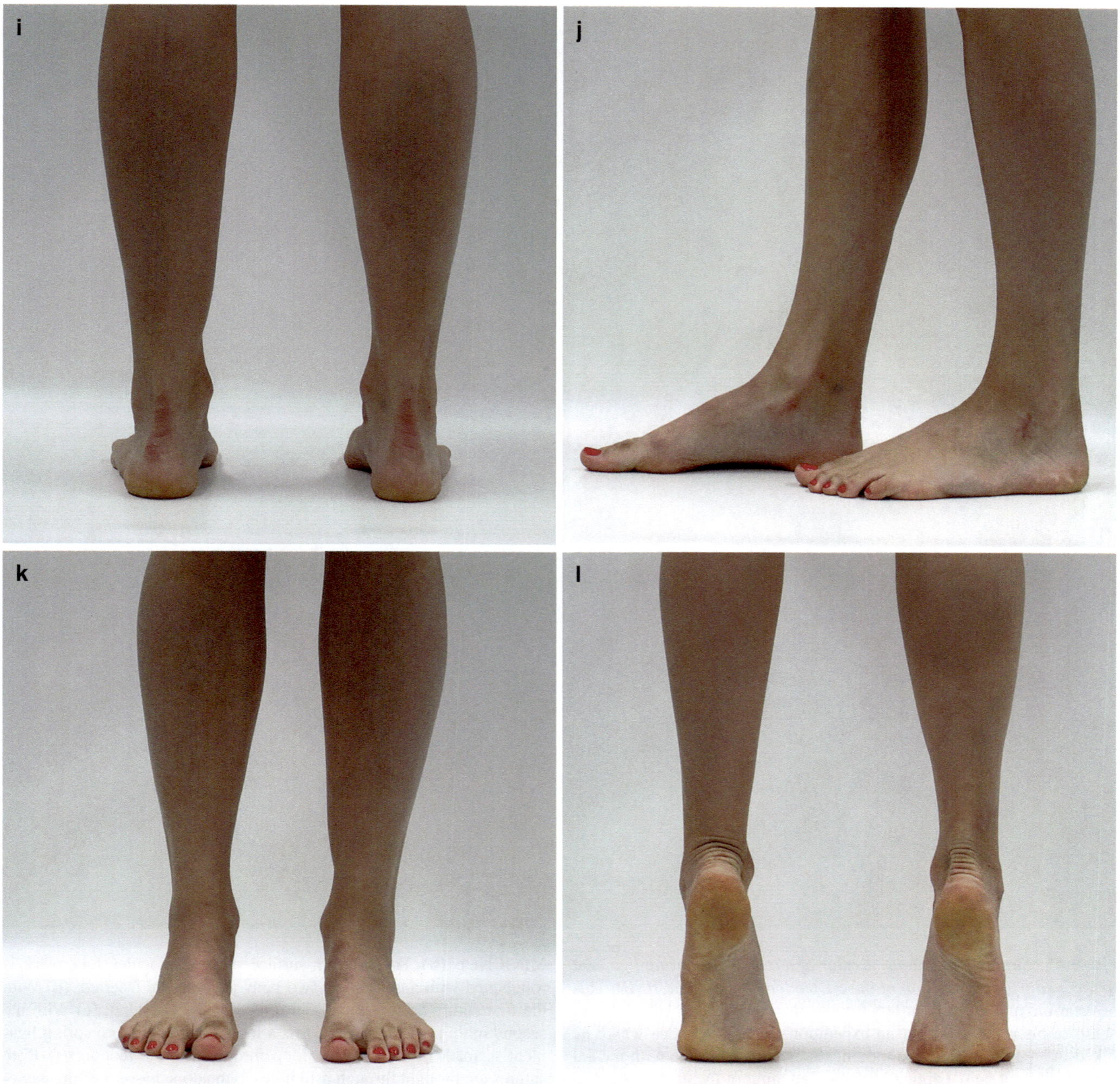

Fig. 5.44 (continued)

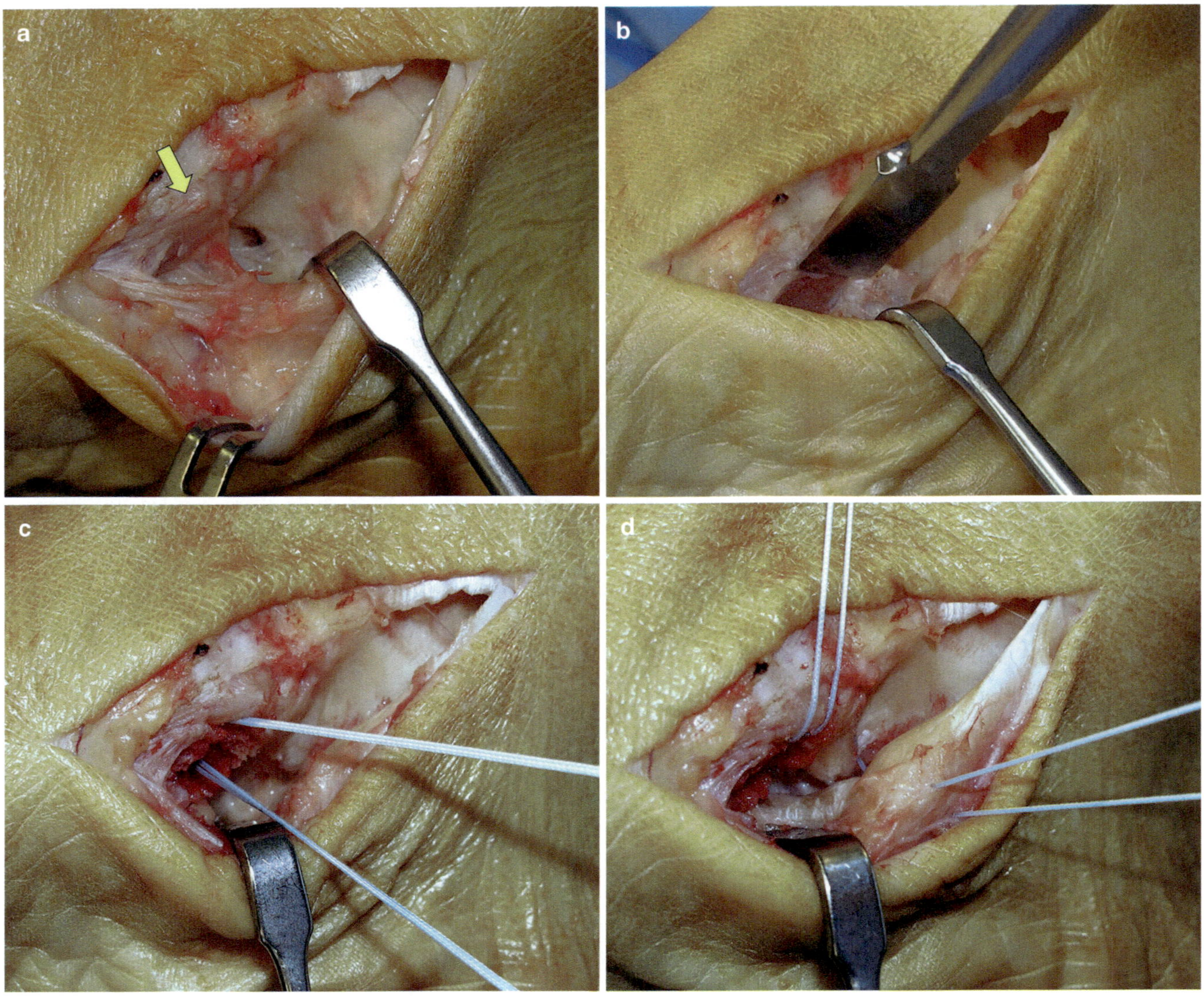

Fig. 5.45 *Surgical Technique: Repair of a tear of the spring ligament associated with an avulsion of the PT tendon (Injury Type III B).* This 56-year-old mountaineer suffers from an increasing painful disability to stabilize his right foot after an expedition to the Antarctica where he hiked in ice and snow. Shoe modifications with an insole with medial support did not help. Clinically, some flattening of the arch was found associated to a valgus deformity of the hindfoot that was not fully corrected in tiptoe position. (**a**) Surgical exploration shows a major avulsion of the PT tendon from the navicular tuberosity (arrow) while the plantar tendon bundle is intact. A rather small tear of the spring ligament is found close to its insertion to the navicular (SMCNL and MPOCNL). (**b**) The inferior surface of the navicular tuberosity is roughened with a chisel. (**c**) Two bony anchors are inserted. (**d**) With the first suture a loop is done into the distal PT tendon. (**e**) With the second more proximal suture, first a loop to catch the torn spring ligament is made followed by a loop through the PT tendon. (**f**) Both sutures are brought through drill holes to the dorsal aspect of the navicular tuberosity. (**g**) While pulling on the sutures, the PT tendon is seen to be reattached firmly to its insertion on the navicular tuberosity. (**h**) Final situation after having made knots. This patient did extremely well, allowing him to practice his sports 4 months later

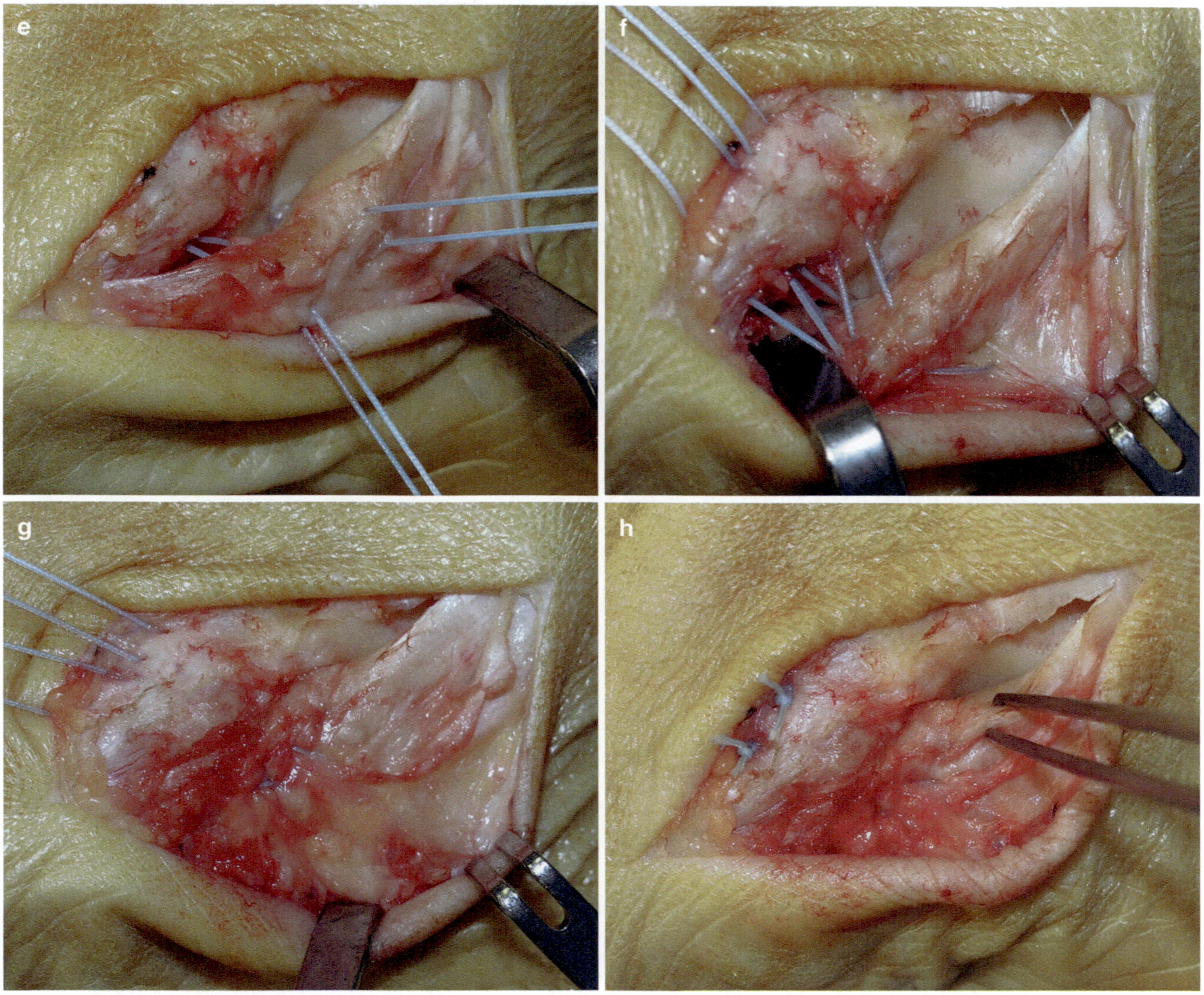

Fig. 5.45 (continued)

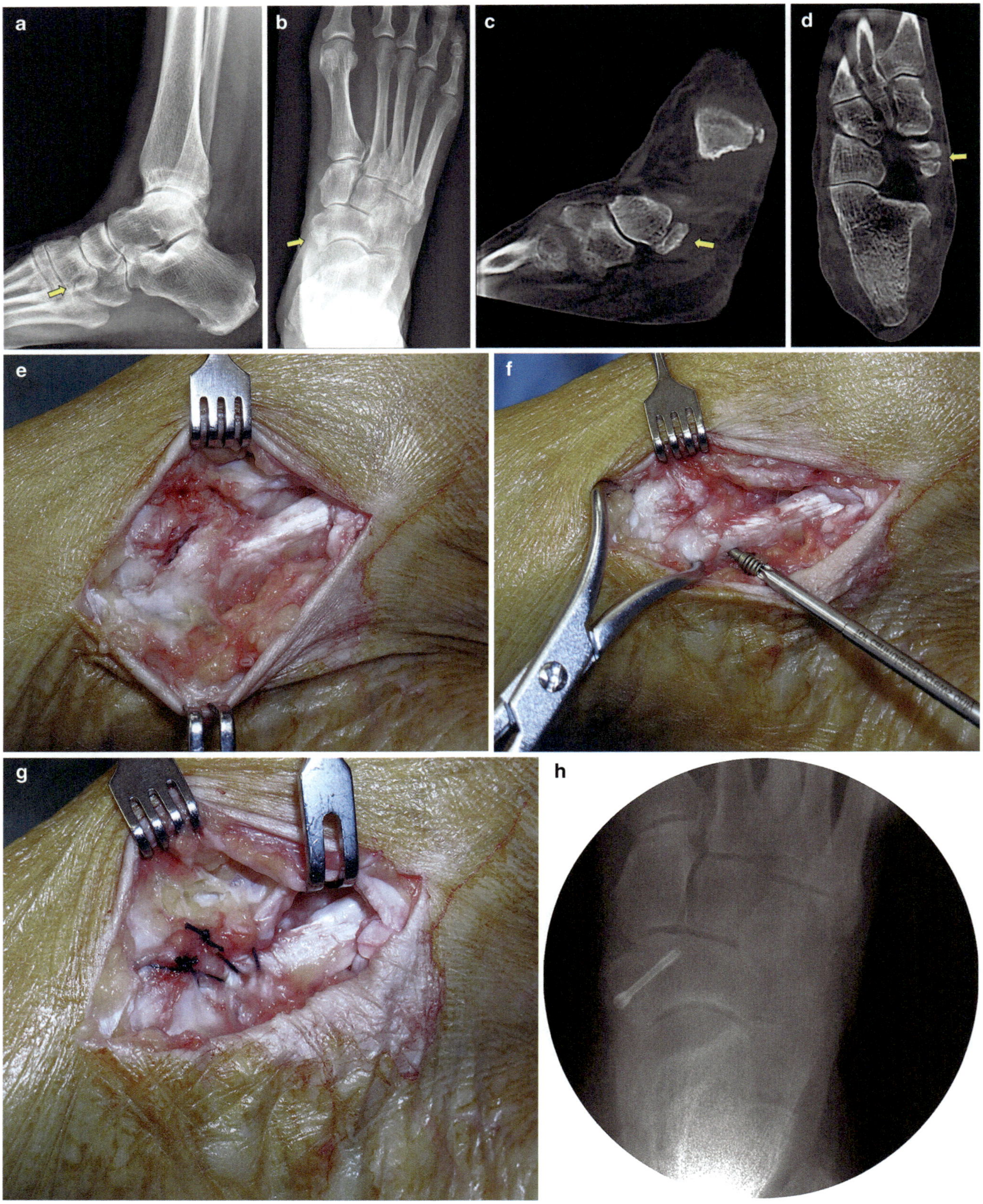

Fig. 5.46 *Surgical Technique: Repair of an acute avulsion fracture of the navicular tuberosity (Injury Type III C).* This 52-year-old female farmer sustained a pronation-abduction trauma when working in a steep slope 3 ½ weeks earlier. Clinically, circumscribed pain at the navicular tuberosity was found with a small local hematoma. The single heel rise test on the affected foot was not possible. Standard radiographs showing the fracture of the medial navicular (arrow): (**a**) lateral view, (**b**) DP view. CT scan confirms the fracture (arrow): (**c**) sagittal plane, (**d**) horizontal plane. (**e**) Surgical exposure of the medial navicular evidences the fracture. (**f**) A 3-mm screw is used for fixation. (**g**) Additional sutures are used to reinforce tendon fixation to the navicular. (**h**) Fluoroscopy showing fracture fixation

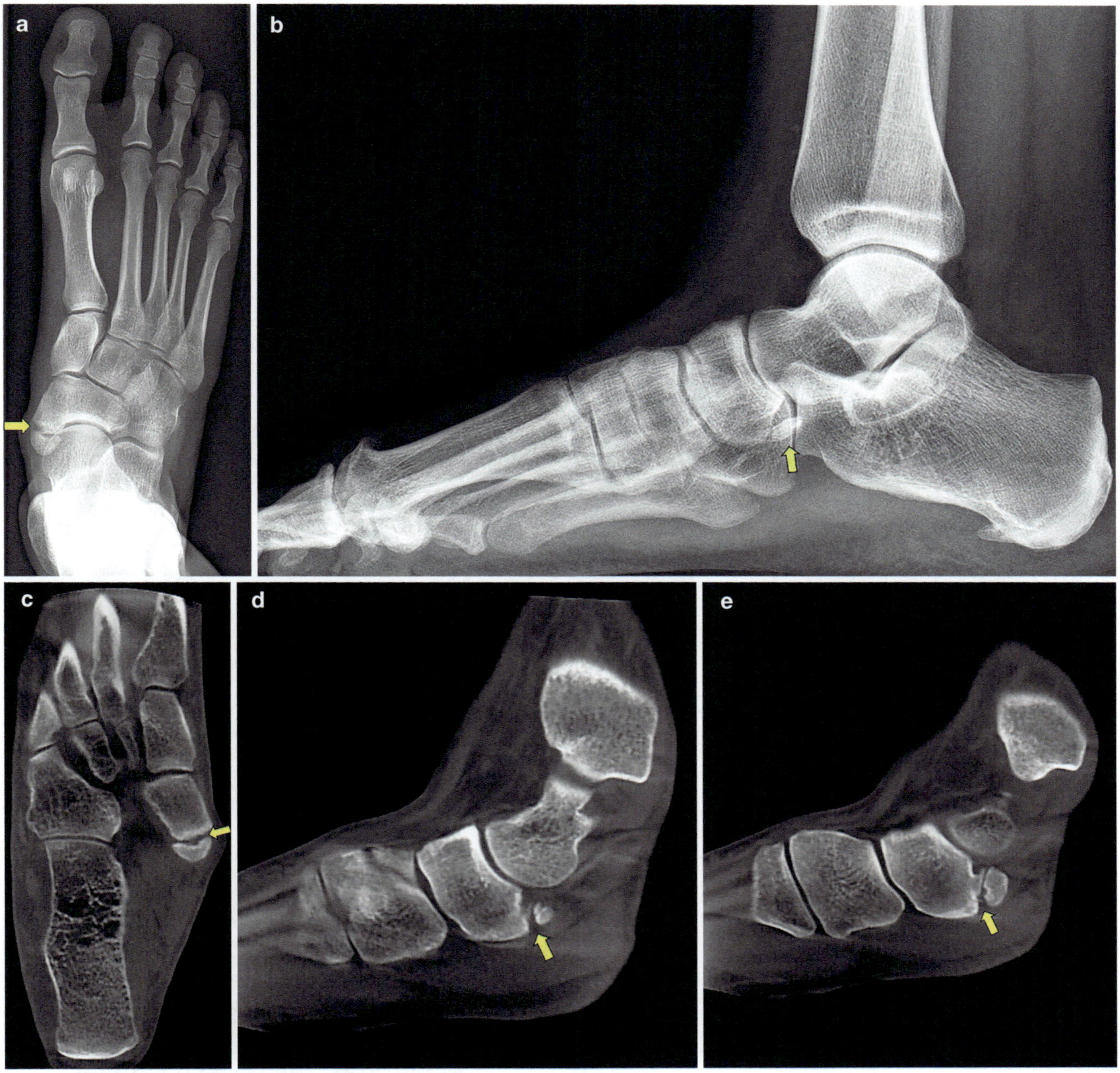

Fig. 5.47 *Surgical Technique: Repair of a disconnected accessory external tibial bone (Injury Type III C)*. This 24-year-old female student complained about sensing persisting pain on the medial aspect of her foot 4 months after falling down the stairs. Clinically, the foot showed a moderate flatfoot deformity with a painful bony prominence over the navicular tuberosity, associated with some pain on palpation along the PT tendon. She reported of having had a prominence on medial aspect of the foot since adolescence, however, never being painful until this accident. Tiptoe position was possible, but with some pain at the navicular. Standard radiographs showing the external accessory bone (arrow). (**a**) DP view, (**b**) lateral view. CT scan confirms the accessory external tibial bone (arrow). (**c**) Horizontal plane, (**d**) and, (**e**) sagittal plane. (**f**) Surgical exploration shows the prominence of navicular with a pseudarthrotic connection to the navicular. Motion between the fragment and the navicular can be seen when moving the foot. (**g**) The partially disrupted pseudarthrosis is dissected by a knife paying attention to preserve the plantar fibers of the PT tendon that run distally to the medial cuneiform and the first metatarsal. (**h**) An osteotomy with the saw is performed to resect the medial navicular while following the spring ligament distally to the naviculocuneiform joint. (**i**) A second osteotomy is performed on the accessory bone site. Notice the preserved plantar fibers of the PT tendon. (**j**) While the foot is held in maximal adduction position, the fragment is pulled distally and then taken by a compression clamp for primary fixation. Notice the achieved tension of the PT tendon. (**k**) The position is checked by fluoroscopy. (**l**) A cannulated 3-mm screw is inserted to fix the fragment. (**m**) The final position is checked by fluoroscopy. (**n**) Additional transosseous non-resorbable sutures are used to enhance the fixation. (**o**) Final resorbable sutures are used for fixation

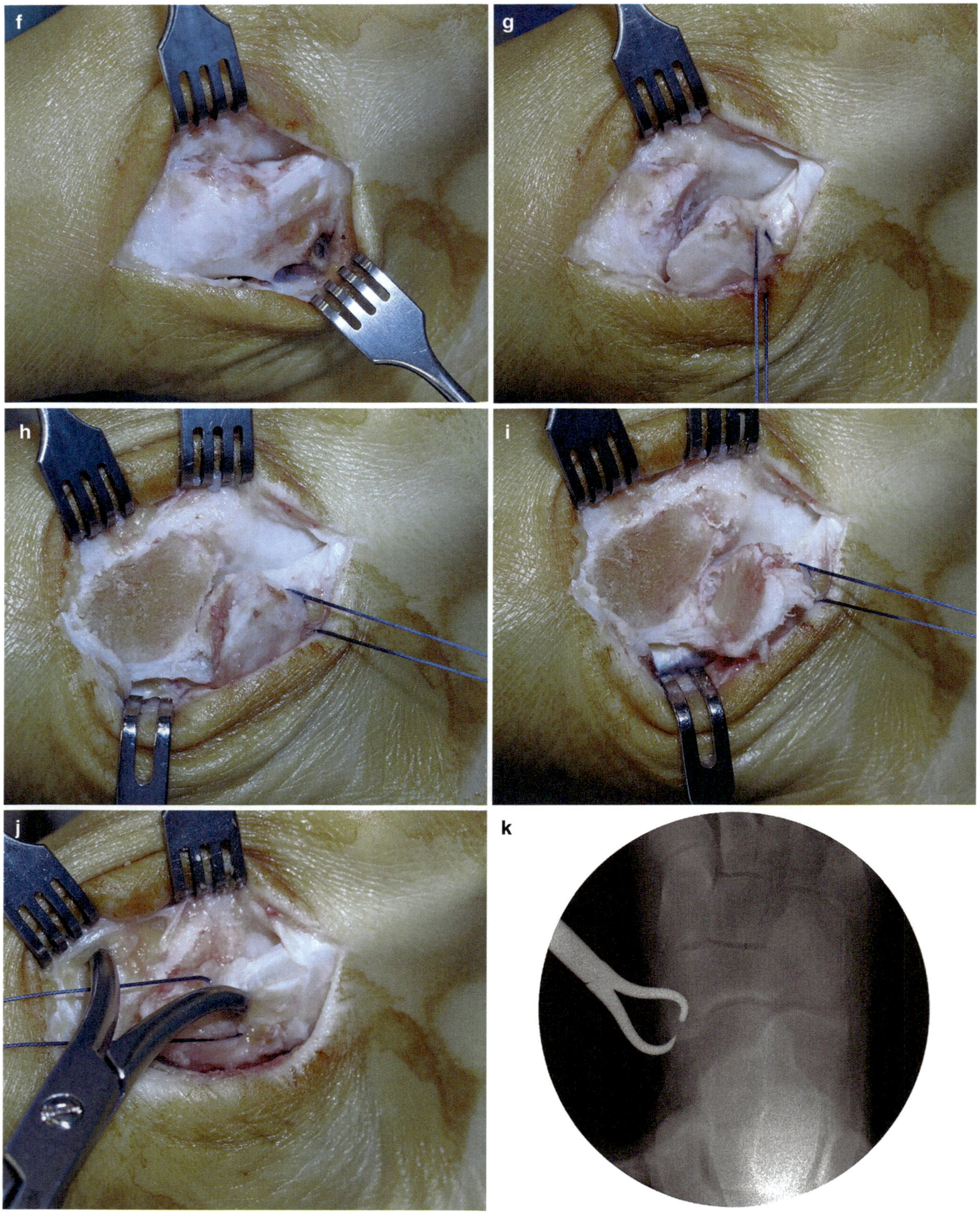

Fig. 5.47 (continued)

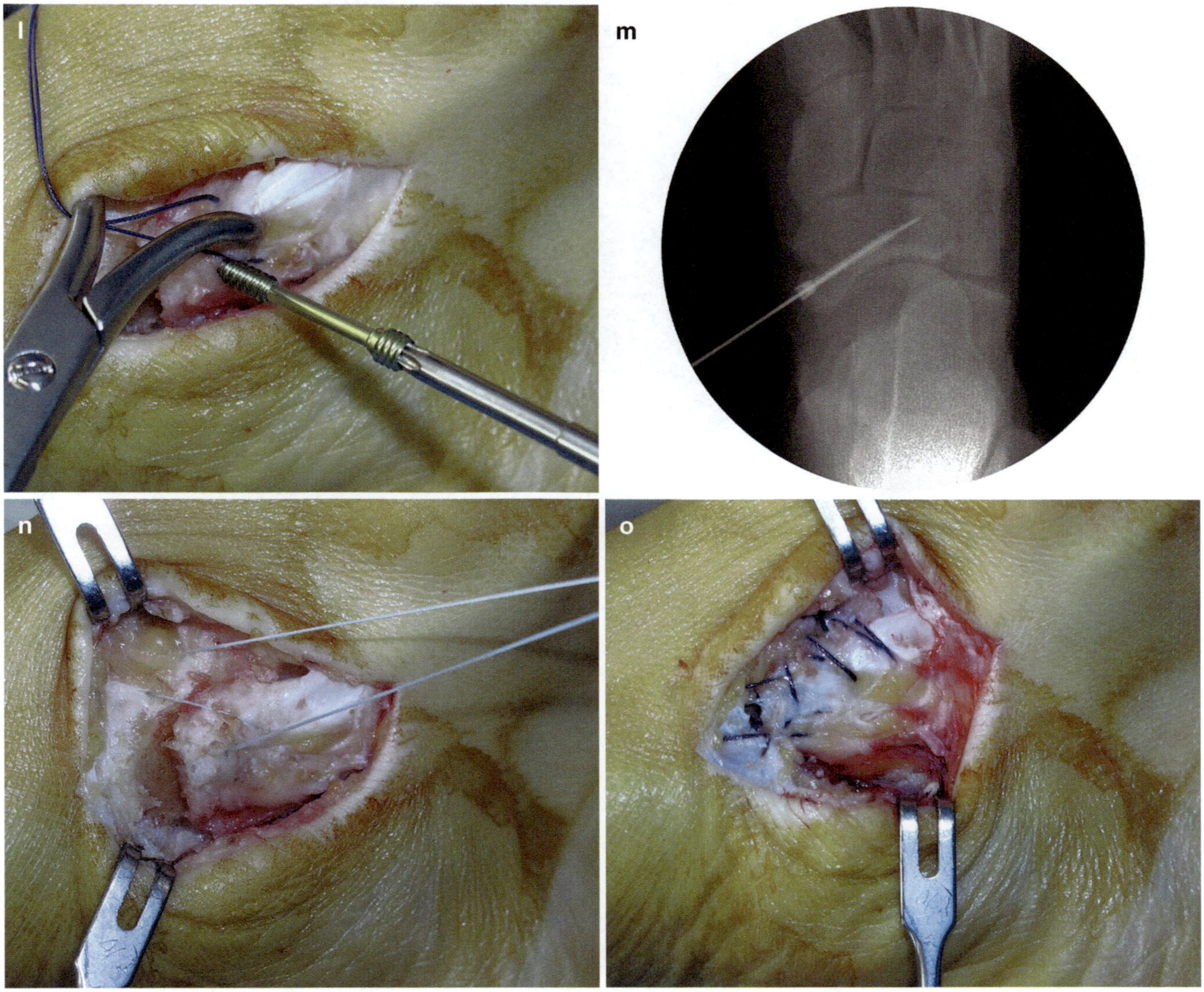

Fig. 5.47 (continued)

reconstruction tunnels [87]. However, the question remains to which extent all these reconstruction techniques perform when used in the impaired deltoid ligament and ankle. And furthermore, it is questionable if they are able to restore its biomechanical characteristics [88].

5.10.4.3 Complete Tear of the Deep Deltoid with a Talar Tilt >10° (Type IV C)

In complete tears of the deep deltoid with a talar tilt >10°, isolated ligament reconstruction without having to perform additional bony procedures, such as fusion of peritalar joints and/or osteotomies, is critical (Fig. 5.55). Alternatively, a tibio-talar-calcaneal (TTC)-fusion can be considered. As the supination deformity will mostly persist, additional correction by stabilizing the medial arch might be necessary to obtain a stable foot.

5.10.5 Additional Procedures

5.10.5.1 Posterior Tibial Tendon Reconstruction

The posterior tibial (PT) tendon is meticulously inspected. If there is secondary degeneration of the tendon due to chronic overload, debridement of the tendon is necessary (Fig. 5.56). A flexor digitorum longus (FDL) tendon transfer should be considered if the tendon is diseased or ruptured (Fig. 5.57) [89, 90]; however, such a tendon condition is rarely found in patients primarily treated for medial ankle instability [10, 11, 60].

5.10.5.2 Posterior Tibial Tendon Shortening

If an incompetent spring ligament results in a chronic overload of the PT tendon, the tendon may undergo a degenerative process with elongation. As repairing the deltoid and spring ligaments alone, without any additional procedures,

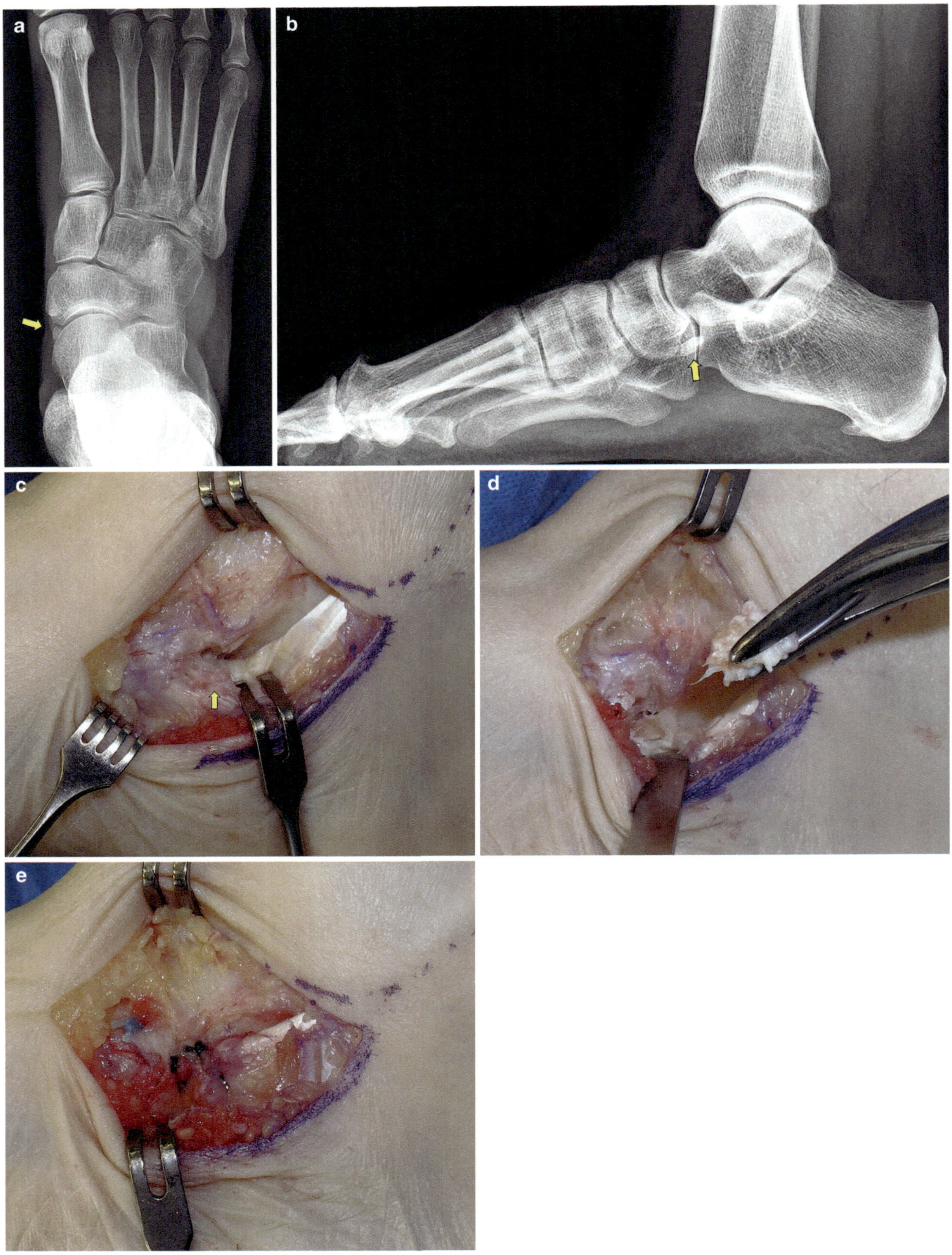

Fig. 5.48 *Surgical Technique: Repair of an acute avulsion of PT tendon (Injury Type III C)*. This 60-year-old female nurse sustained a sprain of her foot while hiking in the forest. Thereafter she senses pain at the insertion site of the PT tendon. Furthermore, she is unable to walk barefoot and on uneven ground. Clinically there is a mild flatfoot deformity with weakness of the medial arch. Pain on palpation is found at the navicular tuberosity. Standard radiographs show the dislocated fracture (arrow): (**a**) DP view, (**b**) lateral view. (**c**) While surgical exploration reveals an intact spring ligament, the avulsion fragment of the PT tendon can be found (arrow). (**d**) Because of the small size, the fragment is resected. (**e**) A suture anchor and multiple transosseous sutures are used for firm reattachment of the PT tendon

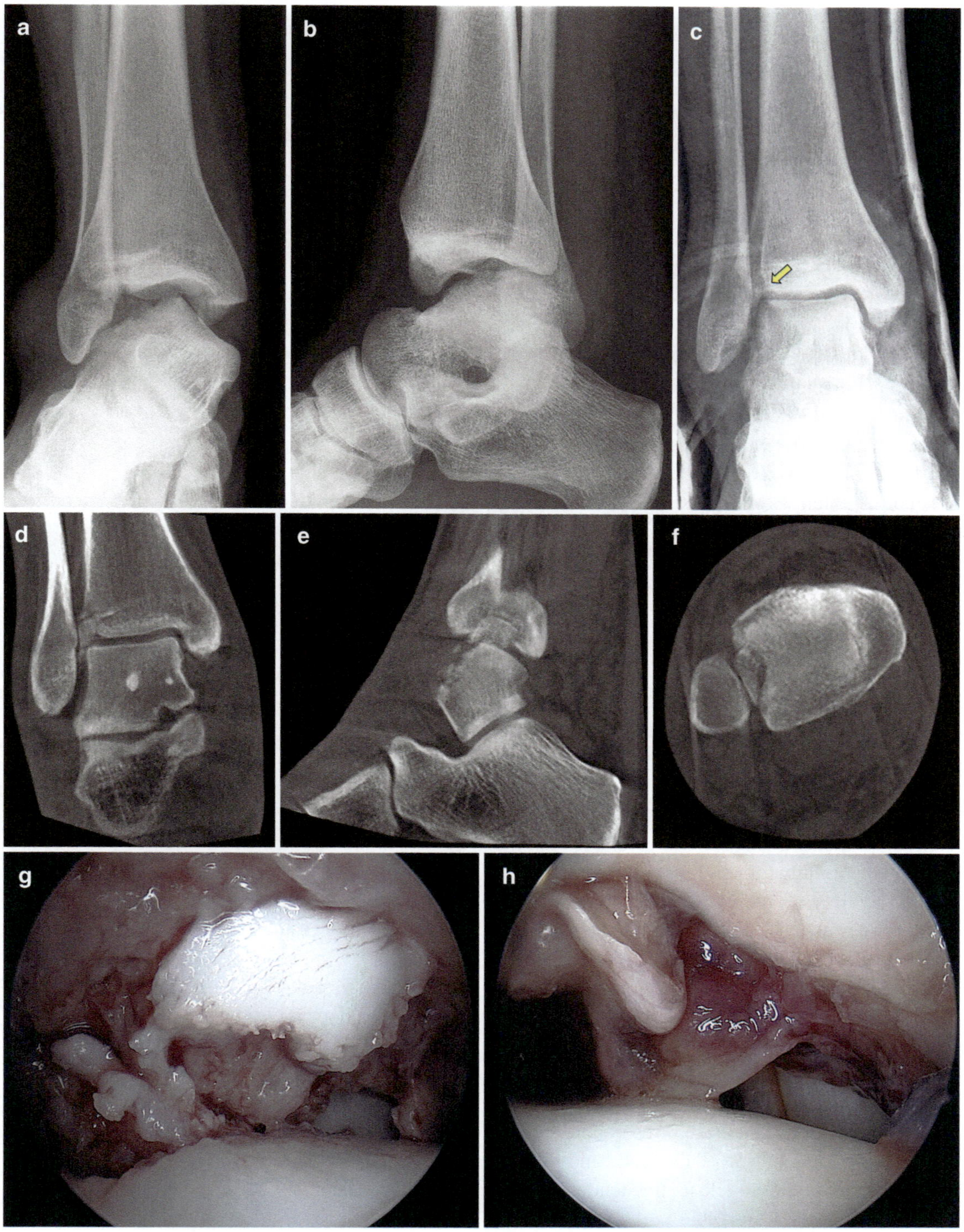

Fig. 5.49 *Surgical Technique: Repair of an acute complete rupture of the deltoid ligament*. This 32-year-old world-class equestrian fell with his horse after a jump and his horse hit his foot on the lateral side. Radiographs taken in the emergency room show a dislocated ankle with complete disruption of the deltoid ligaments: (**a**) AP view, (**b**) lateral view. (**c**) After closed reduction, an osteochondral fracture with a dislocated fragment (arrow) is suspected. (**d–f**) CT scans after reduction show the widening of the syndesmosis with an interposed fragment that originates from the anterolateral talar dome. Preoperative arthroscopy shows the fragment in the incisura (**g**) and a full-thickness rupture of the deltoid allowing to see the flexor digitorum (FDL) and PT tendons (**h**). (**i**) Surgical exposure of the lateral ankle shows the fragment interposed between the fibula and tibia, thus widening the syndesmotic space, while the anterior tibiofibular ligament (ATFL) is seen to be completely torn. The fracture site on the lateral talar dome is also seen. (**j**) The lateral talar dome is reconstructed by reposition and fixation of the osteochondral fragment. (**k**) After the repair of the lateral ankle ligaments, the talus is seen in a correct position. Repair of the syndesmosis by sutures is performed (not shown). (**l**) Surgical exposure of the medial ankle shows the rupture of the distal deep deltoid, close to its insertion on the posteromedial talus. (**m**) A suture anchor is placed into the posteromedial talus and used to repair the deep deltoid. (**n**) The knot is made after tightening the suture. (**o**) A suture anchor on the anterior colliculus is used to reattach the superficial layers of the deltoid that are typically ruptured proximally. The superficial posterior tibiotalar ligament (STTL) that is also disrupted proximally is kept away by the hook. (**p**) The STTL is finally reattached to the medial malleolus by additional transosseous sutures

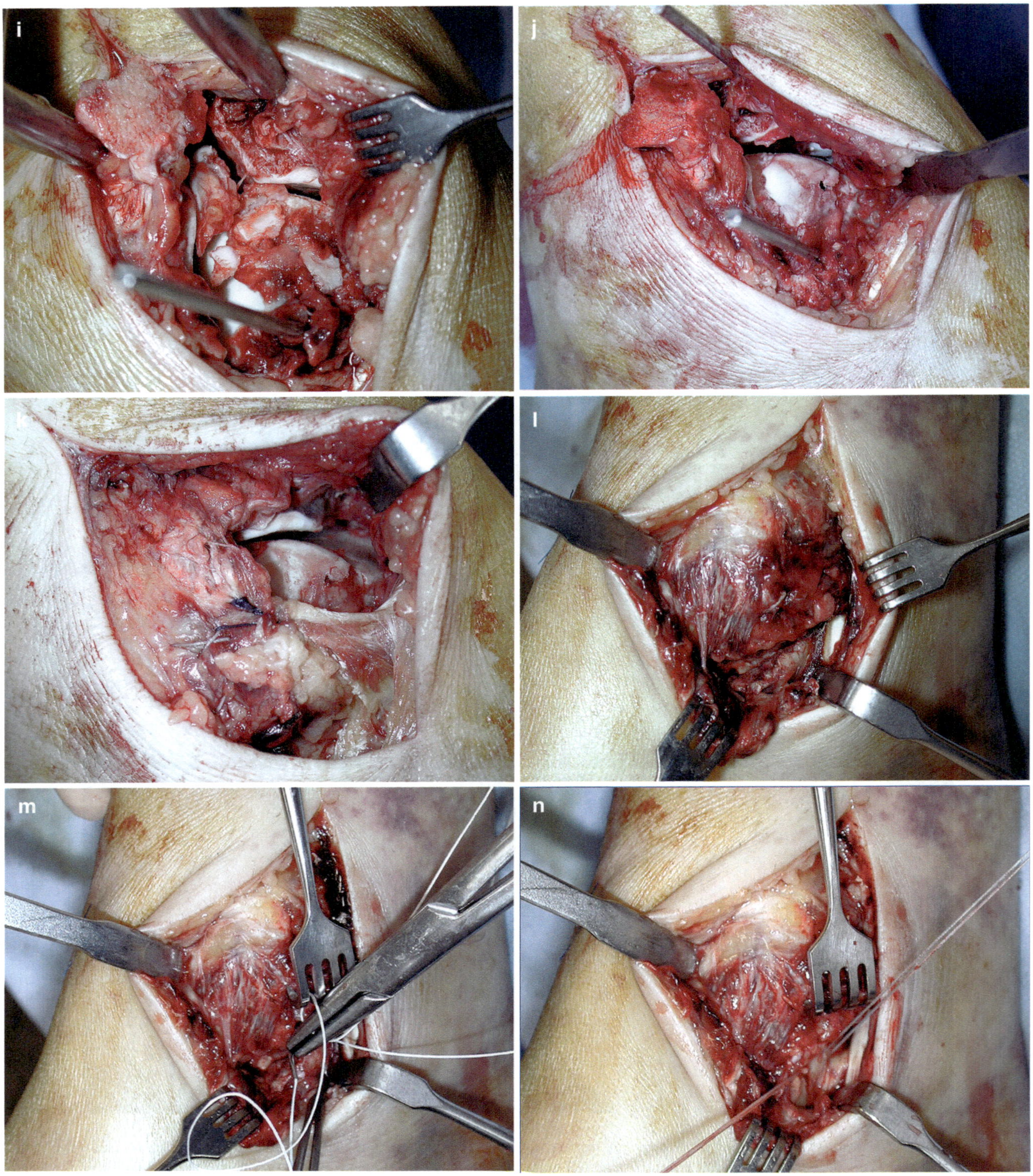

Fig. 5.49 (continued)

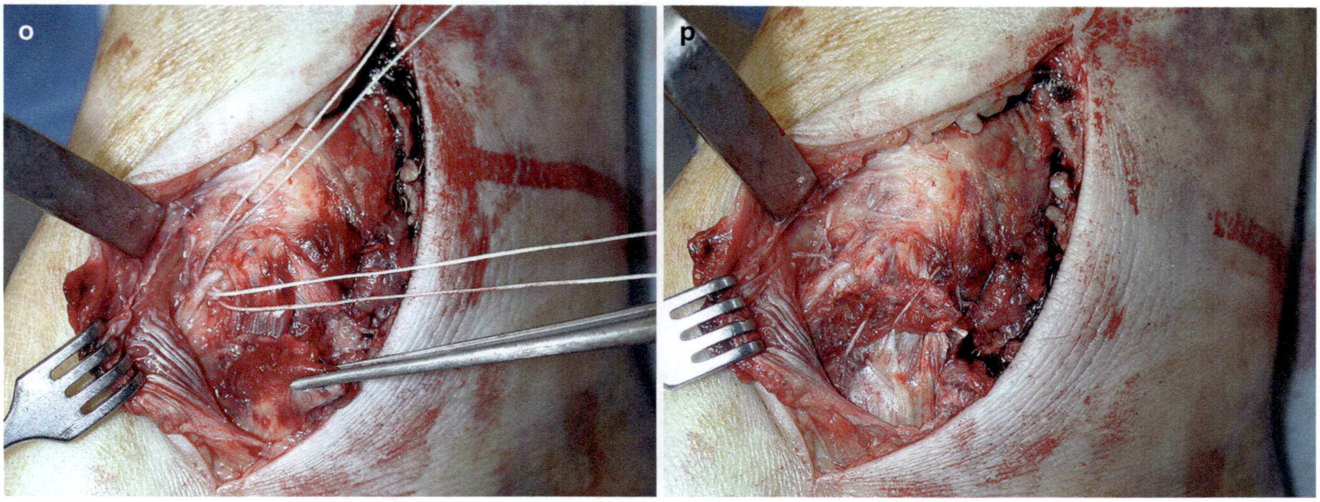

Fig. 5.49 (continued)

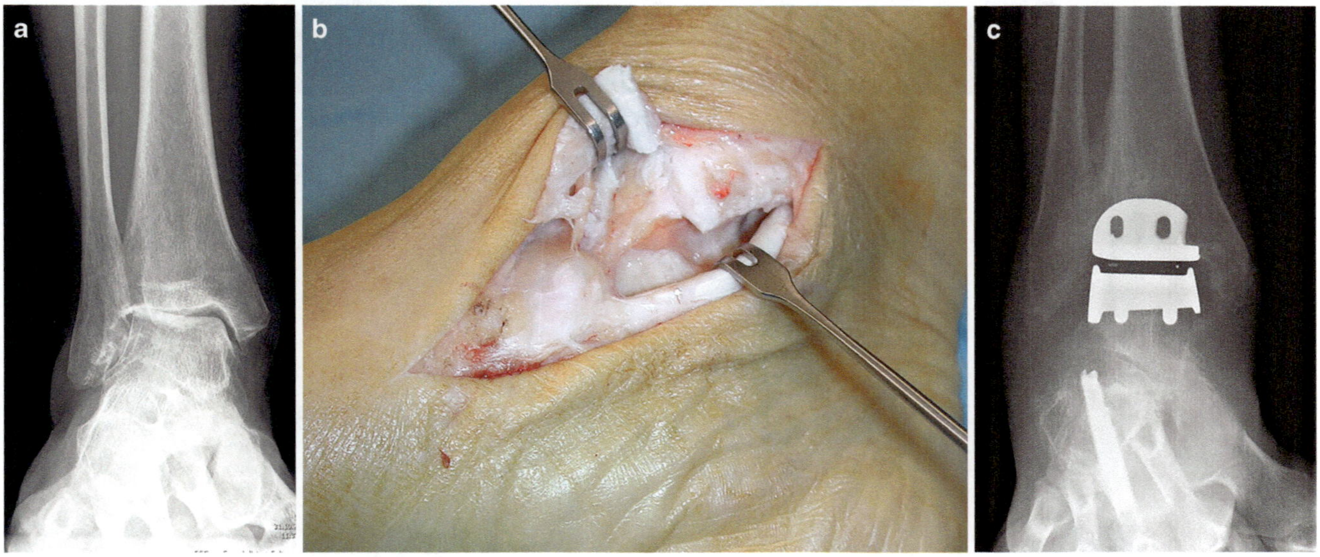

Fig. 5.50 *Surgical Technique: Total ankle replacement for a deep deltoid rupture and peritalar instability*. This 73-year-old active patient is suffering from progressive pain in his lateral right ankle that does not allow him to walk more than 15 min. (**a**) Standard AP radiograph showing a talar valgus tilt of 10° with collapsed lateral tibiotalar joint space and ongoing subchondral changes. (**b**) Surgical exploration reveals a complete rupture of the anterior part of deep deltoid. (**c**) Therefore, a total ankle replacement was done with using the implants as a spacer, thus tensioning the slack ligaments. A medial sliding osteotomy of calcaneus was also done. This radiograph shows the ankle after 10 years well balanced in a very satisfied patient

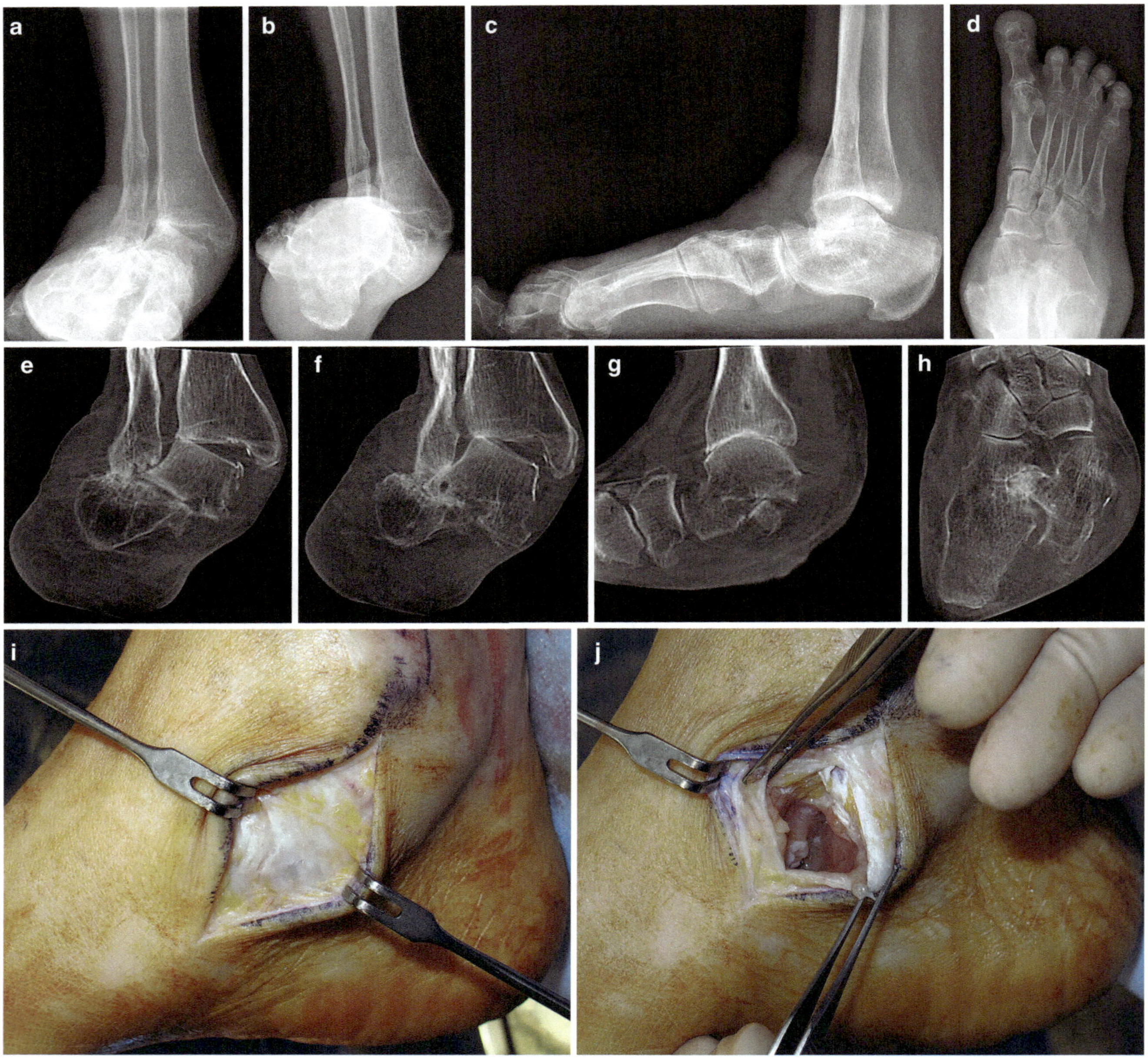

Fig. 5.51 *Surgical Technique: Tibiotalocalcaneal (TTC) fusion for a complete rupture of deltoid and subsequent peritalar subluxation.* This 81-year-old female patient is suffering from massive pain in her lateral ankle that does not allow her to weight-bear her foot. She is using special orthopedic shoes for 6 years. (**a–d**) Standard radiographs showing the deformity in all planes. Notice the stress reaction of fibula. (**e–h**) Weight-bearing CT scans show the peritalar subluxation with sinus tarsi and subfibular impingement, a talar valgus tilt of >20°, and a diastasis of syndesmosis. (**i**) After skin incision, the distracted fascia can be seen. (**j**) Further dissection reveals complete rupture of the whole deltoid-spring ligament complex. Therefore, a TTC-fusion was done (not shown)

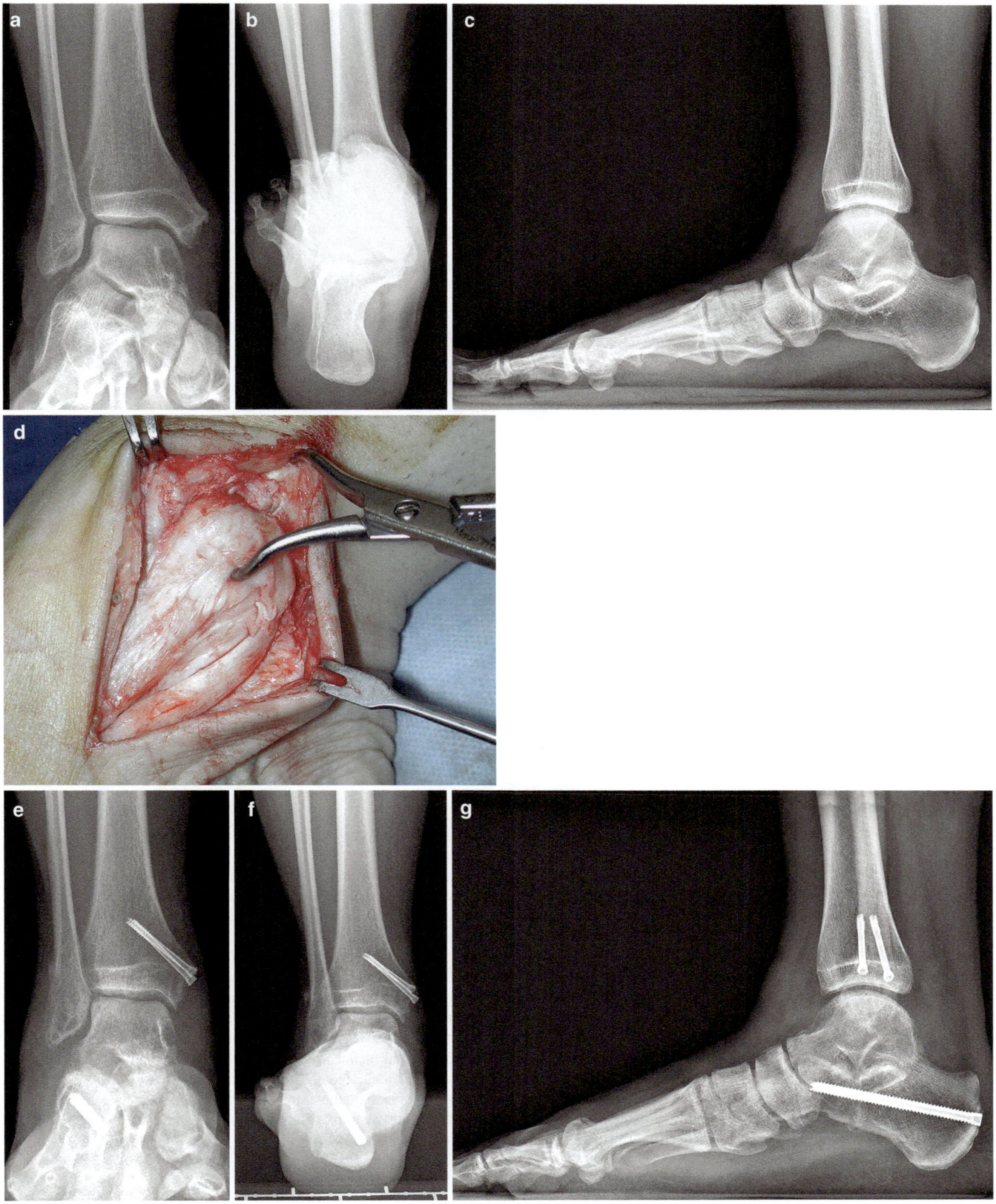

Fig. 5.52 *Surgical Technique: Reconstruction of the deep deltoid ligament with advancement of the deltoid (Injury Type IV A).* This 41-year-old judo fighter is suffering from progressive pain and a feeling of instability of his right ankle. He cannot remember a specific trauma. Clinical investigation reveals a valgus-pronation deformity of both feet that is slightly more pronounced on the right foot. (**a–c**) Standard radiographs show a valgus TAS of 4° and a talar valgus tilt of 3°, resulting in an increased lateral moment arm of the heel (8 mm). The lateral view shows some collapse of the medial arch with a increased navicular coverage. (**d**) As the patient refused the proposed supramalleolar correcting osteotomy, in fear of delayed union, a flip osteotomy of the medial malleolus is performed and the whole deltoid ligament complex is advanced while the foot is held in slight supination. Two screws are used for fixation. Thereafter, a calcaneal lengthening osteotomy is performed (surgical technique see Fig. 5.60). (**e–g**) Five years after surgery, the deformity angles have markedly changed radiographically, as also seen clinically. The patient was able to regain his former level of sports 6 months later and is pain free and very satisfied

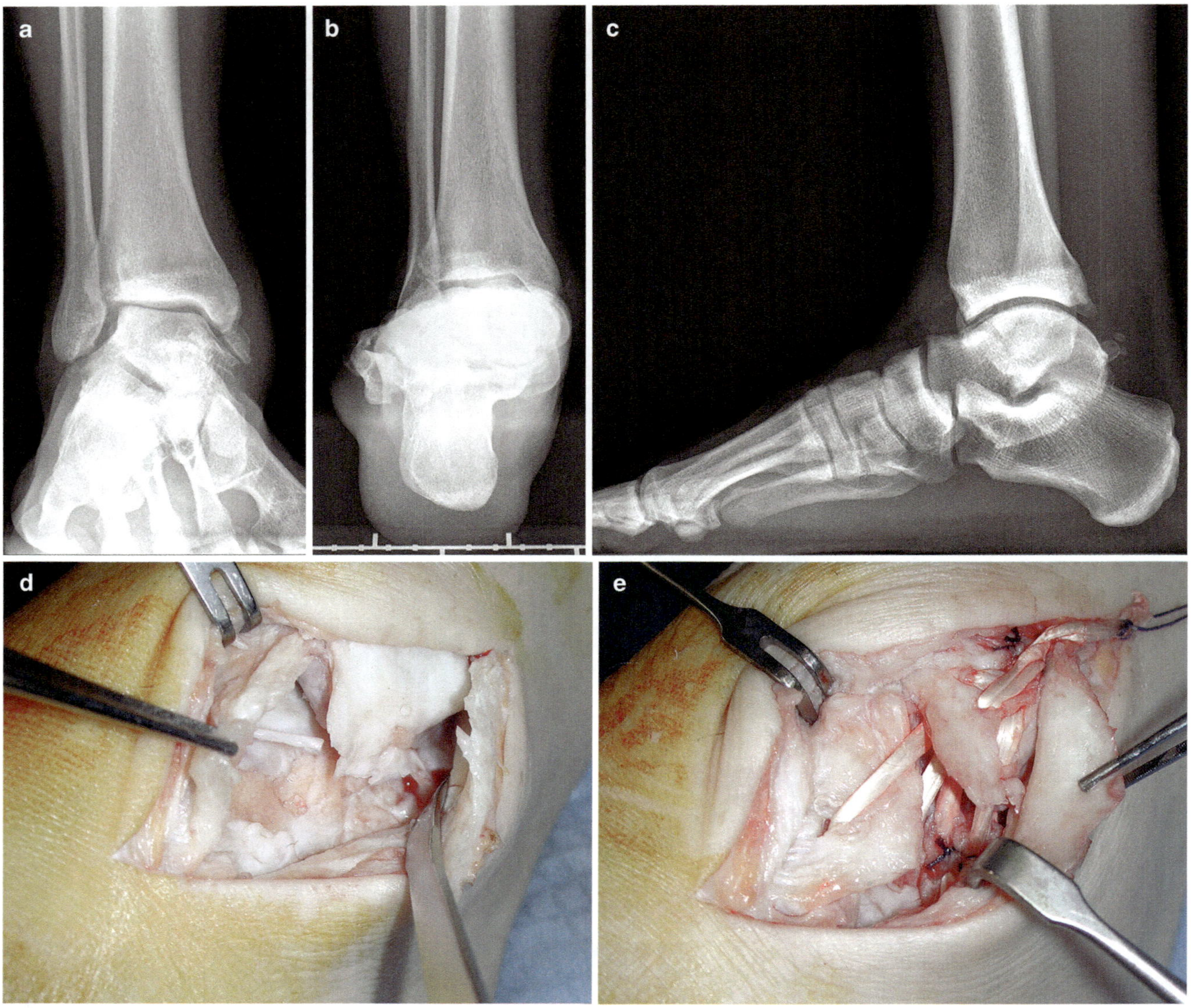

Fig. 5.53 *Surgical Technique: Reconstruction of the deep deltoid ligament with a plantaris tendon graft (Injury Type IV A).* This 24-year-old high-level gymnast sustained a pronation trauma when landing on the floor. Despite conservative treatment measures he has been unable to regain his level of sports activities due to pain and weakness of the medial ankle. Clinically, moderate valgus malalignment of the heel is present. (**a**) AP radiograph shows a bony avulsion of the deltoid with a valgus talar tilt of 5°. (**b**) The hindfoot alignment view confirms a valgus moment arm of approximately 8 mm. (**c**) The lateral view shows the avulsion fragment in the center of medial malleolus. (**d**) Surgical exposure shows the fragment completely detached from the medial malleolus, with only partial remaining attachment of the deltoid to the fragment. Thus, the fragment is removed. Now it can be seen that the whole superficial deltoid, including the TCL, are torn, involving also the deep ligaments. (**e**) 3.5-mm drill holes are made as follows: 2 in the posteromedial aspect of the talus, 2 in the sustentaculum tali, 2 in the central part of the medial malleolus, and 2 in the anterior aspect of the medial malleolus. The free plantaris tendon graft is then first looped from the medial malleolus to the posteromedial talus, and from the medial malleolus to the sustentaculum tali. A third loop is added to grab the distal part of the TSL and the spring ligament. (**f**) A drawing showing the reconstruction with 2 static loops and a dynamic loop anteriorly to avoid a tenodesis effect between the medial malleolus and the navicular. The remaining scarred ligament is used to finalize the reconstruction. No calcaneus osteotomy was added in this high-performance athlete to not change the biomechanics of the foot. The patient returned to full competitive sports activities 6 months later and won an Olympic medal 3 years later

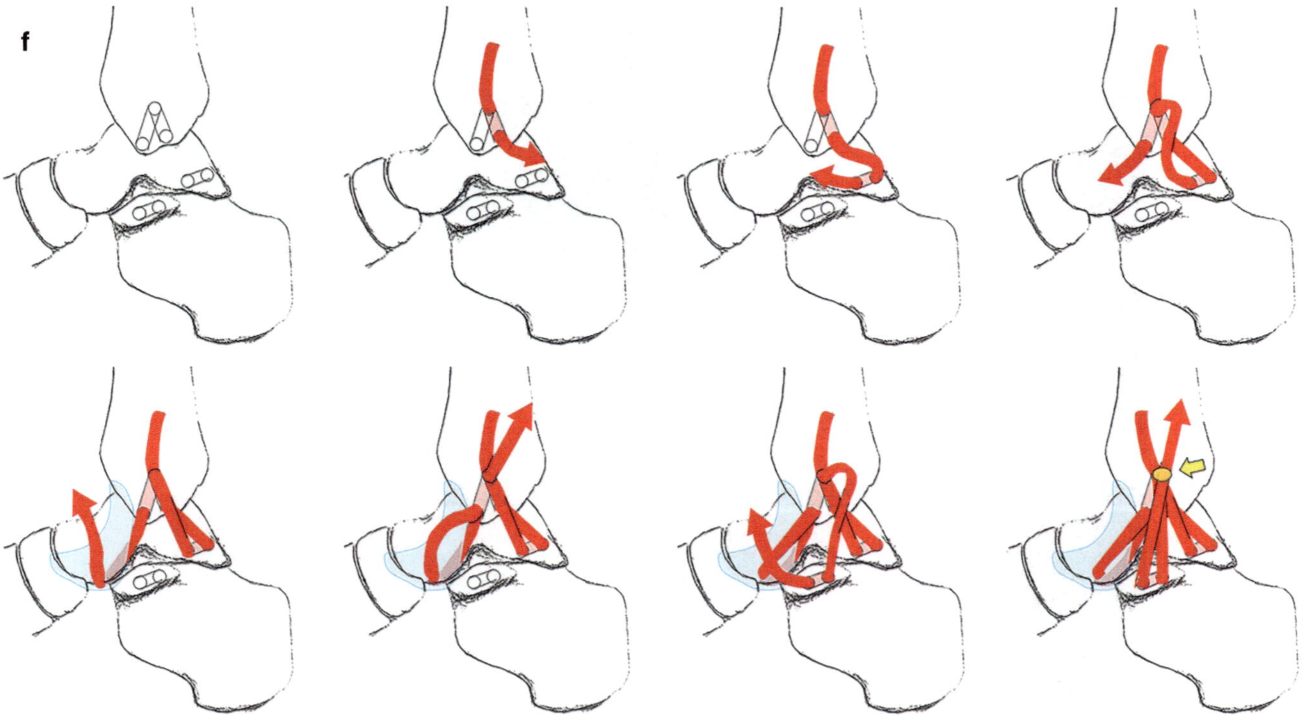

Fig. 5.53 (continued)

would result in an attenuation of the tissue, the outcome could be unpredictable [91]. A Z-shortening tenotomy of the elongated PT tendon [92] can be added to the procedure, to protect the repair (Fig. 5.58).

5.10.5.3 Lateral Ankle Ligament Repair

Reconstruction of the lateral ankle ligaments (surgical technique see Figs. 2.32 and 2.35) is considered when additional lateral instability of the ankle is present. If the condition of the ATFL and CFL is sufficient, ligament repair by reattachment to the fibula is performed. If no substantial ligamentous material is present, augmentation with a free plantaris tendon graft is undertaken.

5.10.5.4 Calcaneal Lengthening Osteotomy

A calcaneal lengthening osteotomy [20, 93] is considered if there is a pre-existing valgus and pronation deformity of the foot (e.g., when a valgus and pronation deformity is also present on the contralateral, asymptomatic foot), and/or if severe attenuation or defect of the deltoid-spring ligament complex is present. Originally, this technique was described for treatment of flatfoot deformities in children where the osteotomy is performed 10 mm proximal to the calcaneocuboid joint (Fig. 5.59a) [93]. In adults, calcaneal osteotomies along and parallel to the posterior facet of the subtalar joint are generally preferred. Since it is performed from lateral to medial, preserving the medial cortex, it is more like an open-

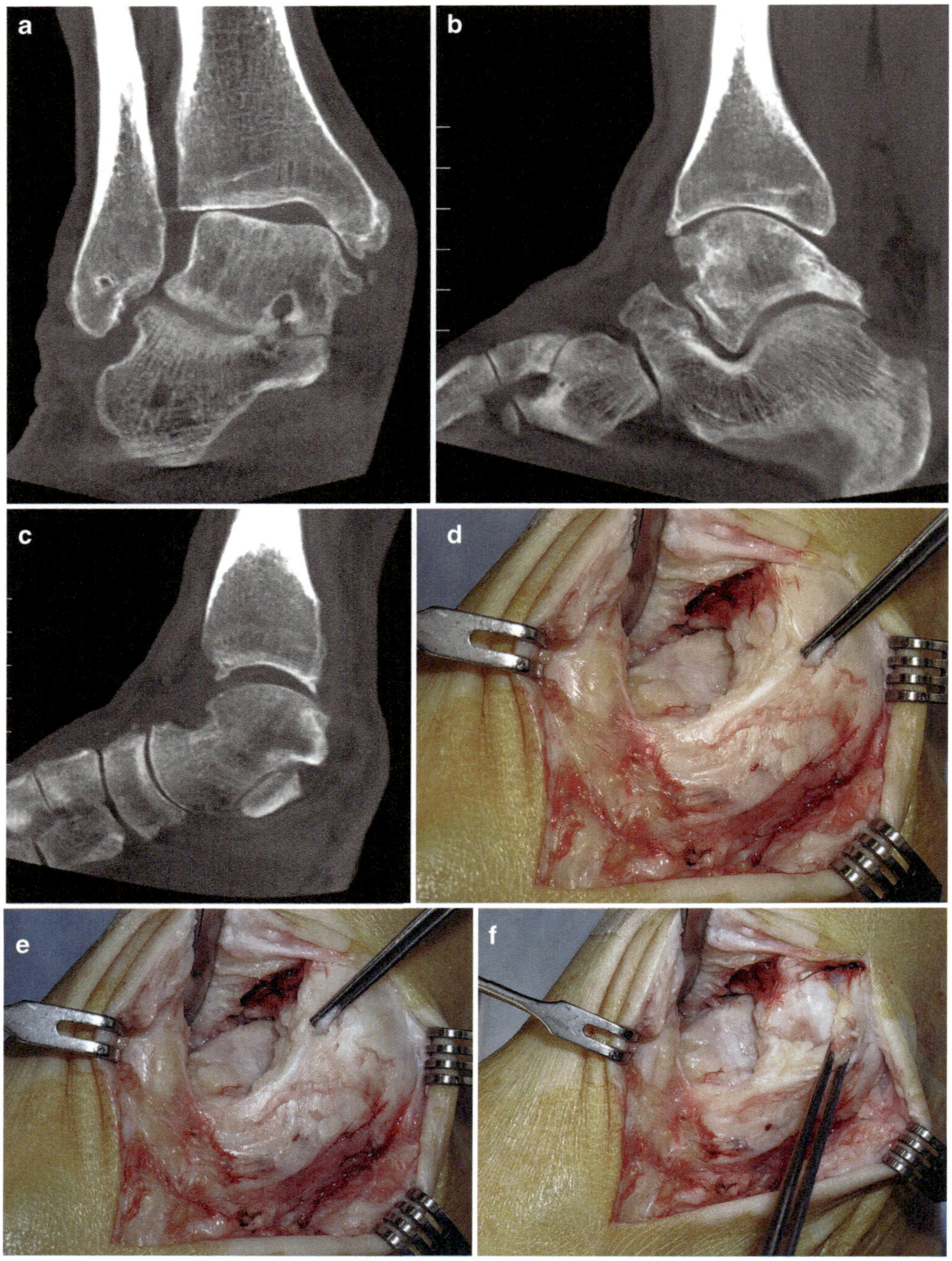

Fig. 5.54 *Surgical Technique: Reconstruction of the deep deltoid ligament with an internal brace (Injury Type IV B).* This 52-year-old former trail runner sustained several ankle sprains that were never specifically treated. In the last 6 months, lateral ankle pain hindered him from running. He wishes to be able to go running again. (**a**) Weight-bearing coronal CT scans show a talar tilt of 10° with a narrowing lateral tibiotalar joint, however, with preserved articular surfaces and no cyst formation. In the sagittal plane, the articular surfaces look preserved as well: (**b**) in the lateral tibiotalar joint, the cartilage is worn out with remaining minimal joint space; (**c**) in the medial tibiotalar joint, there is a marked gapping. (**d**) Surgical exposure evidences a thick, scarred and elongated deltoid ligament that has no connection to the medial malleolus anymore. It can be moved towards posterior, and (**e**) towards anterior, like a wisher. (**f**) After having released the anterior part at its proximal remaining contact area to the tibia, the bald medial malleolus with a smooth surface can be seen. (**g**) First, an internal brace is inserted to the posteromedial aspect of the talus. (**h**) The internal brace is mounted by a strong and sharp needle and then brought through a transosseous suture from the intercollicular groove to the proximal aspect of the medial malleolus where a loop is made to bring the internal brace through a transosseous suture down to the anterior colliculus and from there behind the remaining ligament to the sustentaculum tali. A suture anchor is inserted onto the anterior aspect of the anterior colliculus to reattach the remaining ligament. (**i**) While the foot is held in slight supination, the internal brace is tightened and fixed to the sustentaculum tali. (**j**) The remaining end of the internal brace is used for additional loops to enhance the construct and then finished by a knot. The prepared suture anchor is used to grab the intermediate portion of the superficial deltoid, especially the tibiospring and tibionavicular ligaments. (**k**) The remaining deltoid is finally reattached to the proximal aspect of the medial malleolus with multiple transosseous sutures, thereby advancing it. The stability is checked under fluoroscopy: (**l**) without valgus stress, (**m**) with valgus stress. (**n**) A lateral column lengthening osteotomy (surgical technique see Fig. 5.60) is added to correct the foot position and to protect the reconstructed medial ankle ligaments. The patient was initially very satisfied with the obtained stability and got back to running, however unable to reach his former activity level. Eight years later, he came back with symptomatic valgus osteoarthritis that made total ankle replacement necessary

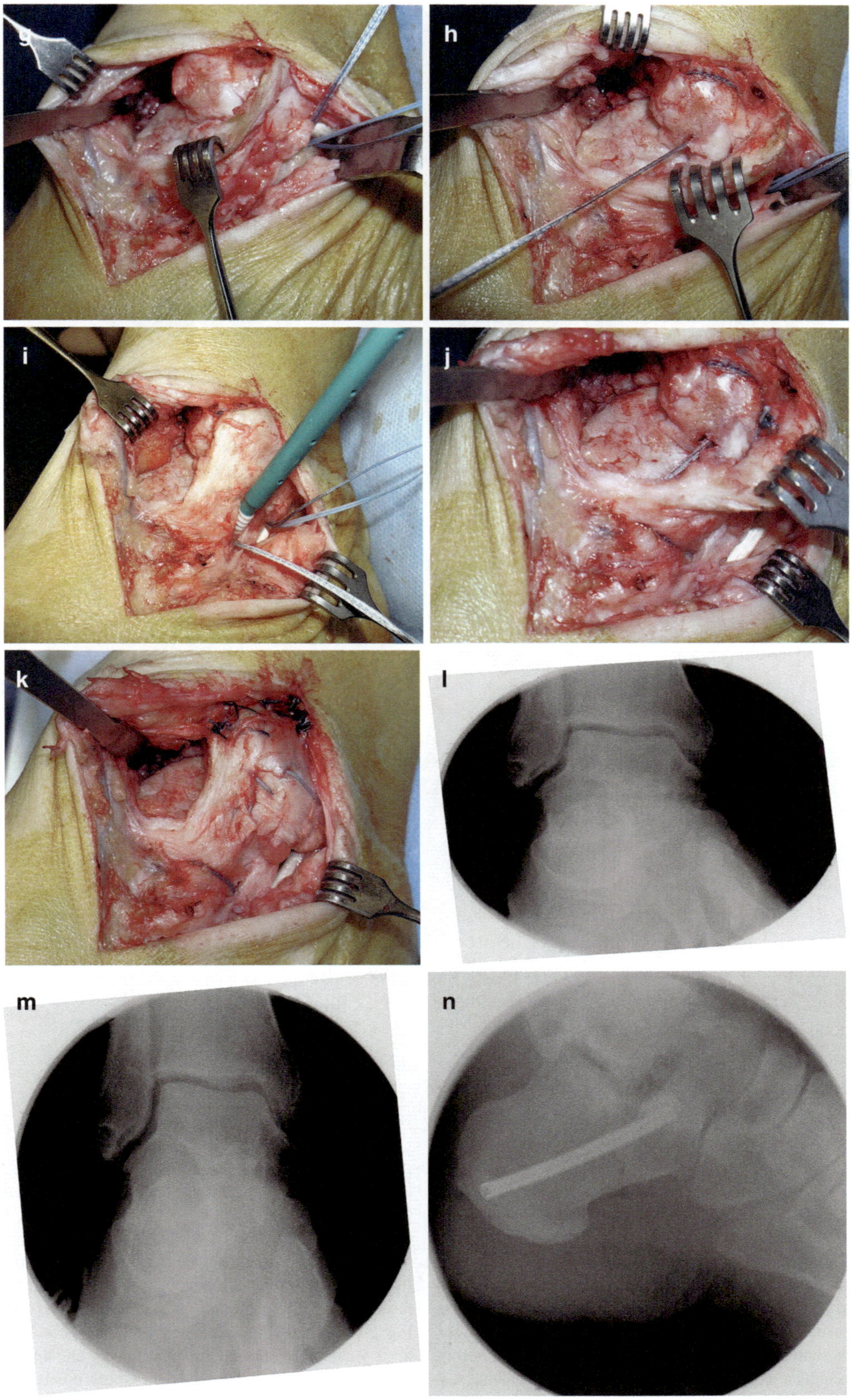

Fig. 5.54 (continued)

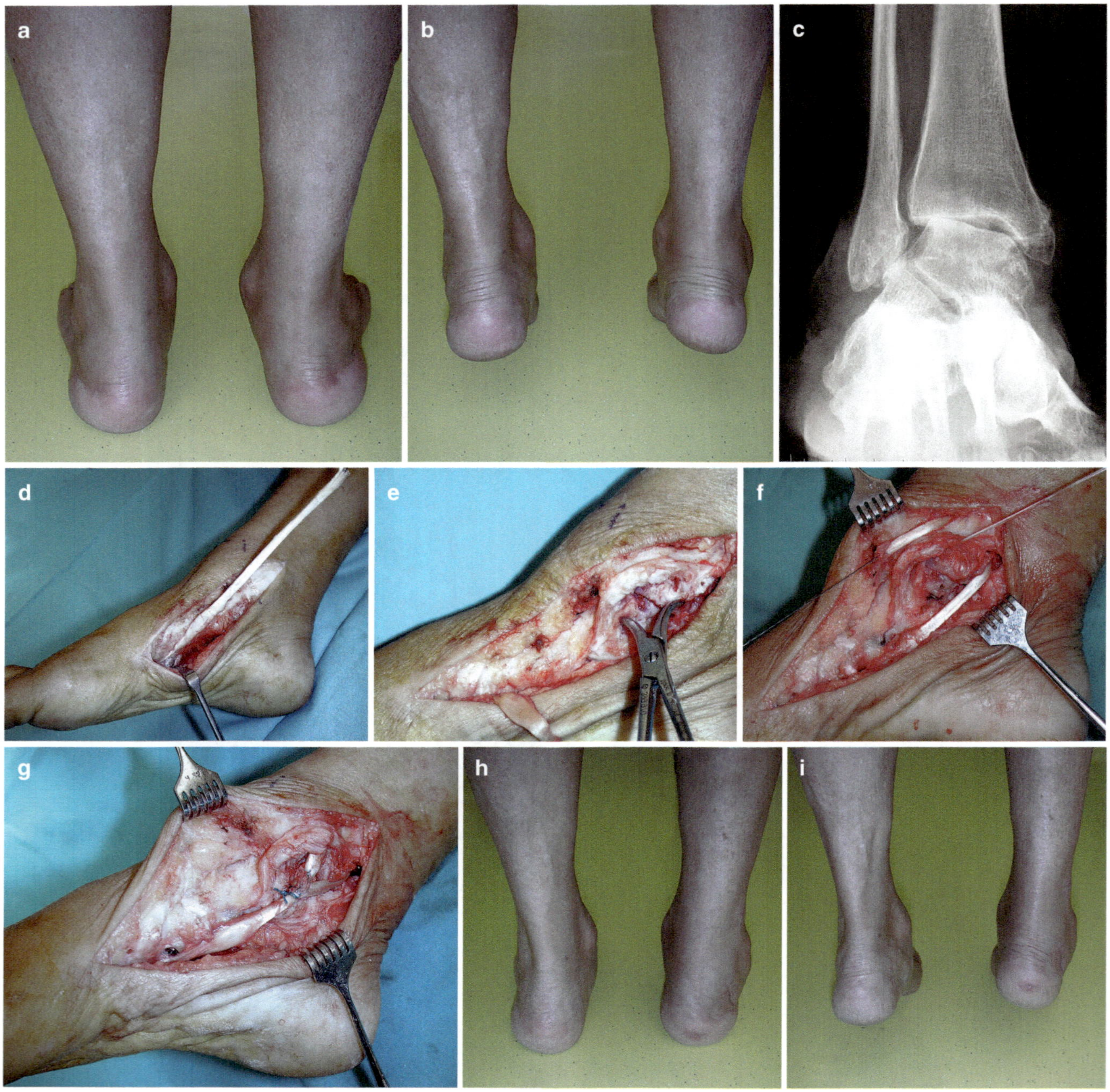

Fig. 5.55 *Surgical Technique: Reconstruction of the deep deltoid ligament with an autograft and bony procedures (Injury Type IV C).* This 56-year-old active female patient sustained a sprain 20 years ago when playing volleyball. While neglecting the injury initially, she regained her activities within some months; however, in the last year she noticed a progressive valgus deformity with an increasing feeling of medial instability. (**a**) From a posterior view, the valgus malalignment can be seen with a medial prominence and a distinct forefoot abduction is present. (**b**) When the patient is asked to go into tiptoe position, the deformity is seen to disappear. (**c**) Standard AP radiograph evidences a valgus tilt of the talus of 18°, furthermore, an old avulsion fragment can be detected. (**d**) The peroneal longus tendon is dissected approximately 10 cm above the ankle and then rerouted to the medial aspect of the foot. (**e**) The avulsion fragment is roughened and then repositioned and fixed by a screw, thereby tightening the remaining ligament structures. (**f**) A tunnel from the intercollicular groove to the anterior aspect of the medial malleolus is created through which the tendon graft is directed. A suture anchor is inserted to reattach the remaining ligament structures later on. (**g**) While the foot is held in slight supination, the end of the graft is sutured to the proximal graft. Thereafter, the remaining ligament structures are taken with the prepared suture anchor to enhance the ligament construct. Notice the screw in the first cuneiform from the fusion of the first naviculocuneiform joint before the tendon graft was inserted. Finally, a medial sliding osteotomy (surgical technique see Fig. 5.61) is performed to realign the heel (not shown). At last follow-up 5 years later, the patient is still very satisfied. (**h**) The foot looks clinically well aligned, and (**i**) in tiptoe position, it is even in slight varus. (**j–m**) The radiographs show a significantly better aligned foot; however, a valgus tilt of the talus persists and the fragment fixation on the medial malleolus failed. Nevertheless, a tiny joint space reappeared in the lateral tibiotalar joint. Fifteen years after surgical reconstruction, the patient is not pain free, however, still satisfied and had no further treatment since

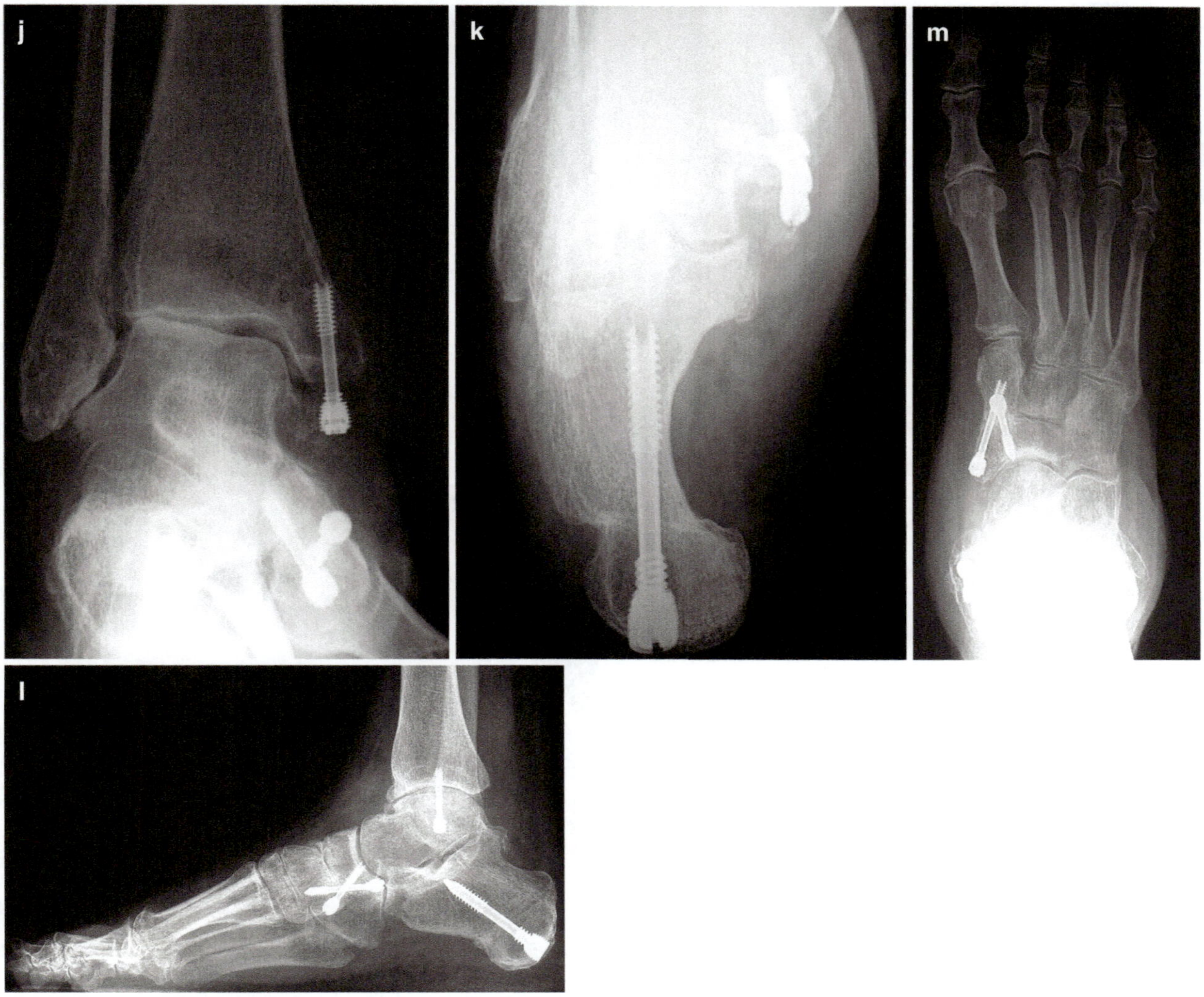

Fig. 5.55 (continued)

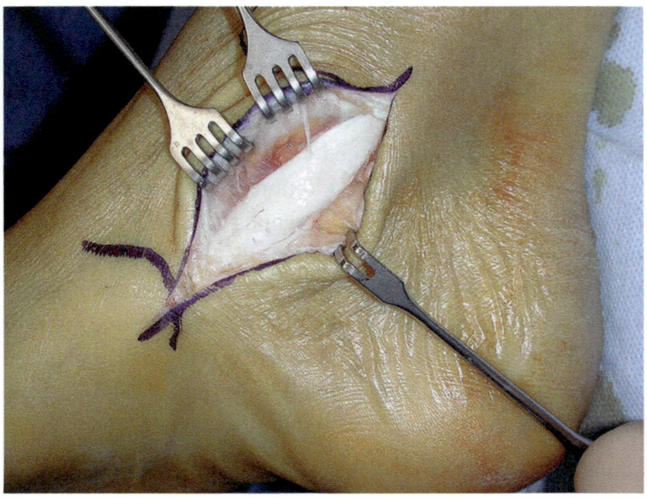

Fig. 5.56 *Surgical Technique: Debridement of the PT tendon.* This PT tendon is thickened and scarred within its sheath; thus, it must first be mobilized and debrided (same patient as Fig. 5.39)

ing wedge osteotomy than a lengthening osteotomy, thus being more stable (Fig. 5.59b) [20]. As the osteotomy is widened, the pronation deformity of the foot is seen to disappear (Fig. 5.60). A correctly sized allograft or a tricortical graft from the iliac crest is placed into the osteotomy site. A screw or a plate may be used to protect the graft from displacing and ensures a stable osteotomy. Radiographically, after the osteotomy is performed, the talar head is re-positioned on the calcaneus and coverage of the talar head is improved (Fig. 5.60o–v).

5.10.5.5 Calcaneal Medial Sliding Osteotomy

A calcaneal sliding osteotomy [94–98] is considered if there is a major coronal plane deformity, as it corrects the hindfoot valgus malalignment, resulting in restoration of the medial arch by a neutral pull of the triceps surae through the ankle. Sliding the tuber of the calcaneus medially corrects the static stability and restores a dynamic balance. In its anatomic

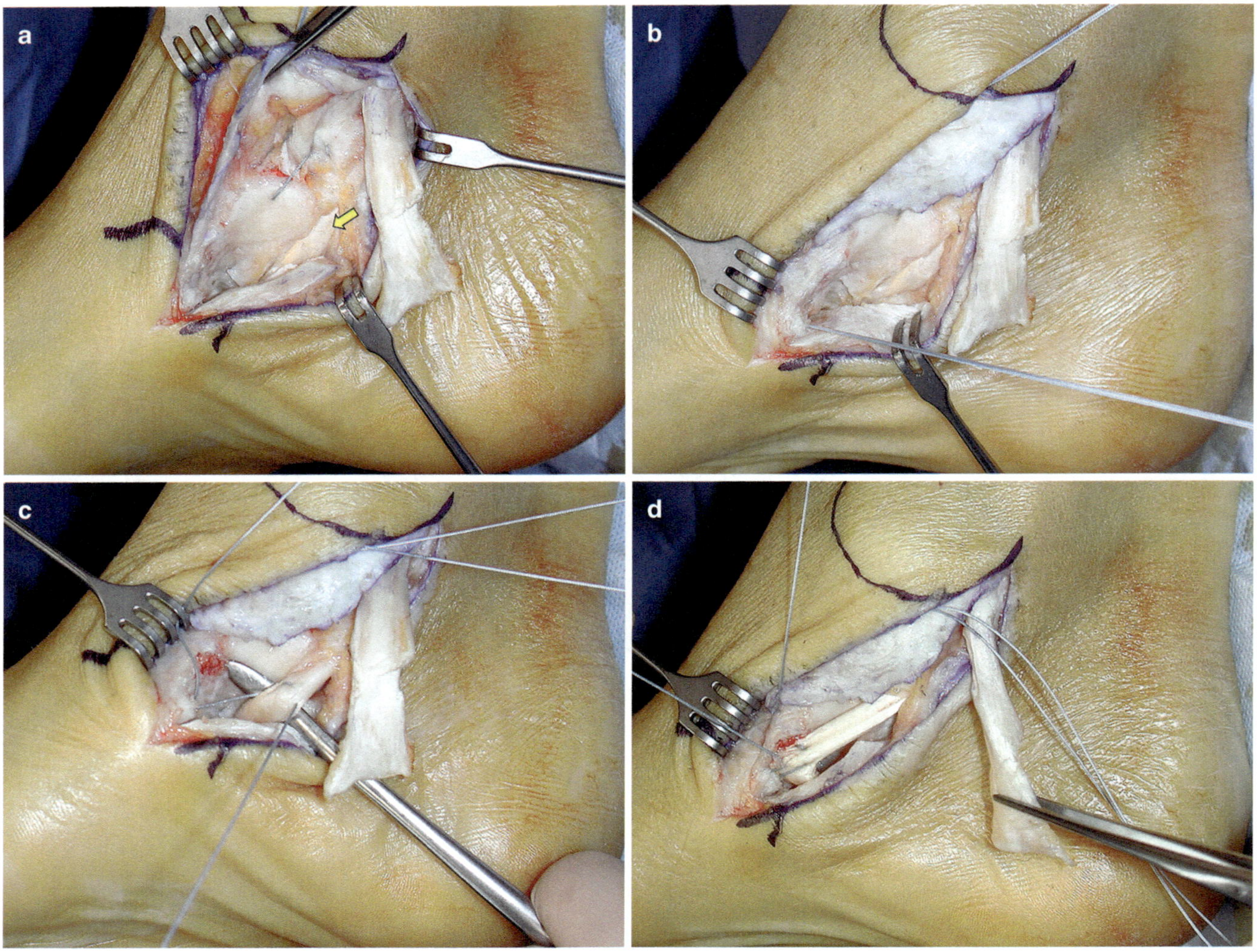

Fig. 5.57 *Surgical Technique: FDL tendon transfer*. If the PT tendon is diseased, an FDL tendon transfer might be considered to replace or enhance the PT tendon (same patient as Fig. 5.39). (**a**) After having done the ligament reconstruction (Fig. 5.39) and debrided the PT tendon and prepared for a shortening by a Z-shaped dissection, the sheath of the FDL tendon is dissected to visualize the tendon (arrow). To preserve the integrity of the sheath and tendon function, the sheath is strictly only opened distally. (**b**) A bony anchor is inserted on the tuberosity of the navicular. (**c**) The FDL tendon is carefully grabbed with an elevatorium and tensioned. Sutures are done with the prepared anchor suture. (**d**) The suture is tightened, and a knot made

alignment, the Achilles tendon pull inverts the hindfoot. When the distal insertion has shifted laterally, as is the case in valgus hindfeet, the resulting vector pulling upwards creates a further eversion force to the hindfoot, additionally contributing to the loss of medial arch stability [99]. By sliding the tuber of the calcaneus medially, this vector is neutralized, and the distal insertion of the Achilles tendon is in line with the tibiotalar and subtalar joints again.

The calcaneal tuber is exposed from lateral and an osteotomy is performed in a slightly oblique direction (Fig. 5.61). Then the calcaneal tuber is shifted medially as much as needed to get a well-aligned hindfoot. The effect can be increased by tilting the tuber additionally in varus. In fear that the tuber may displace towards cranial secondarily by the pull of the Achilles tendon, we adapted the osteotomy technique and perform an incomplete cut, leaving the caudal cortex intact. When opening the osteotomy, the bony bridge left will fracture and form a beak anteriorwards. With this adaptation, we never saw a secondary cranial displacement, although we permit full weight bearing straight after surgery.

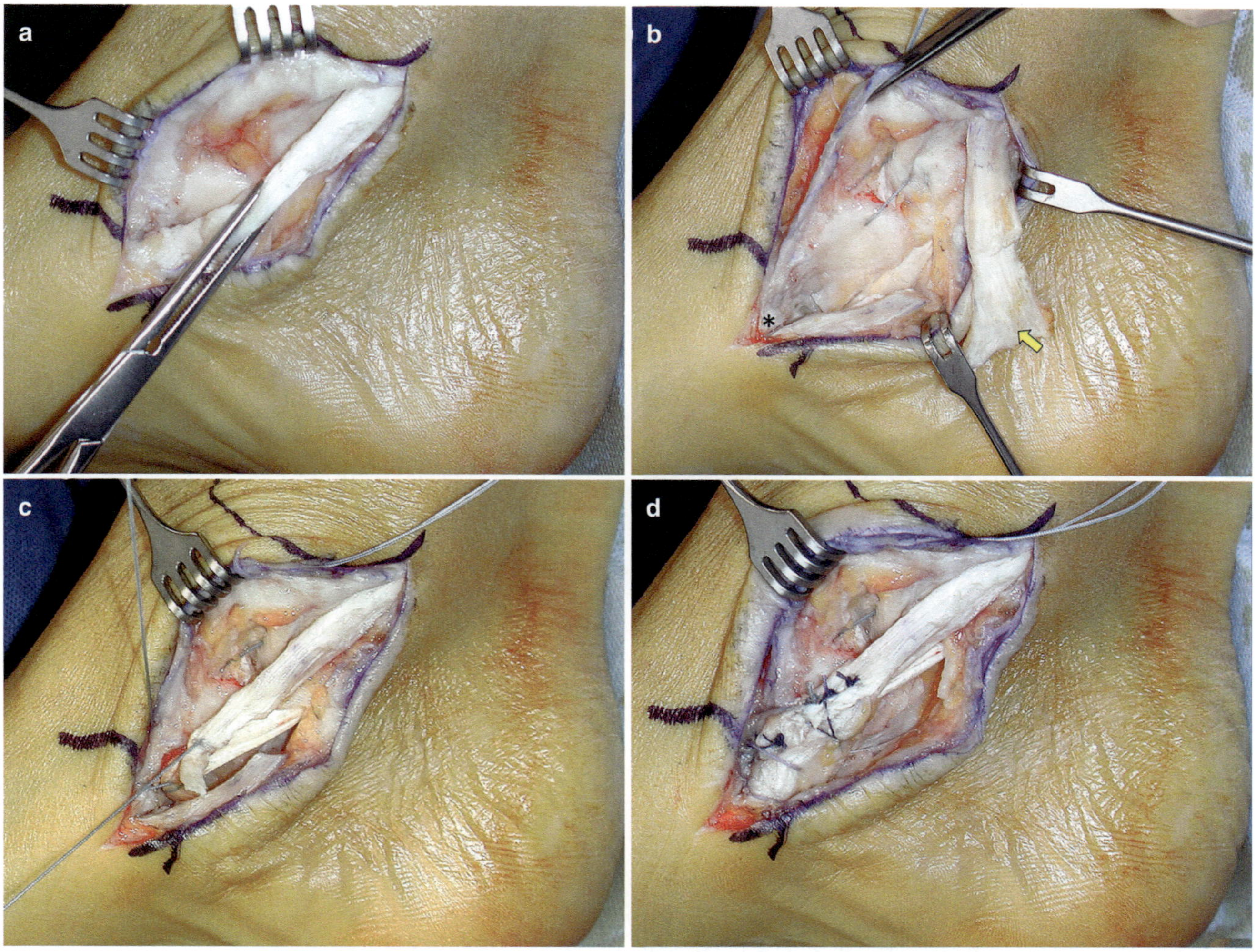

Fig. 5.58 *Surgical Technique: Shortening of the PT tendon.* If the PT tendon is elongated or diseased, a shortening can be considered if the PT muscle is still elastic, e.g., tendon excursion is still present (same patient as Fig. 5.39). (**a**) After debridement of the tendon, the excursion of the PT tendon is checked by pulling with a clamp. In this case, the elasticity of the muscle-tendon unit was preserved. (**b**) The tendon is dissected in a z-shaped fashion such as the proximal stump (arrow) will have the attempted length to reach the navicular tuberosity (asterisk). (**c**) The proximal stump is taken by the suture anchor and inserted to the navicular tuberosity. A suture is made for reattachment. (**d**) The distal stump is then used for additional fixation of the proximal stump, thus enhancing the fixation of the shortened tendon. In this patient, this procedure was combined with an FDL transfer (Fig. 5.57)

5.10.5.6 Combined Calcaneal Lengthening and Medial Sliding Osteotomy

A combined calcaneal lengthening and medial sliding osteotomy is considered if an increased pronation-abduction and heel valgus deformity is present. After being proposed first by Pomeroy and Manoli [100] and called "all-American osteotomy," others reported satisfactory results with this technique (Fig. 5.62) [101, 102]. Later, a calcaneal scarf osteotomy was proposed to combine a sliding and lengthening maneuver with one single osteotomy [101, 103].

5.10.6 Postoperative Management

The foot is protected by a plaster cast or boot for 6 weeks and full weight-bearing is permitted as soon as pain-free

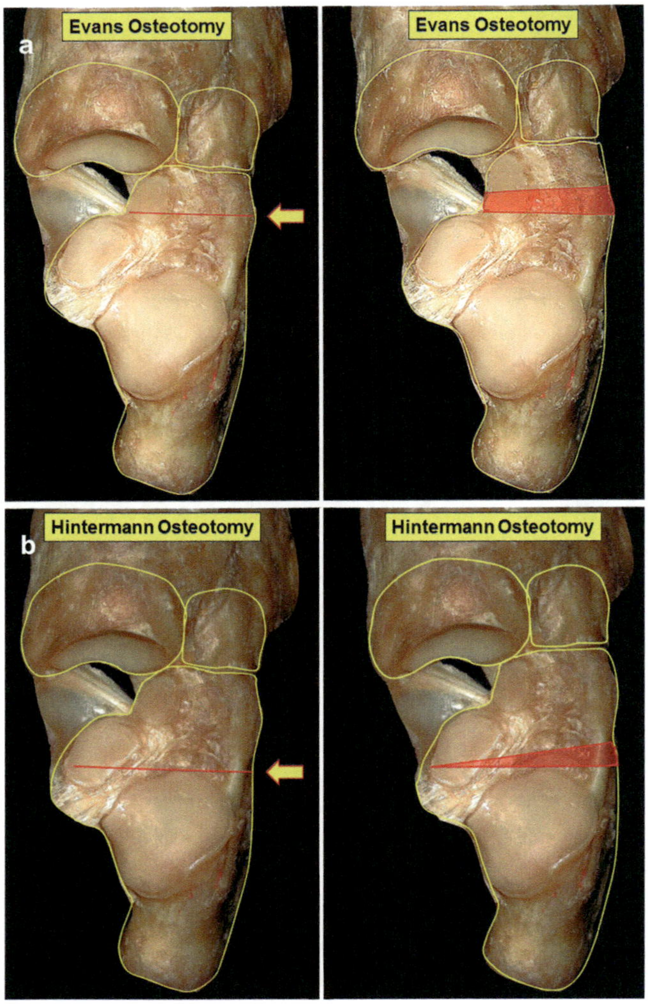

Fig. 5.59 *Surgical Technique: Concept of a lateral column lengthening osteotomy*. (**a**) The Evans osteotomy is performed 1 cm posterior to the calcaneocuboid joint with the aim to lengthen the calcaneus; a quadrangular bone bloc, the size of the space created, is inserted. Specific risks of this procedure are the destabilization of the anterior calcaneus and the possibility of creating an incongruency at the calcaneocuboid joint. (**b**) The Hintermann osteotomy is performed along the anterior border of the posterior subtalar facet and, while preserving the medial cortex, it acts as an open wedge osteotomy. Therefore, it does not destabilize the anterior calcaneus and it does also not create an incongruency at the calcaneocuboid joint

loading is possible. The rehabilitation program including passive and active ankle mobilization and muscular strength training is started thereafter. A stabilizing shoe when walking is used for protection. A walker or stabilizing shoe may be recommended for up to 4–6 weeks after plaster removal, depending on regained muscular balance of the hindfoot. Thereafter, we still recommend the patient to use it for walks on uneven ground, for high-risk sports activities, and for professional work outside. In the case of an arthrodesis, initial plaster or boot immobilization of 8 weeks is recommended.

5.11 Outcome

- The outcome highly depends on the severity of ligament lesions
- The outcome is in general less advantageous than after reconstruction of the lateral ankle ligaments

While good and excellent results have been reported for ligament repair in Type I-injuries [10, 11, 60], the outcome after ligament reconstruction of Type II- and Type III-injuries is less advantageous [10, 62]. Little data exist on the outcome after primary reconstruction of the TSL and spring ligament [104].

Despite the progress made in the understanding and in the improved surgical techniques, surgical treatment of Type IV-injuries is still critical. While techniques which use either an autogenous peroneus longus tendon [78, 105–107], a flexor hallucis longus tendon [108], or a tendon allograft [77, 79] have been proposed, most of them have not shown their efficiency in clinical use yet. Analogously, augmentation techniques with the use of an internal brace for anatomical repair of the medial ankle ligaments have not shown to be efficient at mid- to long term [62, 75].

5.12 Complications

- Inadequate primary treatment and/or reconstruction of the medial ankle ligaments results in persistent instability, which may lead to chronic overload of the PT tendon
- If adequate stability of the medial ankle joint complex is not obtained, the talus will progressively move away from the tibia and the pivoting of the talus along the medial malleolus will be lost

Most complications are a consequence of inadequate reconstruction of the medial ankle ligaments, resulting in persistent instability which may lead to chronic overload of the PT tendon and subsequent degeneration and insufficiency thereof [19, 20, 62]. Not to include reconstruction of the PT tendon in ligament repair of Type III B and III C-injuries may result in chronic pain at the injury site with incomplete recovery despite appropriate rehabilitation.

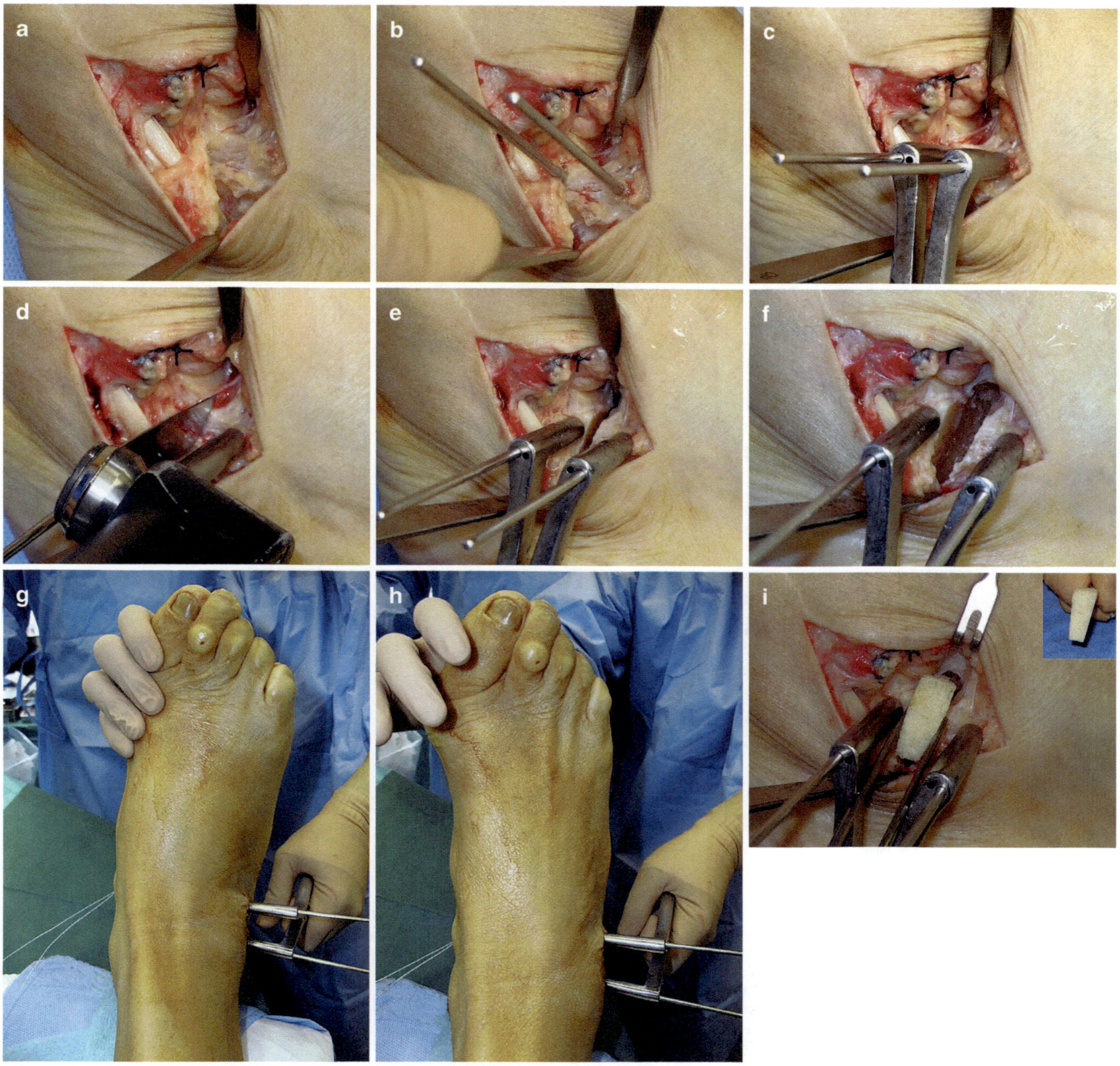

Fig. 5.60 *Surgical Technique: Lateral column lengthening osteotomy.* (**a**) The calcaneal neck is exposed by carefully keeping away the peroneal tendons with two small Hohmann retractors. (**b**) Two parallel K-wires are inserted on each side of the aimed osteotomy, not deeper than 1 cm. (**c**) A Hintermann distractor is mounted over the K-wires. (**d**) The osteotomy is performed along the anterior border of the posterior facet using a saw, preserving the opposite cortex. (**e**) The osteotomy is carefully opened with the distractor. (**f**) The osteotomy is opened as much as needed. In practice, opening of >8 mm is never needed and should be avoided. (**g**) To determine the amount of lengthening, the distraction is released. While the forefoot is held on its medial side, the foot is pronated and abducted as much as possible. (**h**) With these forces applied to the forefoot, distraction is applied until the forefoot is seen to reach a neutral position and the distance of opening is measured. (**i**) A wedge-shaped allograft is prepared accordingly, 1–2 mm smaller as the measured distance, in order to overcorrect the foot especially to preserve little pronation and abduction movement. Because the osteotomy typically opens more cranially than caudally, the wedge is kept a bit larger at its upper part. Then, the graft is inserted. (**j**) An impactor can be used but is usually not necessary as the wedge is a bit smaller. (**k**) When the distractor is removed, the graft is jammed. (**l**) The graft is shaped with a rongeur to prevent impingement with the peroneal tendons and the talus in the sinus tarsi. (**m**) Especially the caudal aspect is smoothened. (**n**) A screw can be used across the osteotomy to protect the graft from displacement. This can be done from posterior, as shown in this case, or from anterior. (**o–v**) The effect of the osteotomy can be seen on standard weight-bearing radiographs, particularly the reduction of the heel valgus (HMA = heel moment arm), the opening of the sinus tarsi (ST, yellow arrow), the reduction of the talocalcaneal overlap (OL, red arrow), the improvement of the Merry-angles (TM-angle), and the improvement of the talonavicular coverage (NC, blue arrow)

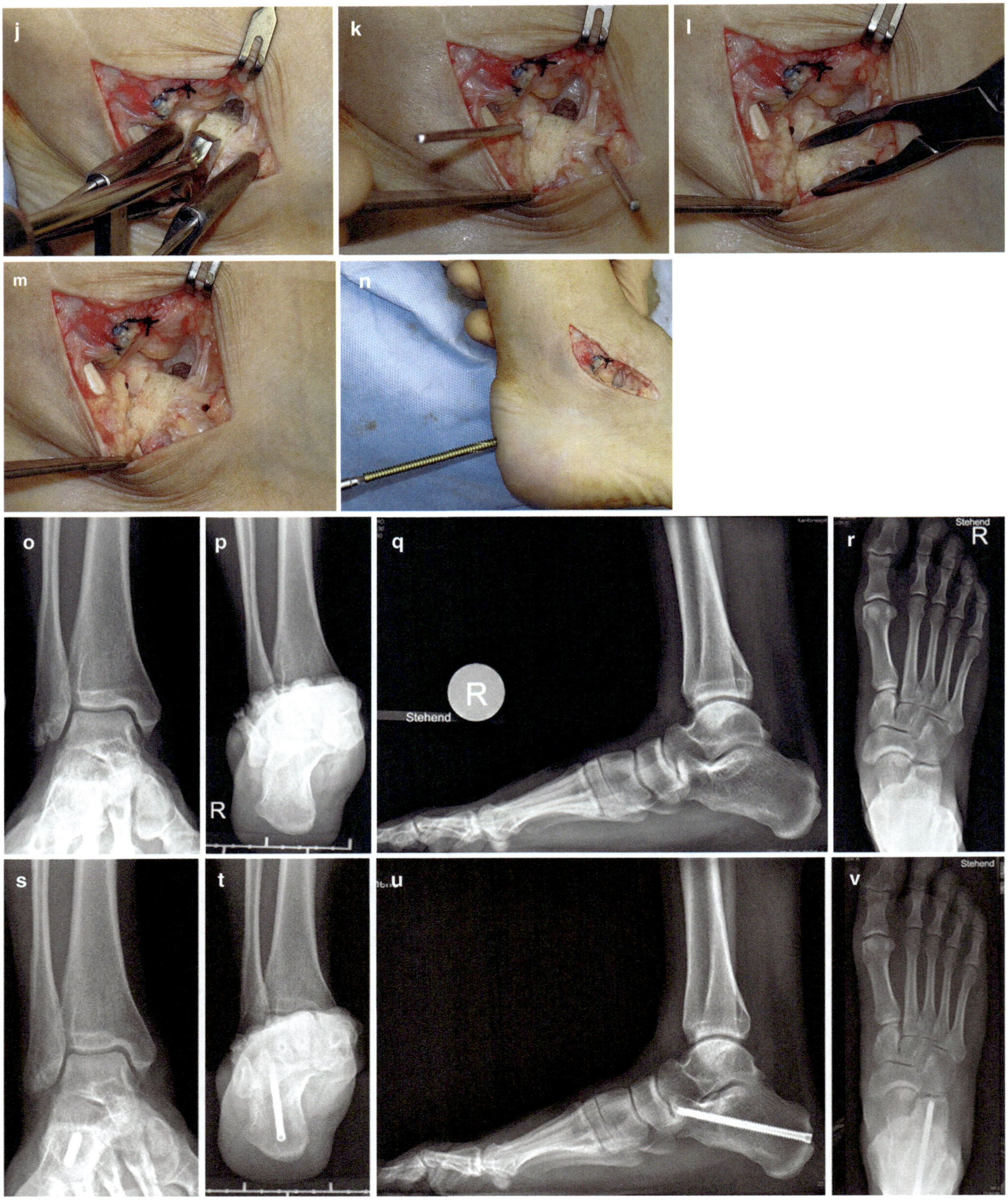

Fig. 5.60 (continued)

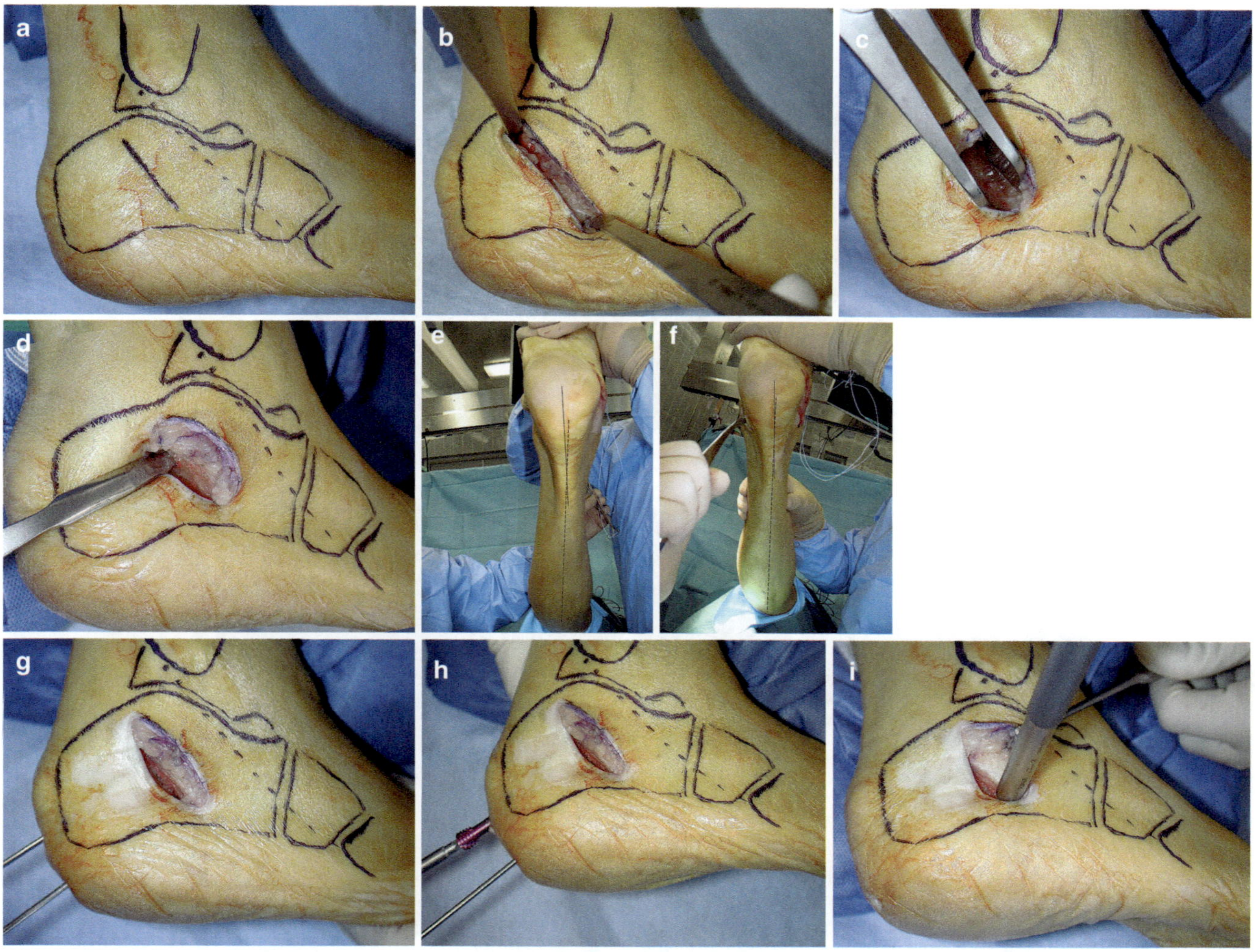

Fig. 5.61 *Surgical Technique: Calcaneal medial sliding osteotomy.* (**a**) A 2–3 cm long oblique incision is made on the lateral aspect of the calcaneal tuber. (**b**) The calcaneus is exposed paying attention not to injure the sural nerve. Two small Hohmann retractors are used to expose the cranial and caudal aspect of the calcaneus. Then, the osteotomy is performed with a saw. Preserving the caudal cortex avoids uncontrolled displacement of the tuber. (**c**) While a flat distractor is used to open the osteotomy by approximately 2 cm, the caudal cortex breaks forming a typical beak towards anterior. The soft tissue on the medial side can typically be seen through the osteotomy. (**d**) While the foot is held in plantarflexion, the tuber is moved medially. The use of one or two Hohmann retractors may facilitate this maneuver. Dorsiflexion of the foot stabilizes the achieved position. (**e**) Hindfoot alignment can be checked by lifting the leg, as shown for the situation before performing the osteotomy. (**f**) The achieved correction is checked while the foot is held in dorsiflexion. One Hohmann retractor may be left in place to ensure for stability. (**g**) Two 2 K-wires are inserted slightly lateral and are used for preliminary fixation to double check the position under fluoroscopy. (**h**) Thereafter, the cannulated screws are inserted. (**i**) The created edge on the calcaneal body is impacted to get a smooth bony surface and to prevent discomfort in the shoe. Fluoroscopy is used to check final position. (**j**) In the lateral view a slight plantarization of the tuber can be seen. This is seen in most patients where the plantar cortex and ligament structures were not cut by the saw. (**k**) The axial view shows the amount of medial translation, the additional effect of varization of the tuber and the screw position as well. It also shows the impacted edge of the calcaneal body (arrow). (**l–s**) The effect of the osteotomy can be seen on standard weight-bearing radiographs, particularly the reduction of the heel valgus (HMA). Though there is still some valgus malalignment of the heel, the talar position improved and a more regular tibiotalar joint space reappeared in both the coronal and sagittal plane

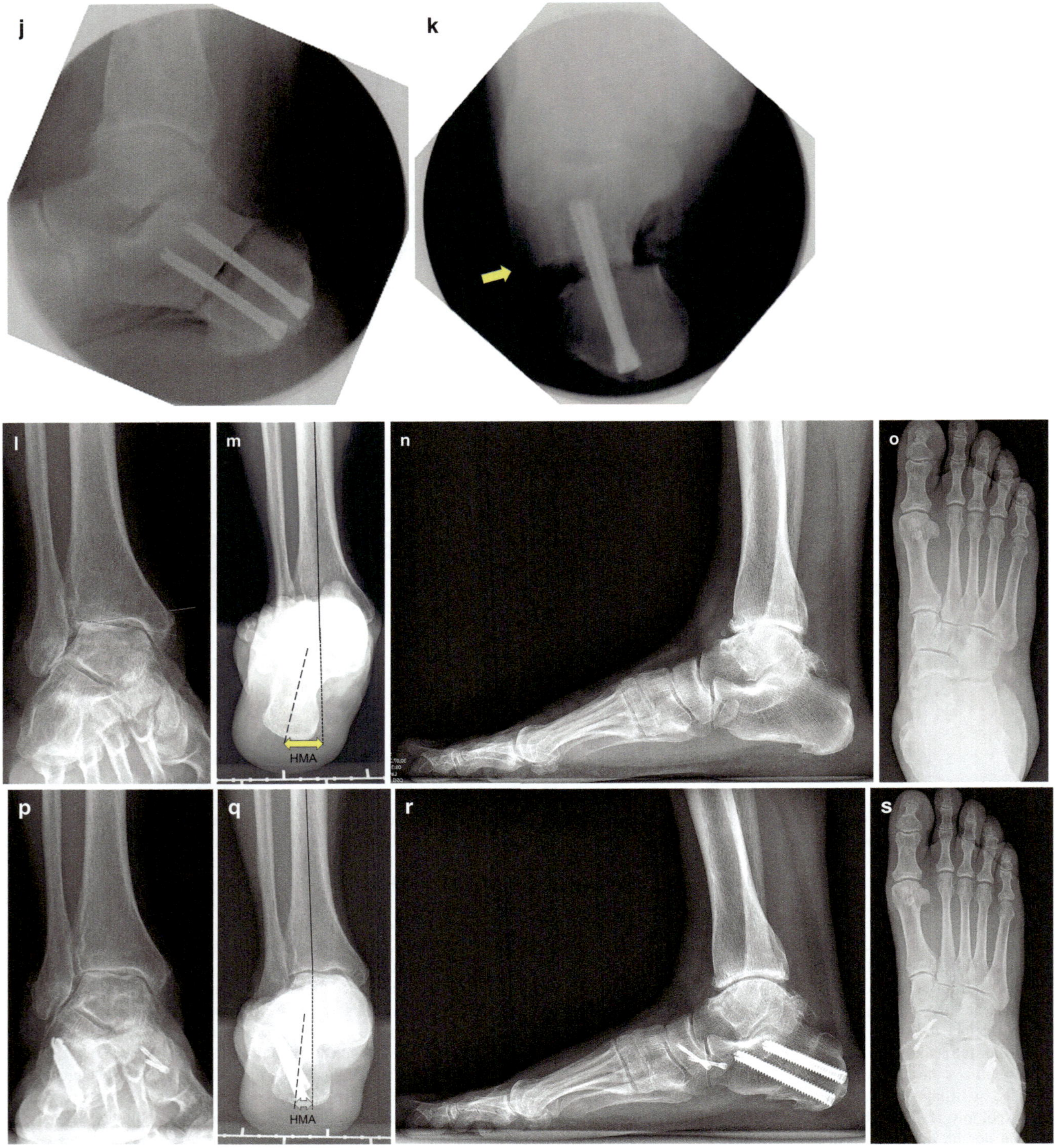

Fig. 5.61 (continued)

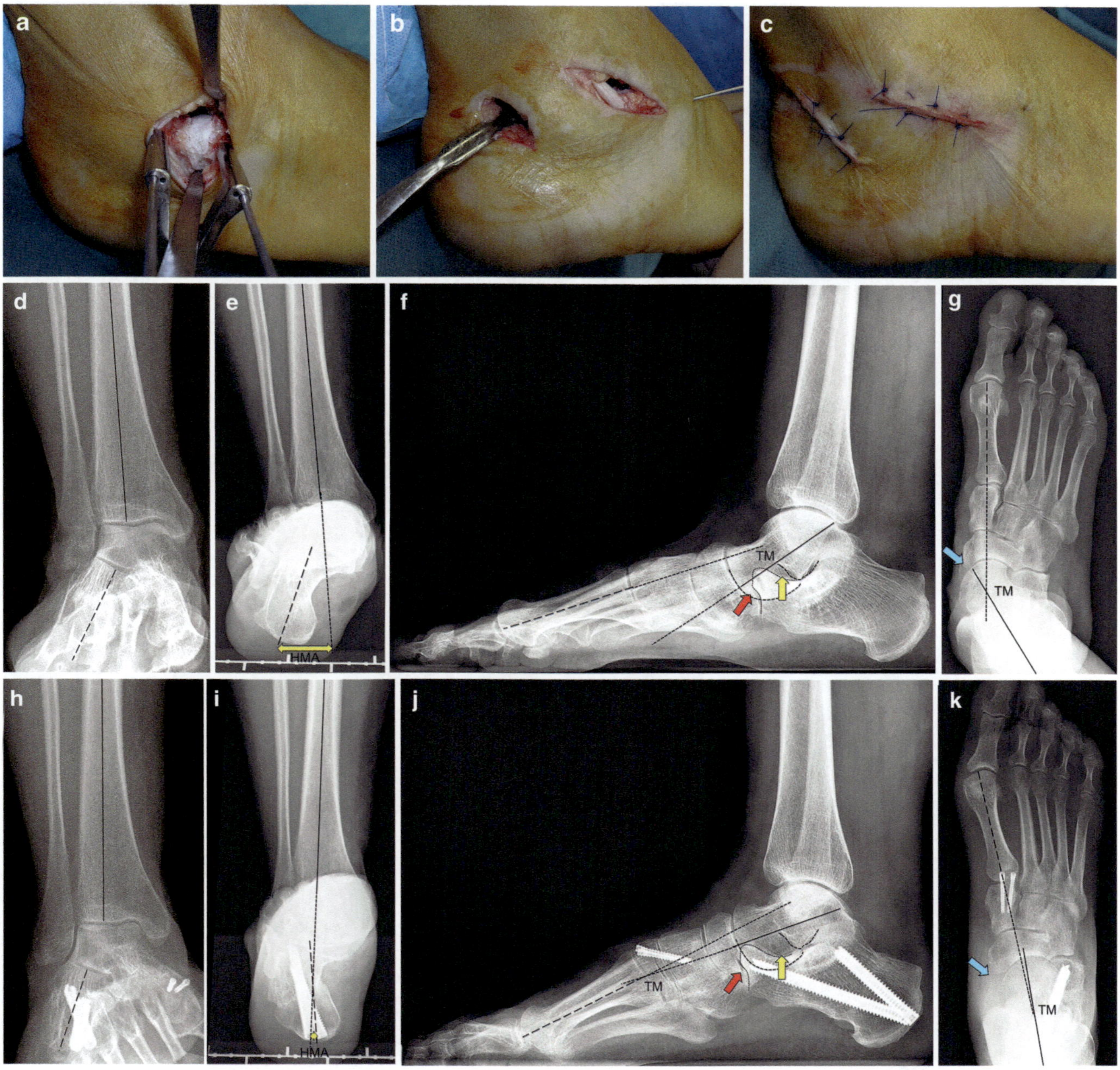

Fig. 5.62 *Surgical Technique: Double calcaneal osteotomy*. (**a**) First, the lateral calcaneal lengthening osteotomy is performed and protected by a K-wire from secondary displacement. (**b**) Thereafter, the medial sliding osteotomy is performed through a separate approach. The screws are inserted in a manner to stabilize both osteotomies. (**c**) The final soft tissue situation after wound closure shows the 2 incisions. (**d–k**) The effect of the osteotomy can be seen on standard weight-bearing radiographs, particularly the reduction of the heel valgus (HMA = heel moment arm), the opening of the sinus tarsi (ST, yellow arrow), the reduction of the talocalcaneal overlap (OL, red arrow), the improvement of the Merry-angles (TM-angle), and the improvement of the talonavicular coverage (NC, blue arrow)

Failure to reroute the used tendon grafts or internal braces onto the anatomic insertion area of the specific tendons on either the medial malleolus, talus, calcaneus, and navicular may change the biomechanics of the ankle joint complex, resulting in motion restriction and laxity of the tibiotalar and peritalar joints. The biomechanics may be altered further, depending on the foot position and increased joint load, leading to subsequent pain [87, 92] (Fig. 5.63). The use of bulky tendon grafts may result in painful soft tissue impingement and swelling, limiting the possibility of wearing normal shoes.

If not addressed by appropriate bony procedures, preexistent plano-valgus, abduction and supination deformity of the foot may result in overload of the reconstructed soft tissues

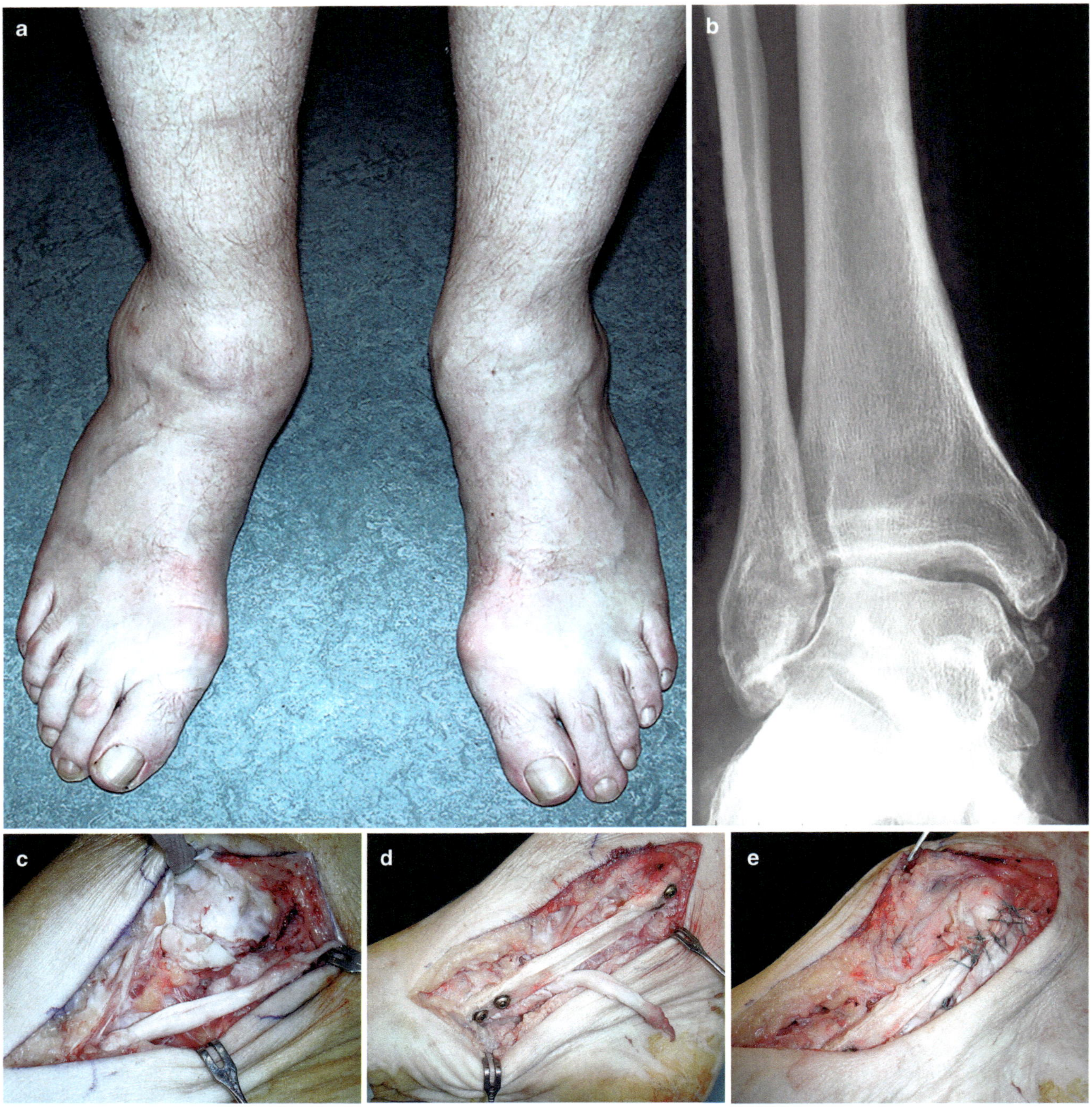

Fig. 5.63 *Surgical Technique: Tibionavicular tenodesis*. This 59-year-old postman is suffering from progressive pain on his lateral ankle. He also reported having had heavy pain on the medial side, that disappeared some weeks ago. (**a**) Clinical presentation with a significant valgus malalignment of the right foot. While the double heel rise test is partially possible, single heel rise is not possible. (**b**) In the AP radiograph, a valgus talar tilt of 12° is found, with little degenerative changes of the tibiotalar joint. (**c**) Surgical exploration reveals a rupture of the PT tendon with an extended avulsion of the deltoid ligament. (**d**) A bone-tendon-bone allograft is used and fixed to the undersurface of the navicular bone and to the posterior aspect of the medial malleolus, respectively. (**e**) The deltoid is reconstructed with the remaining ligaments. Though the foot clinically looked better and the talar valgus tilt was decreased to 7°, the patient was not satisfied. He was not able to walk properly due to pain and discomfort when loading his foot. Therefore, 14 months later, the allograft was removed, and a TTC-fusion was performed with a retrograde nail

with subsequent failure, recurrence of pain, and limited function such as the inability of appropriately loading the foot, particularly during push-off [6].

If adequate stability of the medial ankle joint complex is not obtained, the talus will progressively move away from the tibia and the pivoting of the talus along the medial malleolus will be lost. This leads to a lateral shift of the center of rotation and thus a lateral shift of the articular load. These changes of biomechanics are detrimental for the integrity of the ankle joint complex and will result in progressive deformation and destabilization of the hindfoot, leading to critical overload of the lateral tibiotalar joint [2], which may result in subsequent osteoarthritis [109].

5.13 Conclusions and Future Evolution

- Early diagnosis and appropriate treatment are mandatory for success
- Because isolated injuries to the deltoid and spring ligaments are often primarily missed, the orthopedic surgeon is often faced with the problem after onset of chronic symptoms, destabilization of the medial ankle joint complex, and progressive deformity

Isolated injuries to the deltoid and spring ligaments are often primarily missed, thus the orthopedic surgeon is mostly faced with the problem after onset of chronic symptoms. Meticulous recording of the history and thorough clinical investigation are therefore mandatory to make the diagnosis. Imaging methods may serve to further confirm the diagnosis and to reveal morphological changes subsequent to the initial injury [6, 10].

Though better understanding of medial ankle instability and subsequent biomechanical changes exist, the question remains how an injury to the ligaments of the medial ankle joint complex should be treated best [63, 73, 76]. While primary repair will work for most Type I-injuries, it may not work for Type II- and Type III-injuries [10]. A high incidence of persistent pain and disability is related to injuries with an accessory tibial bone or a detachment of the central slip of the PT tendon insertion at the navicular, such as seen in patients with a spring ligament rupture (Hintermann & Ruiz, *in press*). Therefore, reattachment of the accessory bone or excision thereof with subsequent transosseous fixation of the PT tendon to the navicular is essential for treatment success. In the case of an elongated PT tendon, a Z-shaped PT tendon shortening [92] or a FDL transfer [89, 90] can be added to the procedure, to protect the repair. Controversies still exist however, whether bony procedures should be considered to protect soft tissue reconstructions.

In the last years, the use of tendon autografts and allografts have been proposed to restore adequate stability of the medial ankle joint complex [75–83]. Despite showing acceptable results intraoperatively, studies are needed to examine whether they can resist against applied forces and whether they do not restrict motion over time. Respect of anatomy may thus be crucial, in particular with the use of internal braces [62, 75] and the use of arthroscopic techniques [72].

More studies are necessary to further answer open questions and improve not only the reconstruction techniques, but also to determine the evidence of surgical reconstruction with regard to restoring the stability of the medial ankle joint complex and overall foot function.

References

1. Campbell KJ, Michalski MP, Wilson KJ, Goldsmith MT, Wijdicks CA, Laprade RF, et al. The ligament anatomy of the deltoid complex of the ankle: a qualitative and quantitative anatomical study. J Bone Joint Surg Am. 2014;96(8):e62.
2. Earll M, Wayne J, Brodrick C, Vokshoor A, Adelaar R. Contribution of the deltoid ligament to ankle joint contact characteristics: a cadaver study. Foot Ankle Int. 1996;17(6):317–24.
3. Harper MC. Deltoid ligament: an anatomical evaluation of function. Foot Ankle. 1987;8(1):19–22.
4. Harper MC. The deltoid ligament. An evaluation of need for surgical repair. Clin Orthop Relat Res. 1988;226:156–68.
5. Buchhorn T, Sabeti-Aschraf M, Dlaska CE, Wenzel F, Graf A, Ziai P. Combined medial and lateral anatomic ligament reconstruction for chronic rotational instability of the ankle. Foot Ankle Int. 2011;32(12):1122–6.
6. Hintermann B, Valderrabano V, Boss A, Trouillier HH, Dick W. Medial ankle instability: an exploratory, prospective study of fifty-two cases. Am J Sports Med. 2004;32(1):183–90.
7. Kofotolis ND, Kellis E, Vlachopoulos SP. Ankle sprain injuries and risk factors in amateur soccer players during a 2-year period. Am J Sports Med. 2007;35(3):458–66.
8. Waterman BR, Belmont PJ Jr, Cameron KL, Svoboda SJ, Alitz CJ, Owens BD. Risk factors for syndesmotic and medial ankle sprain: role of sex, sport, and level of competition. Am J Sports Med. 2011;39(5):992–8.
9. Crim JR, Beals TC, Nickisch F, Schannen A, Saltzman CL. Deltoid ligament abnormalities in chronic lateral ankle instability. Foot Ankle Int. 2011;32(9):873–8.
10. Hintermann B. Medial ankle instability. Foot Ankle Clin. 2003;8(4):723–38.
11. Hintermann B, Knupp M, Pagenstert GI. Deltoid ligament injuries: diagnosis and management. Foot Ankle Clin. 2006;11(3):625–37.
12. Dabash S, Elabd A, Potter E, Fernandez I, Gerzina C, Thabet AM, et al. Adding deltoid ligament repair in ankle fracture treatment: is it necessary? A systematic review. Foot Ankle Surg. 2019;25(6):714–20.

13. Lee S, Lin J, Hamid KS, Bohl DD. Deltoid ligament rupture in ankle fracture: diagnosis and management. J Am Acad Orthop Surg. 2019;27(14):e648–e58.
14. Lee TH, Jang KS, Choi GW, Jeong CD, Hong SJ, Yoon MA, et al. The contribution of anterior deltoid ligament to ankle stability in isolated lateral malleolar fractures. Injury. 2016;47(7):1581–5.
15. Sun X, Li T, Sun Z, Li Y, Yang M, Li S, et al. Does routinely repairing deltoid ligament injuries in type B ankle joint fractures influence long term outcomes? Injury. 2018;49(12):2312–7.
16. Hintermann B, Regazzoni P, Lampert C, Stutz G, Gachter A. Arthroscopic findings in acute fractures of the ankle. J Bone Joint Surg Br. 2000;82(3):345–51.
17. Tornetta P 3rd. Competence of the deltoid ligament in bimalleolar ankle fractures after medial malleolar fixation. J Bone Joint Surg Am. 2000;82(6):843–8.
18. Deland JT. The adult acquired flatfoot and spring ligament complex. Pathology and implications for treatment. Foot Ankle Clin. 2001;6(1):129–35, vii.
19. Deland JT, de Asla RJ, Sung IH, Ernberg LA, Potter HG. Posterior tibial tendon insufficiency: which ligaments are involved? Foot Ankle Int. 2005;26(6):427–35.
20. Hintermann B, Valderrabano V, Kundert HP. Lengthening of the lateral column and reconstruction of the medial soft tissue for treatment of acquired flatfoot deformity associated with insufficiency of the posterior tibial tendon. Foot Ankle Int. 1999;20(10):622–9.
21. Nelson DR, Younger A. Acute posttraumatic planovalgus foot deformity involving hindfoot ligamentous pathology. Foot Ankle Clin. 2003;8(3):521–37.
22. Boss AP, Hintermann B. Anatomical study of the medial ankle ligament complex. Foot Ankle Int. 2002;23(6):547–53.
23. Hintermann B, Golanó P. The anatomy and function of the deltoid ligament. Tech Foot Ankle Surg. 2014;13(2):67–72.
24. Milner CE, Soames RW. Anatomy of the collateral ligaments of the human ankle joint. Foot Ankle Int. 1998;19(11):757–60.
25. Pankovich AM, Shivaram MS. Anatomical basis of variability in injuries of the medial malleolus and the deltoid ligament. I. Anatomical studies. Acta Orthop Scand. 1979;50(2):217–23.
26. Sarrafian SK. Anatomy of foot and ankle. 2nd ed. Philadelphia: Lippincott Williams and Wilkins; 1993.
27. Siegler S, Block J, Schneck CD. The mechanical characteristics of the collateral ligaments of the human ankle joint. Foot Ankle. 1988;8(5):234–42.
28. Won HJ, Koh IJ, Won HS. Morphological variations of the deltoid ligament of the medial ankle. Clin Anat. 2016;29(8):1059–65.
29. Milner CE, Soames RW. The medial collateral ligaments of the human ankle joint: anatomical variations. Foot Ankle Int. 1998;19(5):289–92.
30. Yammine K. The morphology and prevalence of the deltoid complex ligament of the ankle. Foot Ankle Spec. 2017;10(1):55–62.
31. Davis WH, Sobel M, DiCarlo EF, Torzilli PA, Deng X, Geppert MJ, et al. Gross, histological, and microvascular anatomy and biomechanical testing of the spring ligament complex. Foot Ankle Int. 1996;17(2):95–102.
32. Mengiardi B, Pinto C, Zanetti M. Medial collateral ligament complex of the ankle: MR imaging anatomy and findings in medial instability. Semin Musculoskelet Radiol. 2016;20(1):91–103.
33. Patil V, Ebraheim NA, Frogameni A, Liu J. Morphometric dimensions of the calcaneonavicular (spring) ligament. Foot Ankle Int. 2007;28(8):927–32.
34. Rule J, Yao L, Seeger LL. Spring ligament of the ankle: normal MR anatomy. AJR Am J Roentgenol. 1993;161(6):1241–4.
35. Taniguchi A, Tanaka Y, Takakura Y, Kadono K, Maeda M, Yamamoto H. Anatomy of the spring ligament. J Bone Joint Surg Am. 2003;85(11):2174–8.
36. Melao L, Canella C, Weber M, Negrao P, Trudell D, Resnick D. Ligaments of the transverse tarsal joint complex: MRI-anatomic correlation in cadavers. AJR Am J Roentgenol. 2009;193(3):662–71.
37. Golano P, Farinas O, Saenz I. The anatomy of the navicular and periarticular structures. Foot Ankle Clin. 2004;9(1):1–23.
38. Hardy RH. Observations on the structure and properties of the plantar calcaneo-navicular ligament in man. J Anat. 1951;85(2):135–9.
39. Gray H. In: Williams PL, Warwick R, Dyson M, Bannister LH, editors. Gray's anatomy. 37th ed. Edinburgh: Churchill Livingstone; 1989. p. 459–544.
40. Close JR. Some applications of the functional anatomy of the ankle joint. J Bone Joint Surg Am. 1956;38-A(4):761–81.
41. Rasmussen O, Kromann-Andersen C, Boe S. Deltoid ligament. Functional analysis of the medial collateral ligamentous apparatus of the ankle joint. Acta Orthop Scand. 1983;54(1):36–44.
42. Nigg BM, Skarvan G, Frank CB, Yeadon MR. Elongation and forces of ankle ligaments in a physiological range of motion. Foot Ankle. 1990;11(1):30–40.
43. Lapidus PW. Kinesiology and mechanical anatomy of the tarsal joints. Clin Orthop Relat Res. 1963;30:20–36.
44. Bruns J, Rehder U. Ligament kinematics of the ankle joint. An experimental study. Z Orthop Ihre Grenzgeb. 1993;131(4):363–9.
45. Luo ZP, Kitaoka HB, Hsu HC, Kura H, An KN. Physiological elongation of ligamentous complex surrounding the hindfoot joints: in vitro biomechanical study. Foot Ankle Int. 1997;18(5):277–83.
46. Quiles M, Requena F, Gomez L, Garcia-Sancho L. Functional anatomy of the medial collateral ligament of the ankle joint. Foot Ankle. 1983;4(2):73–82.
47. Hintermann B, Sommer C, Nigg BM. Influence of ligament transection on tibial and calcaneal rotation with loading and dorsi-plantarflexion. Foot Ankle Int. 1995;16(9):567–71.
48. Sommer C, Hintermann B, Nigg BM, van den Bogert AJ. Influence of ankle ligaments on tibial rotation: an in vitro study. Foot Ankle Int. 1996;17(2):79–84.
49. Borton DC, Saxby TS. Tear of the plantar calcaneonavicular (spring) ligament causing flatfoot. A case report. J Bone Joint Surg Br. 1997;79(4):641–3.
50. Tryfonidis M, Jackson W, Mansour R, Cooke PH, Teh J, Ostlere S, et al. Acquired adult flat foot due to isolated plantar calcaneonavicular (spring) ligament insufficiency with a normal tibialis posterior tendon. Foot Ankle Surg. 2008;14(2):89–95.
51. Weerts B, Warmerdam PE, Faber FW. Isolated spring ligament rupture causing acute flatfoot deformity: case report. Foot Ankle Int. 2012;33(2):148–50.
52. Grath GB. Widening of the ankle mortise. A clinical and experimental study. Acta Chir Scand Suppl. 1960;Suppl 263:1–88.
53. Hintermann B. Bandverletzung der Sprunggelenke (Teil1) [Ligament injury of the ankle joint (I)]. Sportverletz Sportschaden. 1996;10(3):47.
54. Cifuentes-De la Portilla C, Larrainzar-Garijo R, Bayod J. Biomechanical stress analysis of the main soft tissues associated with the development of adult acquired flatfoot deformity. Clin Biomech (Bristol, Avon). 2019;61:163–71.
55. Kelly M, Masqoodi N, Vasconcellos D, Fowler X, Osman WS, Elfar JC, et al. Spring ligament tear decreases static stability of the ankle joint. Clin Biomech (Bristol, Avon). 2019;61:79–83.
56. Smyth NA, Aiyer AA, Kaplan JR, Carmody CA, Kadakia AR. Adult-acquired flatfoot deformity. Eur J Orthop Surg Traumatol. 2017;27(4):433–9.
57. Hintermann B, Nigg BM, Sommer C. Foot movement and tendon excursion: an in vitro study. Foot Ankle Int. 1994;15(7):386–95.
58. Silver RL, de la Garza J, Rang M. The myth of muscle balance. A study of relative strengths and excursions of normal muscles about the foot and ankle. J Bone Joint Surg Br. 1985;67(3):432–7.

59. Jeong MS, Choi YS, Kim YJ, Kim JS, Young KW, Jung YY. Deltoid ligament in acute ankle injury: MR imaging analysis. Skelet Radiol. 2014;43(5):655–63.
60. Hintermann B, Boss A, Schafer D. Arthroscopic findings in patients with chronic ankle instability. Am J Sports Med. 2002;30(3):402–9.
61. Kitaoka HB, Luo ZP, An KN. Reconstruction operations for acquired flatfoot: biomechanical evaluation. Foot Ankle Int. 1998;19(4):203–7.
62. Nery C, Lemos A, Raduan F, Mansur NSB, Baumfeld D. Combined spring and deltoid ligament repair in adult-acquired flatfoot. Foot Ankle Int. 2018;39(8):903–7.
63. Bastias GF, Dalmau-Pastor M, Astudillo C, Pellegrini MJ. Spring ligament instability. Foot Ankle Clin. 2018;23(4):659–78.
64. Chun TH, Park YS, Sung KS. The effect of ossicle resection in the lateral ligament repair for treatment of chronic lateral ankle instability. Foot Ankle Int. 2013;34(8):1128–33.
65. Hintermann B. What the orthopaedic foot and ankle surgeon wants to know from MR imaging. Semin Musculoskelet Radiol. 2005;9(3):260–71.
66. Khor YP, Tan KJ. The anatomic pattern of injuries in acute inversion ankle sprains: a magnetic resonance imaging study. Orthop J Sports Med. 2013;1(7):2325967113517078.
67. Ormsby N, Jackson G, Evans P, Platt S. Imaging of the tibionavicular ligament, and its potential role in adult acquired flatfoot deformity. Foot Ankle Int. 2018;39(5):629–35.
68. Warner SJ, Garner MR, Fabricant PD, Schottel PC, Loftus ML, Hentel KD, et al. The diagnostic accuracy of radiographs and magnetic resonance imaging in predicting deltoid ligament ruptures in ankle fractures. HSS J. 2019;15(2):115–21.
69. Crim J, Longenecker LG. MRI and surgical findings in deltoid ligament tears. AJR Am J Roentgenol. 2015;204(1):W63–9.
70. Komenda GA, Ferkel RD. Arthroscopic findings associated with the unstable ankle. Foot Ankle Int. 1999;20(11):708–13.
71. Schafer D, Hintermann B. Arthroscopic assessment of the chronic unstable ankle joint. Knee Surg Sports Traumatol Arthrosc. 1996;4(1):48–52.
72. Lui TH, Mak CYD. Arthroscopic approach to the spring (calcaneonavicular) ligament. Foot Ankle Surg. 2018;24(3):242–5.
73. Alshalawi S, Galhoum AE, Alrashidi Y, Wiewiorski M, Herrera M, Barg A, et al. Medial ankle instability: the deltoid dilemma. Foot Ankle Clin. 2018;23(4):639–57.
74. Czajka CM, Tran E, Cai AN, DiPreta JA. Ankle sprains and instability. Med Clin North Am. 2014;98(2):313–29.
75. Acevedo J, Vora A. Anatomical reconstruction of the spring ligament complex: "internal brace" augmentation. Foot Ankle Spec. 2013;6(6):441–5.
76. Brodell JD Jr, MacDonald A, Perkins JA, Deland JT, Oh I. Deltoid-spring ligament reconstruction in adult acquired flatfoot deformity with medial peritalar instability. Foot Ankle Int. 2019:1071100719839176.
77. Deland JT, de Asla RJ, Segal A. Reconstruction of the chronically failed deltoid ligament: a new technique. Foot Ankle Int. 2004;25(11):795–9.
78. Ellis SJ, Williams BR, Wagshul AD, Pavlov H, Deland JT. Deltoid ligament reconstruction with peroneus longus autograft in flatfoot deformity. Foot Ankle Int. 2010;31(9):781–9.
79. Haddad SL, Dedhia S, Ren Y, Rotstein J, Zhang LQ. Deltoid ligament reconstruction: a novel technique with biomechanical analysis. Foot Ankle Int. 2010;31(7):639–51.
80. Jeng CL, Bluman EM, Myerson MS. Minimally invasive deltoid ligament reconstruction for stage IV flatfoot deformity. Foot Ankle Int. 2011;32(1):21–30.
81. Jung HG, Park JT, Eom JS, Jung MG, Lee DO. Reconstruction of superficial deltoid ligaments with allograft tendons in medial ankle instability: a technical report. Injury. 2016;47(3):780–3.
82. Oburu E, Myerson MS. Deltoid ligament repair in flatfoot deformity. Foot Ankle Clin. 2017;22(3):503–14.
83. Xu C, Zhang MY, Lei GH, Zhang C, Gao SG, Ting W, et al. Biomechanical evaluation of tenodesis reconstruction in ankle with deltoid ligament deficiency: a finite element analysis. Knee Surg Sports Traumatol Arthrosc. 2012;20(9):1854–62.
84. Gougoulias N, Sakellariou A. When is a simple fracture of the lateral malleolus not so simple? How to assess stability, which ones to fix and the role of the deltoid ligament. Bone Joint J. 2017;99-B(7):851–5.
85. Yu GR, Zhang MZ, Aiyer A, Tang X, Xie M, Zeng LR, et al. Repair of the acute deltoid ligament complex rupture associated with ankle fractures: a multicenter clinical study. J Foot Ankle Surg. 2015;54(2):198–202.
86. Zeegers AV, van der Werken C. Rupture of the deltoid ligament in ankle fractures: should it be repaired? Injury. 1989;20(1):39–41.
87. Clanton TO, Williams BT, James EW, Campbell KJ, Rasmussen MT, Haytmanek CT, et al. Radiographic identification of the deltoid ligament complex of the medial ankle. Am J Sports Med. 2015;43(11):2753–62.
88. Ji Y, Tang X, Li Y, Xu W, Qiu W. Analysis of 3-dimensional finite element after reconstruction of impaired ankle deltoid ligament. Exp Ther Med. 2016;12(6):3913–6.
89. Backus JD, McCormick JJ. Tendon transfers in the treatment of the adult flatfoot. Foot Ankle Clin. 2014;19(1):29–48.
90. Pihl CM, Stender CJ, Balasubramanian R, Edinger KM, Sangeorzan BJ, Ledoux WR. Passive engineering mechanism enhancement of a flexor digitorum longus tendon transfer procedure. J Orthop Res. 2018;36(11):3033–42.
91. Steginsky B, Vora A. What to do with the spring ligament. Foot Ankle Clin. 2017;22(3):515–27.
92. Vadell AM, Peratta M. Calcaneonavicular ligament: anatomy, diagnosis, and treatment. Foot Ankle Clin. 2012;17(3):437–48.
93. Evans D. Calcaneo-valgus deformity. J Bone Joint Surg Br. 1975;57(3):270–8.
94. Chan JY, Williams BR, Nair P, Young E, Sofka C, Deland JT, et al. The contribution of medializing calcaneal osteotomy on hindfoot alignment in the reconstruction of the stage II adult acquired flatfoot deformity. Foot Ankle Int. 2013;34(2):159–66.
95. Greenfield S, Cohen B. Calcaneal osteotomies: pearls and pitfalls. Foot Ankle Clin. 2017;22(3):563–71.
96. Nyska M, Parks BG, Chu IT, Myerson MS. The contribution of the medial calcaneal osteotomy to the correction of flatfoot deformities. Foot Ankle Int. 2001;22(4):278–82.
97. Stufkens SA, Knupp M, Hintermann B. Medial displacement calcaneal osteotomy. Tech Foot Ankle Surg. 2009;8(2):85–90.
98. Weinfeld SB. Medial slide calcaneal osteotomy. Technique, patient selection, and results. Foot Ankle Clin. 2001;6(1):89–94, vii.
99. Trnka HJ, Easley ME, Myerson MS. The role of calcaneal osteotomies for correction of adult flatfoot. Clin Orthop Relat Res. 1999;365:50–64.
100. Pomeroy GC, Manoli A 2nd. A new operative approach for flatfoot secondary to posterior tibial tendon insufficiency: a preliminary report. Foot Ankle Int. 1997;18(4):206–12.
101. Aly AS, Abdel Rahman AF, Mahmoud S. Double calcaneal osteotomy in treatment of flexible planovalgus foot deformity in ambulatory cerebral palsy. A case series study. Foot Ankle Surg. 2019;25(5):640–5.
102. Didomenico LA, Haro AA 3rd, Cross DJ. Double calcaneal osteotomy using single, dual-function screw fixation technique. J Foot Ankle Surg. 2011;50(6):773–5.
103. Feuerstein CA, Weil L Jr, Weil LS Sr, Klein EE, Agerakis NG, Akram U. The calcaneal scarf osteotomy: surgical correction of the adult acquired flatfoot deformity and radiographic results. Foot Ankle Spec. 2013;6(5):367–71.

104. Palmanovich E, Shabat S, Brin YS, Feldman V, Kish B, Nyska M. Anatomic reconstruction technique for a plantar calcaneonavicular (spring) ligament tear. J Foot Ankle Surg. 2015;54(6):1124–6.
105. Choi K, Lee S, Otis JC, Deland JT. Anatomical reconstruction of the spring ligament using peroneus longus tendon graft. Foot Ankle Int. 2003;24(5):430–6.
106. Lui TH. Technical tips: reconstruction of deep and superficial deltoid ligaments by peroneus longus tendon in stage 4 posterior tibial tendon dysfunction. Foot Ankle Surg. 2014;20(4):295–7.
107. Williams BR, Ellis SJ, Deyer TW, Pavlov H, Deland JT. Reconstruction of the spring ligament using a peroneus longus autograft tendon transfer. Foot Ankle Int. 2010;31(7):567–77.
108. Lee KT, Park YU, Jegal H, Park JW, Choi JP, Kim JS. New method of diagnosis for chronic ankle instability: comparison of manual anterior drawer test, stress radiography and stress ultrasound. Knee Surg Sports Traumatol Arthrosc. 2014;22(7):1701–7.
109. Horisberger M, Valderrabano V, Hintermann B. Posttraumatic ankle osteoarthritis after ankle-related fractures. J Orthop Trauma. 2009;23(1):60–7.

6 Deltoid Ligament Injuries in Ankle Fractures

Medial ankle instability after a lateral malleolar fracture has its origin in either a medial malleolar fracture, a deltoid ligament lesion, or a combination hereof. The diagnostic procedure regarding evaluation of deltoid ligament lesions in supination-exorotation (SE) fractures (Weber Type B) has its limitations and thus, these lesions may remain unrecognized [1–5]. In pronation-exorotation (PE) fractures (Weber Type C) including Maisonneuve fractures, in contrast, the medial ankle must always be considered to be potentially unstable; thus here, the question remains whether the injured deltoid ligament should be addressed during surgical treatment of the fracture [6].

6.1 Trauma Mechanism

- Pronation or rotation movements of the hindfoot are the main cause for deltoid ligament lesions in ankle fractures.
- Deltoid ligament injuries in ankle fractures are more often seen after a pronation-external rotation trauma than after a supination-external rotation trauma.

The main cause for deltoid ligament lesions is pronation or rotation movements of the hindfoot [1, 2, 5, 7–11]. Lauge-Hansen [8] simulated several rotational, ab- and adductional movements of the lower leg with a fixed foot in pronation or in supination and hereby developed a system to classify ankle fractures. With an SE fracture mechanism in stage 1, a rupture or avulsion of the ATFL occurs, followed by an increased pressure of the talus against the fibula, which results in a twisting motion of the fibula around its longitudinal axis, producing the typical spiral (Weber Type B) fracture at the level of the syndesmosis (stage 2). When the exorotation is continued, the talus is subluxated and the hindfoot adopts a valgus position. During this movement the tip of the fractured fibula and the talus can collide with the posterior tibial tubercle, resulting in a splitting off of a triangular shaped piece of bone, also known as Volkmann's fracture (stage 3). With ongoing exorotation, in stage 4, a fracture of the medial malleolus or a rupture of the deltoid ligament results. This however was questioned by others who believe that based on the fracture mechanism, avulsion fractures should occur at the same rate as deltoid ligament ruptures [1, 5, 9, 12, 13]. Others have reported that especially the deep portions of the deltoid ligament rupture in exorotation trauma while superficial components remaining intact [14]. Some have also reported the deep deltoid being ruptured in combination with a medial fracture [15, 16]. Fixation of small anterior fractures of the medial malleolus, to which only the superficial portion of the ligament attaches, may therefore not be sufficient to restore medial stability [15, 17, 18]. In 60–70% of the avulsion fractures of the posterior colliculus, the strong posterior tibiotalar ligament remains intact and attached to the fractured fragment, while the other weaker components are torn [16, 19, 20]. The frequency of damage to the deltoid ligament in SE fractures is higher than previously expected and ranges from 20 to 50% [9, 21]. These numbers could still be underestimating the true amount, due to the lack of diagnostic reliability.

The trauma mechanism of SE fractures and of pronation-exorotation (PE) fractures is the same. The difference between the two is the position of the foot at the moment of impact which leads to the fracture. With a foot in pronation there is initial tension on the medial structures. A lateral fracture resulting from PE is unstable as it is associated with a medial fracture or deltoid rupture. However, it was also hypothesized that high fibular fractures can occur without any injury to the medial side [17, 22].

B. Hintermann, R. Ruiz, *Foot and Ankle Instability*, https://doi.org/10.1007/978-3-030-62926-7_6

6.2 Diagnosis

- In medial ligament injuries, clinical features of the injured ankle are inadequate predictors of the involvement of the deep deltoid.

While in the past orthopedic surgeons mainly relied on clinical signs such as ecchymosis, swelling, and tenderness to evaluate integrity of the medial structures (Fig. 6.1) [23–25], this may have changed with the availability of new imaging modalities [26]. In lateral ligament injuries, clinical evaluation has been a great value; moreover, additional (imaging) investigation has shown little or no contribution to accurately determine the diagnosis [27]. In medial ligament injuries, in contrast, clinical features of the injured ankle are inadequate predictors of the involvement of the deep deltoid injuries in SE type ankle fractures, with the exception of medial tenderness [28, 29].

As a primary measure, standard radiographs and/or CT scans are used to make the diagnosis of an ankle fracture. They may enable the orthopedic surgeon to differentiate between a medial malleolar fracture, a deltoid ligament injury, and a combination thereof (Fig. 6.2). Furthermore, they are the basis for injury classification.

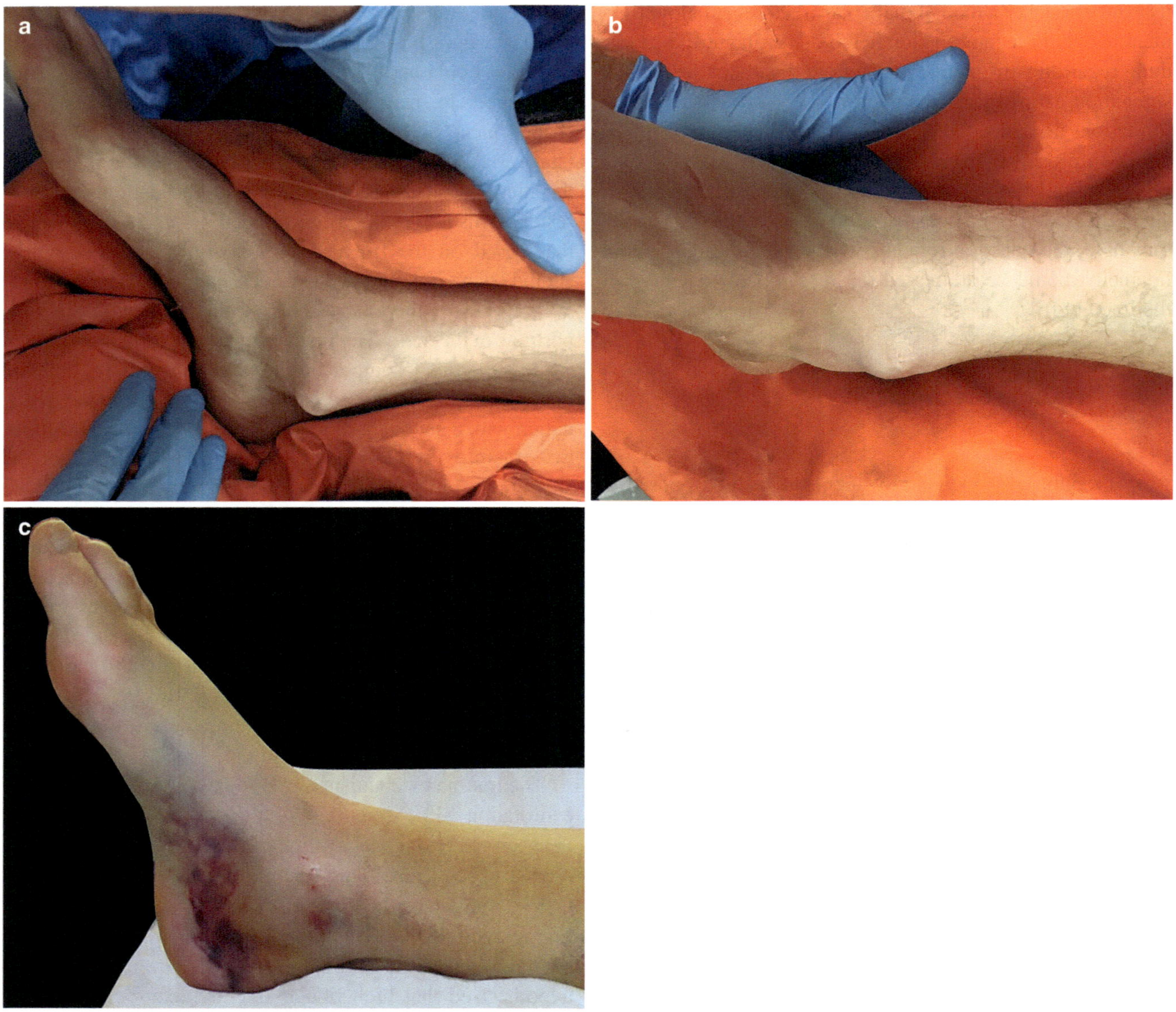

Fig. 6.1 Acute ankle fracture, medial view. (**a**) Acute dislocation fracture of the ankle with lateral translation of talus putting at risk the skin over the medial malleolus, indicating a complete rupture of deltoid ligament. (**b**) After closed reposition of the ankle, a deltoid ligament injury may be hidden to clinical assessment. (**c**) In this case, 3 days after the injury, ecchymosis, swelling, and tenderness over the medial ankle indicate an injury to the deltoid ligament

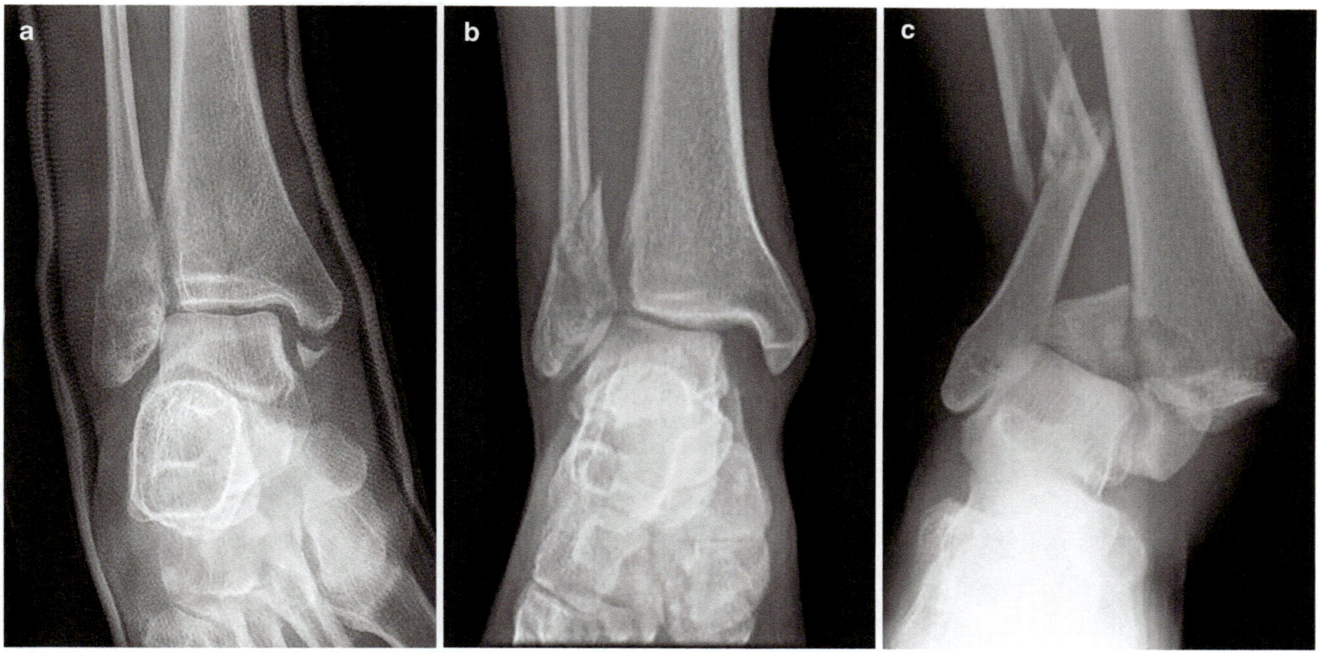

Fig. 6.2 Standard AP radiographs of acute injured ankles. (**a**) Avulsion fracture of the medial malleolus. (**b**) Deltoid ligament rupture. (**c**) Combined fracture and deltoid ligament injury

The Lauge-Hansen classification that takes ligamentous injuries into account is more difficult to use than the Weber classification [5, 8, 9]. Furthermore, its application showed only poor to fair interobserver reliability [30–35]. A specific problem with the Lauge-Hansen classification is that it considers some fractures stable despite the deep deltoid being injured [36, 37]. Therefore, the diagnostic value of the Lauge-Hansen classification, for ligamentous injuries in SE fractures, seems limited.

Weight-bearing radiographs (Fig. 6.3), external rotation (Fig. 6.4), or gravity stress (Fig. 6.5) tests have been proposed as an indirect measure of deltoid injury or deltoid insufficiency. However, the amount of medial clear space widening, indicative for a positive test, was defined variably [16, 29, 36, 38–44]. A medial clear space of ≥4 mm, with that value being at least 1 mm greater than the superior tibiotalar space, is a value that is accepted in the literature to represent a deep deltoid ligament rupture [32, 38, 44, 45]. However, the direction of rotational stress applied to the foot [29, 40, 46], the flexion position of the foot [43], and the amount of applied force [18, 41, 47] may influence the result. Patients may experience pain during an ankle stress test and thus activate muscles to resist against the applied force [29], thus a gravity stress test without manual stress application might be superior [41]. The main limitation of the gravity stress radiograph is the inability to control dorsiflexion and plantar flexion.

6.3 Imaging

- Standard radiographs and/or CT scans, as used to make the diagnosis of an ankle fracture, enable the orthopedic surgeon to differentiate between a medial malleolar fracture, a deltoid ligament injury, and a combination thereof.
- A medial clear space of ≥4 mm, with that value being at least 1 mm greater than the superior tibiotalar space, is a value that is accepted in the literature to represent a deep deltoid ligament rupture.
- MRI, though not as a routine, could be helpful in determining deltoid ligament integrity.

Ultrasonography proved to be an accurate tool, allowing the identification of deltoid ligament disruptions and the involved components, in a more dynamic fashion (Fig. 6.6) [48–51]. The major advantages of ultrasound include dynamic evaluation of structures, low cost, and wide availability; its accuracy, however, depends on the investigator's experience.

Magnetic resonance imaging (MRI) could be helpful in determining deltoid ligament integrity directly after trauma and could be useful in individual cases in which doubt on joint stability and soft tissue integrity exists (Fig. 6.7) [37,

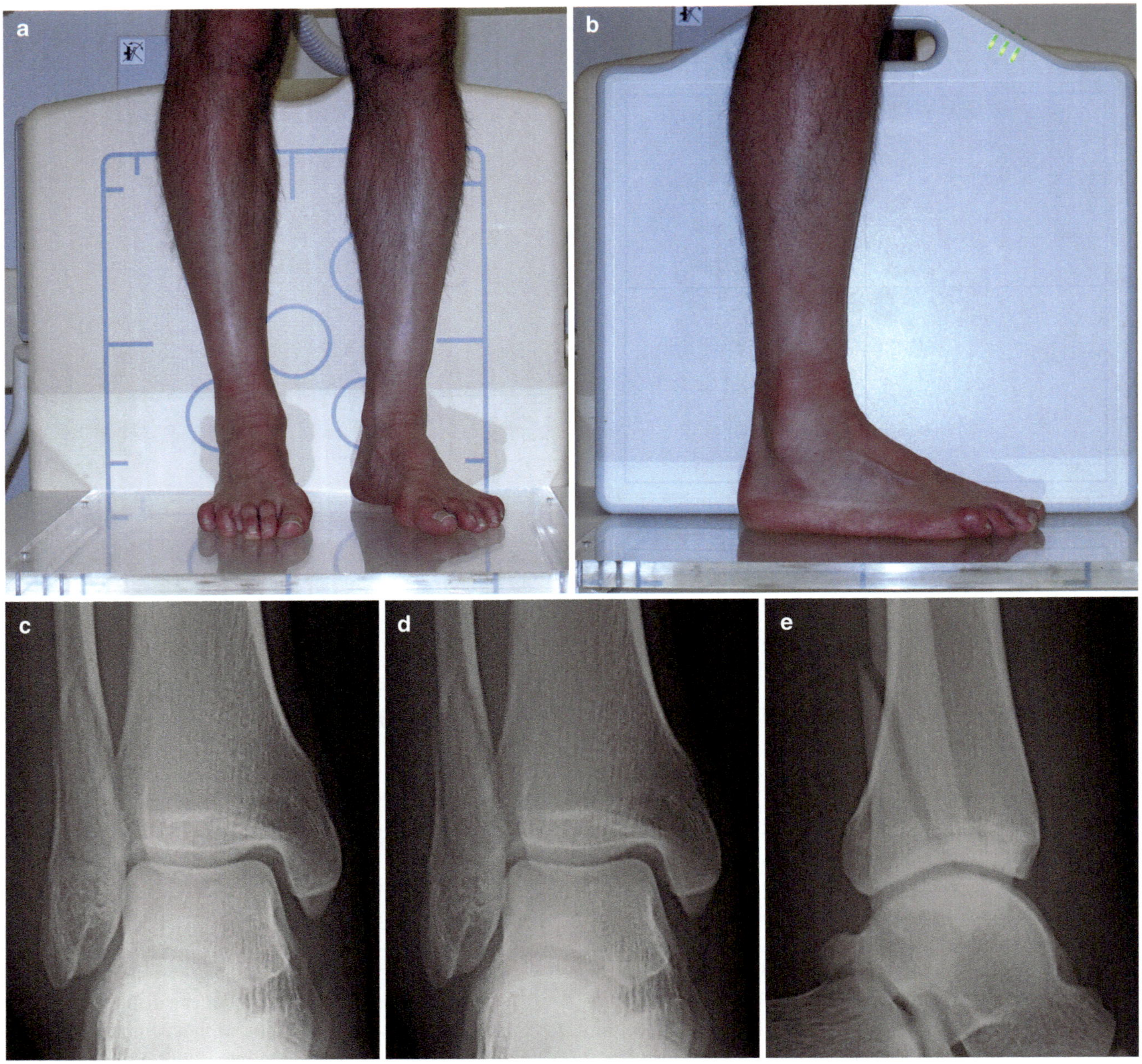

Fig. 6.3 *Set-up for taking weight-bearing radiographs*. The patient is standing with his/her weight equally distributed on both legs, as comfortably as possible. (**a**) For the AP view, the foot is internally rotated 10° by the patient turning the entire body, not only the leg. (**b**) The lateral view is taken lateromedially accordingly. (**c**) A medial clear space <4 mm is considered as being a stable fracture. (**d**) A medial clear space >4 mm in width is considered as radiographic instability. (**e**) An opening of the fracture of >2 mm is considered as radiographic instability

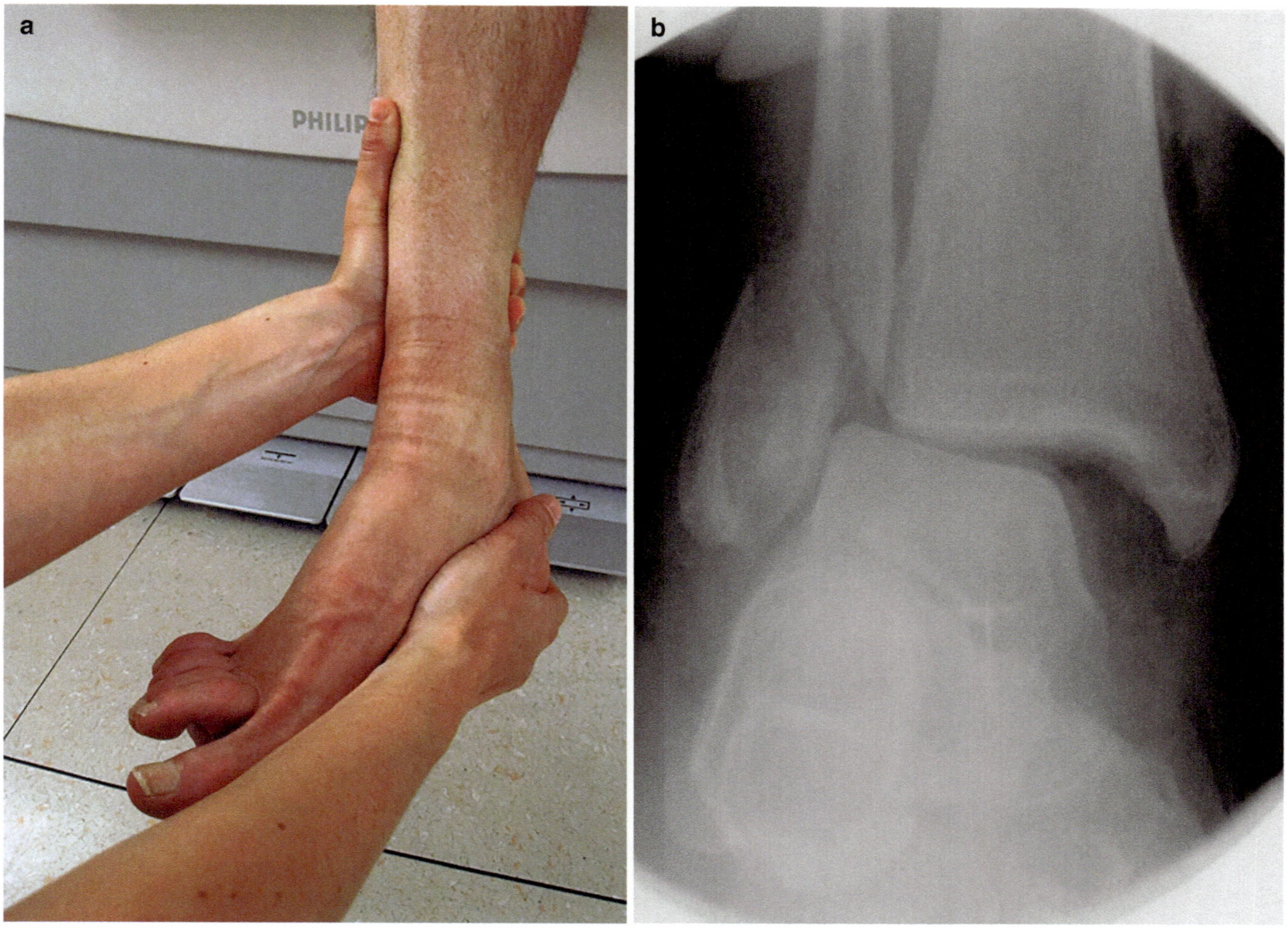

Fig. 6.4 *Manual stress test*. (**a**) The examiner stabilizes the leg with one hand and with the other, applies an external rotation load to the foot, with the ankle in neutral flexion. (**b**) A lateral shift >2 mm is considered as radiographic instability. A medial clear space of ≥4 mm, with that value being at least 1 mm greater than the superior tibiotalar space, is a value that is accepted to represent an unstable ankle fracture

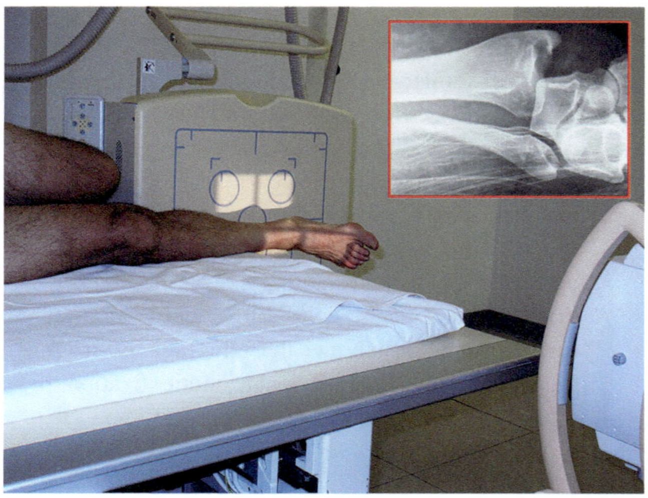

Fig. 6.5 *Gravity stress test*. Clinical photograph demonstrating the optimal positioning of the ankle for the gravity stress radiograph. A lateral shift >2 mm is considered as radiographic instability. A medial clear space of ≥4 mm, with that value being at least 1 mm greater than the superior tibiotalar space, is a value that is accepted to represent an unstable ankle fracture

52–54]. In cases where the medial clear space was less than 5 mm on injury radiographs, stress test measurements were much less accurate than MRI in predicting deltoid ruptures (46% vs. 79%, respectively) with a high false positive rate (80%) [54]. In contrast, a medial clear space measurement of greater than 5 mm on injury radiographs was a strong predictor of deep deltoid ligament rupture (accuracy of 95%).

6.4 Arthroscopy

- Direct arthroscopic visualization ensures detection and evaluation of intra-articular fractures, osteochondral lesions, loose bodies, and associated ligamentous injuries.

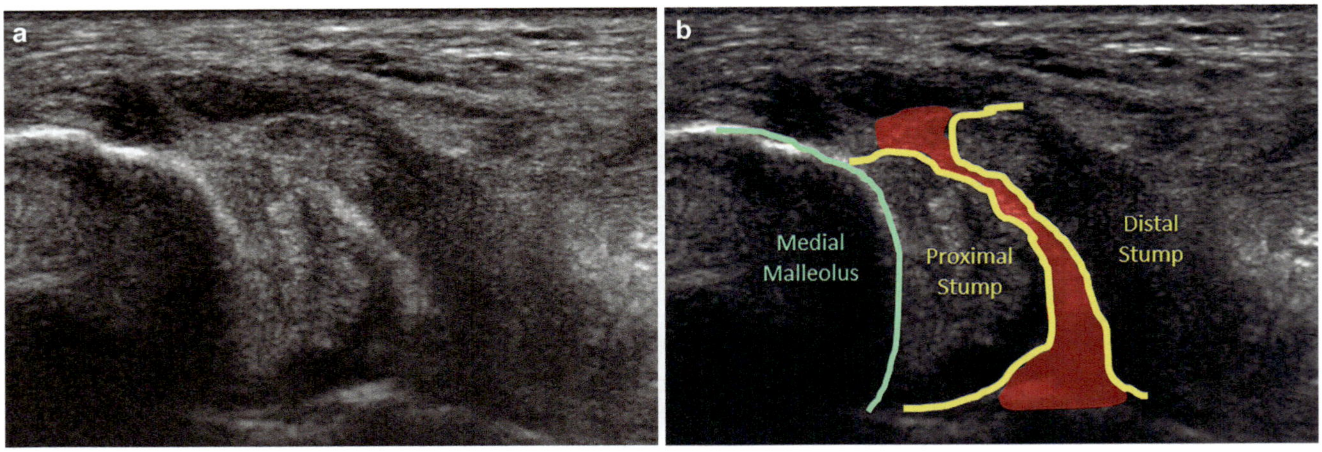

Fig. 6.6 *Ultrasonography*. (**a**) Complete rupture of the deltoid ligament. (**b**) Same image with explanations

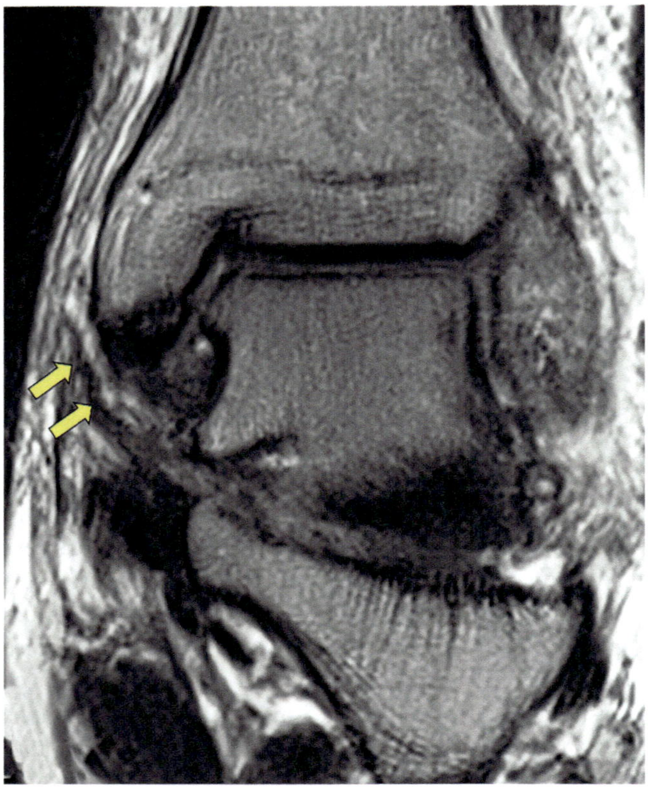

Fig. 6.7 *Magnetic resonance imaging (MRI)*. The rupture of the deltoid can be seen as an avulsion along its insertion onto the medial malleolus (arrows)

Ankle arthroscopy was found to be a useful adjuvant tool to understand the severity and complexity of acute ankle fractures (Fig. 6.8), as direct arthroscopic visualization ensures detection and evaluation of intra-articular fractures (Fig. 6.9), associated osteochondral lesions (Fig. 6.10), loose bodies (Fig. 6.11), syndesmosis disruption (Fig. 6.12), and ligamentous injuries (Fig. 6.13) [21, 55, 56]. While lateral ligamentous injuries were found more often in Type B than in Type C-fractures, no difference was noted in the frequency of deltoid ligamentous lesions [57]. The association between the presence of deep deltoid ligament tears and syndesmosis disruption in Weber B cases was statistically significant but not in Weber C cases [21, 55].

6.5 Treatment

- The indication to perform deltoid ligament repair in ankle injuries with widened medial clear space without a medial malleolus fracture being present remains controversial; however, there is evidence that primary repair is helpful to restore the integrity of the medial ankle, especially to stabilize the talus against anterolateral rotation.
- Primary repair of the deltoid ligament is an effective measure to stabilize the talus against lateral translation, thus making syndesmotic fixation in most cases unnecessary.

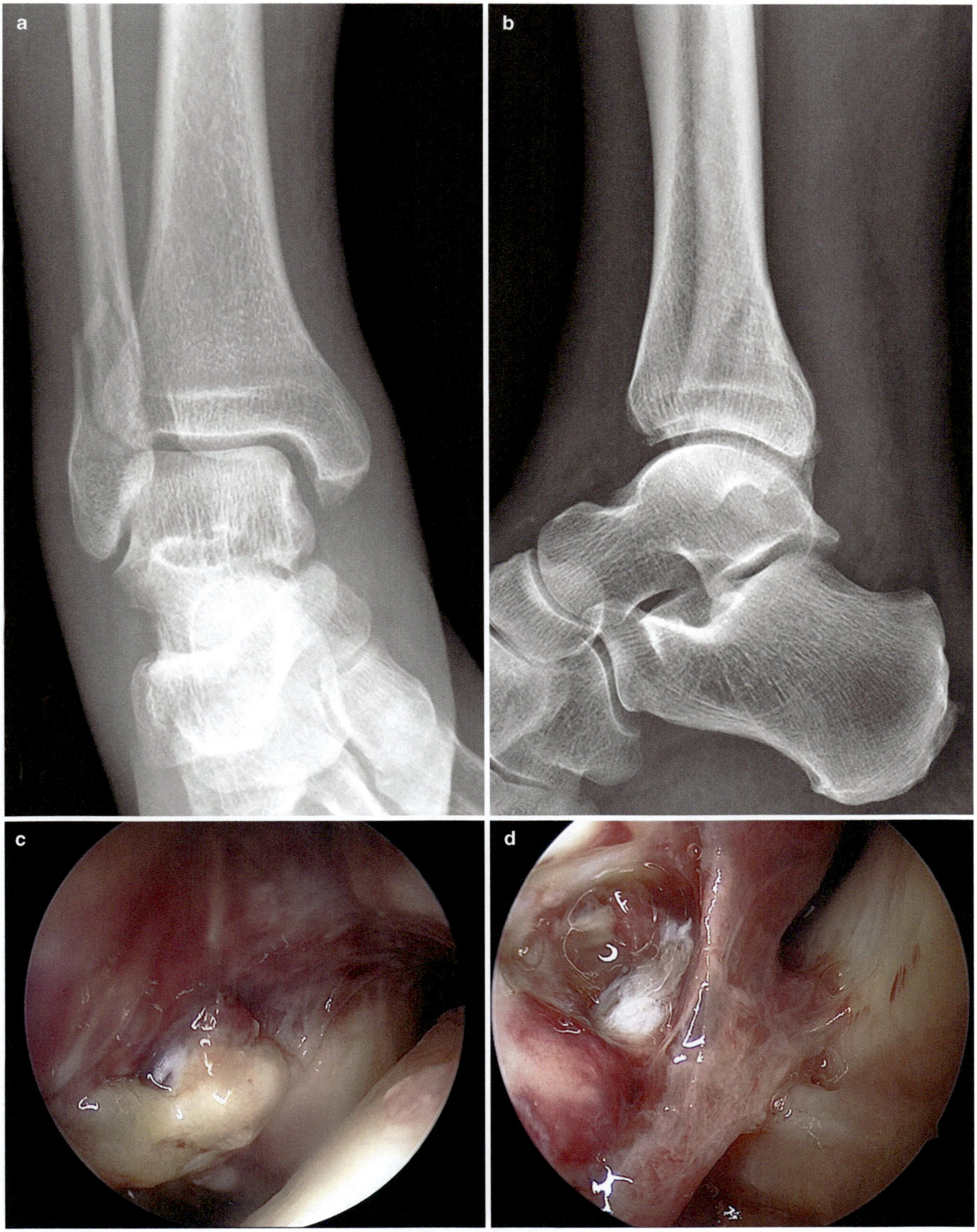

Fig. 6.8 Preoperative arthroscopy is a useful adjuvant tool to understand the severity and complexity of acute ankle fractures and to detect associated lesions. This 36-year-old female patient sustained a Weber type B-fracture while walking in the snow. (**a**) Non-weight-bearing AP radiograph showing the fracture with minimal widening of the medial clear space; the talar shift cannot be assessed in this, not ideally exposed, radiograph. (**b**) The lateral radiograph shows a well-aligned ankle with gapping of the fracture being present. (**c**) Anterolateral view showing a partial rupture of the syndesmosis, without displacement of the fibula in the incisura. (**d**) Further distally the partial rupture can be better visualized and ATFL injury can be identified. (**e**) Medially, a significant opening of the medial clear space can be seen. (**f**) More distally, the deep deltoid is seen attenuated, but not ruptured

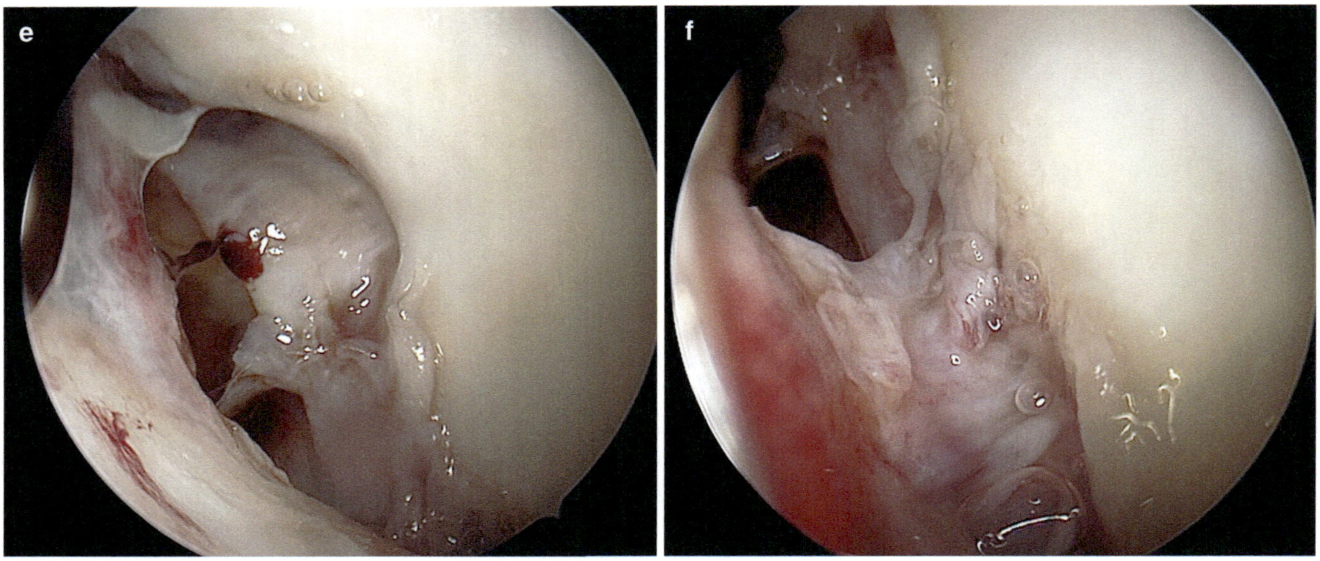

Fig. 6.8 (continued)

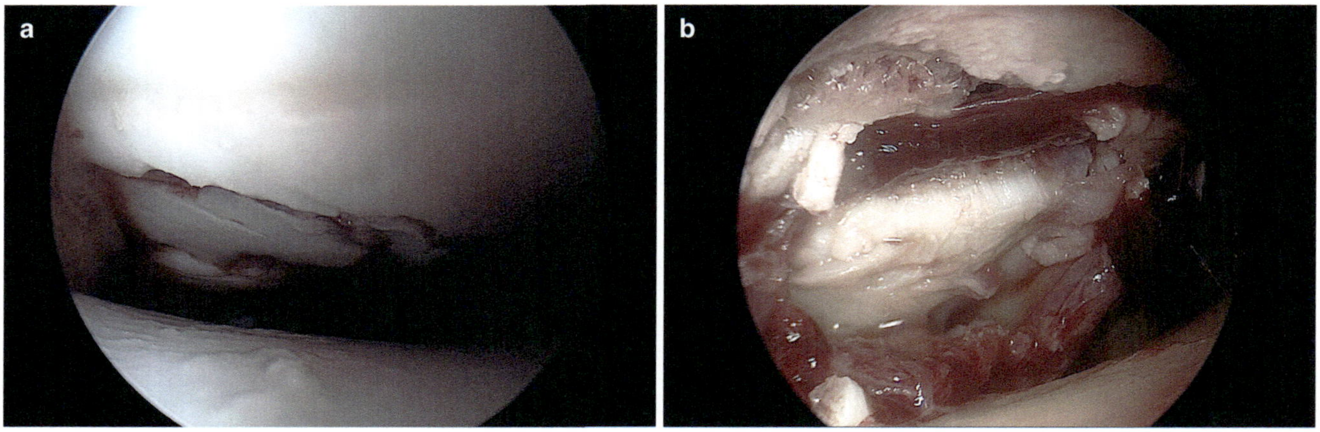

Fig. 6.9 *Intra-articular fractures*. (**a**) A posterior malleolar (Volkmann) fracture with intermediate fragmentation showing minimal displacement of the articular surface. (**b**) A posterior malleolar (Volkmann) fracture with multiple osteochondral fractures and loose bodies with major displacement

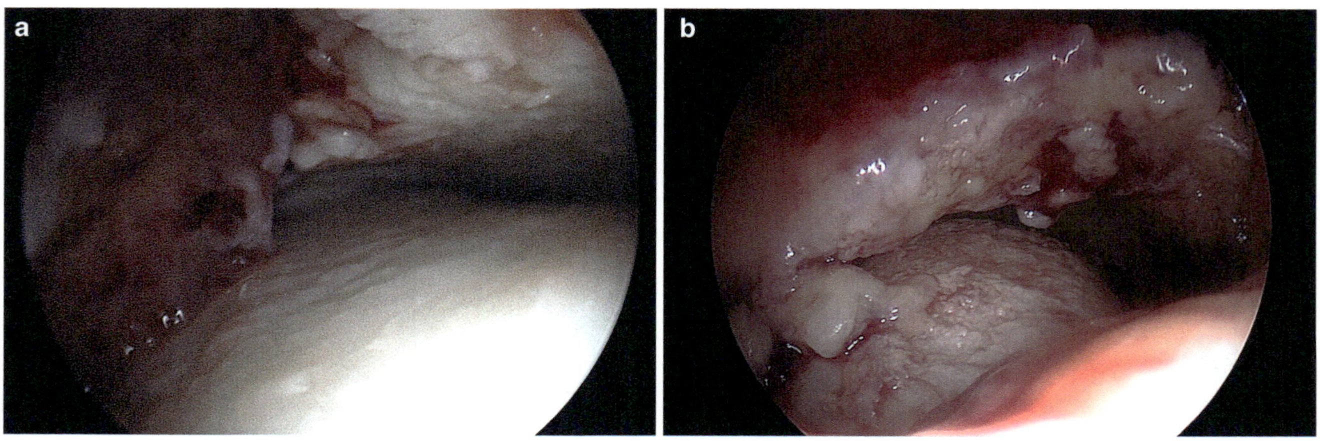

Fig. 6.10 *Osteochondral lesions*. (**a**) A deep osteochondral lesion on the anterolateral tibia, with fragmentation and some impaction of the subchondral bone. (**b**) Deep osteochondral lesions mainly on the medial talus with some involvement of the opposite articular tibial surface

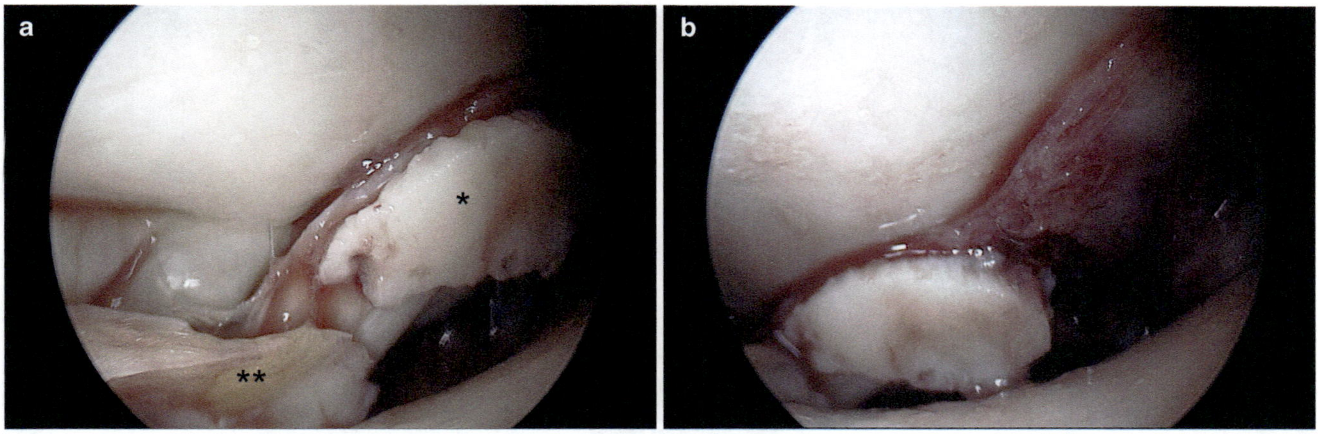

Fig. 6.11 *Loose bodies*. (**a**) Cartilage fragment (asterisk) and bigger osteochondral fragment (double asterisk) in the posterolateral corner of the tibiotalar joint. (**b**) Osteochondral fragment in the posterior aspect of the tibiotalar joint

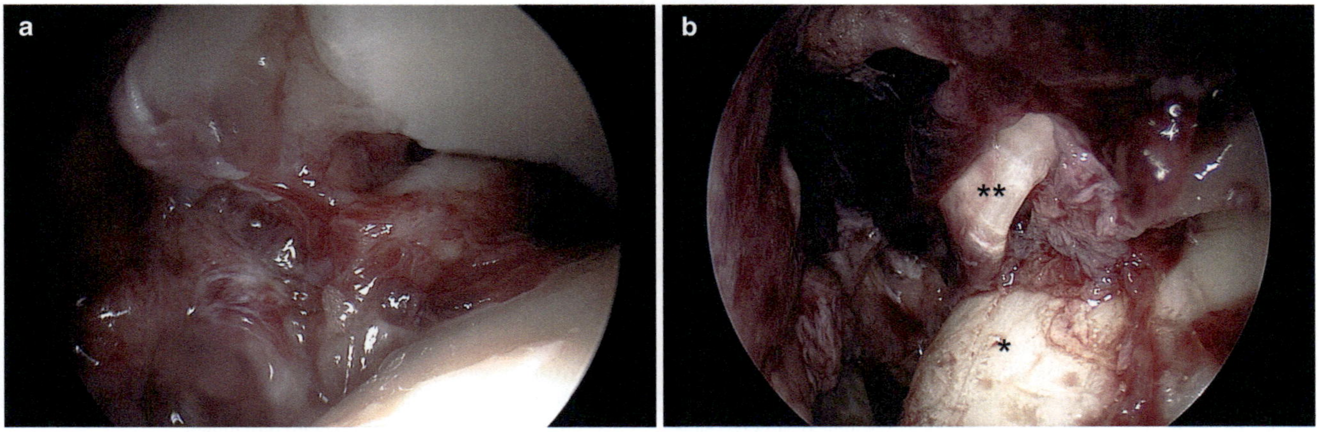

Fig. 6.12 *Syndesmotic disruption*. (**a**) The anterior inferior tibiofibular ligament (AITFL) is completely disrupted, but the fibula is only minimally displaced. (**b**) Complete avulsion of the AITFL (asterisk) with a small bony fragment (double asterisk) from tibia, with associated tear of the lateral ankle ligaments and capsular; the fibula is displaced and cannot be seen

The indication to perform deltoid ligament repair in ankle injuries with widened medial clear space without a medial malleolus fracture being present remains controversial (Fig. 6.14). While no difference in long-term functional outcome was reported, persistent medial clear space widening and malreduction are seen more frequently without deltoid repair [58–63]. In cases with high-grade unstable fractures of the lateral malleolus, repair of the anterior deltoid ligament is advised to restore medial ankle stability [59, 64]. Combined repair of the posterior inferior tibiofibular ligament and deltoid ligament was found to restore an equivalent amount of ankle and syndesmotic rotational stability (Fig. 6.15). When compared to trans-syndesmotic screw fixation, ligamentous repair can potentially be a viable treatment alternative in patients with an unstable ankle fracture with syndesmotic disruption [65–67].

With the belief that the ruptured ends of the deltoid ligament retract and are not apposed, and that disrupted ligaments heal better when they are surgically approximated, some authors have advocated surgical repair of the ligament

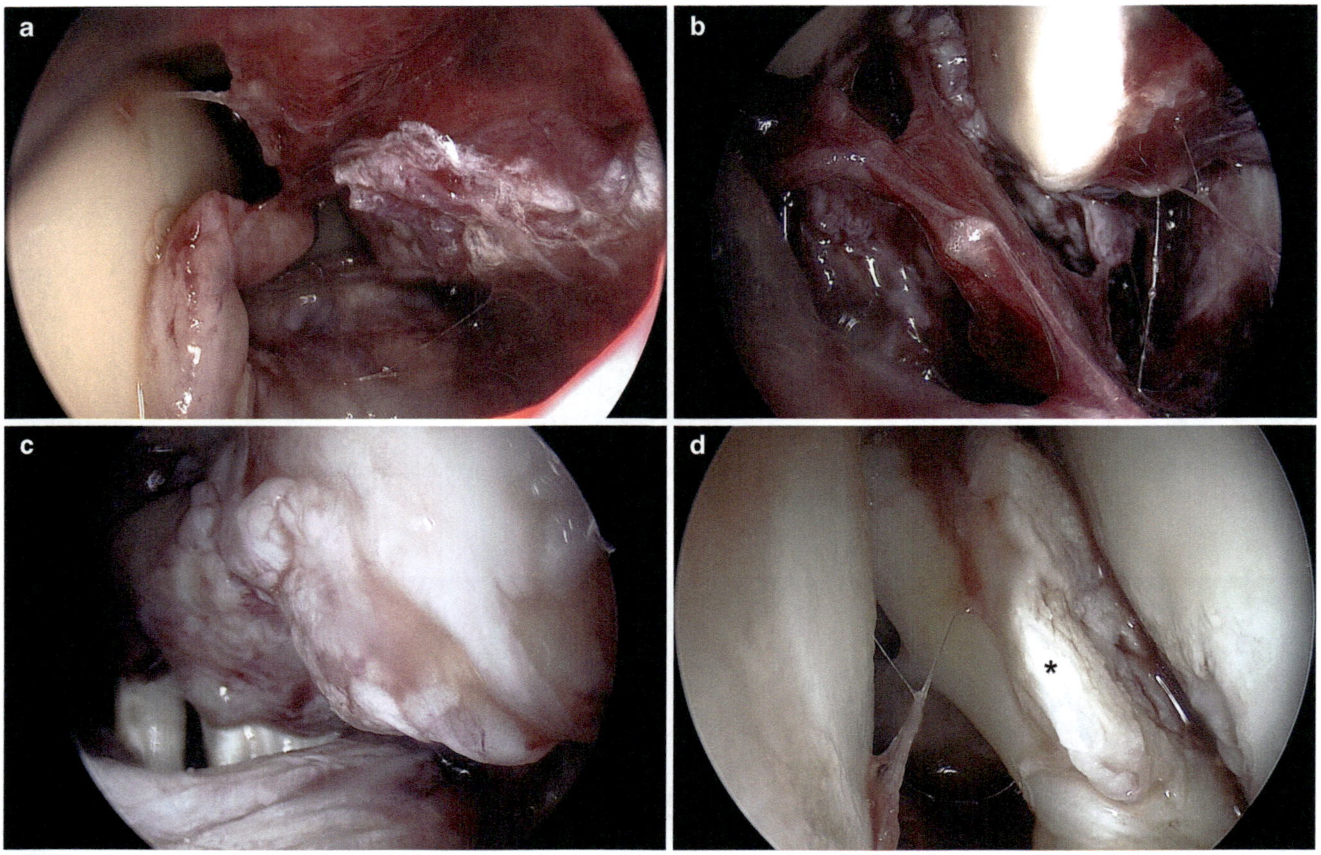

Fig. 6.13 *Ligamentous injuries*. (**a**) Widening of the medial clear space with interposed superficial deltoid ligament that is completely ruptured; the deep deltoid looks intact in its proximal part, but it must be injured distally. (**b**) Complete avulsion of the superficial deltoid, involving also the deep part; the medial clear space is markedly widened. (**c**) Free view of the FDL and PT tendons indicating a complete rupture of the deltoid ligament; some tissue is left at the site of origin site on the medial malleolus. (**d**) Free view of the PT tendon that is dislocated in posterior medial clear space beneath the deep deltoid ligament (asterisk) indicating a complete rupture of the deep deltoid ligament

in conjunction with reduction of the fibular fracture (Fig. 6.16) [5, 25, 68–76]. Others however have reported adequate results without surgical repair of the deltoid ligament, thus relying on restoration of the normal osteoligamentous anatomy of the lateral structures of the ankle joint to achieve stability of the ankle [35, 77–81].

Unfortunately, there are only a few studies in which the need for exploration and suturing of the deltoid ligament after ankle fractures was the primary interest [23, 58, 61, 63, 82–86]. Of those that are found in the literature, all came to similar conclusions: that if adequate reduction of the fractured fibula and normalization of the medial clear space is achieved, it is not necessary to explore the medial clear space and to reconstruct the deltoid ligament. Only if there is interposition on the medial side after adequate reduction of the fibular fracture, an exploration of the medial clear space is required.

Rupture of the deep deltoid ligament combined with a displaced lateral malleolar fracture is the biomechanical equivalent of a bimalleolar fracture [14, 16, 87] and therefore is best treated with open reduction and internal fixation of the fibula, to restore mortise anatomy (Fig. 6.17).

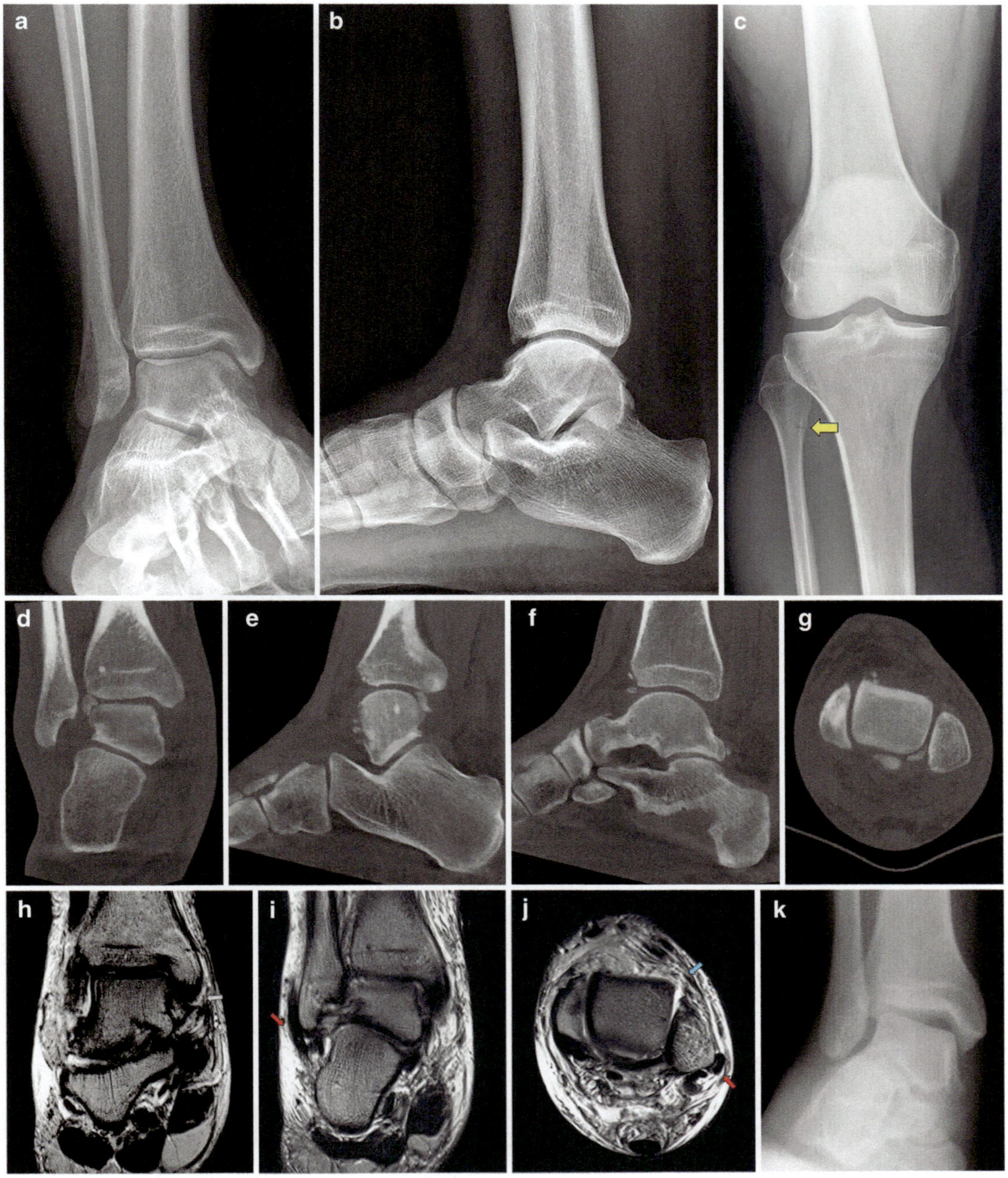

Fig. 6.14 *Surgical Technique: Deltoid ligament reconstruction in a Maisonneuve fracture*. This 26-year-old soccer player sustained an eversion-abduction trauma, with subsequent massive pain, hematoma, and tenderness over the medial ankle ligaments as well as pain over the syndesmosis. Standard radiographs show a congruent ankle: (**a**) AP view and (**b**) lateral view. (**c**) AP of the knee shows an incomplete high fibula fracture (arrow). Based on these radiographs, one might consider conservative treatment. However, due to the impressive clinical symptoms and the need for best treatment in this professional soccer player, further investigations are indicated. (**d**–**g**) CT scans showing a major fragment in the posterolateral ankle and some damage to the anterolateral talus. (**h**–**j**) MRI showing a complete avulsion of the deltoid (yellow arrow), a dislocation of the peroneal tendons (red arrow), and a disruption of the ATFL (blue arrow) and potentially also of the AITFL. (**k**) Preoperative eversion stress test under fluoroscopy evidences a complete rupture of the deltoid ligament with a talar tilt of 24°. Preoperative arthroscopy: (**l**) View of the posterolateral tibiotalar joint shows the free fragment (asterisk) as well as the intact posterior syndesmotic ligaments. (**m**) View of the lateral part of the ankle shows a complete avulsion of the lateral ankle ligaments, e.g., ATFL and CFL (asterisk) as well as the dislocated PL and PB tendons. Double asterisk = tip of fibula. First, the lateral ankle ligaments are repaired through a lateral incision and the fibular retinaculum is reconstructed (not shown). The free fragment is grabbed and reattached to the anterolateral talus with two 2.5-mm screws. Thereafter the medial ankle ligaments are repaired: (**n**) Approach to the medial ankle ligaments. (**o**) After the skin incision, the fascia is found to be only minimally disrupted, indicating that the continuity of the deltoid ligament might be preserved. The tendon sheath of the PT and FDL tendons is disrupted and shows subluxation of the tendons. (**p**) After dissection of the fascia, the tear of the superficial deltoid along the medial malleolus can be seen (yellow arrow), while the superficial deltoid is kept away (red arrow). (**q**) The deep deltoid is disrupted distally, close to its insertion (arrow). (**r**) First, the posterior deltoid is repaired with a bony anchor inserted to the posteromedial talus (arrow); thereafter, a suture anchor is inserted to the anterior colliculus. (**s**) Both sutures are tightened. (**t**) The tendon sheath of the PT tendon is then identified and repaired. (**u**) Final reconstruction before skin closure. This patient could return to a regular training program after 8 weeks and he regained his former activity level 6.5 months after surgery

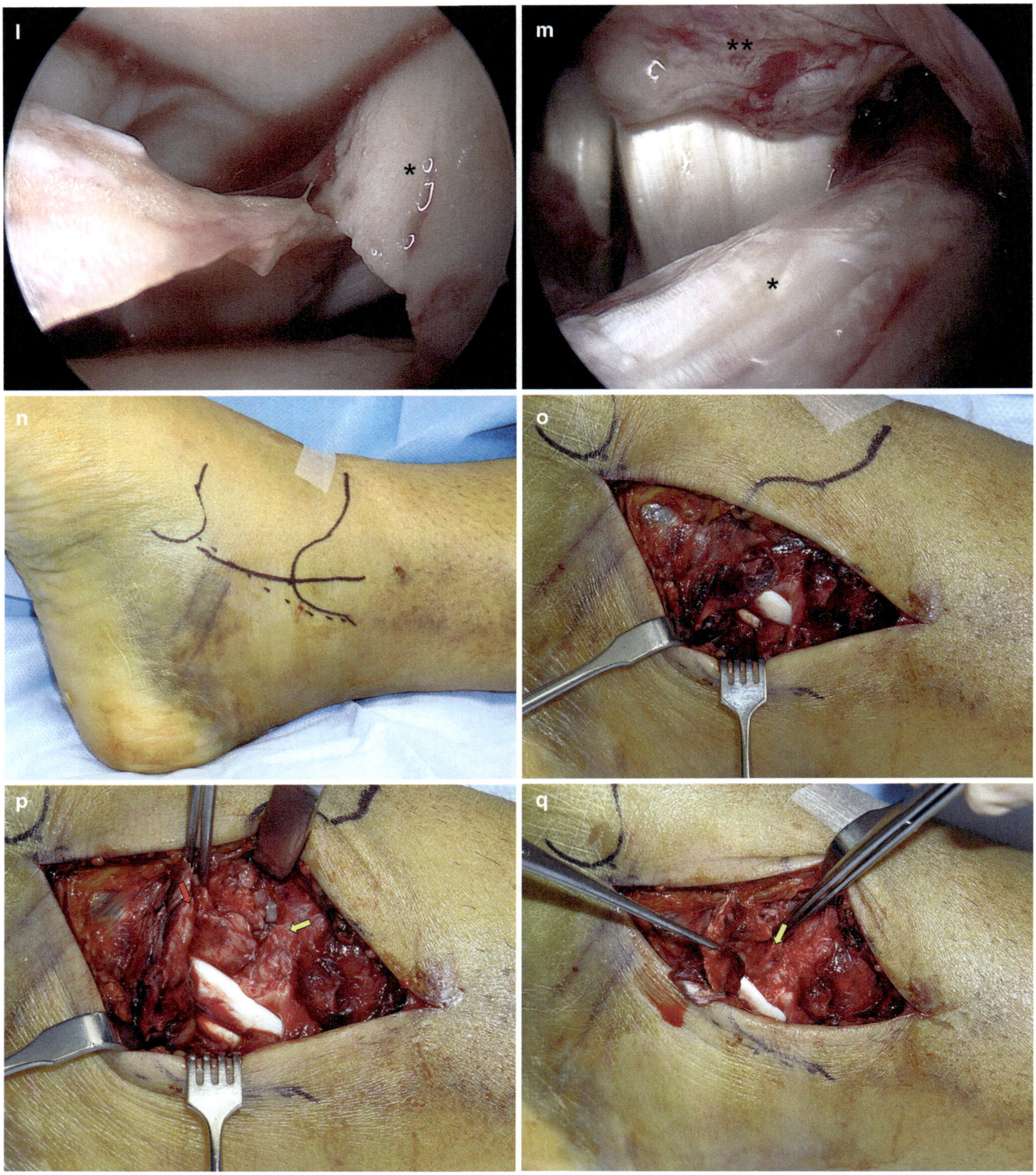

Fig. 6.14 (continued)

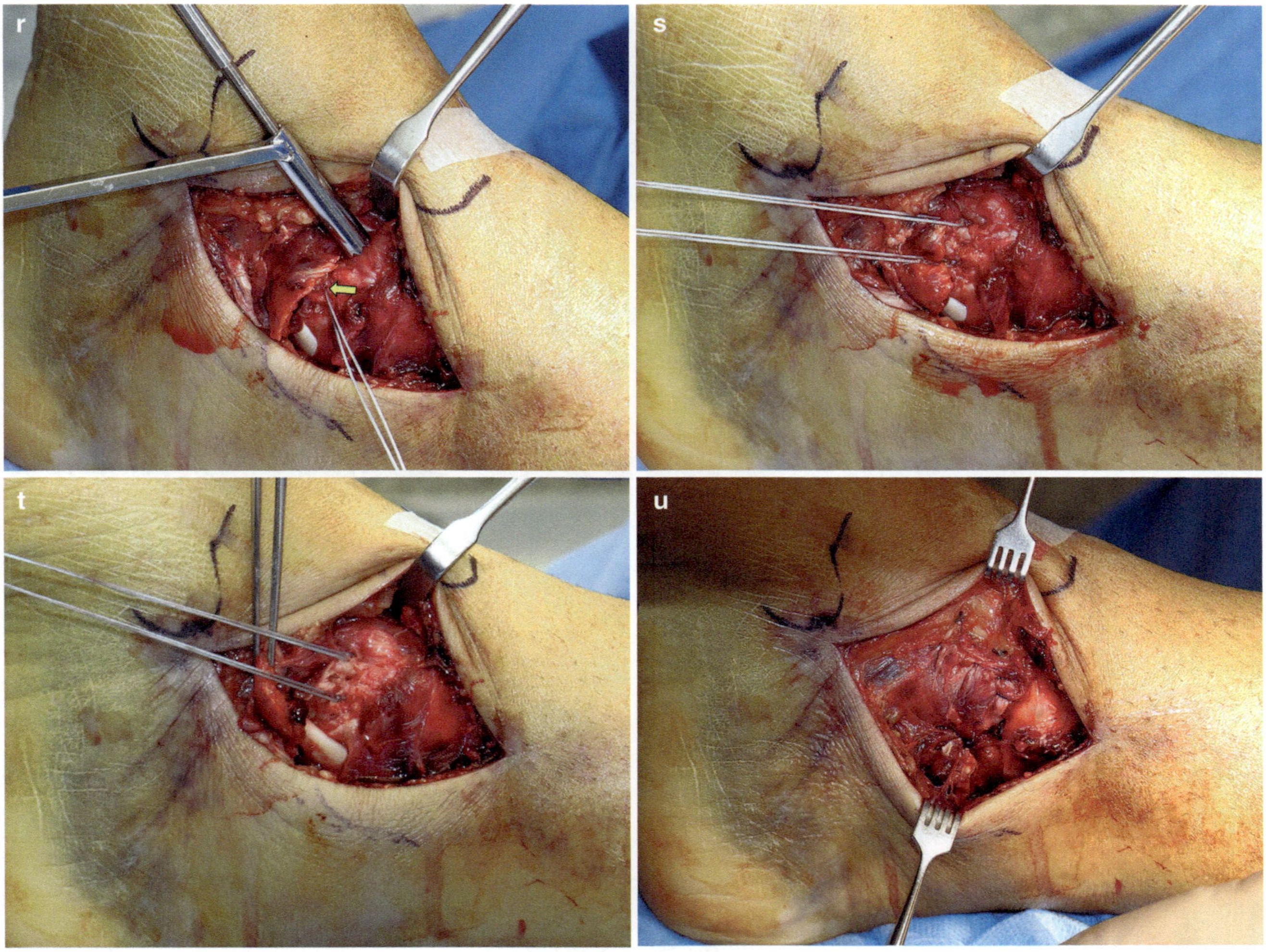

Fig. 6.14 (continued)

6.6 Outcome

- Little data exist on the outcome of patients with nonoperatively managed deltoid ruptures compared to those treated surgically.
- Persistent medial clear space widening and malreduction were reported more frequently without deltoid repair.
- Lower pain scores were reported in patients who had deltoid ligament repair.

There is limited data reporting the outcome of patients with nonoperatively managed deltoid ruptures compared to those treated surgically in the presence of fibular stabilization for unstable fractures of the ankle. Persistent medial clear space widening and malreduction were reported more frequently without deltoid repair [58–63]. Restoration of the medial clear space was found to have a significant influence on clinical outcome [62]. Whereas, no data exist on the role played by the fracture type, particularly whether there is a difference in the need to restore the deltoid in SE- compared to PE-fractures. Though not statistically evaluated, conservative management of deltoid ruptures in ankle fractures could

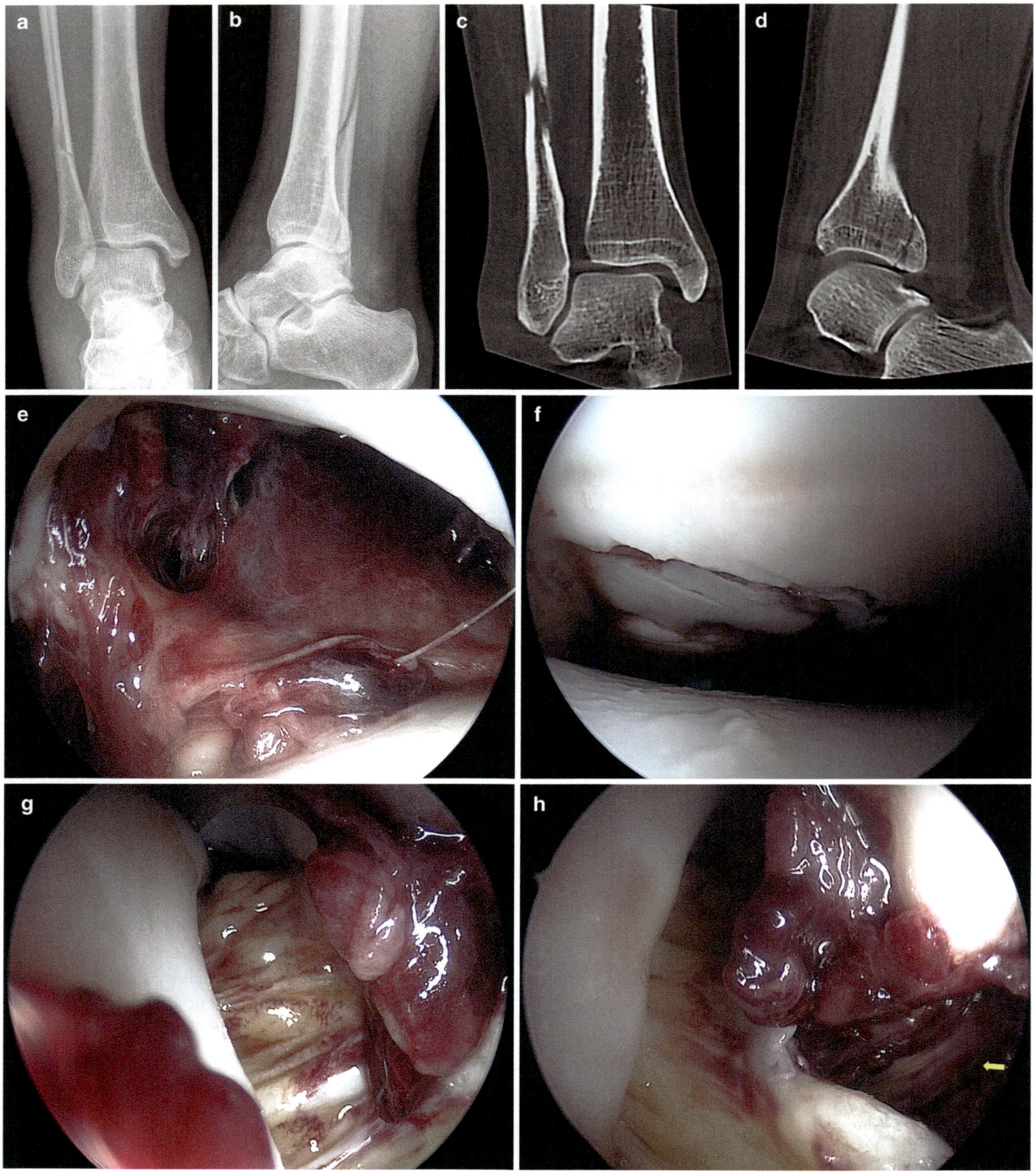

Fig. 6.15 *Surgical Technique: Deltoid ligament reconstruction in a Weber C-fracture without syndesmotic stabilization.* This 29-year-old handball player sustained this fracture during a training session. (**a**) Standard radiograph, AP view, showing the fibula fracture approximately 10 cm above the ankle with widening of the syndesmosis and medial clear space, as well as a talar translation. (**b**) The lateral view evidences a fracture of the posterior malleolus (Volkmann). (**c** and **d**) These findings are confirmed with CT scan. (**e**) Arthroscopy shows a complete rupture of the syndesmotic ligaments, the empty incisura tibialis, whereas the dislocated fibula is not visible. (**f**) A posterolateral avulsion fracture (Volkmann) connected to the posterior fibula showing a minimal displacement of the interfragmentary fracture. (**g**) The medial clear space is markedly widened; the deep deltoid ligament is elongated but its continuity is preserved. (**h**) More anteriorly a complete disruption of the superficial deltoid (asterisk) is seen, allowing the view of the intact fibers of deep deltoid ligament beneath (arrow). (**i**) After open reduction and internal fixation of the fibula, the talus looks well repositioned with regained congruity and alignment of the ankle under fluoroscopy. (**j**) However, while applying lateral stress to the foot, the talus is seen to translate laterally with disruption of the tibiotalar alignment. (**k**) Lateral stress test after deltoid ligament reconstruction shows a stable joint, without any talar translation within the mortise. (**l**) The hook test confirms achieved stability of the fibula, making additional measures unnecessary. This patient was able to return to his former activity level. At his 10-year follow-up control, he was very pleased with the ankle, allowing unlimited physical activity

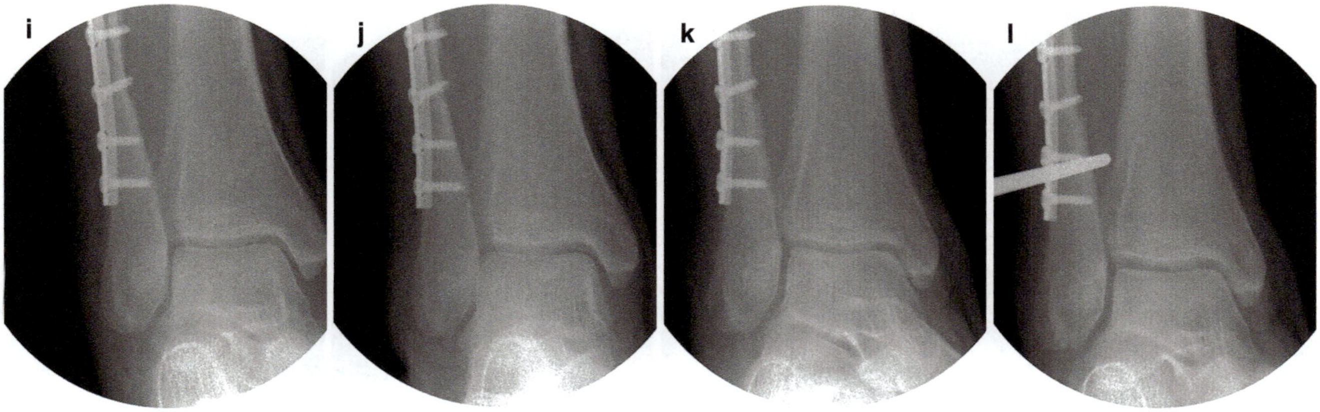

Fig. 6.15 (continued)

result in fewer complications, reduced surgical time, and lower cost [58, 61, 82–86].

6.7 Complications

- Persisting anteromedial rotation instability of the ankle can result in a progressive valgus and pronation deformity.
- Ankle mortise malreduction can lead to chronic ankle instability, ankle pain, and subsequent posttraumatic arthritis.

The problem of SE fractures is the medial "invisible injury" [81]. The decision to treat a seemingly stable SE stage 2 fracture conservatively, without accurate assessment of the deltoid ligament injury, may predispose a patient to early posttraumatic osteoarthritis [5, 9, 16, 88, 89].

In PE injuries that are seen mostly in feet with a valgus and pronation configuration, insufficient treatment of the deltoid injury may result in persistent anteromedial rotation instability of the ankle, with subsequent increase of valgus and pronation deformity (Fig. 6.18). The pivoting of the talus along the medial malleolus will be lost, which will lead to a lateral shift of the center of rotation of the ankle and thus a lateral shift of the articular load. These changes of biomechanics are detrimental for the integrity of the ankle joint complex and will result in progressive deformation and destabilization of the hindfoot, leading to critical overload of the lateral tibiotalar joint and overuse of the PT tendon.

In ankle fractures with a widened medial clear space, deltoid ligament repair was associated with superior and long-term reduction of the ankle, evident by the immediate postoperative difference in the medial clear space, as well as maintenance of the medial clear space over time [60]. Ankle mortise malreduction can lead to chronic ankle instability and ankle pain, and subsequent posttraumatic arthritis [89–91]. With as little as 1-mm talar shift, a 49% increase in ankle joint pressure was found [91]. There is also evidence that postoperative ankle malalignment is a prognostic factor for developing posttraumatic arthritis [90]. This was consistent with the obtained results of lower pain scores in patients who had deltoid ligament repair [62, 63, 92].

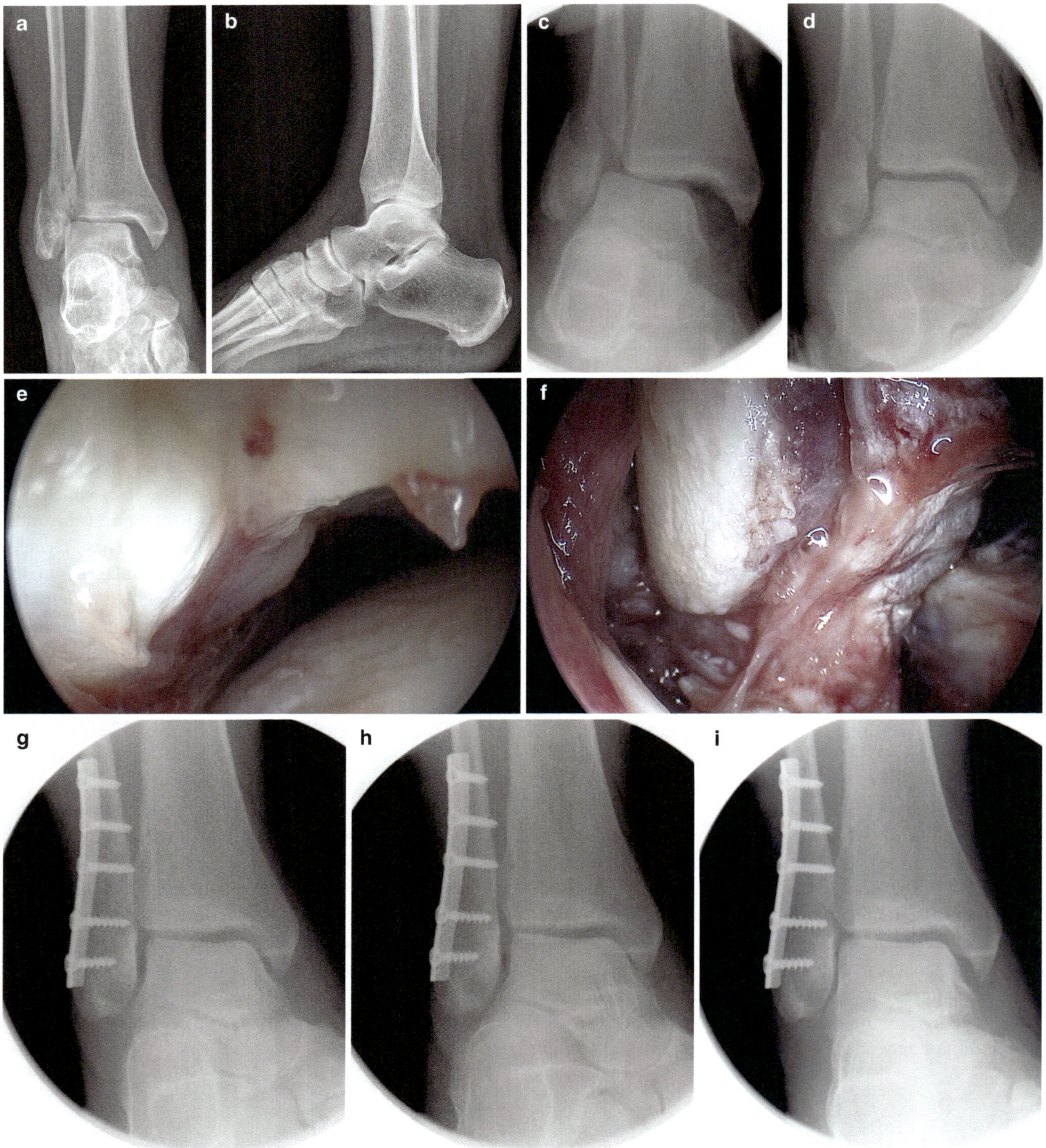

Fig. 6.16 *Surgical Technique: Deltoid ligament reconstruction in a Weber B-fracture*. This 51-year-old female patient twisted her ankle in the snow. (**a**) AP view evidences a Weber Type B-fracture with a massive widening of the medial clear space and lateral translation of talus, indicating a deltoid ligament rupture. (**b**) Lateral view showing the oblique fibular fracture. Preoperative fluoroscopy. (**c**) When applying lateral stress to the foot, the lateral talar shift is seen to increase significantly, and the medial clear space is widened accordingly. (**d**) When applying medial stress to the foot, the talus is seen to be reduced, and the medial clear space is closed. (**e**) Preoperative arthroscopy evidences a partial rupture of the AITFL. (**f**) On the medial side, the medial clear space is widened, associated with interposed ligaments and deep cartilage lesions to the medial malleolus. The superficial deltoid is completely torn, whereas the continuity of the deep deltoid, though elongated, seems to be preserved. (**g**) After open reduction and internal fixation of the fibula, there is still some valgus talar tilt with the talus slightly externally rotated within the mortise. (**h**) When applying abduction stress to the forefoot, the external rotation of talus is slightly increased, while there is no talar translation. (**i**) When applying lateral stress to the foot, some talar translation is seen, associated to a widening of the medial clear space as well as also distinct widening of the syndesmotic space. (**j**) Surgical exploration shows the complete avulsion of the superficial deltoid, whereas the deep deltoid seems to be preserved (arrow). Asterisk = anterior colliculus of medial malleolus. (**k**) When pulling the ligament (arrow), the deep deltoid is found to be extensively damaged. (**l**) Now the disruption of PT tendon sheath can be seen. (**m**) Deltoid ligament repair using the same technique as shown in Fig. 6.15 is done; the ligament repair is strong when tightening the 2 sutures. (**n**) Situation after final repair. (**o**) Stress test under fluoroscopy showing a stable and well-aligned ankle

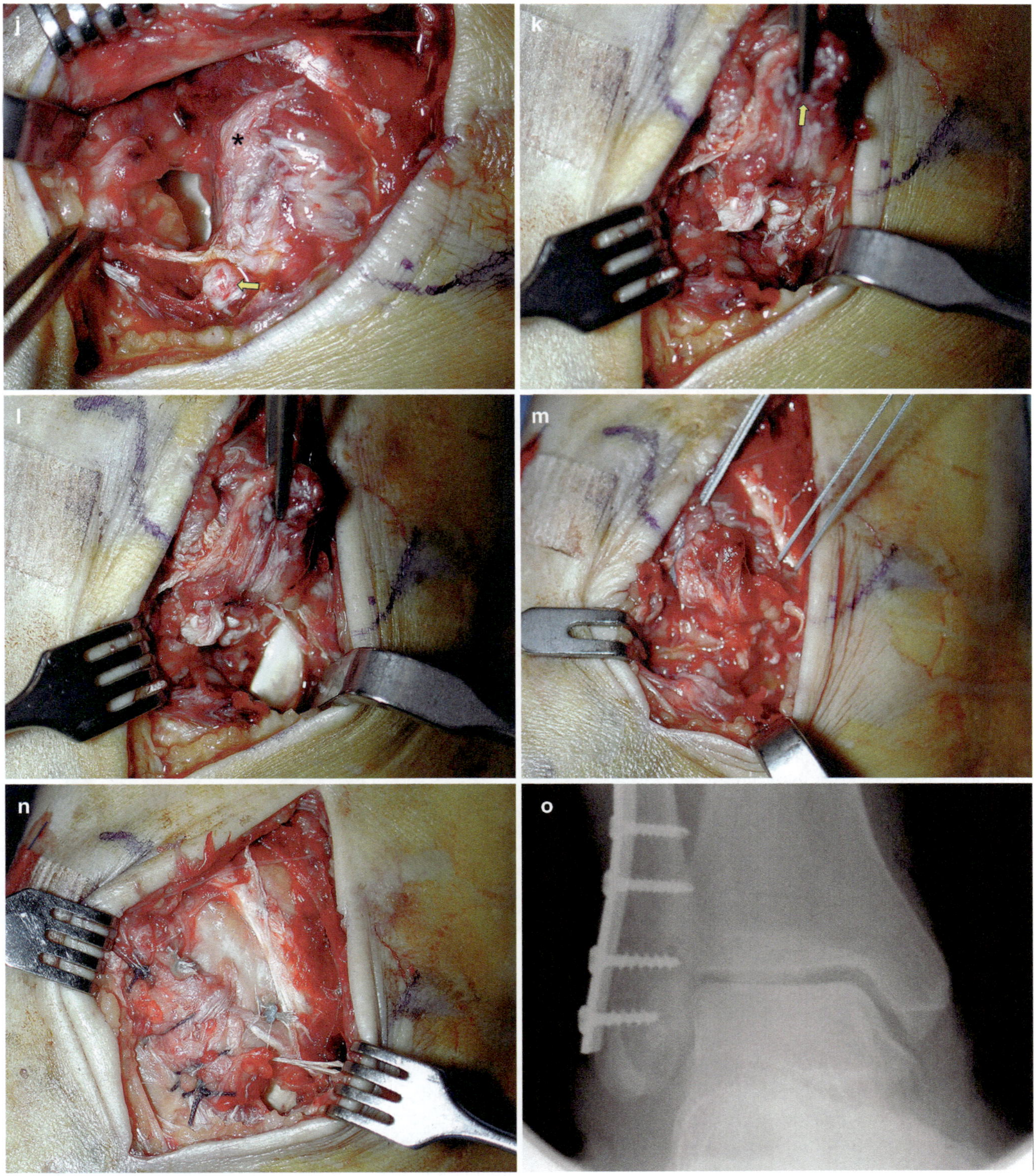

Fig. 6.16 (continued)

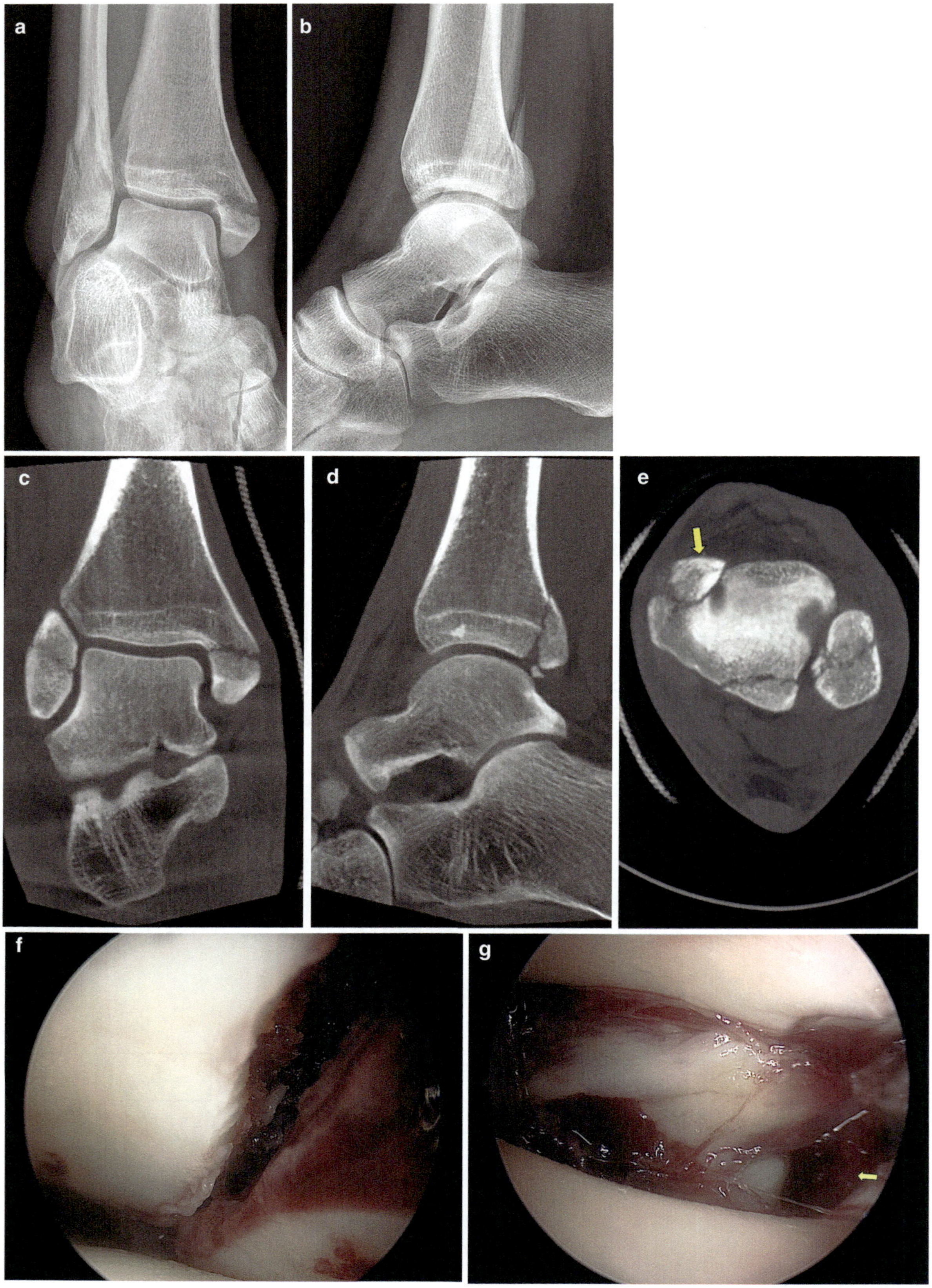
a
b
c
d
e
f
g

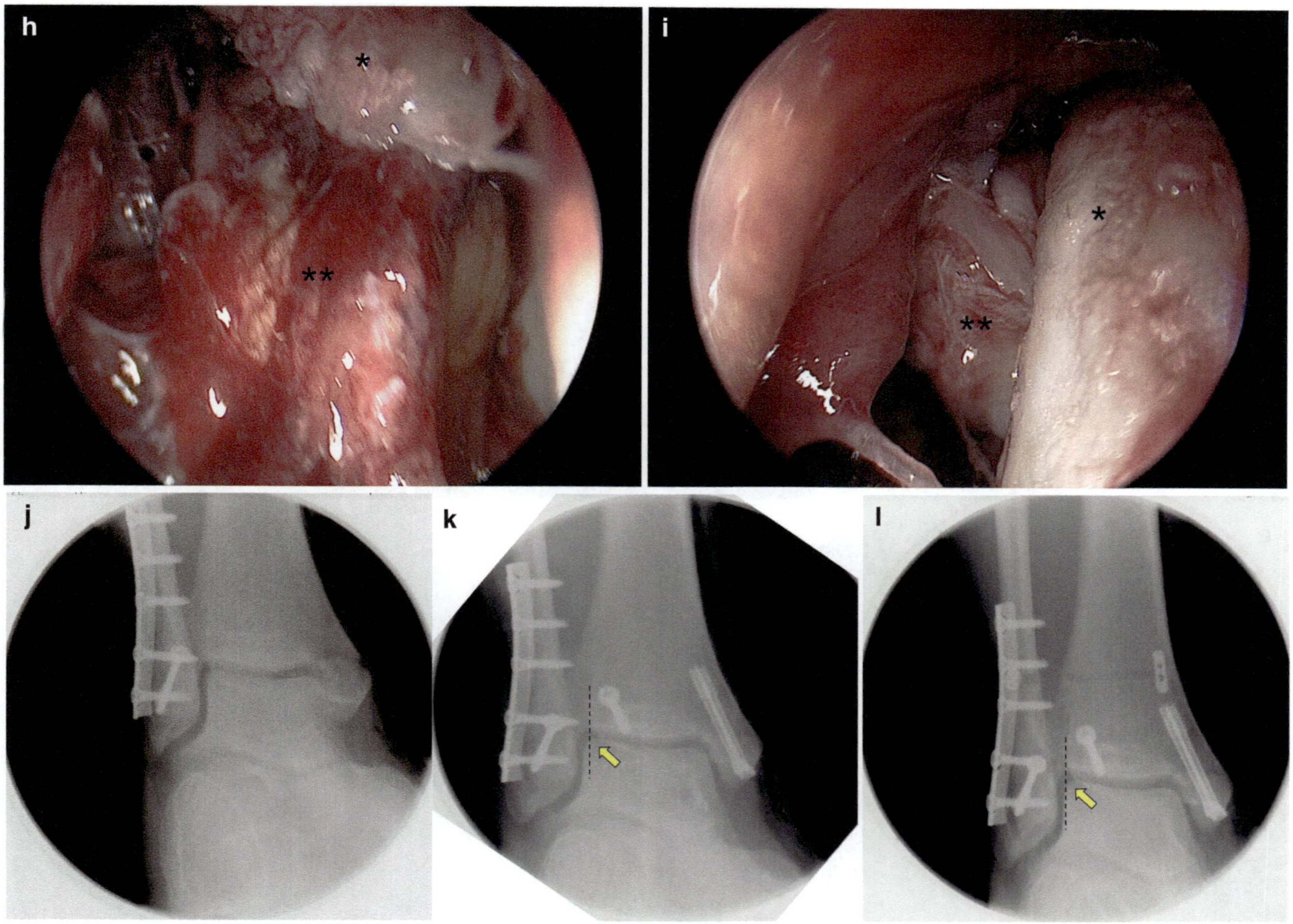

Fig. 6.17 (continued)

Fig. 6.17 *Surgical Technique: Surgical treatment of a trimalleolar fracture*. This 49-year-old male patient sustained this fracture while hiking. Standard radiographs evidence a minimally displaced trimalleolar fracture with aligned talus: (**a**) AP view, (**b**) lateral view. (**c–e**) CT scans show a fracture of the anterior part of the medial malleolus with some malrotation of the fragment (arrow), whereas the posterior part seems intact. Preoperative arthroscopy: (**f**) medial view shows a fracture of the medial malleolus. (**g**) posteromedial view shows the PT tendon subsequent to a disruption of its tendon sheath. (**h**) Lateral view shows a complex injury to the ATFL (Asterisk) and AITFL (double Asterisk). (**i**) The lateral shoulder of the talus evidences deep cartilage lesions (Asterisk); the proximal stump of the AITFL can be seen (double Asterisk). (**j**) After internal fixation of the fibula, the anteromedial instability persists. (**k**) With additional fixation of the medial and posterior malleoli, medial instability of the malleolus is successfully addressed; however, lateral stress indicates some lateral translation (arrow) and widening of the syndesmotic space without widening of the medial clear space. (**l**) Therefore, a suture button is used for transfixation of the syndesmosis which results in a well-aligned talus (arrow) and a congruent ankle joint

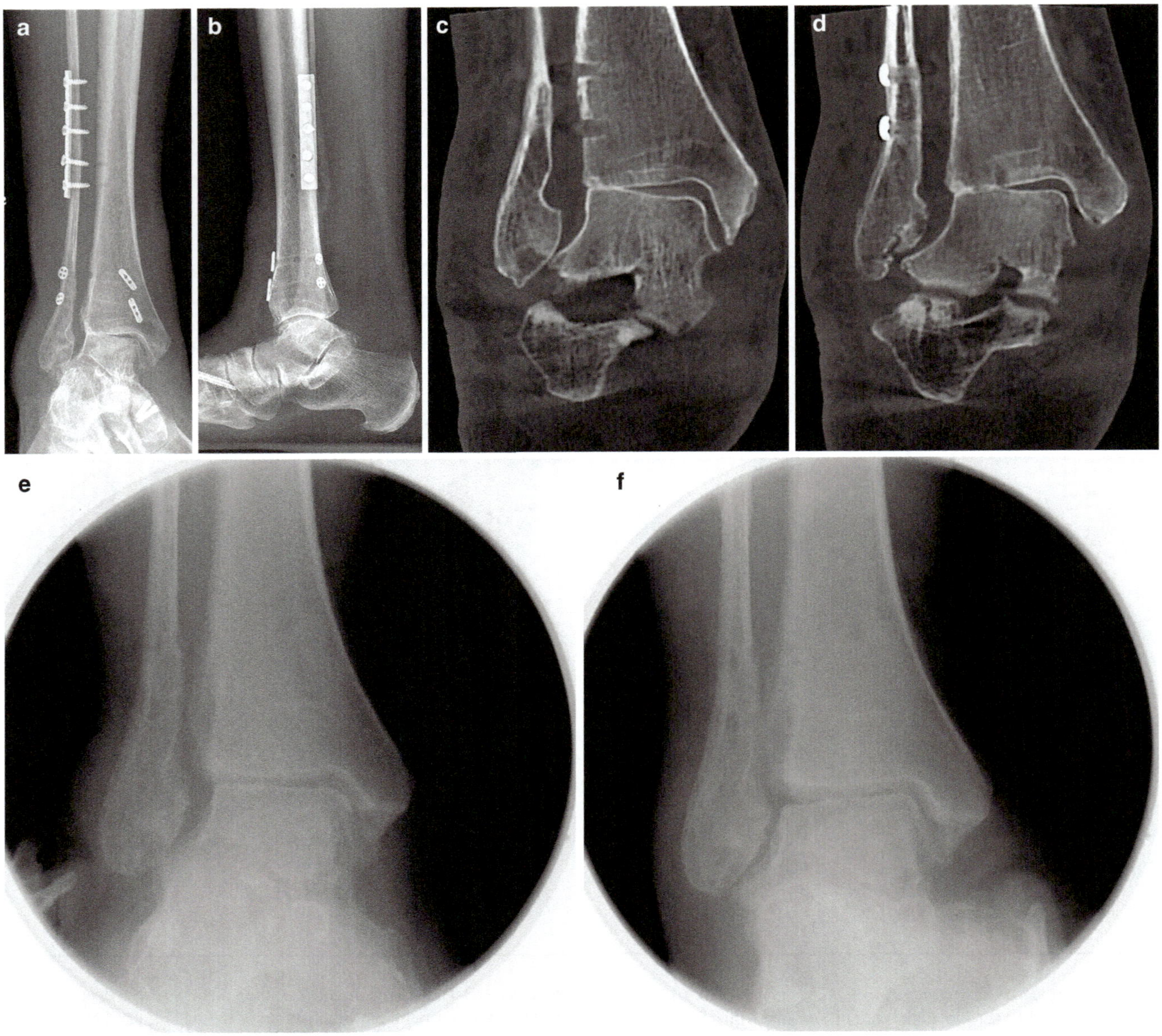

Fig. 6.18 *Surgical Technique: Supramalleolar osteotomy and distal tibiofibular (syndesmotic) fusion for failed treatment.* This 68-year-old active female patient sustained a mid-shaft fibular fracture (Weber Type C) which was initially treated by internal fixation and additional transfixation of the syndesmosis with 2 suture buttons. The deltoid ligament was not repaired. Nineteen months later the patient shows up complaining of progressive lateral ankle pain and a feeling of instability. (**a**) The AP view of standard radiographs shows a valgus tilt of the talus with a syndesmosis diastasis. (**b**) Lateral view shows a distinct posterior translation of the talus indicating an instability of the tibiotalar joint. CT scans confirm these findings. (**c**) They reveal an increased widening of the medial clear space in the anterior tibiotalar joint when compared to (**d**) more posterior, indicating the external rotation position of talus in the mortise. (**e**) The valgus tilt of talus is removed after hardware removal. (**f**) However, when applying lateral stress to the foot, the talus is translated towards lateral with some widening of the medial clear space. (**g**) A moderate medial closing wedge osteotomy of the distal tibia is performed to address the slightly impacted lateral tibial surface with subsequent valgus TAS and to compensate for the wear of lateral tibiotalar joint. (**h**) With this angular correction, the fibula has become shorter, enabling anatomic reduction of the tibiofibular joint. In this position, a distal tibiofibular (syndesmotic) fusion is performed using a plate over the fibula to enhance the primary compression force of the screws. (**i**) Final result in AP view, and (**j**) lateral view showing a well-balanced ankle joint. At the 10-year follow-up control, the patient is very satisfied reporting no pain and no limitations in her daily life. (**k**) Weight-bearing radiographs show a balanced ankle although some heel valgus is present seen in the AP view, and (**l**) a distinctly increased posterior malalignment of tibiotalar joint in the lateral view. (**m** and **n**) WB CT scans also show a slightly valgus talar position with a solid tibiofibular fusion. As compared with the preoperative situation (**c** and **d**), the lateral tibiotalar joint space recovered, but the talar tilt persists with the same pattern as preoperatively. Retrospectively, adding a medial sliding osteotomy might have avoided progressive valgus malalignment of the heel

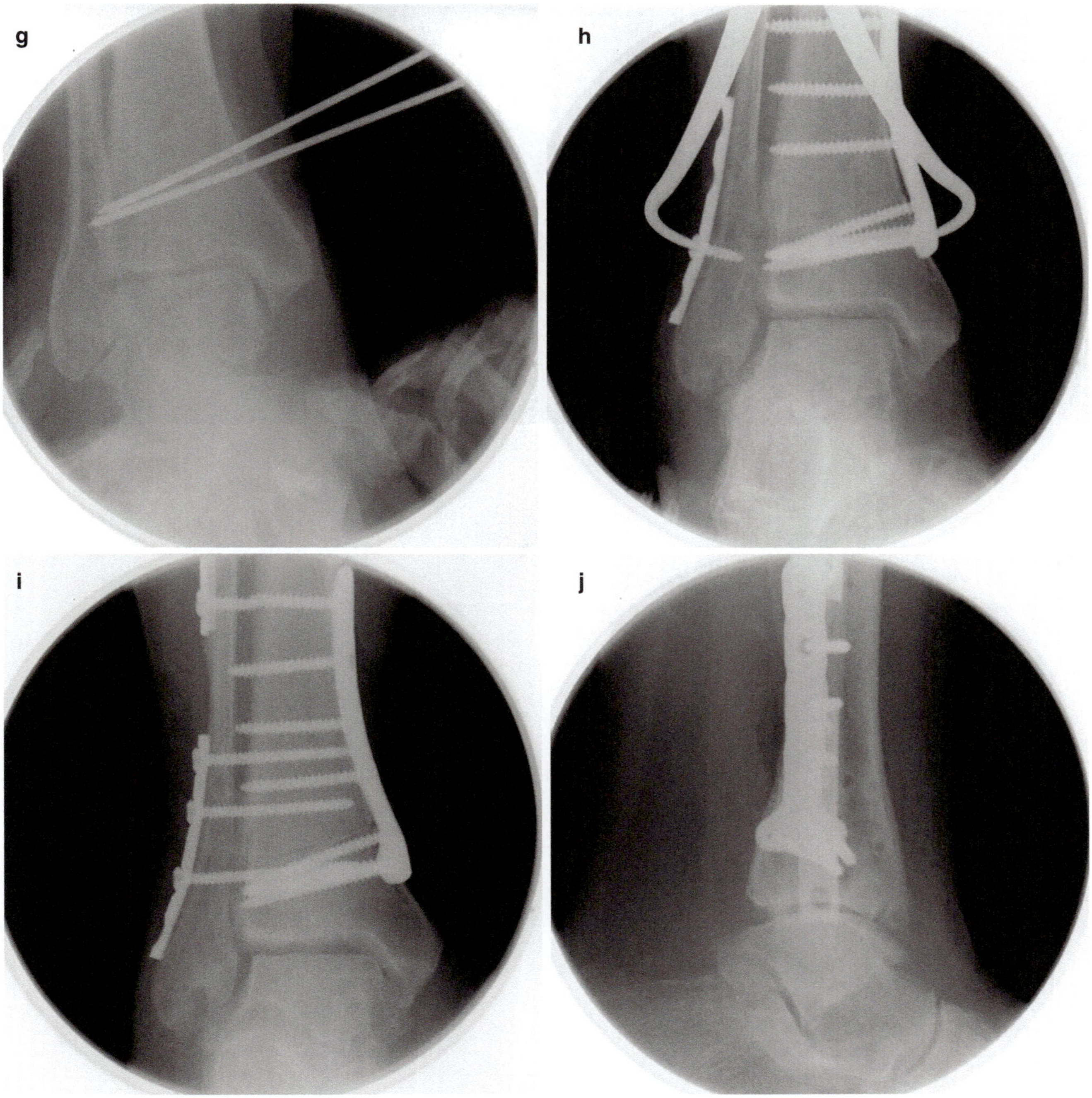

Fig. 6.18 (continued)

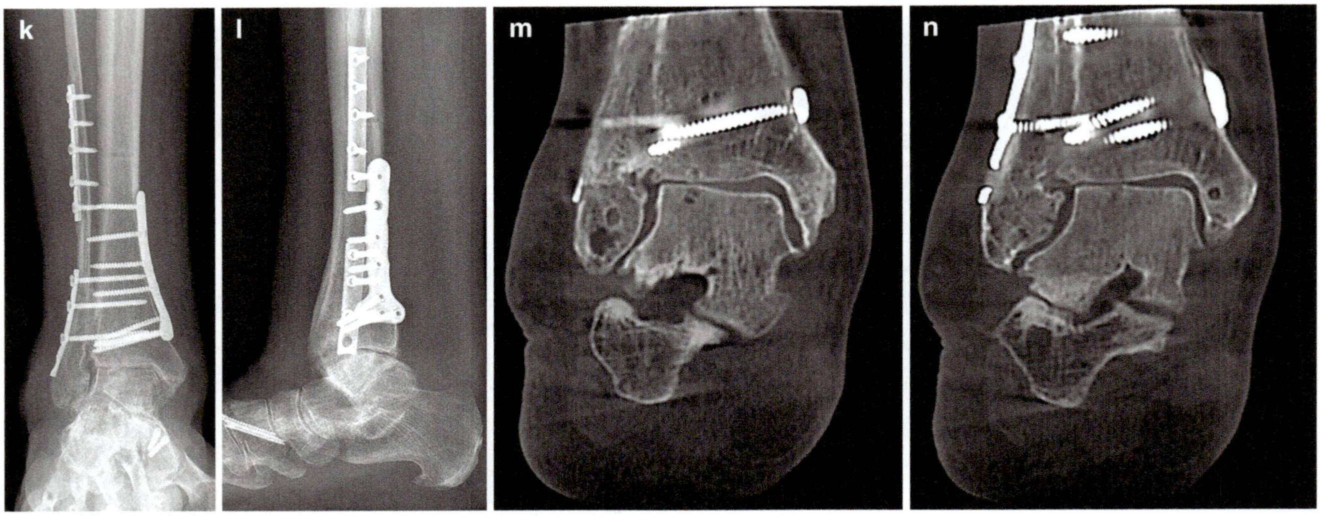

Fig. 6.18 (continued)

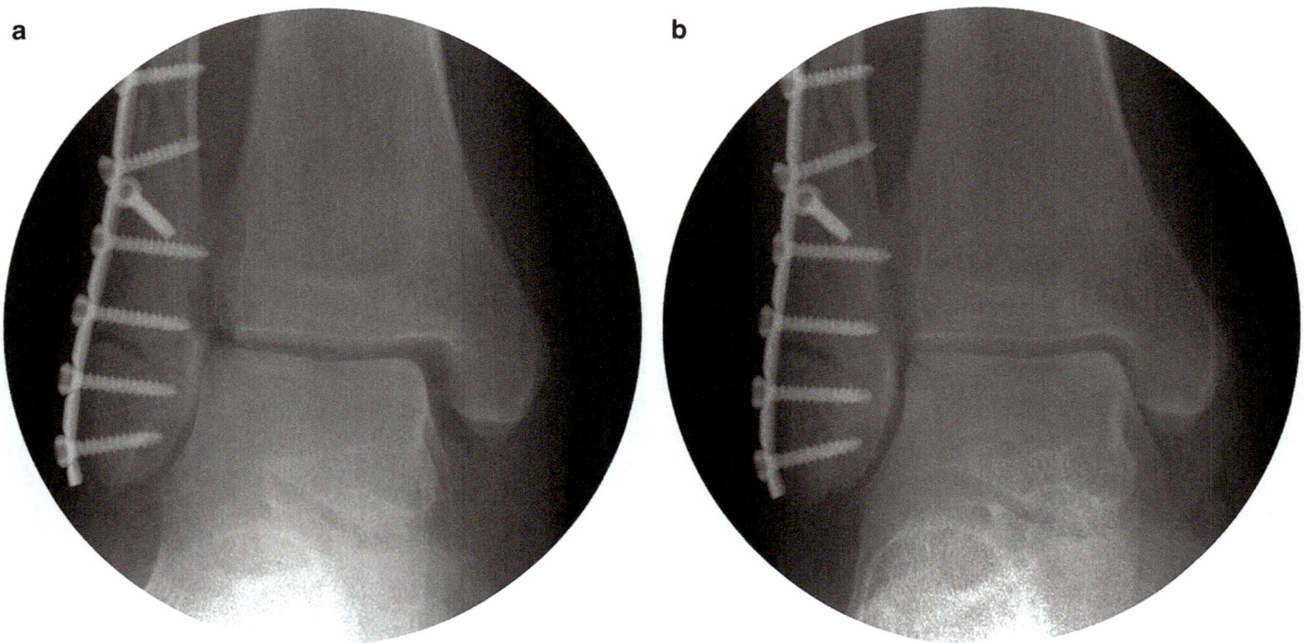

Fig. 6.19 *Surgical Technique: Effect of deltoid ligament repair to coronal plane stability of the ankle.* Weber Type B-fracture in a 52-year-old patient. Lateral stress test (**a**) before and (**b**) after deltoid repair, indicating that deltoid repair was sufficient to restore coronal plane stability of the injured ankle, thus making additional syndesmotic transfixation unnecessary

6.8 Conclusions

- Interposition of the deltoid ligament in the medial clear space is generally accepted to indicate surgical exploration and repair of the deltoid ligament.
- The paradigm to primarily reconstruct the lateral pillar of the ankle to create a buttress to keep the talus in place and to neglect the medial side, as long as the medial clear space is normal, should be critically questioned.

Although there is common agreement on treating unstable fractures with open reduction and internal fixation, for stable fractures this is not the case. Some authors have reported unsatisfying results with conservative treatment of seemingly stable fractures. The crucial problem may be that the radiographs show no displacement despite the presence of a deltoid ligament rupture, with subsequent inadequate treatment. Therefore, the question remains which diagnostic tool is best to validate the integrity of the deep portion of the deltoid ligament. To date, gravity stress radiographs have provided the best results in detecting deltoid ligament ruptures in acute ankle fractures. A medial clear space of >4 mm, seen after a fibular fracture (4 mm being at least 1 mm greater than the superior tibiotalar space), is a value that is widely accepted to represent a ruptured deep deltoid ligament. Clinical diagnostic criteria, such as pain over the deltoid ligament, swelling, ecchymosis, or combinations hereof, do not have enough sensitivity and specificity to rule out instability of the ankle joint. Both, ultrasonography and MRI, have potential to predict a deep deltoid rupture, but their use is limited by its availability and accuracy.

Exploration and reconstruction of the deltoid ligament is generally thought to be necessary if the medial clear space has not returned to its normal width after adequate reduction and fixation of the fibular fracture, indicating interposition of the deltoid ligament. Arthroscopy can be helpful in determining interposition when the medial clear space remains wide after proper reduction.

Normalization of the medial clear space is obviously the main criteria used by orthopedic surgeons to decide whether the medial side of the ankle is adequately restored in conservatively or surgically treated ankle fractures. Remaining rotational instability resulting in exorotation of the talus within the reconstructed ankle mortise is generally neglected. It can be typically seen as lateral tibiotalar misalignment in the mortise view (Fig. 6.19a) that disappears after repair of the superficial deltoid ligament (Fig. 6.19b). Restoration of the medial pillar, ensuring stability and motion of the talus about the helical axis of the ankle joint, might be fundamental in restoring an ankle to function normally and to preserve it from osteoarthritic changes in the near future.

The paradigm to primarily reconstruct the lateral pillar of the ankle to create a buttress to keep the talus in place and to neglect the medial side, as long as the medial clear space is normal, should be critically questioned. Despite providing stability to the lateral ankle, the talus will remain disconnected from the tibia, thereby the pivoting of the talus along the medial malleolus will be lost. This leads to a lateral shift of the center of rotation of the ankle joint and thus a lateral shift of the articular load. These changes of biomechanics are detrimental for the integrity of the ankle joint complex and will result in progressive deformation and destabilization of the hindfoot, leading to critical overload of the lateral tibiotalar joint and subsequent osteoarthrosis.

References

1. Bauer M, Bergstrom B, Hemborg A, Sandegard J. Malleolar fractures: nonoperative versus operative treatment. A controlled study. Clin Orthop Relat Res. 1985;199:17–27.
2. Kristensen KD, Hansen T. Closed treatment of ankle fractures. Stage II supination-eversion fractures followed for 20 years. Acta Orthop Scand. 1985;56(2):107–9.
3. Ponzer S, Nasell H, Bergman B, Tornkvist H. Functional outcome and quality of life in patients with type B ankle fractures: a two-year follow-up study. J Orthop Trauma. 1999;13(5):363–8.
4. Stufkens SA, Knupp M, Lampert C, van Dijk CN, Hintermann B. Long-term outcome after supination-external rotation type-4 fractures of the ankle. J Bone Joint Surg Br. 2009;91(12):1607–11.
5. Yde J. The Lauge Hansen classification of malleolar fractures. Acta Orthop Scand. 1980;51(1):181–92.
6. Stufkens SA, van den Bekerom MP, Knupp M, Hintermann B, van Dijk CN. The diagnosis and treatment of deltoid ligament lesions in supination-external rotation ankle fractures: a review. Strategies Trauma Limb Reconstr. 2012;7(2):73–85.

7. Hönigschmied J. Leichenexperimente über die zerreissungen der bänder im sprunggelenk mit rücksicht auf die entstehung der indirecten knöchelfracturen. Deutsch Zschr Chir. 1877;8: 239–60.
8. Lauge-Hansen N. Fractures of the ankle. II. Combined experimental-surgical and experimental-roentgenologic investigations. Arch Surg. 1950;60(5):957–85.
9. Lindsjo U. Operative treatment of ankle fracture-dislocations. A follow-up study of 306/321 consecutive cases. Clin Orthop Relat Res. 1985;(199):28–38.
10. Maissonneuve MJG. Recherches sur la fracture du pérone. Arch Gen Med. 1840;52:165–87.
11. Weber BG. Injuries of the ankle. Bern: Hans Huber; 1972.
12. Cedell CA. Rupture of the posterior talotibial ligament with the avulsion of a bone fragment from the talus. Acta Orthop Scand. 1974;45(3):454–61.
13. Tejwani NC, McLaurin TM, Walsh M, Bhadsavle S, Koval KJ, Egol KA. Are outcomes of bimalleolar fractures poorer than those of lateral malleolar fractures with medial ligamentous injury? J Bone Joint Surg Am. 2007;89(7):1438–41.
14. Rasmussen O. Stability of the ankle joint. Analysis of the function and traumatology of the ankle ligaments. Acta Orthop Scand Suppl. 1985;211:1–75.
15. Pai VS. Medial malleolar fracture associated with deltoid ligament rupture. J Foot Ankle Surg. 1999;38(6):420–2.
16. Schuberth JM, Collman DR, Rush SM, Ford LA. Deltoid ligament integrity in lateral malleolar fractures: a comparative analysis of arthroscopic and radiographic assessments. J Foot Ankle Surg. 2004;43(1):20–9.
17. Gardner MJ, Demetrakopoulos D, Briggs SM, Helfet DL, Lorich DG. Malreduction of the tibiofibular syndesmosis in ankle fractures. Foot Ankle Int. 2006;27(10):788–92.
18. Tornetta P 3rd. Competence of the deltoid ligament in bimalleolar ankle fractures after medial malleolar fixation. J Bone Joint Surg Am. 2000;82(6):843–8.
19. Klein MA. MR imaging of the ankle: normal and abnormal findings in the medial collateral ligament. AJR Am J Roentgenol. 1994;162(2):377–83.
20. Siegler S, Block J, Schneck CD. The mechanical characteristics of the collateral ligaments of the human ankle joint. Foot Ankle. 1988;8(5):234–42.
21. Hintermann B, Regazzoni P, Lampert C, Stutz G, Gachter A. Arthroscopic findings in acute fractures of the ankle. J Bone Joint Surg Br. 2000;82(3):345–51.
22. Michelson JD, Waldman B. An axially loaded model of the ankle after pronation external rotation injury. Clin Orthop Relat Res. 1996;328:285–93.
23. Baird RA, Jackson ST. Fractures of the distal part of the fibula with associated disruption of the deltoid ligament. Treatment without repair of the deltoid ligament. J Bone Joint Surg Am. 1987;69(9):1346–52.
24. Ebraheim NA, Elgafy H, Padanilam T. Syndesmotic disruption in low fibular fractures associated with deltoid ligament injury. Clin Orthop Relat Res. 2003;409:260–7.
25. Pankovich AM, Shivaram MS. Anatomical basis of variability in injuries of the medial malleolus and the deltoid ligament. I Anatomical studies. Acta Orthop Scand. 1979;50(2):217–23.
26. van den Bekerom MP, Mutsaerts EL, van Dijk CN. Evaluation of the integrity of the deltoid ligament in supination external rotation ankle fractures: a systematic review of the literature. Arch Orthop Trauma Surg. 2009;129(2):227–35.
27. van Dijk CN, Mol BW, Lim LS, Marti RK, Bossuyt PM. Diagnosis of ligament rupture of the ankle joint. Physical examination, arthrography, stress radiography and sonography compared in 160 patients after inversion trauma. Acta Orthop Scand. 1996;67(6): 566–70.
28. Baumhauer JF, Geppert MJ, Michelson JD, Walling AK. Ankle and foot: trauma. Orthopaedic knowledge update. 7. Rosemont: American Academy of Orthopaedic Surgeons; 2002. p. 548.
29. DeAngelis NA, Eskander MS, French BG. Does medial tenderness predict deep deltoid ligament incompetence in supination-external rotation type ankle fractures? J Orthop Trauma. 2007;21(4):244–7.
30. Arimoto HK, Forrester DM. Classification of ankle fractures: an algorithm. AJR Am J Roentgenol. 1980;135(5):1057–63.
31. Michelson J, Solocoff D, Waldman B, Kendell K, Ahn U. Ankle fractures. The Lauge-Hansen classification revisited. Clin Orthop Relat Res. 1997;345:198–205.
32. Michelson JD. Fractures about the ankle. J Bone Joint Surg Am. 1995;77(1):142–52.
33. Nielsen JO, Dons-Jensen H, Sorensen HT. Lauge-Hansen classification of malleolar fractures. An assessment of the reproducibility in 118 cases. Acta Orthop Scand. 1990;61(5):385–7.
34. Rasmussen S, Madsen PV, Bennicke K. Observer variation in the Lauge-Hansen classification of ankle fractures. Precision improved by instruction. Acta Orthop Scand. 1993;64(6):693–4.
35. Yablon IG, Heller FG, Shouse L. The key role of the lateral malleolus in displaced fractures of the ankle. J Bone Joint Surg Am. 1977;59(2):169–73.
36. Carr JB, Trafton P. Malleolar and soft tissue injuries of the ankle. In: Browner B, Jupiter JB, Levine AM, Trafton P, editors. Skeletal trauma. Philadelphia: Saunders; 1998. p. 2357.
37. Gardner MJ, Demetrakopoulos D, Briggs SM, Helfet DL, Lorich DG. The ability of the Lauge-Hansen classification to predict ligament injury and mechanism in ankle fractures: an MRI study. J Orthop Trauma. 2006;20(4):267–72.
38. Gill JB, Risko T, Raducan V, Grimes JS, Schutt RC Jr. Comparison of manual and gravity stress radiographs for the evaluation of supination-external rotation fibular fractures. J Bone Joint Surg Am. 2007;89(5):994–9.
39. Harper MC. Deltoid ligament: an anatomical evaluation of function. Foot Ankle. 1987;8(1):19–22.
40. Jeong BO, Kim TY, Baek JH, Song SH, Park JS. Assessment of ankle mortise instability after isolated supination-external rotation lateral malleolar fractures. J Bone Joint Surg Am. 2018;100(18):1557–62.
41. Michelson JD, Varner KE, Checcone M. Diagnosing deltoid injury in ankle fractures: the gravity stress view. Clin Orthop Relat Res. 2001;387:178–82.
42. Nortunen S, Flinkkila T, Lantto I, Kortekangas T, Niinimaki J, Ohtonen P, et al. Diagnostic accuracy of the gravity stress test and clinical signs in cases of isolated supination-external rotation-type lateral malleolar fractures. Bone Joint J. 2015;97-B(8):1126–31.
43. Park SS, Kubiak EN, Egol KA, Kummer F, Koval KJ. Stress radiographs after ankle fracture: the effect of ankle position and deltoid ligament status on medial clear space measurements. J Orthop Trauma. 2006;20(1):11–8.
44. Pitakveerakul A, Kungwan S, Arunakul P, Arunakul M. Radiographic parameters in gravity stress view of the ankle: normative data. Foot Ankle Surg. 2019;25(6):819–25.
45. van Leeuwen C, Haak T, Kop M, Weil N, Zijta F, Hoogendoorn J. The additional value of gravity stress radiographs in predicting deep deltoid ligament integrity in supination external rotation ankle fractures. Eur J Trauma Emerg Surg. 2019;45(4):727–35.
46. Ashraf A, Murphree J, Wait E, Winston T, Wooldridge A, Meriwether M, et al. Gravity stress radiographs and the effect of ankle position on deltoid ligament integrity and medial clear space measurements. J Orthop Trauma. 2017;31(5):270–4.
47. McConnell T, Creevy W, Tornetta P 3rd. Stress examination of supination external rotation-type fibular fractures. J Bone Joint Surg Am. 2004;86(10):2171–8.
48. Chen PY, Wang TG, Wang CL. Ultrasonographic examination of the deltoid ligament in bimalleolar equivalent fractures. Foot Ankle Int. 2008;29(9):883–6.

49. Lechner R, Richter H, Friemert B, Palm HG, Gottschalk A. The value of ultrasonography compared with magnetic resonance imaging in the diagnosis of deltoid ligament injuries—is there a difference? Z Orthop Unfall. 2015;153(4):408–14.
50. Peetrons P, Creteur V, Bacq C. Sonography of ankle ligaments. J Clin Ultrasound. 2004;32(9):491–9.
51. Rosa I, Rodeia J, Fernandes PX, Teixeira R, Saldanha T, Consciencia JG. Ultrasonographic assessment of deltoid ligament integrity in ankle fractures. Foot Ankle Int. 2020;41(2):147–53.
52. Hintermann B. What the orthopaedic foot and ankle surgeon wants to know from MR imaging. Semin Musculoskelet Radiol. 2005;9(3):260–71.
53. Mengiardi B, Pinto C, Zanetti M. Medial collateral ligament complex of the ankle: MR imaging anatomy and findings in medial instability. Semin Musculoskelet Radiol. 2016;20(1):91–103.
54. Warner SJ, Garner MR, Fabricant PD, Schottel PC, Loftus ML, Hentel KD, et al. The diagnostic accuracy of radiographs and magnetic resonance imaging in predicting deltoid ligament ruptures in ankle fractures. HSS J. 2019;15(2):115–21.
55. Chan KB, Lui TH. Role of ankle arthroscopy in management of acute ankle fracture. Art Ther. 2016;32(11):2373–80.
56. Loren GJ, Ferkel RD. Arthroscopic assessment of occult intra-articular injury in acute ankle fractures. Arthroscopy. 2002;18(4):412–21.
57. Hintermann B, Boss A, Schafer D. Arthroscopic findings in patients with chronic ankle instability. Am J Sports Med. 2002;30(3):402–9.
58. Dabash S, Elabd A, Potter E, Fernandez I, Gerzina C, Thabet AM, et al. Adding deltoid ligament repair in ankle fracture treatment: is it necessary? A systematic review. Foot Ankle Surg. 2019;25(6):714–20.
59. Lee TH, Jang KS, Choi GW, Jeong CD, Hong SJ, Yoon MA, et al. The contribution of anterior deltoid ligament to ankle stability in isolated lateral malleolar fractures. Injury. 2016;47(7):1581–5.
60. Salameh M, Alhammoud A, Alkhatib N, Attia AK, Mekhaimar MM, D'Hooghe P, et al. Outcome of primary deltoid ligament repair in acute ankle fractures: a meta-analysis of comparative studies. Int Orthop. 2020;44(2):341–7.
61. Sun X, Li T, Sun Z, Li Y, Yang M, Li S, et al. Does routinely repairing deltoid ligament injuries in type B ankle joint fractures influence long term outcomes? Injury. 2018;49(12):2312–7.
62. Woo SH, Bae SY, Chung HJ. Short-term results of a ruptured deltoid ligament repair during an acute ankle fracture fixation. Foot Ankle Int. 2018;39(1):35–45.
63. Zhao HM, Lu J, Zhang F, Wen XD, Li Y, Hao DJ, et al. Surgical treatment of ankle fracture with or without deltoid ligament repair: a comparative study. BMC Musculoskelet Disord. 2017;18(1):543.
64. Yu GR, Zhang MZ, Aiyer A, Tang X, Xie M, Zeng LR, et al. Repair of the acute deltoid ligament complex rupture associated with ankle fractures: a multicenter clinical study. J Foot Ankle Surg. 2015;54(2):198–202.
65. Butler BA, Hempen EC, Barbosa M, Muriuki M, Havey RM, Nicolay RW, et al. Deltoid ligament repair reduces and stabilizes the talus in unstable ankle fractures. J Orthop. 2020;17:87–90.
66. Jones CR, Nunley JA 2nd. Deltoid ligament repair versus syndesmotic fixation in bimalleolar equivalent ankle fractures. J Orthop Trauma. 2015;29(5):245–9.
67. Schottel PC, Baxter J, Gilbert S, Garner MR, Lorich DG. Anatomic ligament repair restores ankle and syndesmotic rotational stability as much as syndesmotic screw fixation. J Orthop Trauma. 2016;30(2):e36–40.
68. Anderson LD. In: Crenshaw AH, editor. Fractures. 5th ed. St. Louis: Mosby; 1971.
69. Braunstein PW, Wade PA. Treatment of unstable fractures of the ankle. Ann Surg. 1959;149(2):217–26.
70. Close JR. Some applications of the functional anatomy of the ankle joint. J Bone Joint Surg Am. 1956;38-A(4):761–81.
71. Dziob JM. Ligamentous injuries about the ankle joint. Am J Surg. 1956;91(4):692–7; discussion, 7–8.
72. Klossner O. Late results of operative and non-operative treatment of severe ankle fractures. A clinical study. Acta Chir Scand Suppl. 1962;(Suppl 293):1–93.
73. Purvis GD. The unstable oblique distal fibular fracture. Clin Orthop Relat Res. 1973;92:330–7.
74. Quigley TB. Fractures and ligament injuries of the ankle. Am J Surg. 1959;98:477–83.
75. Ryan JR. Fracture of the lateral malleolus with associated tear of the medical collateral ligament of the ankle. Ann Emerg Med. 1981;10(4):211–2.
76. Solonen KA, Lauttamus L. Operative treatment of ankle fractures. Acta Orthop Scand. 1968;39(2):223–37.
77. Bonnin JG. Injury to the ligaments of the ankle. J Bone Joint Surg Br. 1965;47(4):609–11.
78. de Souza LJ, Gustilo RB, Meyer TJ. Results of operative treatment of displaced external rotation-abduction fractures of the ankle. J Bone Joint Surg Am. 1985;67(7):1066–74.
79. Denham RA. Internal fixation for unstable ankle fractures. J Bone Joint Surg Br. 1964;46:206–11.
80. Mast JW, Teipner WA. A reproducible approach to the internal fixation of adult ankle fractures: rationale, technique, and early results. Orthop Clin North Am. 1980;11(3):661–79.
81. Staples OS. Injuries to the medial ligaments of the ankle. J Bone Joint Surg Am. 1960;42A:1287–307.
82. Harper MC. The deltoid ligament. An evaluation of need for surgical repair. Clin Orthop Relat Res. 1988;226:156–68.
83. Maynou C, Lesage P, Mestdagh H, Butruille Y. Is surgical treatment of deltoid ligament rupture necessary in ankle fractures? Rev Chir Orthop Reper App Mot. 1997;83(7):652–7.
84. Stromsoe K, Hoqevold HE, Skjeldal S, Alho A. The repair of a ruptured deltoid ligament is not necessary in ankle fractures. J Bone Joint Surg Br. 1995;77(6):920–1.
85. Tourne Y, Charbel A, Picard F, Montbarbon E, Saragaglia D. Surgical treatment of bi- and trimalleolar ankle fractures: should the medial collateral ligament be sutured or not? J Foot Ankle Surg. 1999;38(1):24–9.
86. Zeegers AV, van der Werken C. Rupture of the deltoid ligament in ankle fractures: should it be repaired? Injury. 1989;20(1):39–41.
87. Clarke HJ, Michelson JD, Cox QGK, Jinnah RH. Tibio-Talar stability in bimalleolar ankle fractures: a dynamic in vitro contact area study. Foot Ankle Int. 1991;11(4):222–7.
88. Bauer M, Johnell O, Redlund-Johnell I, Johnsson K. Ankle fractures. Foot Ankle. 1987;8(1):23–5.
89. Pettrone FA, Gail M, Pee D, Fitzpatrick T, Van Herpe LB. Quantitative criteria for prediction of the results after displaced fracture of the ankle. J Bone Joint Surg Am. 1983;65(5):667–77.
90. Horisberger M, Valderrabano V, Hintermann B. Posttraumatic ankle osteoarthritis after ankle-related fractures. J Orthop Trauma. 2009;23(1):60–7.
91. Ramsey PL, Hamilton W. Changes in tibiotalar area of contact caused by lateral talar shift. J Bone Joint Surg Am. 1976;58(3):356–7.
92. Gu G, Yu J, Huo Y, Xu G, Yin Z, Yu J, Sheng L, Li L. Efficacy of deltoid ligament reconstruction on the curative effect, complication and long-term prognosis in ankle fracture-dislocation with deltoid ligament injury. Int J Clin Exp Med. 2017;10(9):13778–83.

7 Peritalar Instability

Loss of peritalar stability allows the talus to rotate and translate on the calcaneal and navicular bone surfaces, thereby resulting in a three-dimensional positional change and various talar malpositions. Typically, the tibiotalar (ankle) joint has lost its intrinsic stability, allowing the talus to tilt into valgus or varus, or to move anteriorwards while the foot is loaded. To date, little is known about the underlying causes. However, peritalar instability may result from differences in articular geometry, instability pattern of ligaments, and applied forces to the hindfoot complex.

7.1 Anatomy of the Peritalar Joint

- Being interposed between other bones and having no insertion of tendons, the talus moves due to the movement of peritalar structures.
- The subtalar joint has two to three articular facets; however, there is a considerable variation in shape and size of the facets.
- The anterior subtalar joint also contributes to the formation of the coxa pedis, along with the posterior surface of the navicular.

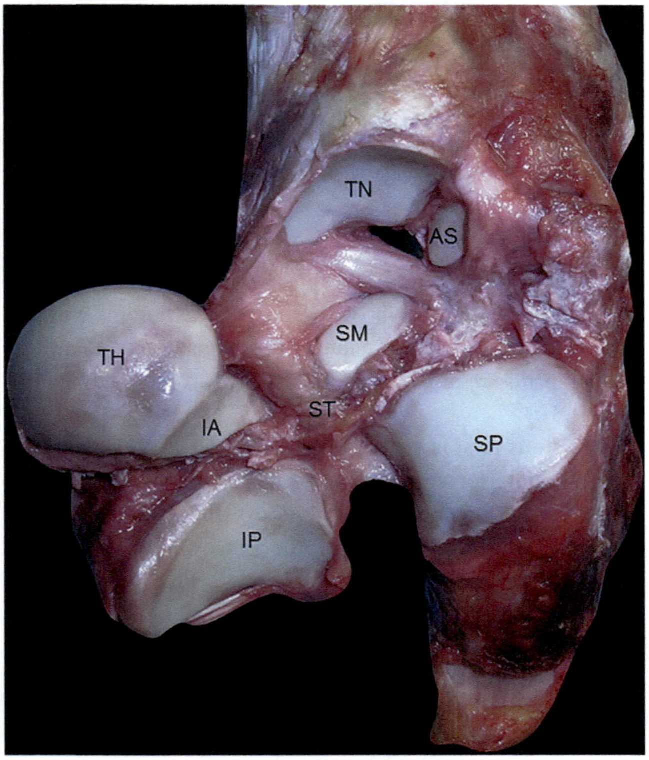

Fig. 7.1 The subtalar joint is formed by the articulations between the talus and the calcaneus and consists of an intricate structure with two separate joint cavities. The posterior subtalar joint is formed between the inferior posterior facet (IP) of the talus and the superior posterior (SP) facet of the calcaneus. The anterior subtalar, or talocalcaneonavicular, joint is formed from the head (TH) of the talus, the anterior-superior (AS) facets, the sustentaculum tali (ST) of the calcaneus, and the concave proximal surface of the tarsal navicular (TN). The superior medial (SM) facet of calcaneus articulates with the inferior anterior facet (IA) of the talus

The talus is covered by articular cartilage on more than 60% of its surface and has no muscle insertions. Thus, the talus moves due to the movement of peritalar structures [1]. The subtalar joint usually has three articular facets on the inferior part of the talus and the superior part of the calcaneus (Fig. 7.1). The posterior facet is the largest and forms a saddle-like joint under the talus, with a concave shape in the long axis. There is considerable variation in shape and size of the facets. The posterior facet is separated from the anterior and middle facets. The anterior and middle facets are often continuous.

Two or three articular facets mirror those of the talus. The posterior facet is in the middle third of the calcaneus. The anterior third of the calcaneus supports the anterior and middle facets. The calcaneal surface contributes to the formation of the sustentaculum tali over which the talus leans (Fig. 7.2). The sustentaculum tali provides a sliding surface for the posterior tibial tendon, the flexor hallucis longus tendon, and the

B. Hintermann, R. Ruiz, *Foot and Ankle Instability*, https://doi.org/10.1007/978-3-030-62926-7_7

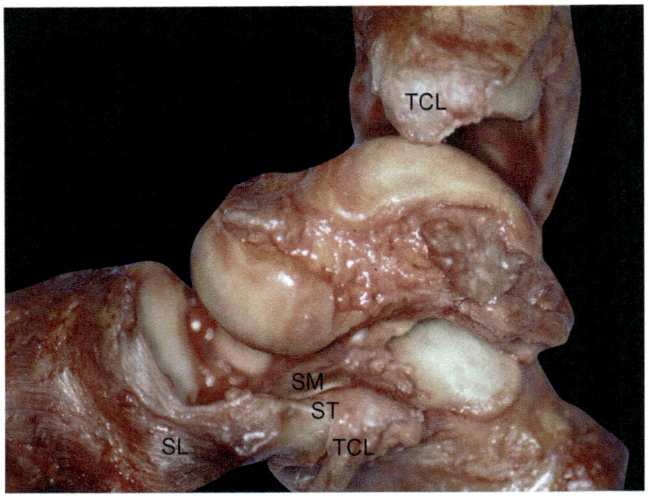

Fig. 7.2 Medial view after transection of the deltoid ligament, showing the sustentaculum tali (ST) over which the talus leans. It contains the medial (SM) facet of the subtalar joint and serves at its anterior border as the insertion area of the spring ligament (SL) complex. The tibiocalcaneal ligament (TCL) also has its distal insertion on the sustentaculum tali

flexor digitorum tendon. The anterior subtalar joint also contributes to the formation of the coxa pedis, along with the posterior surface of the navicular, the calcaneonavicular ligament (spring ligament), and the fibrocartilago navicularis (Fig. 7.3).

The sinus tarsi is situated between the talocalcaneonavicular joint anteriorly and the posterior talocalcaneal joint posteriorly. The wide anterolateral part of this conical cavity is the sinus tarsi itself, whereas the narrower posteromedial part is known as the canalis tarsi (Fig. 7.4) [2].

7.2 Anatomy of the Peritalar Ligaments

- The subtalar ligaments form a complex ligamentous complex that is divided into intrinsic and extrinsic ligaments.
- The ligaments of the deltoid-spring ligament complex contribute to the coxa pedis and ensure for the dynamic stability of the talar head.

The major subtalar ligaments are divided into two groups: (1) the *intrinsic* (sinus tarsi) ligaments, including the interosseous talocalcaneal ligament (ITCL) and the cervical ligament, and (2) the *extrinsic* ligaments, including the calcaneofibular ligament (CFL) and the tibiocalcaneal fascicle of the deltoid ligament (Fig. 7.5).

There is a great variability of descriptions about shape, orientation, and location of the intrinsic (sinus tarsi) ligaments [3–7]. They were described to consist of three different ligaments [8]: (1) the posterior band of the ITCL, (2) the anterior band of the ITCL (also known as the cervical ligament), and (3) the inferior extensor retinaculum.

Together the ITCL and cervical ligament stabilize the subtalar joint and form a barrier between the anterior and posterior joint capsules. These ligaments, which cross obliquely through the canalis tarsi, have been described as the "cruciate ligaments of the subtalar joint" [9].

7.2.1 The Cervical Ligament

The cervical ligament lies anterior and lateral to the interosseous ligament and runs from the cervical tubercle of the calcaneus anteriorly and medially to the talar neck (Fig. 7.5a). The cervical ligament lies within the sinus tarsi and provides support to both the anterior and posterior joints [10]. It is the strongest of the subtalar ligaments and has been shown to resist supination during in vitro kinematic experiments [5, 9, 11].

7.2.2 The Interosseous Talocalcaneal Ligament

The interosseous talocalcaneal ligament (ITCL) lies just posterior to, and courses more medially than, the cervical ligament (Fig. 7.5a). The ITCL originates on the calcaneus just anterior to the posterior subtalar joint capsule and runs superiorly and medially to its insertion on the talar neck. Because of its diagonal orientation and oblique fiber arrangement across the joint, portions of the ITCL are taut throughout pronation and supination [7, 9, 11]. This ligament is sometimes called the ligament of the canalis tarsi [7].

7.2.3 The Inferior Extensor Retinacula

Fibers of the inferior extensor retinacula have also been proposed to provide support to the lateral aspect of the subtalar joint [5] (Fig. 7.6).

7.2.4 The Peripheral Ligaments of the Subtalar Joint

The peripheral ligaments of the subtalar joint include the calcaneofibular (CFL), lateral talocalcaneal (LTCL), and fibulotalocalcaneal (FTCL) ligaments.

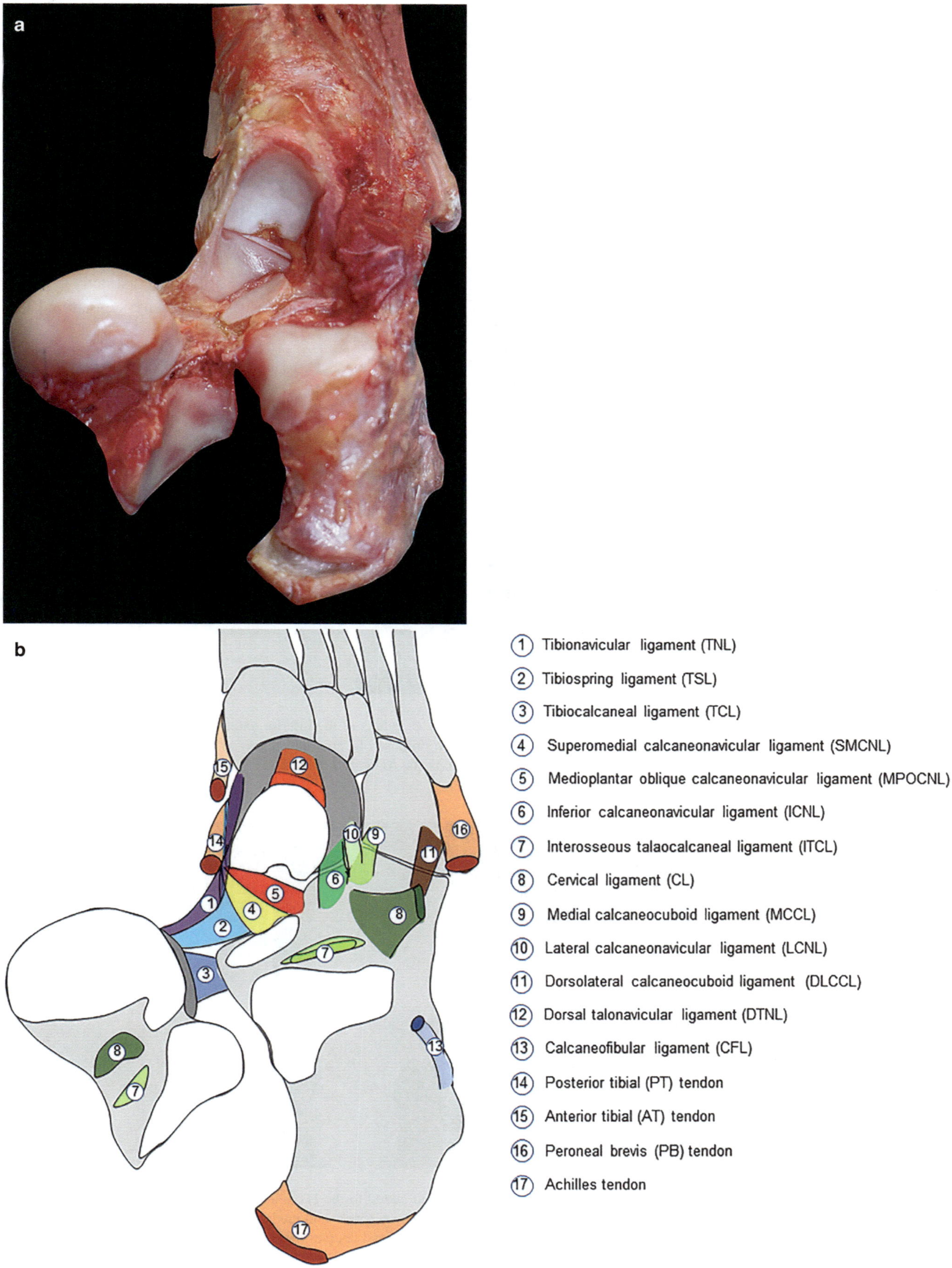

Fig. 7.3 Superior view of the subtalar and talocalcaneonavicular joints. This articulation is similar to a ball-and-socket joint, with the talar head being the ball and the anterior calcaneal and proximal navicular surfaces forming the socket in conjunction with the spring ligament. (**a**) Photograph; (**b**) Drawing

7.2.4.1 The Calcaneofibular Ligament

The calcaneofibular ligament (CFL) is integral in preventing excessive inversion and internal rotation of the calcaneus in relation to the talus [7, 11, 12] (Fig. 7.5a, b). While the CFL does not normally connect the calcaneus to the talus, various attachments of the anterior aspect of the CFL to the talus have been reported [5].

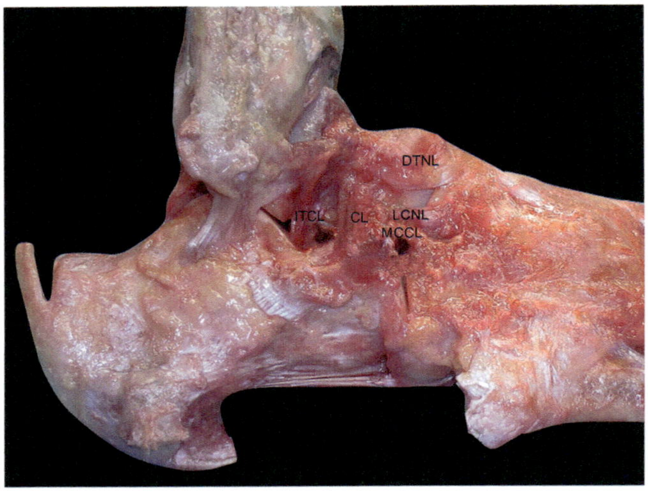

Fig. 7.4 The anterior and posterior subtalar joints have separate ligamentous joint capsules (removed in this picture) and are separated from each other by the sinus tarsi and canalis tarsi. The cervical ligament (CL) and interosseous talocalcaneal ligament (ITCL) form a barrier between the anterior and posterior joint capsules as well as stabilize the subtalar joint. The medial calcaneocuboid (MCCL) and lateral calcaneonavicular (LCNL) ligaments form the bifurcatum ligament. *DTNL* dorsal talonavicular ligament

7.2.4.2 The Lateral Talocalcaneal Ligament

The lateral talocalcaneal ligament (LTCL) runs parallel and anterior to the CFL but only crosses the posterior subtalar joint (Fig. 7.5a). While the LTCL is smaller and weaker than the CFL, it helps prevent excessive supination of the subtalar joint [7, 9, 13].

7.2.4.3 The Fibulotalocalcaneal Ligament

The fibulotalocalcaneal ligaments (FTCL), or ligament of Rouvière, run from the posterior surface of the lateral malleolus to the posterolateral surface of the talus and then to the posterolateral calcaneus (Fig. 7.5b). It lies distinctly posterior to the CFL and assists in resisting excessive supination [9].

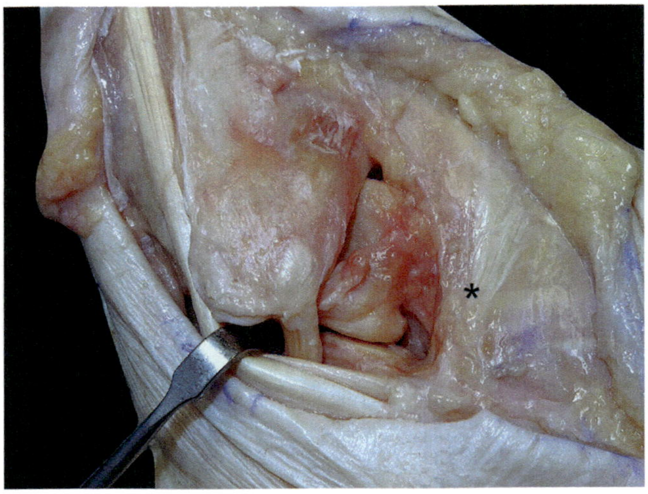

Fig. 7.6 Fibers of the inferior extensor retinacula (asterisk) have also been proposed to provide support to the lateral aspect of the subtalar joint. The ATFL is dissected

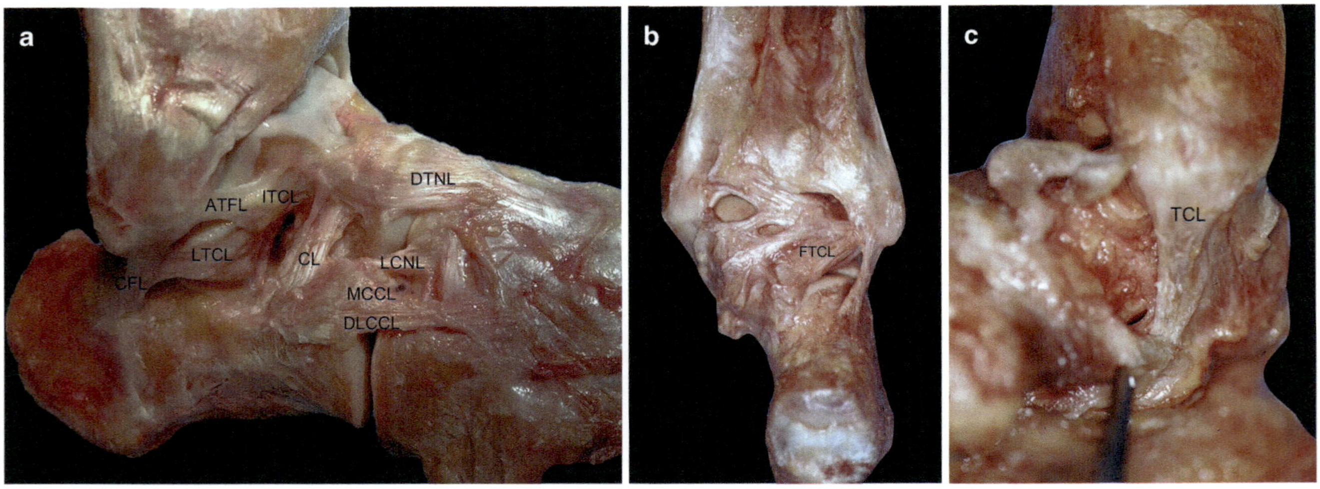

Fig. 7.5 (**a**) Lateral, (**b**) posterior, and (**c**) medial view of the ankle joint: The deep ligaments consist of the cervical (CL) and interosseous talocalcaneal (ITCL) ligaments, whereas the peripheral ligaments of the subtalar joint include the calcaneofibular (CFL), lateral talocalcaneal (LTCL), and fibulotalocalcaneal (FTCL) ligaments. The CL lies anterior and lateral to the ITCL and runs from the cervical tubercle of the calcaneus anteriorly and medially to the talar neck. The ITCL lies just posterior to and courses more medially than the cervical ligament. The tibiocalcaneal ligament (TCL) runs from the anterior colliculus of the medial malleolus to the sustentaculum tali

7.3 Joint Axis and Motion

- Due to the complex joint anatomy and the difficulties in precise measurements of bone motion, determining the axis of rotation and specific joint motion is difficult.
- For pronation-supination, more motion occurs at the talonavicular than at the subtalar joint.

Due to the complex joint anatomy and the difficulties in precise measurement of bone motion (particularly for the talus), the details of subtalar joint motion has not been well documented [3, 14–16]. Although the primary motion of this joint has been described as hinge-like, screw-like, or multiaxial [6], it has been well recognized that the axis of subtalar joint shows some variations. Should the subtalar joint act as a mitered hinge connecting the talus and the calcaneus, and be inclined 45° from transverse, a simple torque converter is created. Meaning, rotation of the vertical member is coupled to equal rotation of the horizontal member. A vertically aligned subtalar joint axis (over 45°), such as that of a cavus foot, causes less rotation of the horizontal segment for a given rotation of the vertical one. A more horizontally aligned axis (as in a flatfoot) causes a greater rotation of the horizontal member for a given rotation of the vertical member [17].

The sagittal plane is the least dominant plane in the subtalar joint motion so that subtalar joint impairments may not affect progression of gait, which depends on sagittal plane motion. Therefore the subtalar joint was considered a nonessential joint for gait and posture as long as it is properly aligned [18]. This may explain why subtalar arthrodesis works quite well when compared with fusion of the ankle or the talonavicular joints [17].

During foot pronation/supination, the largest amount of motion occurs at the talonavicular joint followed by the talocalcaneal joint; in the latter, motion occurs mainly by supination [19, 20]. Fusion of the talonavicular joint completely blocks motion at the subtalar joint, but not oppositely: fusion of the subtalar joint allows for significant motion at the neighboring joints, including the talonavicular joint [21]. During pronation, the sinus tarsi closes because the lateral process of the talus glides anteriorly towards the prethalamic surface of the calcaneus. During foot supination, the sinus tarsi opens.

7.4 Biomechanics of Peritalar Instability

- Under physiological conditions there is an equilibrium of the acting forces, supported by the intrinsic stability of the tibiotalar (ankle) joint, thus stabilizing the talus on top of the calcaneus.
- With loss of stability of the tibiotalar (ankle) joint, the subtalar joint does not seem to be able to compensate for the instability and starts to tilt.
- This tilting leads to the primary loss of subtalar stability which may result in peritalar instability, typically seen as an instability in the sagittal plane.

7.4.1 Stable Tibiotalar (Ankle) Joint

The highly congruent talocrural joint was found to provide as much as 100% talar frontal plane stability while the foot is loaded [22], suggesting that incompetence of the collateral ligaments will not affect talar position within the ankle (Fig. 7.7). As the talus does not have direct muscle attachments, this bone has a "sandwich"-like position, which is controlled and manipulated by forces applied through the proximal and distal segments.

Under physiological conditions there is equilibrium of the acting forces supported by the intrinsic stability of tibiotalar joint. The posterior facet of the subtalar joint has a convex/concave surface like a ball-and-socket type joint. The configuration of the posterior facet allows rotational movements which especially support the accommodation during walking or running on uneven ground (Fig. 7.7b). The anterior facet of the subtalar joint has a more flat configuration, therefore translational movements in the subtalar joint occur more through this joint facet (Fig. 7.7c). The contour of osseous structures from the lateral view is oblique meaning that the talus has a general tendency to slide anteriorly under higher ankle loading.

7.4.2 Unstable Tibiotalar (Ankle) Joint

In cases without the contribution of intrinsic stability of the tibiotalar joint, the subtalar joint does not seem to be able to compensate for the instability and starts to tilt, resulting in peritalar instability [23] (Fig. 7.8). In some cases, the calcaneus follows the orientation of talus; in the majority of cases

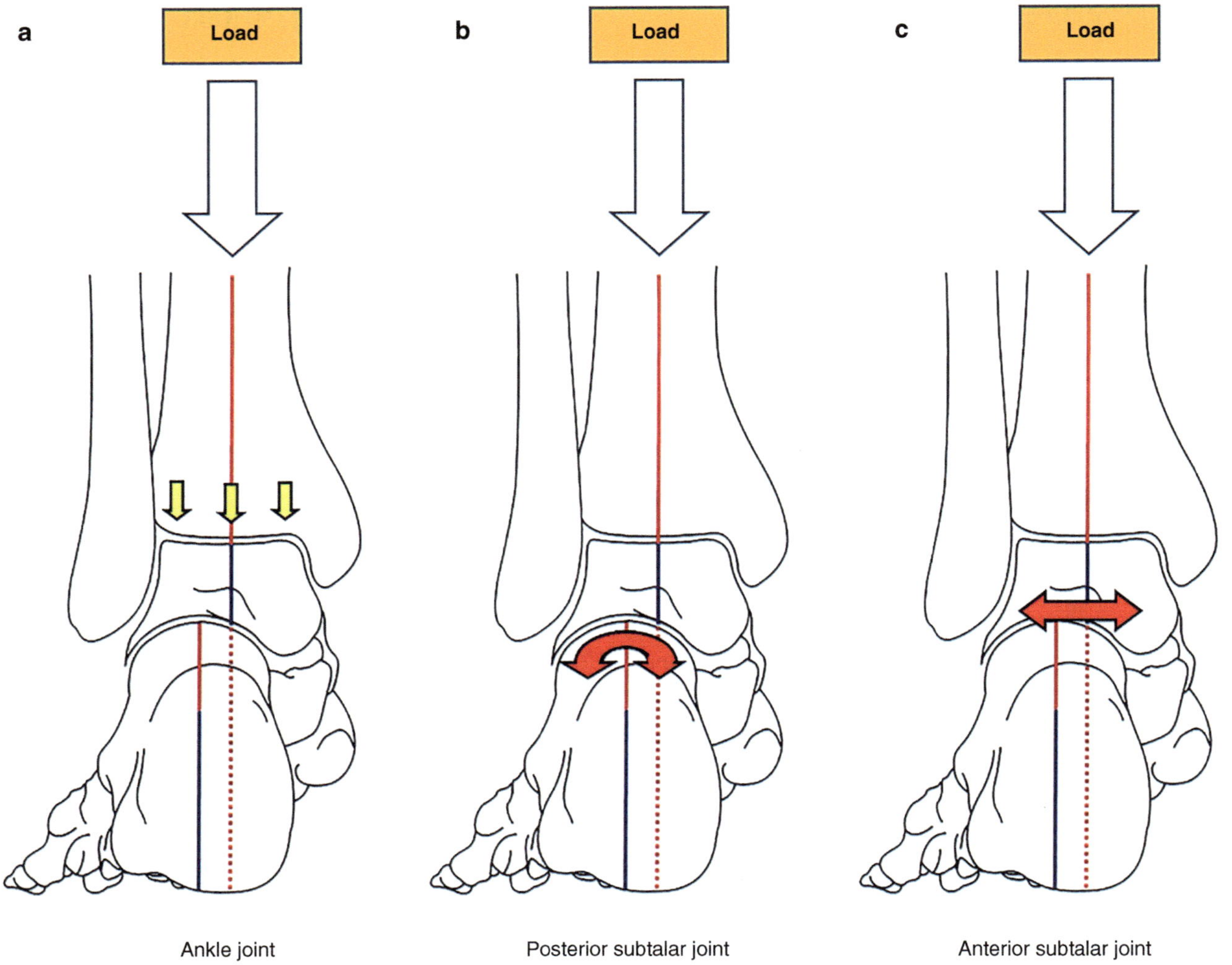

Fig. 7.7 Loading pattern and joint forces found in a physiologically balanced ankle joint complex: **a**) tibiotalar joint, **b**) posterior talocalcaneal joint, and **c**) anterior talocalcaneal joint. The tibiotalar joint load is symmetric (yellow arrows). "Reproduced with permission from Hintermann B, Knupp M, Barg A. Peritalar instability. Foot Ankle Int. 2012 May;33(5):450–4. doi: https://doi.org/10.3113/FAI.2012.0450. PMID: 22735291

the calcaneus goes in the opposite direction, resulting in a so-called "zigzag" or "z-shaped" deformity [23] (Fig. 7.9). Such contradictory movement of the calcaneus may often result in a clinical appearance of a well-aligned hindfoot. As its height has decreased, the surrounding soft tissue structures do typically demonstrate additional loss of tension with clinical appearance of a "floppy hindfoot."

Subsequentially, the forces of the tibialis posterior and peroneus brevis that act distally in the functional hindfoot chain [24–26] may influence the deformity process, as both muscles cause a pulling effect especially at the distal segment of the foot/hindfoot complex.

7.4.3 Unstable Peritalar Joints

If the instability originates primarily from the peritalar joints, while intrinsic stability of the ankle is preserved, a complex translational movement of the talus in the sagittal plane occurs along the posterior facet, associated with a dorsiflexion movement, which results in a decreased talocalcaneal angle (Fig. 7.10). The integrity of the tibiotalar (ankle) joint remains intact (Fig. 7.11). The effect of loading the foot on unstable peritalar joint can be seen when comparing a standard non-weight-bearing with weight-bearing radiographs (Fig. 7.12).

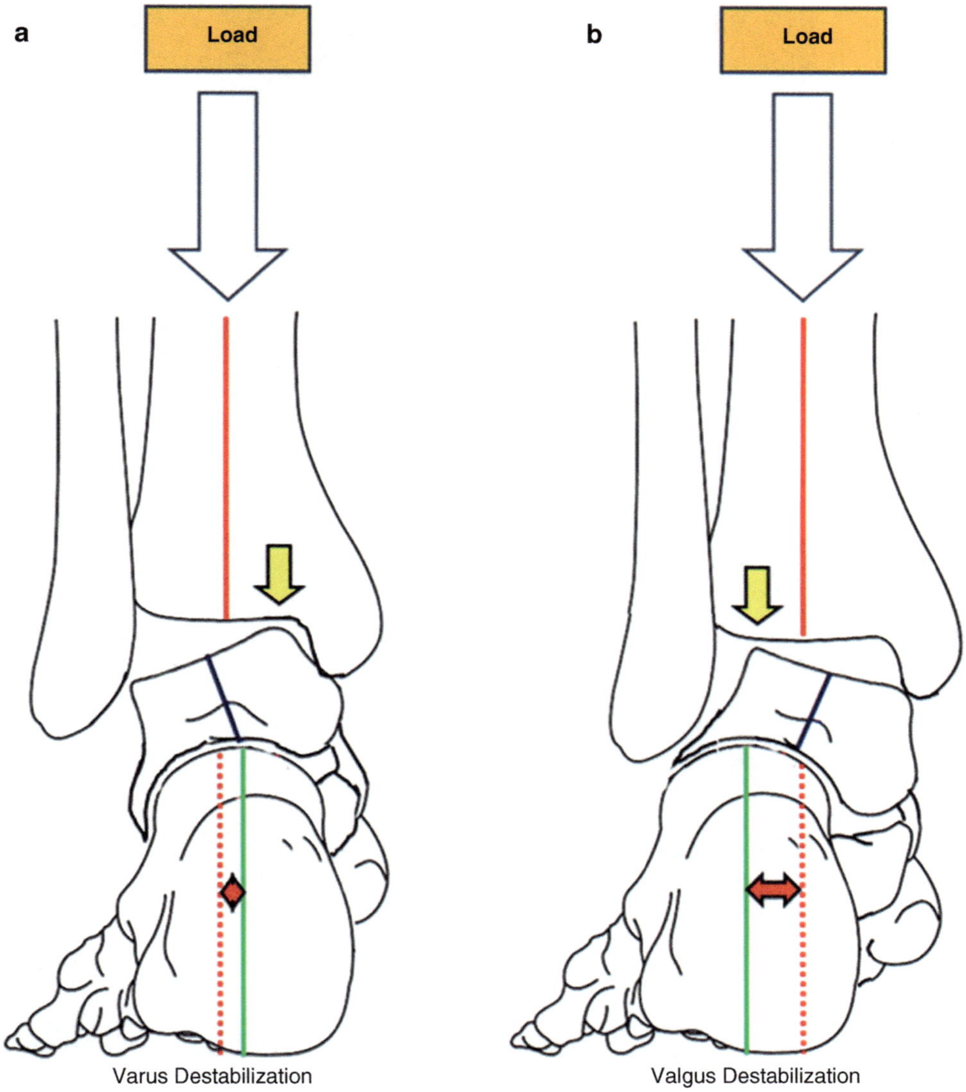

Fig. 7.8 With loss of intrinsic stability of the tibiotalar joint, the talus tilts into (**a**) varus or (**b**) valgus, whereas the subtalar joint can compensate for the instability by an opposing movement. The calcaneus remains aligned, but it typically moves more towards lateral in a valgus ankle as it does towards medially in a varus ankle (red arrows). Peak joint load in a varus tilted talus is found in the medial tibiotalar joint and in a valgus tilted talus in the lateral tibiotalar joint (yellow arrows)

7.5 Conclusions and Clinical Implications

Peritalar instability is the result of a complex destabilization of the talus on top of the calcaneal surfaces that results in a varus or valgus tilt movement, and/or translational and rotational movements of the talus on top of the calcaneus. Typically, the deformity increases when the foot is loaded. The calcaneus may follow the movement and orientation of the talus; however, in most cases, the calcaneus goes in the opposite direction, resulting in a clinical appearance of a well-aligned hindfoot.

7.6 History and Clinical Findings

- Patients often cannot report on the precise injury mechanism.
- Clinical symptoms of an instability at either the ankle or peritalar level are very similar, therefore it is often hard to distinguish between the two.

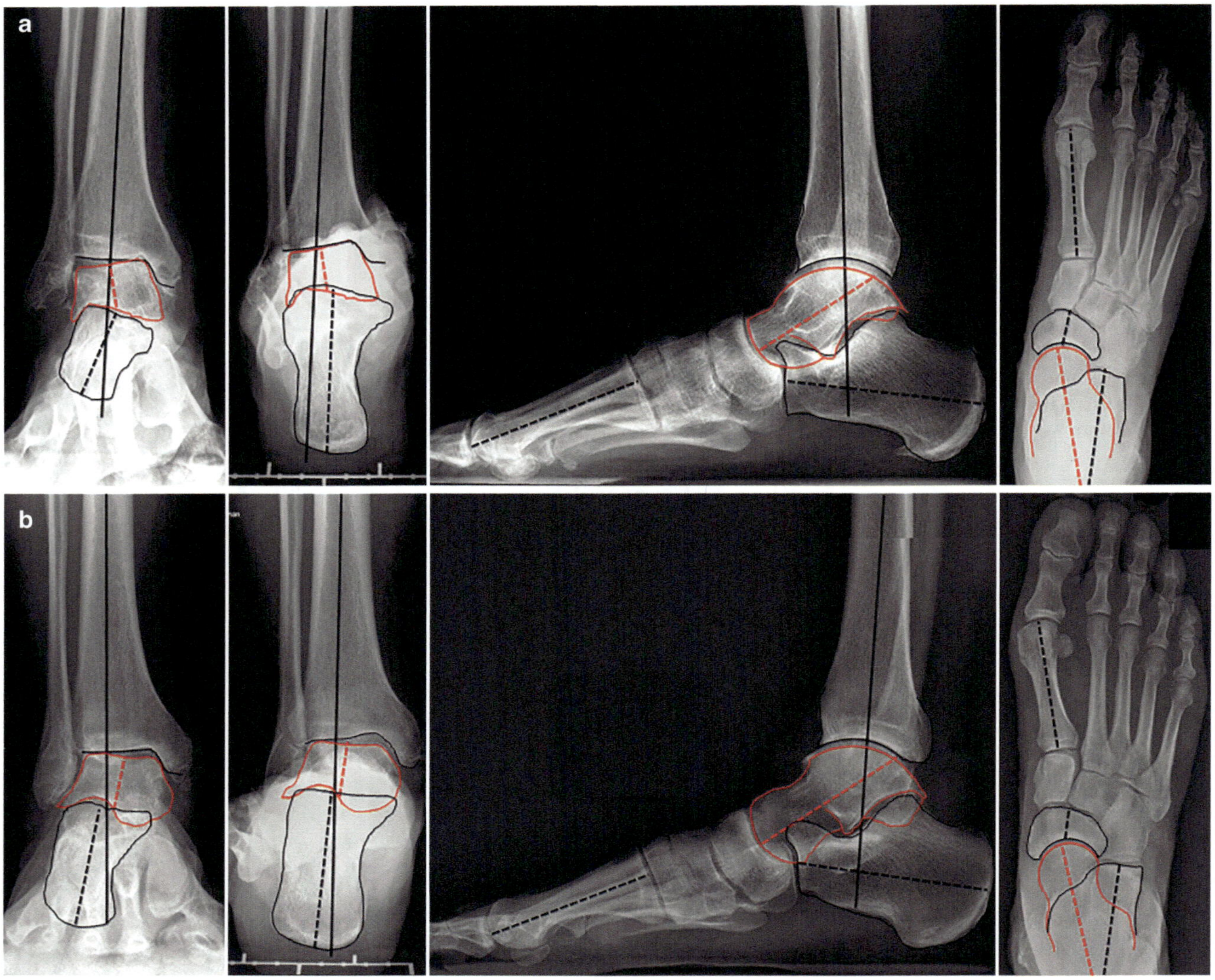

Fig. 7.9 Standard weight-bearing radiographs (AP, hindfoot, lateral, and DP view) of a (**a**) varus-valgus deformity, and (**b**) valgus-varus deformity, showing a contradictory movement of the calcaneus (see text). In the varus-valgus deformity, the sinus tarsi is typically closed which may result in sinus tarsi impingement (see lateral view of Fig. 7.9a)

7.6.1 History

Most patients give a history of an acute sprain in the past, but often they cannot report on the precise injury mechanism. They typically complain about permanent or recurrent feeling of instability of the ankle like "rolling over" or "giving away" [3, 23, 27–29]. Because the clinical symptoms of an instability at either the ankle or peritalar level are very similar, it is often hard to distinguish between the two [3, 27, 30]. Additional symptoms include recurrent swelling, painful stiffness of the subtalar joint, and diffuse pain in the hindfoot with significant aggravation during sports activities or walking on uneven ground [27, 29]. Furthermore, some patients stated that they must look at the ground constantly or feel insecure while walking in the night [30]. Patients with peritalar instability prefer to wear high top shoes, or a hindfoot stabilizing orthotic.

7.6.2 Clinical Presentation

In the acute phase after injury to the peritalar joints, the clinical findings are similar to those in patients with severe ankle sprain: ecchymosis/hematoma, swelling, and tenderness, often localized laterally in the area of the sinus tarsi or medially in the area of the deltoid/spring ligament complex. In the chronic phase, lower limb and hindfoot alignment may show a wide variation of abnormalities, such as pronation or supination which are often associated to a neutral heel alignment that can result in a zigzag position of the hindfoot [23](Fig. 7.13). While the patient is sitting with hanging feet, manual stress testing may reveal rotational and translational instability of the calcaneus that can be associated with increased varus or valgus talar tilt (Fig. 2.14).

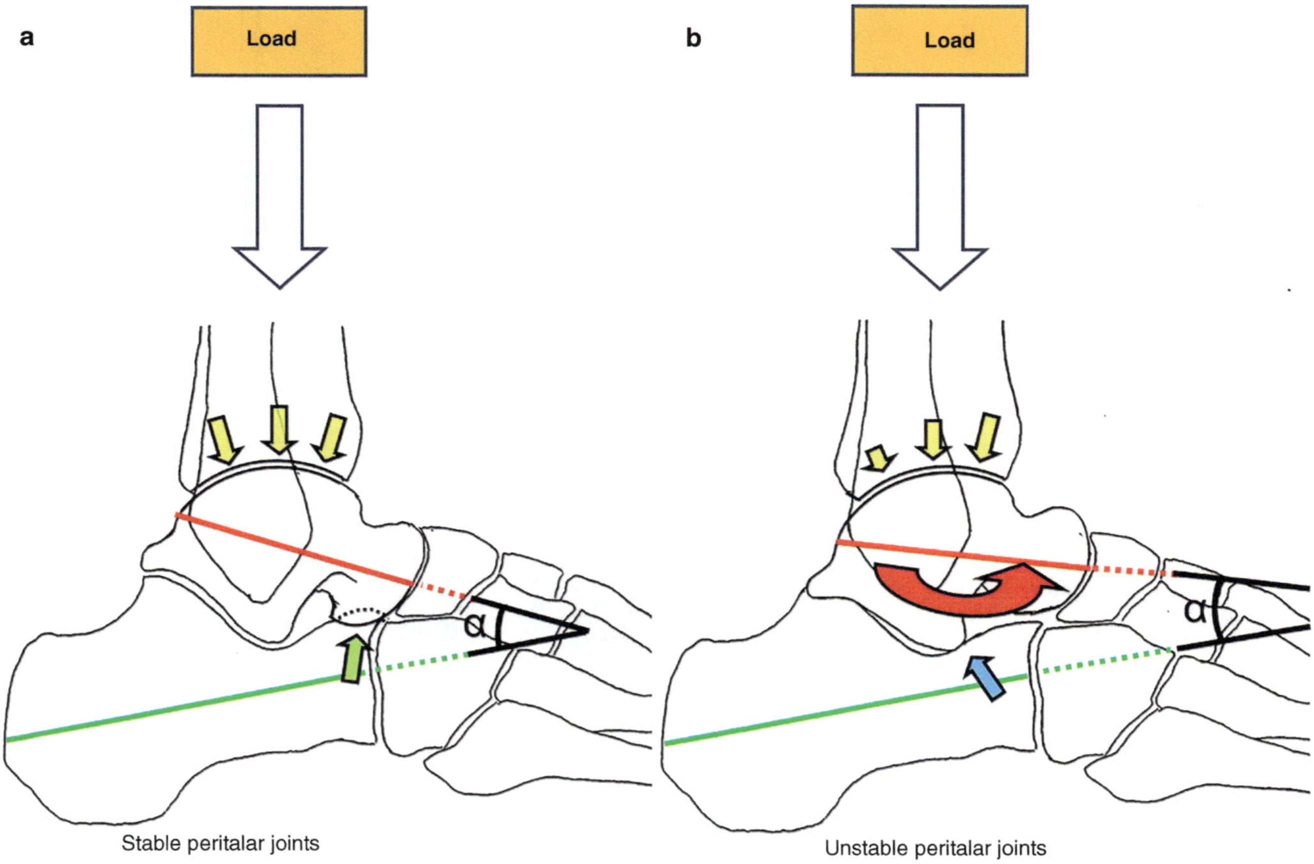

Fig. 7.10 (**a**) An illustration showing loading pattern and joint forces in a physiologically balanced ankle joint complex in the sagittal plane. There exists a symmetrical tibiotalar joint load and a talocalcaneal angle (α) of 25–35°. Typically, there is an overlap of anterior process of calcaneus to the talar head (green arrow). (**b**) In the case of primary instability of the peritalar joints, the talus translates towards anterior along the oblique posterior facet of the calcaneus and the talar head moves up, resulting in an increased tibiotalar joint load at its anterior part and a decreased talocalcaneal angle. Typically, sinus tarsi impingement occurs (blue arrow). As the intrinsic stability of the tibiotalar joint is preserved, the talus does not tilt in the frontal plane

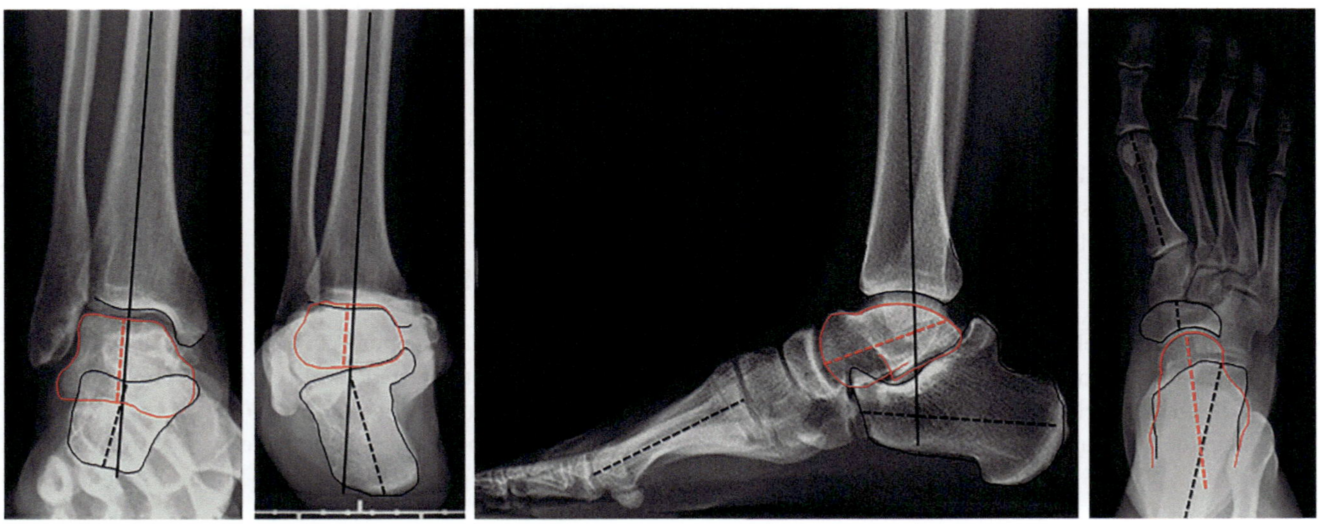

Fig. 7.11 Standard weight-bearing radiographs (AP, hindfoot, lateral, and DP view) of a patient with primary peritalar instability. This results in a complex translational and rotational movement of the talus in the sagittal plane during foot loading, whereas the stability of tibiotalar joint in coronal plane remains preserved. The talus may rotate externally in the horizontal plane, and the calcaneus may tilt into varus

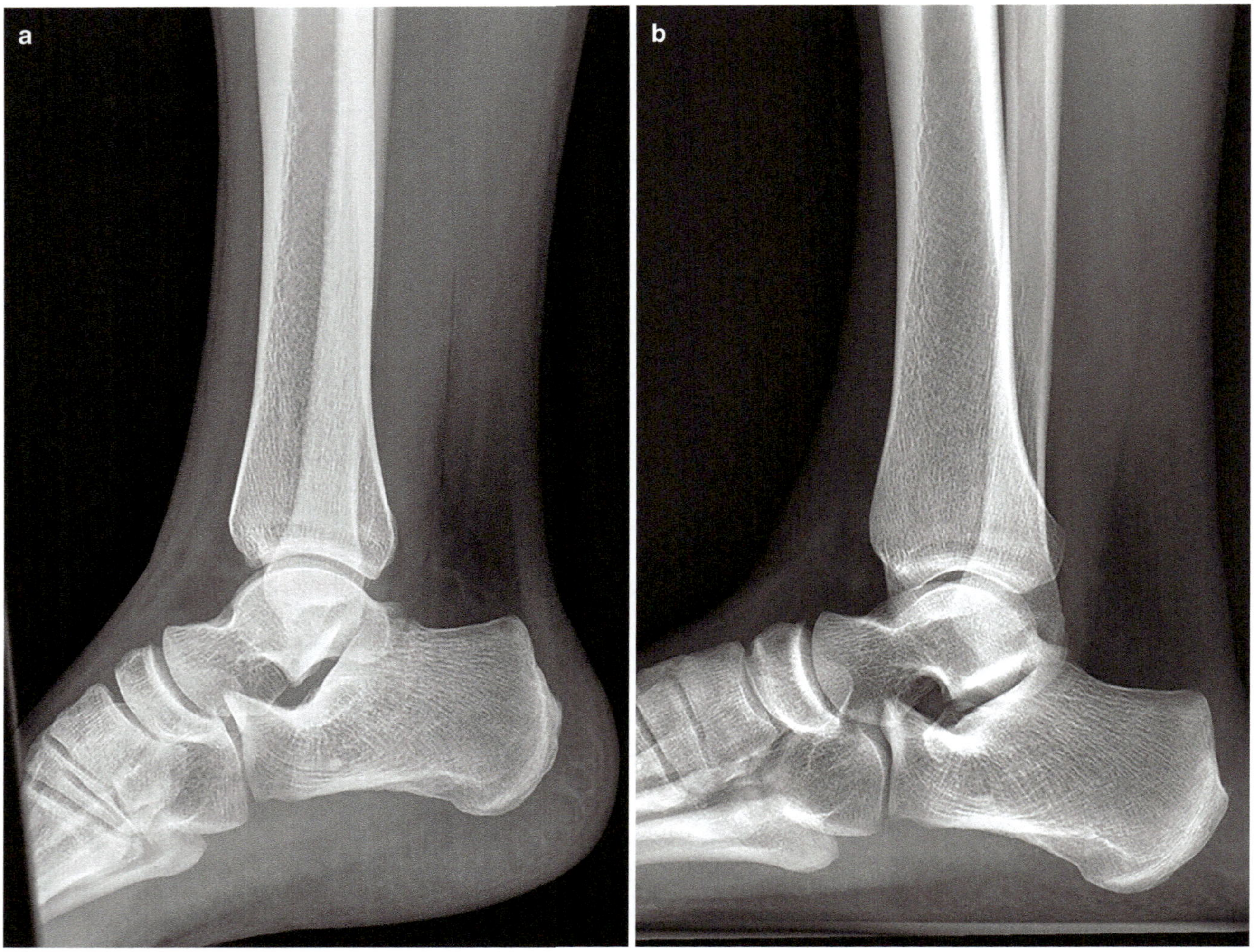

Fig. 7.12 Effect of weight-bearing of a foot with peritalar instability shown in a standard lateral radiograph. (**a**) Without weight bearing: The talus is in a moderate dorsiflexion position of talus associated with a symmetric gapping in the subtalar joint. (**b**) With weight-bearing: The talus has shifted anteriorly, and the dorsiflexion has increased, resulting in a limited contact area in the posterior subtalar joint

7.7 Imaging

- Separation of the posterior facet of the calcaneus and talus, the subtalar tilt angle, and the anterior displacement of the calcaneus on the talus are the main radiological findings indicating chronic subtalar instability.
- MRI may be helpful to detect ligament injuries and associated osteochondral lesions.
- CT scan, especially with weight-bearing, allows a more detailed analysis of the subtalar joint.

Peritalar instability allows the talus to rotate and translate on the calcaneal and navicular bone surfaces, thereby resulting in a 3-D positional change. Progresses in imaging modalities, particularly weight-bearing CT scan, have brought more insight in this pathology.

7.7.1 Radiography

Radiographic assessment of the peritalar instability includes AP, lateral, and mortise views of the ankle and the dorsoplantar view of the foot (Fig. 7.14). All radiographs should be performed with weight-bearing to assess the functional deformities of the hindfoot. In order to

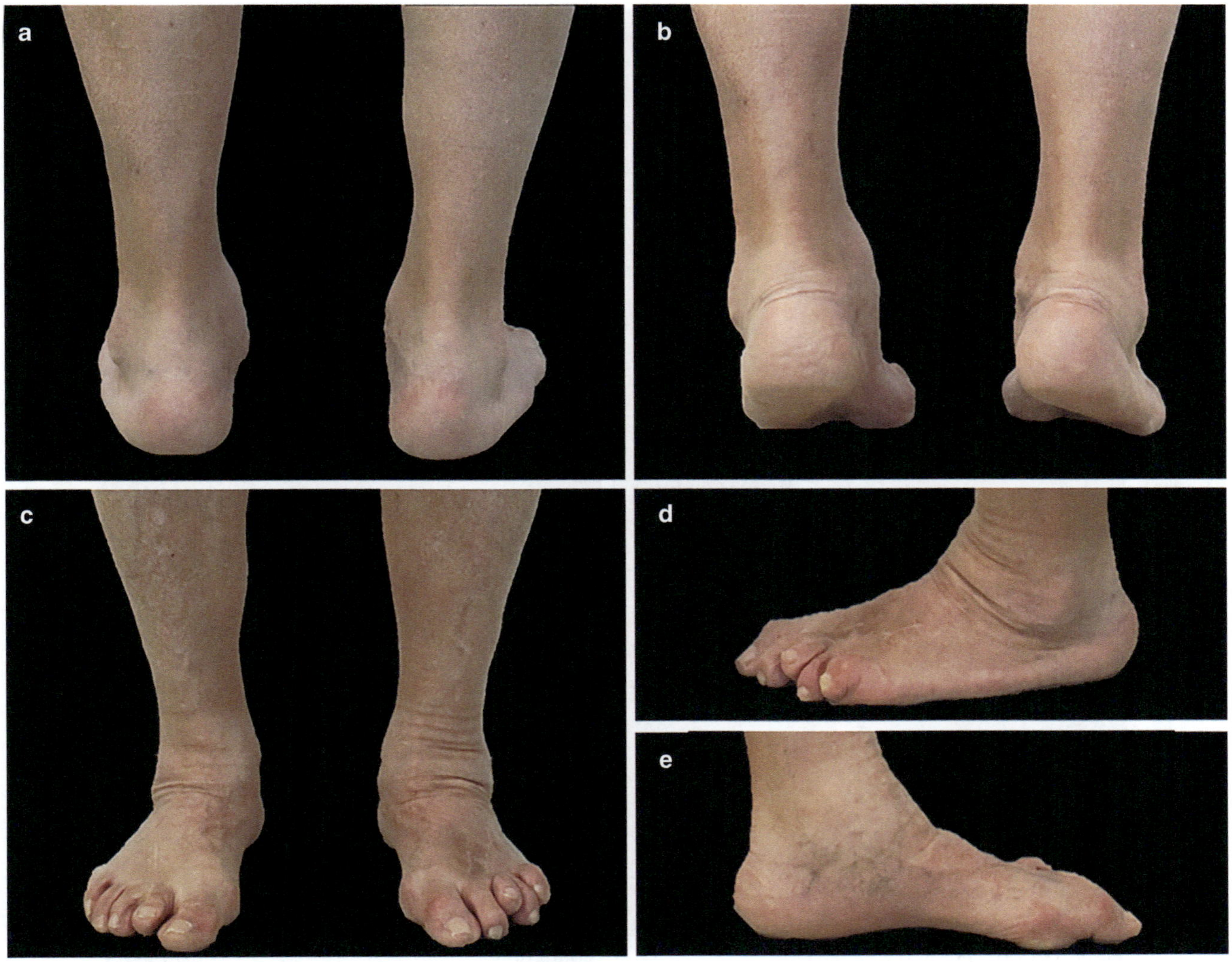

Fig. 7.13 A 67-year-old former soccer player with peritalar instability associated to valgus destabilization of the right ankle joint. (**a**) Viewed from posterior, the foot looks aligned, but slightly externally rotated and thickened when compared to the contralateral side; (**b**) in tiptoe position, there is less varization movement; (**c**) Viewed from anterior, the foot looks symmetrical with a slight internal rotation; Viewed from (**d**) lateral and (**e**) medial, the foot does not show significant changes

assess the calcaneus position in relationship to the longitudinal axis of the tibia, the Saltzman view (hindfoot alignment view) should be performed [31] (Fig. 7.15). Bilateral radiographic assessment may be helpful for comparison.

Separation of the posterior facet of the calcaneus and talus [32] (Fig. 7.16), the subtalar tilt angle [33] (Fig. 7.17), and the anterior displacement of the calcaneus on the talus [28] (Fig. 7.18) have been described to indicate chronic subtalar instability. Subtalar stress radiography can also be used to quantify subtalar instability. Subtalar arthrography, in contrast, can help to identify and quantify ligament lesions [34, 35].

7.7.2 MRI

With MRI, it is possible to document structural alterations of the ligaments and chondral lesions in correlation with acute or chronic trauma (Fig. 7.19). Arthro-MRI of the posterior subtalar joint allows to see little bone insertional detachments of the interosseous talocalcaneal ligament. MRI has been shown to have a statistically significant relationship between detection of injured structures and symptoms including giving way and pain [36], and to assess abnormalities of the ligaments [37]. It was also reported that painful intra-articular talocalcaneal impingement can be detected with the use of MRI [38]. Furthermore, degenerative pathol-

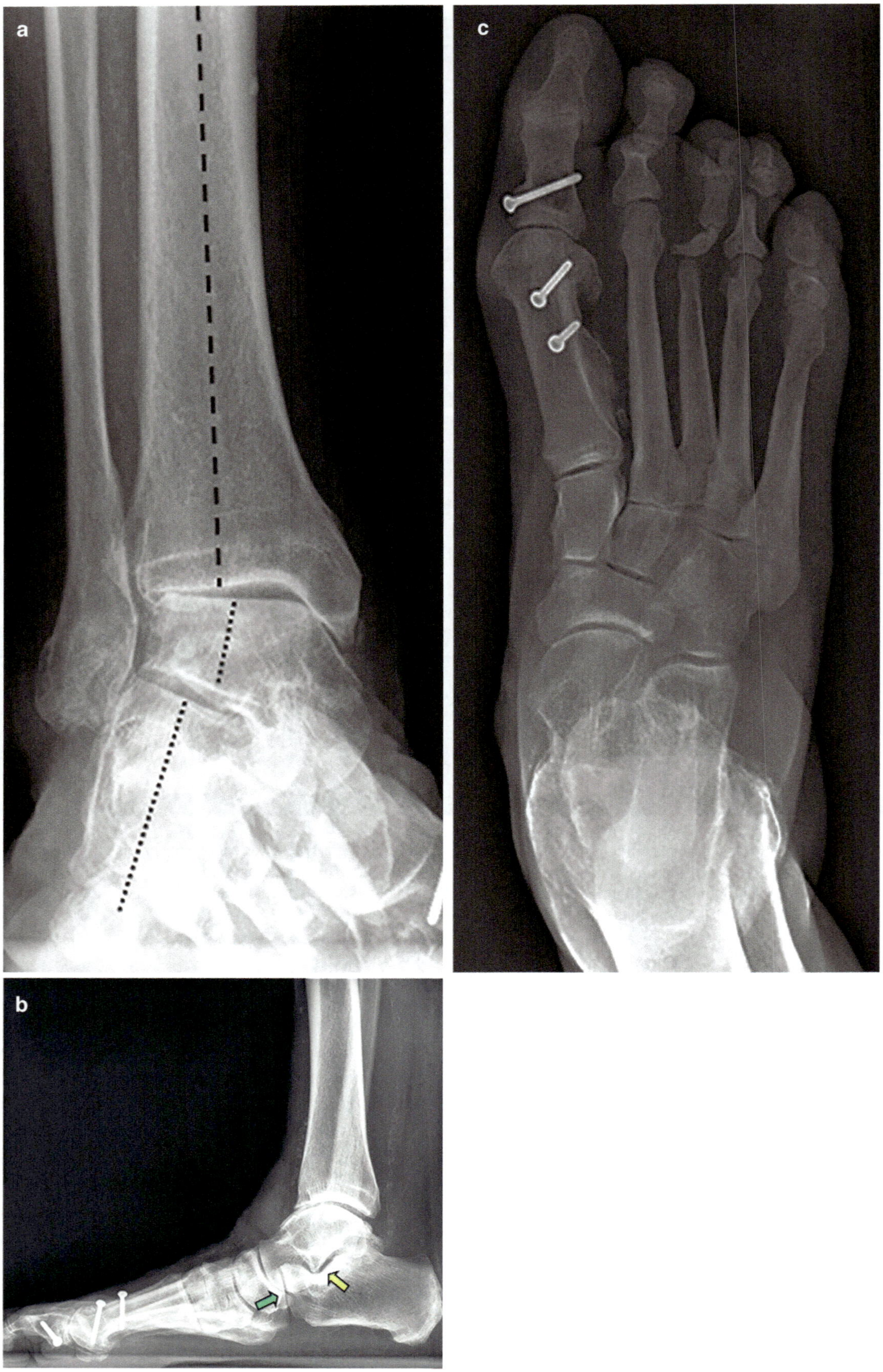

Fig. 7.14 Standard weight-bearing radiographs (same patient as Fig. 7.13): (**a**) AP view of the ankle showing valgus destabilization at the tibiotalar (ankle) joint; (**b**) lateral view of the foot showing a distinct anterior translation of the talus at the tibiotalar joint and an anterior translation of the talus at the talocalcaneal joint with closed sinus tarsi (yellow arrow) and substantial overlap of the anterior calcaneus (green arrow); (**c**) DP view of the foot showing regular position of the foot

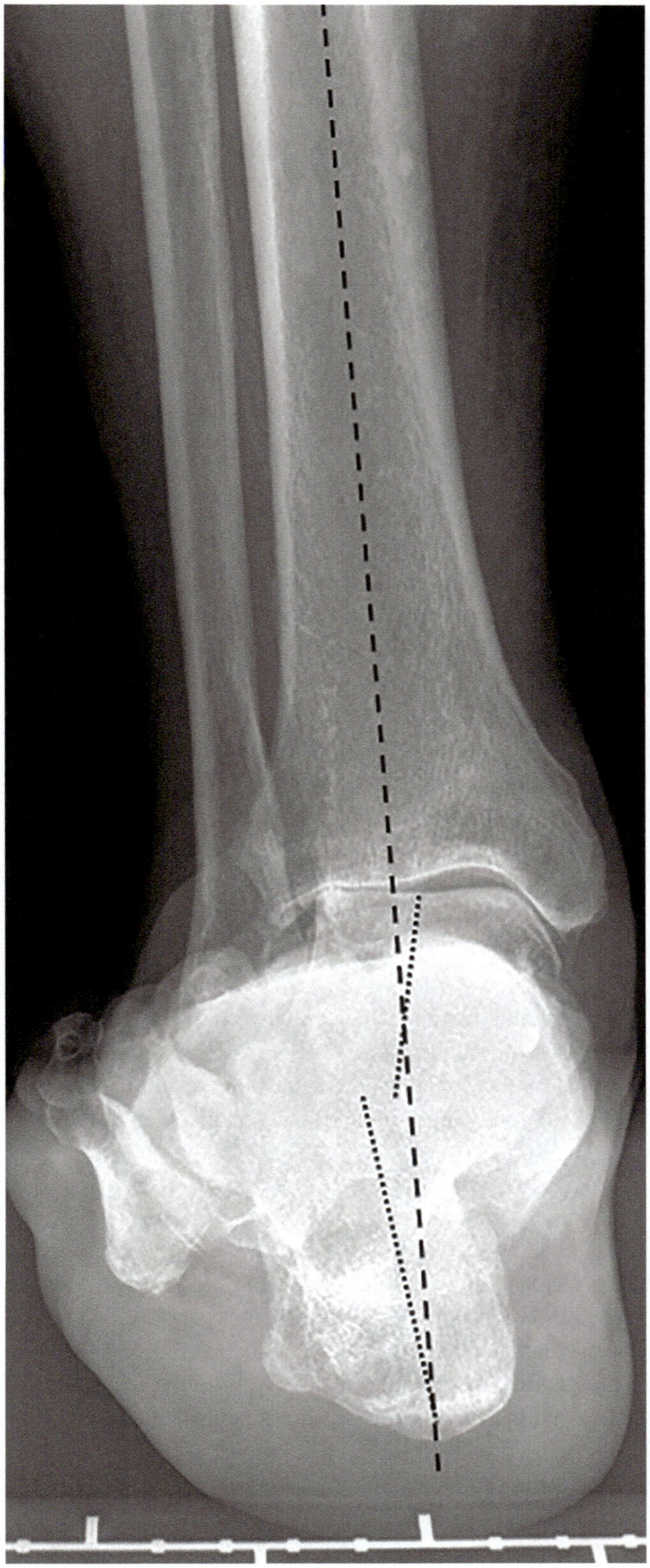

Fig. 7.15 A Saltzman hindfoot alignment view (same patient as Fig. 7.13) showing a neutral alignment, despite the presence of a valgus tilt at the tibiotalar joint. This is due to a compensatory varus tilt at the talocalcaneal (subtalar) joint

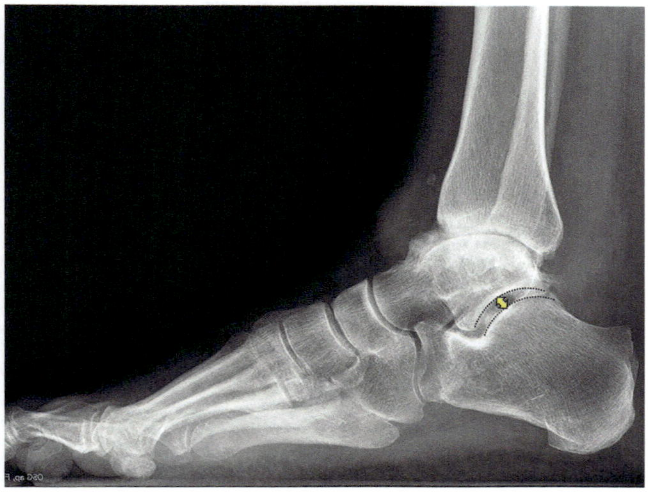

Fig. 7.16 Lateral view showing the separation of the posterior facet of the calcaneus and the talus (arrow)

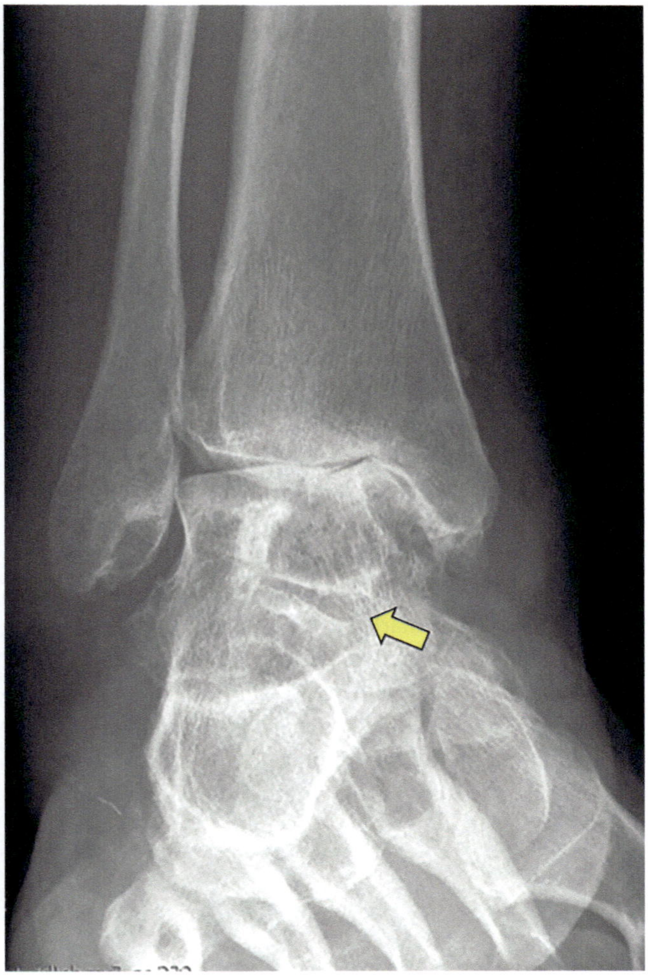

Fig. 7.17 AP view showing the subtalar tilt angle (arrow)

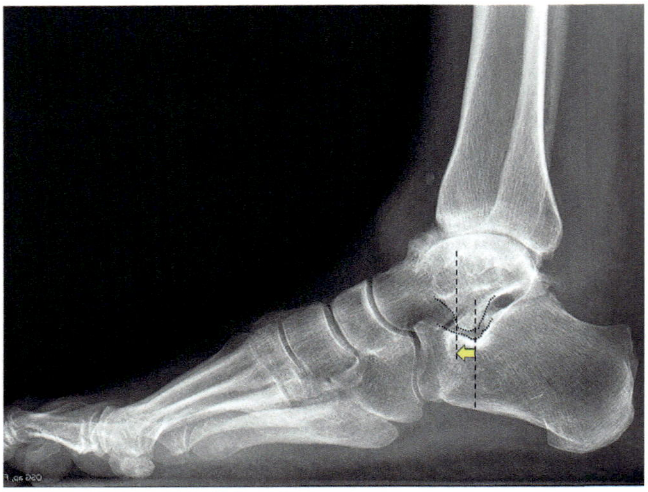

Fig. 7.18 Lateral view showing the anterior displacement of the calcaneus on the talus (arrow)

ogy of the subtalar joint that may develop in patients with chronic laxity [39] can also be seen with MRI.

7.7.3 CT Scan

With the introduction of weight-bearing CT scans, a more detailed analysis of the subtalar joint during loading became possible [40, 41]. Recent studies using weight-bearing CT have shown that the morphology of the posterior facet in the coronal plane differs between individuals [41–48] (Fig. 7.20).

Weight-bearing CT images have been established as a great dynamic imaging tool to demonstrate increased deformity in the acquired flatfoot deformity (AAFD) [40, 49, 50]. An increased subluxation among the patients with AAFD of 56% was reported versus 13% among the controls at the anterior and middle facets and 30% versus 11% at the posterior facet [51]. Currently, the middle facet is used as an isolated marker for peritalar instability, with a mean subluxation (uncoverage) of approximately 45% in symptomatic patients with AAFD and 5% among the controls [52] (Fig. 7.21). Measurement of the amount of linear subluxation of the subtalar joint at the posterior facet in the coronal plane was also proposed to indicate peritalar instability [43, 48–50, 53, 54]; however, it was found to be less reliable [52] (Fig. 7.22). Lateral subluxation was reported to cause sinus tarsi (Fig. 7.23) and subfibular impingement [55] (Fig. 7.24).

Although a promising technology for imaging the subtalar joint, weight-bearing CT scans have yet to become a clinical standard.

7.8 Arthroscopy

- Arthroscopy may also be used for assessing injuries to the ligaments and articular surfaces in subtalar instability.

Arthroscopy has become an important diagnostic and therapeutic procedure and may also be used in the diagnosis of subtalar instability [56] (Fig. 7.25). It allows evaluation of the ITCL and allows for stress investigation under direct visualization [57]. A tear of the ITCL has been identified as a cause for subtalar instability [58]. Arthroscopy can also be used to assess sinus tarsi impingement [38].

7.9 Classification of Peritalar Instability

- Often it remains unclear why the talus tilts into varus or valgus.
- Classification thus describes the resulting deformity, but cannot be used to explain the underlying cause.

It remains unclear as to why the talus tilts into various malpositions. Subtalar joint congruency and contact area are low [59] as the talus rests on the convex posterior and flat intermediate and anterior calcaneal facets [23].

To classify the peritalar instability, the first major step of classification is based on the assessment of the talus in the

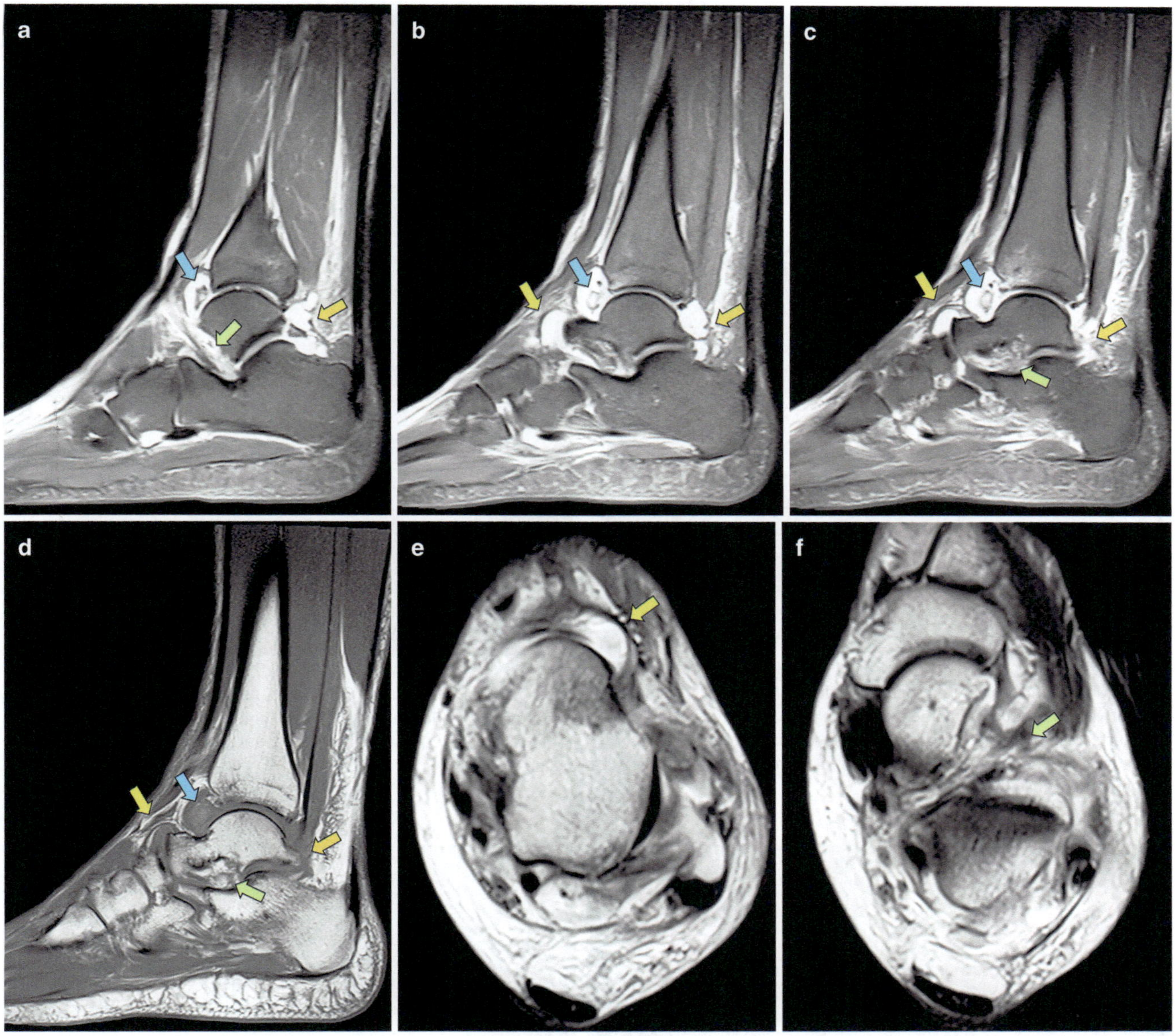

Fig. 7.19 MR imaging in a 32-year-old male patient after an acute sprain of his left hindfoot while bouldering. (**a**) Lateral view (T1) showing bony avulsion of the posterior process of the talus (orange arrow), a fragment from the anterior rim of the tibia (blue arrow) and partial lesion with bony avulsion of the ITCL (green arrow); (**b**) this lateral view (T1) additionally shows the rupture of the dorsal talonavicular ligament with the dorsal capsular of the talonavicular joint (yellow arrow); (**c**) further laterally (T1) an incomplete lesion of the ITLC can be seen (green arrow); (**d**) in a T2 weighted image, the partial lesion of the ITCL can be seen more clearly (green arrow); (**e**) in this horizontal view (T1), the distension of the anterolateral capsular of the talonavicular joint can be seen (yellow arrow); (**f**) more caudally (T1), partial lesion of the ITCL can be seen (green arrow)

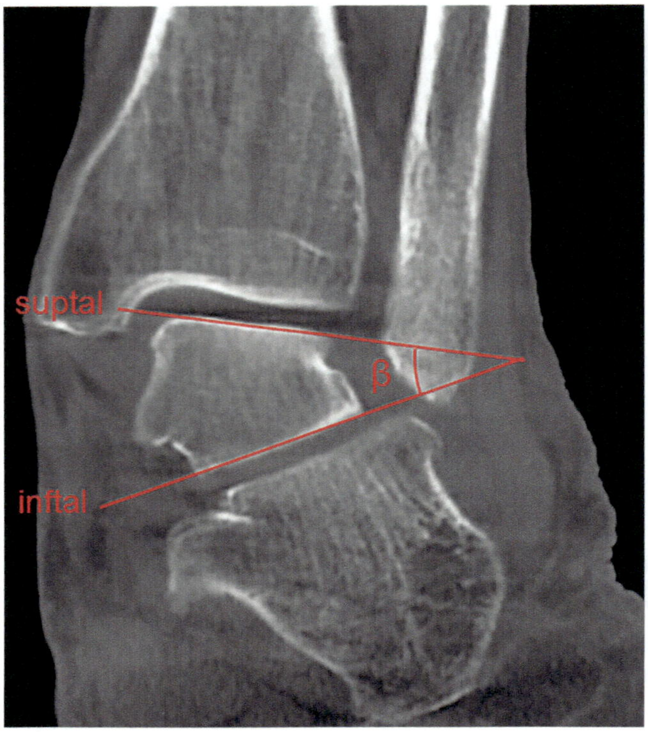

Fig. 7.20 Weight-bearing CT scan: Peritalar instability was found significantly more frequent in patients with an angle between the superior talar surface (suptal) and inferior talar surface (inftal) of more than 17°, indicating that a suptal-inftal angle of >17° is a predisposition for developing peritalar instability

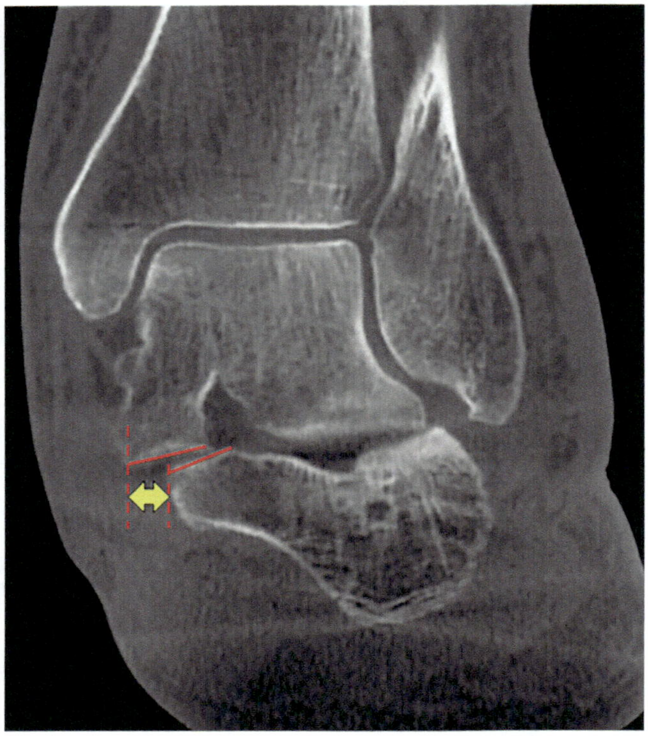

Fig. 7.21 Weight-bearing CT scan: A percentage of uncoverage of the middle facet (yellow arrow) of >18% and an incongruence angle of the middle facet of >8° were found to be a strong predictor of peritalar instability

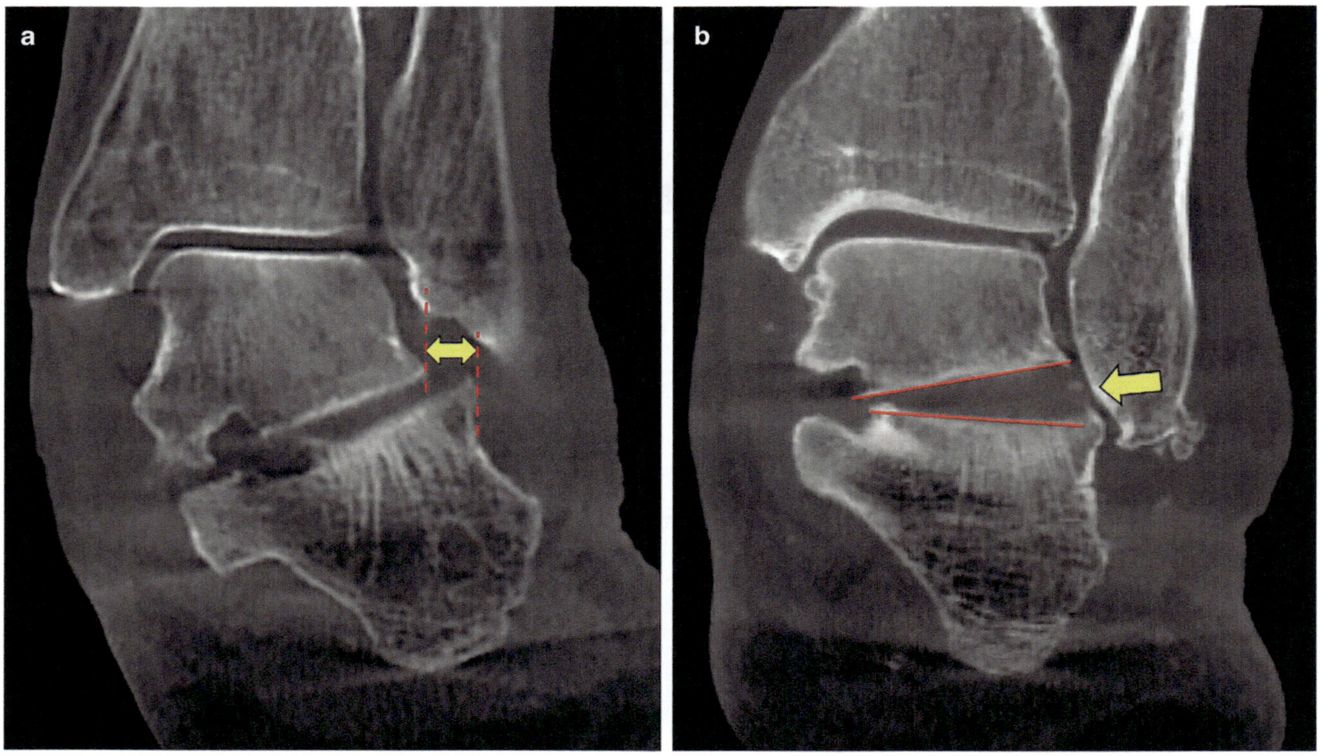

Fig. 7.22 Weight-bearing CT scan: (**a**) Linear and (**b**) angular subluxation at the posterior facet in the coronal plane may also indicate peritalar instability

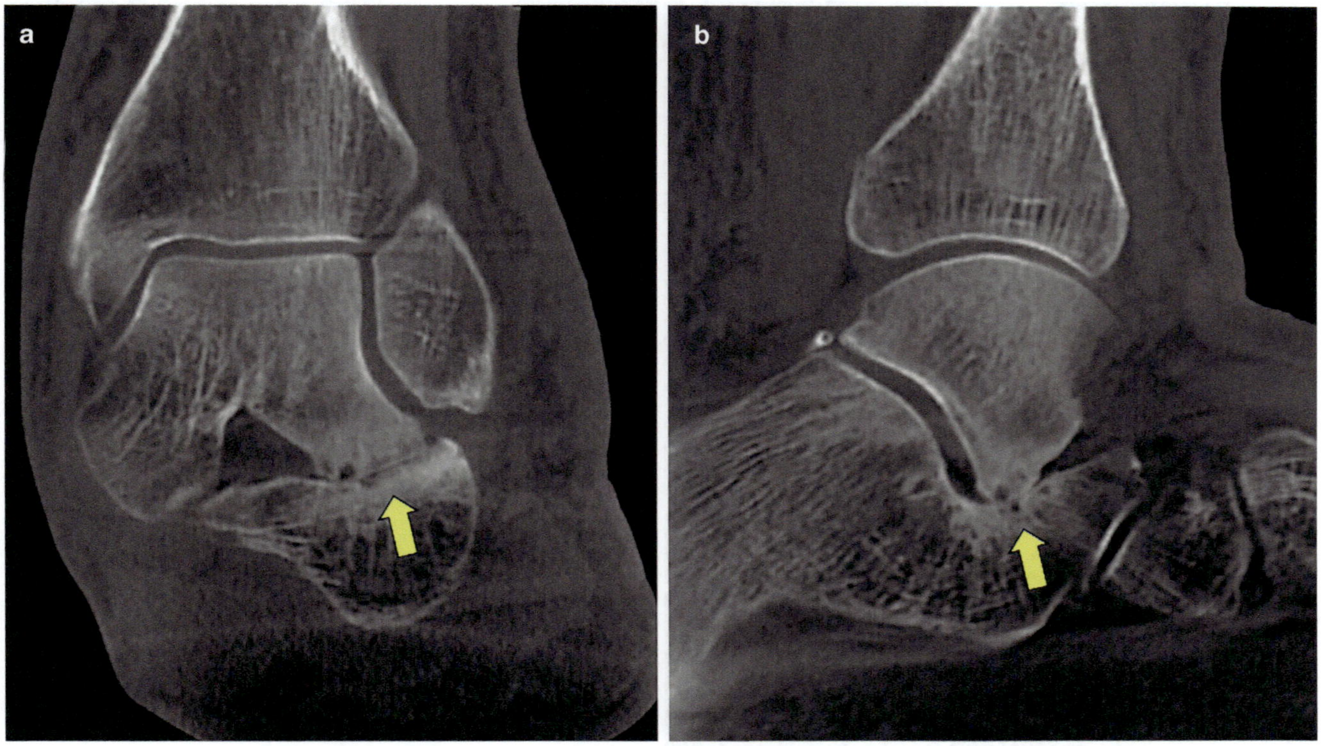

Fig. 7.23 Weight-bearing CT scan: Lateral subluxation causes sinus tarsi impingement, indicated by the yellow arrow. (**a**) coronal plane; (**b**) sagittal plane

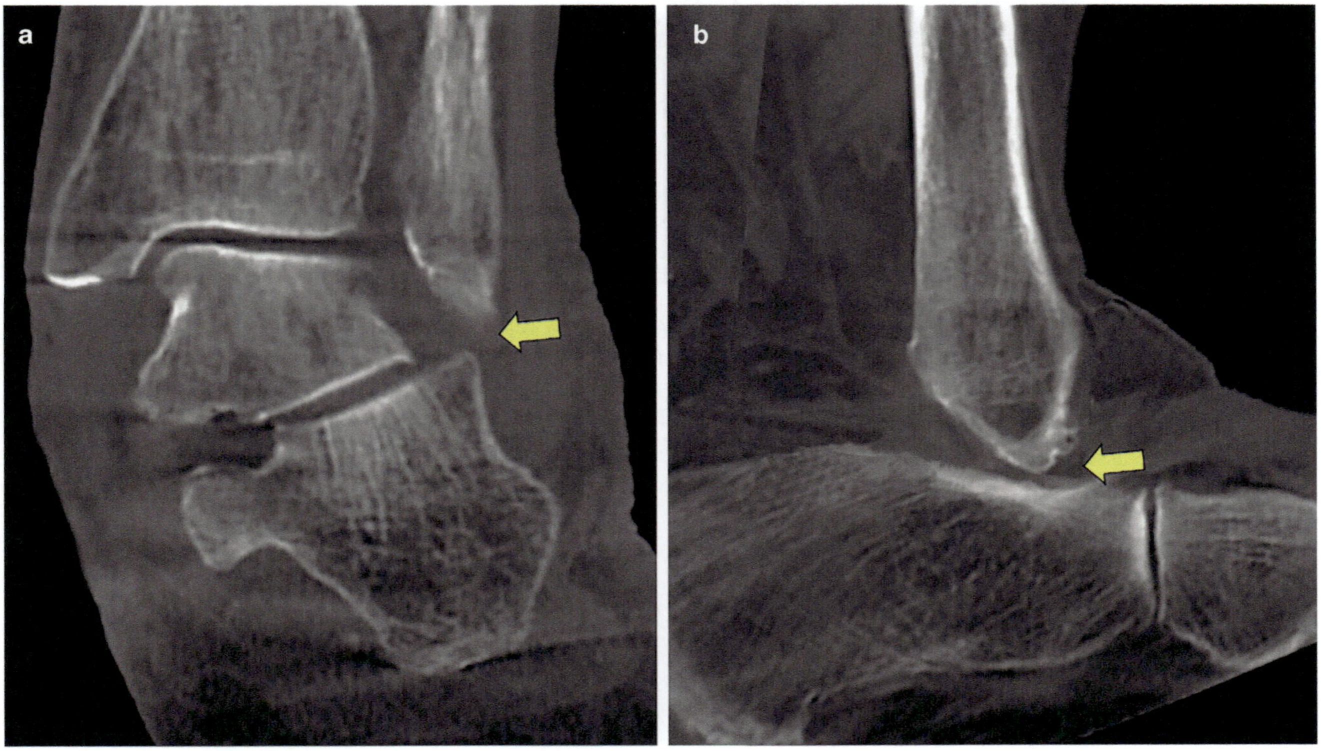

Fig. 7.24 Weight-bearing CT scan: If lateral subluxation further progresses, subfibular impingement will occur (yellow arrow), shown here in the (**a**) coronal plane and (**b**) sagittal plane, with the typical sign of a "missed talus"

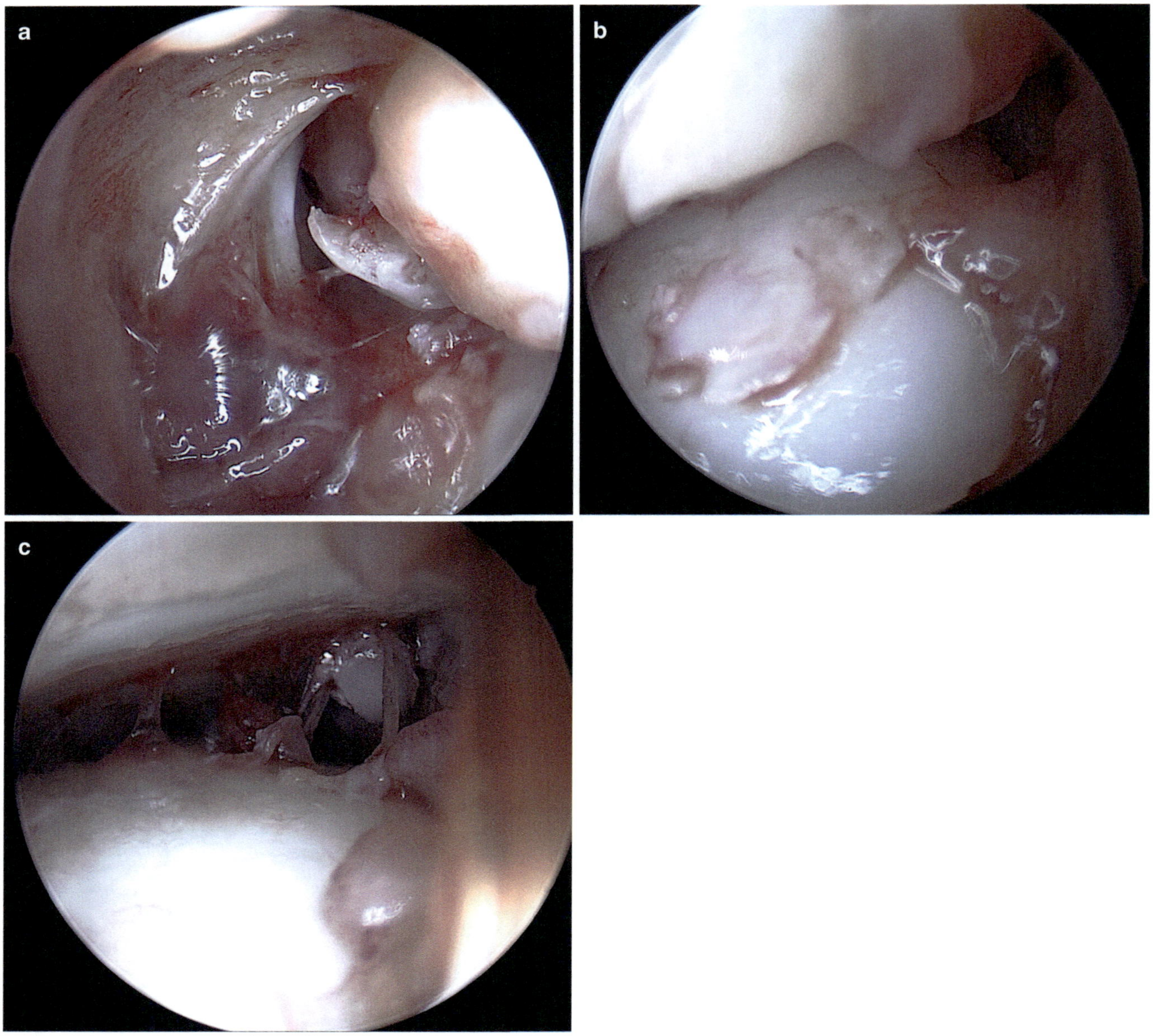

Fig. 7.25 Arthroscopy of the subtalar joint through a sinus tarsi portal (same patient as Fig. 7.19). (**a**) incomplete rupture of the ITCL; (**b**) cartilage lesions on the posterior facet of the calcaneal articular surface; and (**c**) fracture of the posterior process of the talus

frontal plane: neutral, valgus or varus deformity [60], and thereafter on the assessment of the talus in the sagittal and horizontal plane (Fig. 7.26).

The four predominant varus malposition configurations were dorsiflexion (sagittal plane) combined with neutral or external rotation (horizontal plane) and neutral (sagittal plane) combined with neutral or internal rotation (horizontal plane), accounting for 89.7% of all ankles, whereas the three predominant valgus malposition configurations were neutral (sagittal plane) combined with neutral or external rotation (horizontal plane) and plantar flexion (sagittal plane) combined with neutral (horizontal plane), accounting for 95% of all ankles [60]. This indicates that in varus and valgus tilted ankles, malposition of the talus in the coronal plane does not reliably predict malposition in the sagittal or horizontal planes, as loss of peritalar stability leads to various talar malposition configurations.

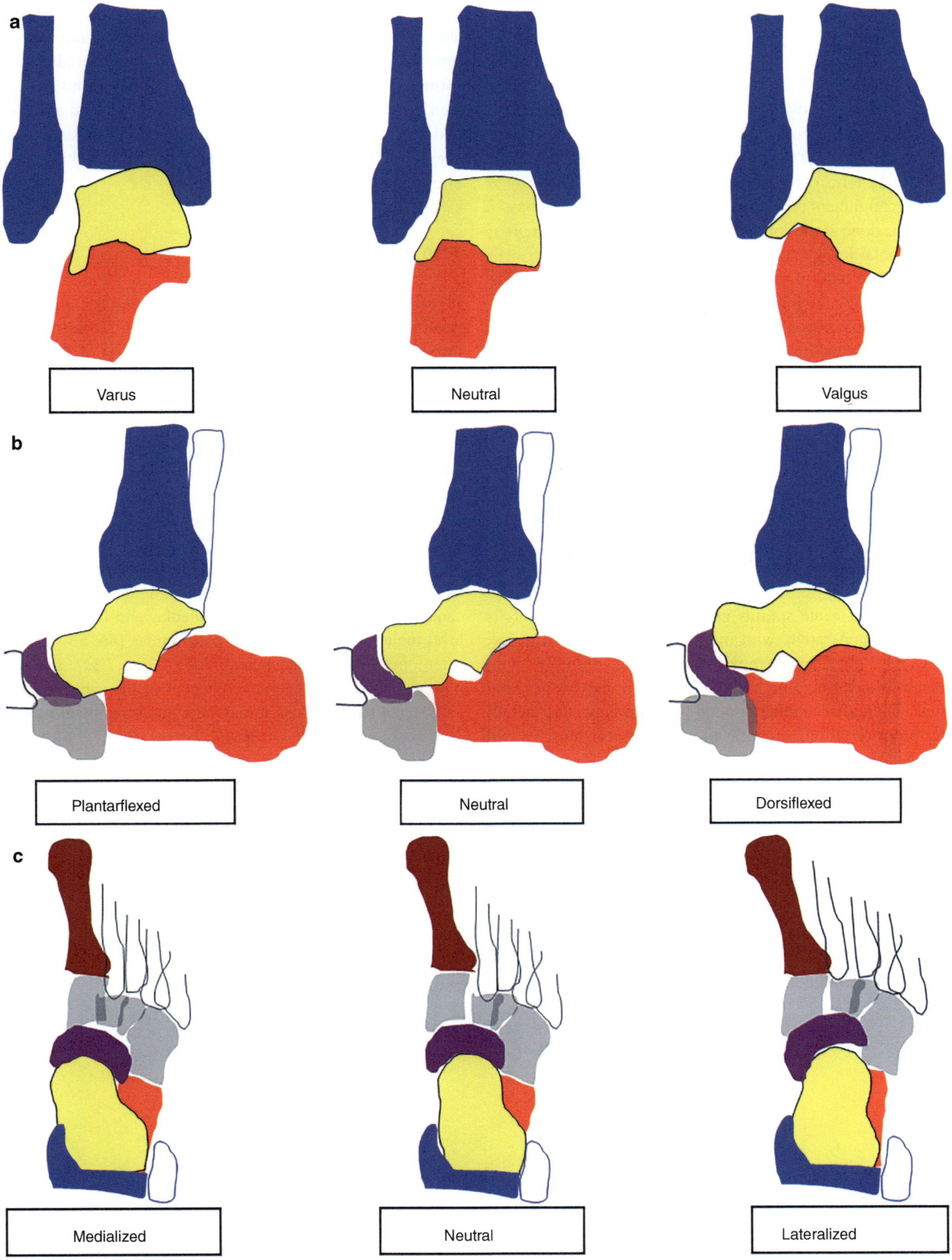

Fig. 7.26 An illustration showing various possible changes of the talar position in peritalar instability: (**a**) in the coronal plane; (**b**) the sagittal plane; and (**c**) horizontal plane (see text)

7.10 Treatment of Peritalar Instability

- Treatment of acute injuries is usually nonoperative; in the case of major avulsion fragments, surgical reconstruction may be indicated.
- As soft tissue reconstruction alone may not result in long-term peritalar stability, osseous balancing by realignment procedures may be indicated; they may be done at the supramalleolar level, at the inframalleolar level, or both levels.
- In the case of progressive degenerative changes of the subtalar joint, a distraction arthrodesis of the subtalar fusion might be advised, allowing also to tension the ligamentous apparatus.

As in acute or chronic ankle instability, nonoperative measures are considered prior to surgical treatment. An exception is peritalar dislocation that might need immediate surgical intervention.

7.10.1 Acute Injury

Treatment of acute sprains involving the peritalar joints is usually nonoperative, with immobilization and/or rest, ice, elevation, physical therapy, and bracing. Initially, non-weight-bearing may be advised until pain and swelling are gone. Thereafter, a rehabilitation program may start including proprioception, strengthening of peroneal muscles and coordination exercises.

Treatment of acute peritalar dislocations (Fig. 7.27), in contrast, need surgical intervention when closed reduction is not possible and reposition cannot be secured by immobilization with a plaster or boot. Most avulsion fractures of the dorsal talonavicular ligament or the posteromedial talar process involve sizable articular components with displacement of the ankle, subtalar, and talonavicular joints (Fig. 7.28a–c). These injuries should be treated with open reduction internal fixation to anatomically restore the articular surfaces of the talus and to restore the stability of the peritalar joints [61] (Fig. 7.28d, e). An attempt to treat severely comminuted injuries with open reduction internal fixation should be performed, keeping in mind that remaining defects and/or excision of major articular fragments can lead to rapid arthrosis and joint instability [62] (Fig. 7.29). Concern exists regarding fracture excision leading to hindfoot instability and altered biomechanics [63].

7.10.2 Chronic Instability

In cases with failure of conservative measures, operative treatment may be considered (Fig. 7.30). Regarding the importance of the ITCL as a primary stabilizer of the subtalar joint, the idea of ITCL reconstruction appears reasonable and promising. The use of a partial Achilles tendon graft [28] and the anterior half of peroneus brevis tendon [39] has been proposed. Recently, an arthroscopic approach was described with an improved visualization for tunnel placement of a gracilis tendon graft from the ipsilateral knee [64].

Soft tissue reconstruction alone may not result in long-term peritalar stability (Fig. 7.31). Surgical procedures addressing osseous balancing by realignment procedures may be a better treatment option. Realignment procedures can be performed at the supramalleolar and inframalleolar level including supramalleolar osteotomies [46, 65–72] and osteotomies of the calcaneus [73–77] (Fig. 7.32). In cases with progressive degenerative changes of the subtalar joint, an isolated subtalar fusion may be a good treatment option. A distraction arthrodesis through lateral (Fig. 7.33) or posterolateral (Fig. 7.34) might be necessary to tension the ligaments and thereby realign the bony structures. In patients with concomitant degenerative changes of the tibiotalar joint, total ankle replacement may resolve the peritalar instability by restoring the biomechanics of the subtalar joint resulting in stability within the mortise. This can be especially the case in patients with valgus deformity of the hindfoot (Fig. 7.35). A distraction arthrodesis of the subtalar joint may also serve to restore medial ankle stability and to reposition the talus.

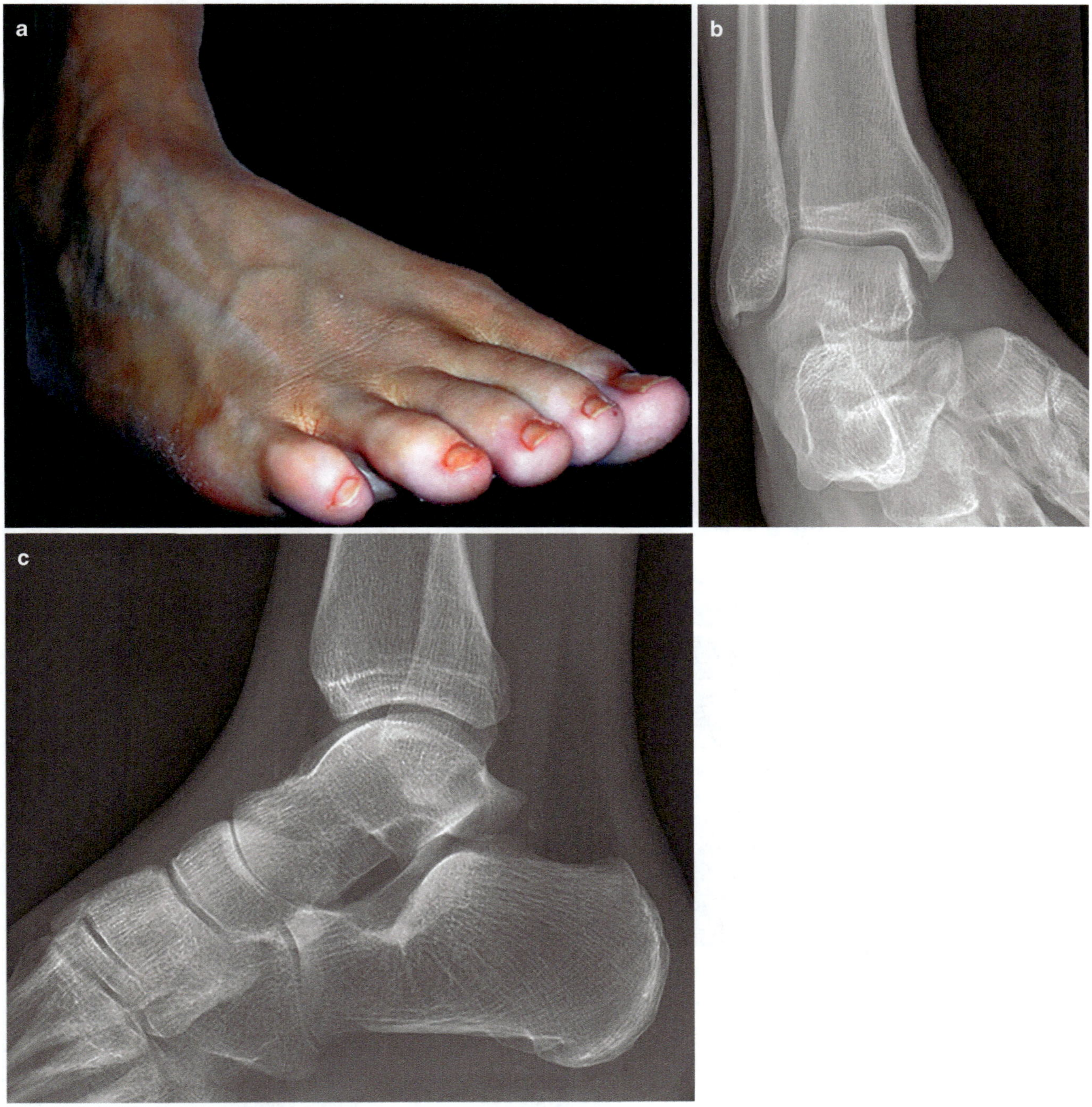

Fig. 7.27 Acute peritalar dislocation in a 19-year-old male patient. (**a**) Clinical presentation showing the foot adduction and the prominence of the talar head on the lateral aspect of the foot. Radiographic view: (**b**) AP view; (**c**) lateral view

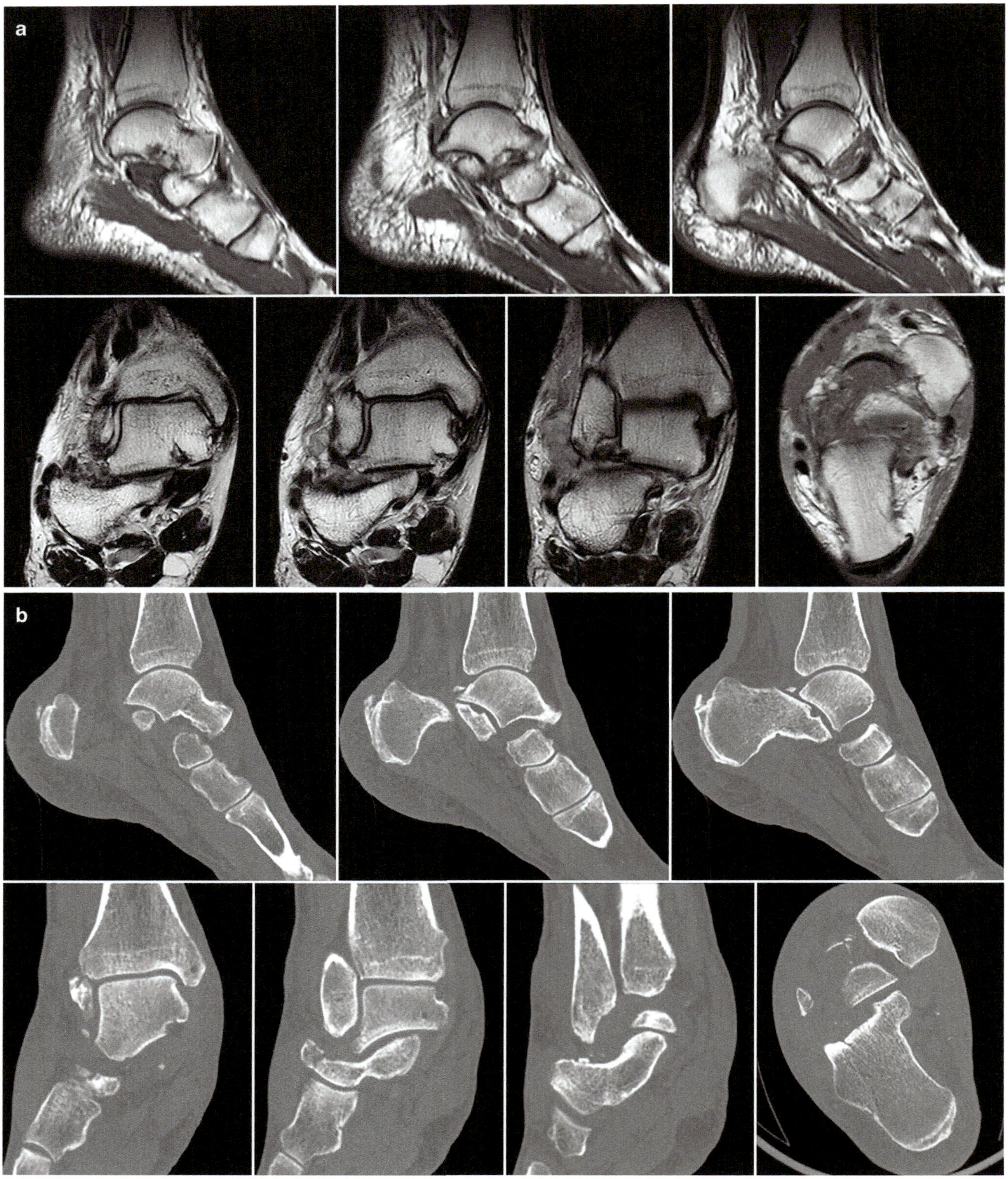

Fig. 7.28 *Surgical technique: surgical treatment of acute peritalar dislocation*. This 57-year-old male patient suffered an acute peritalar dislocation after fall from a ladder. (**a**) MRI showing the dislocation of the talus with extrusion of the talar head out of the coxa pedis. While the ITCL, LTCL, FTCL, and CFL were completely disrupted, the ATFL, the deep deltoid and syndesmotic ligaments remained intact. The spring ligament generally remains intact in these injury mechanisms. (**b**) A CT scan showing the dislocation with avulsion of the posteromedial talar process and a non-dislocated lateral fracture of the calcaneus. (**c**) 3-D view showing the dislocation in more detail. (**d**) Standard radiographs, AP, lateral, and DP view just after closed reduction of the talar head. After insertion of a K-wire for transfixation of the talonavicular joint, thus keeping the talar head in position, the posteromedial ligaments are reconstructed with the use of an anchor. The K-wire is removed 4 weeks later. (**e**) Standard weight-bearing radiographs after 4 months, showing a stable situation and an anatomic position of the talus

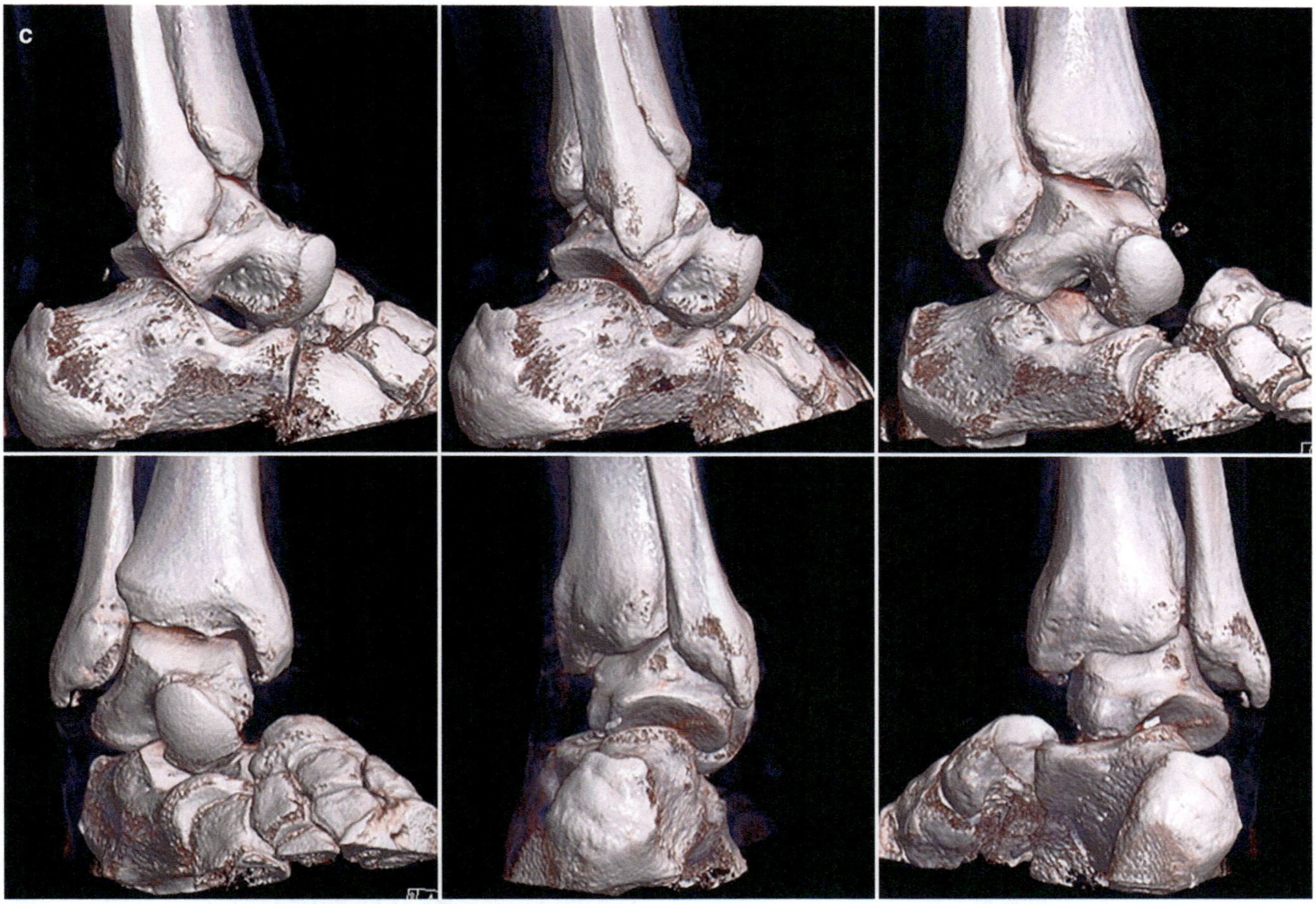

Fig. 7.28 (continued)

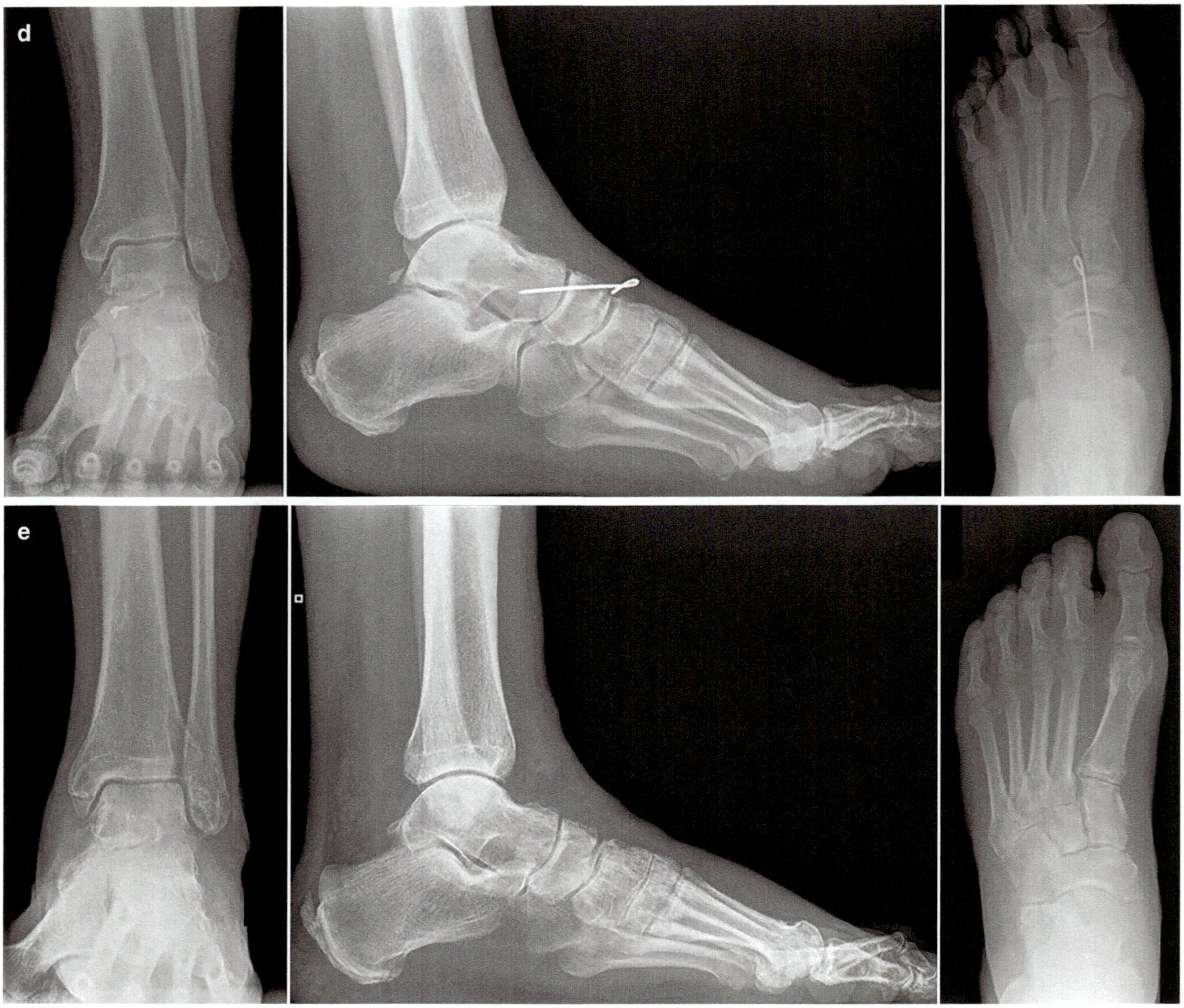

Fig. 7.28 (continued)

7.11 Results

- Little is known on the outcome after surgical treatment of peritalar instability.
- Subtalar arthrodesis seems to provide the best results regarding repositioning of the talus on top of the calcaneus.

Satisfactory to good results have been reported with surgical reconstruction of the ITCL with the use of a tendon graft [28, 39]; however, the literature is still spare and no mid- to long-term survival outcome is available. While several reports have shown good to excellent survival rates and improvement in clinical outcomes after correcting osteotomies [59, 67, 70, 78, 79], none of these reports have focused on the loss of peritalar stability. This loss allows the talus to rotate and translate on the calcaneal and navicular bone surfaces, thereby resulting in a three-dimensional positional change of the talus, leading to various possible mispositioning of the talus, this being the origin of the problem being treated. No report exists about reconstructive surgery of talar malposition after loss of peritalar stability without supramalleolar correction.

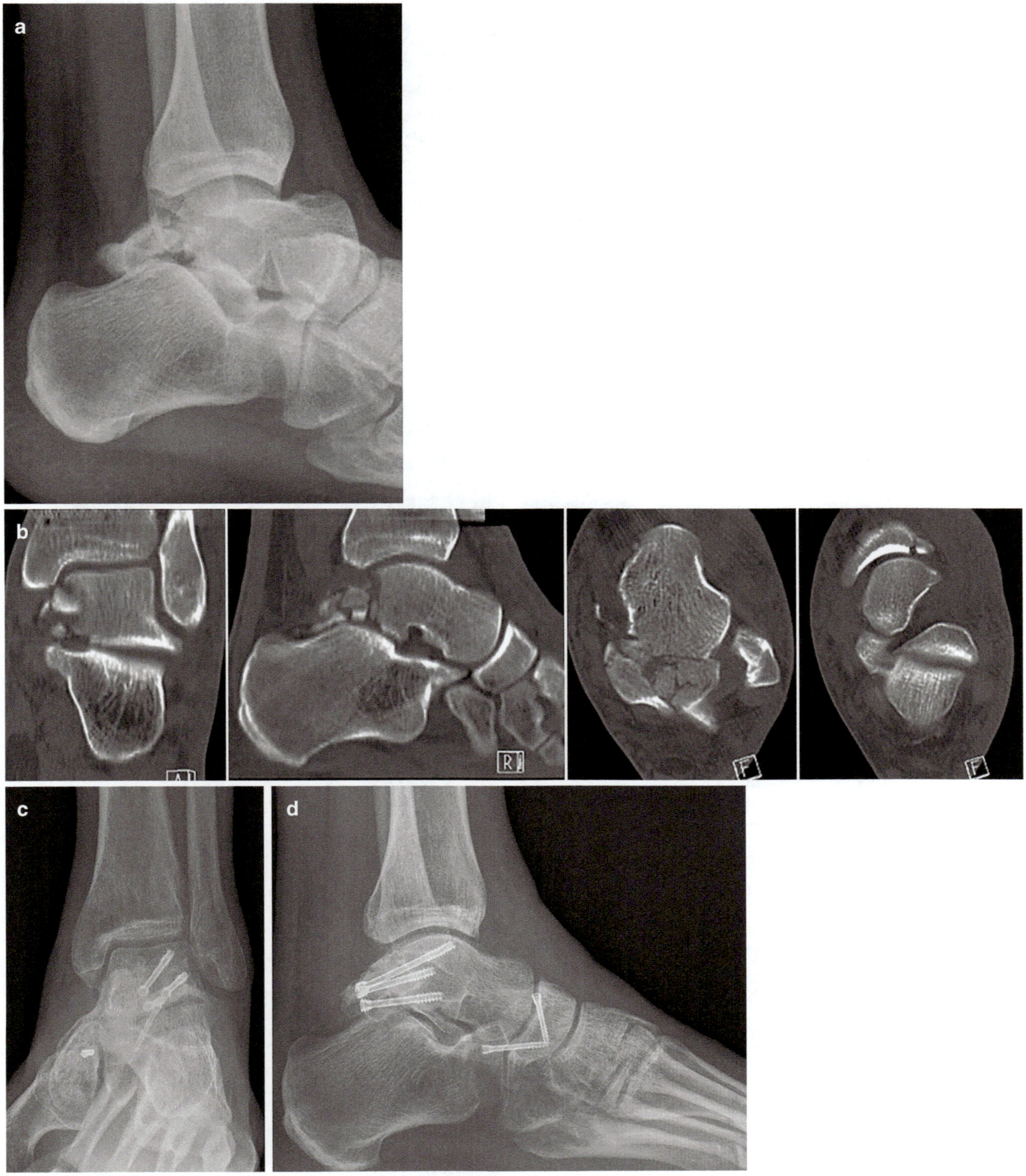

Fig. 7.29 *Surgical technique: surgical treatment of acute peritalar dislocation with communitive fracture*. This 39-year-old male patient suffered an acute peritalar dislocation after a moto-scouter accident. (**a**) Primary radiographic assessment shows the dislocated head with a communitive fracture of the posterior talus. (**b**) CT scans show the communitive fracture of the posterior talar process with involvement of the medial talar body and, in addition, a fracture of the navicular bone. (**c**) AP and (**d**) lateral weight-bearing standard radiographs 12 weeks after open reduction and internal fixation of the posteromedial talus and percutaneous screw fixation of the navicular. The peritalar joints are anatomically restored and the fractures healed

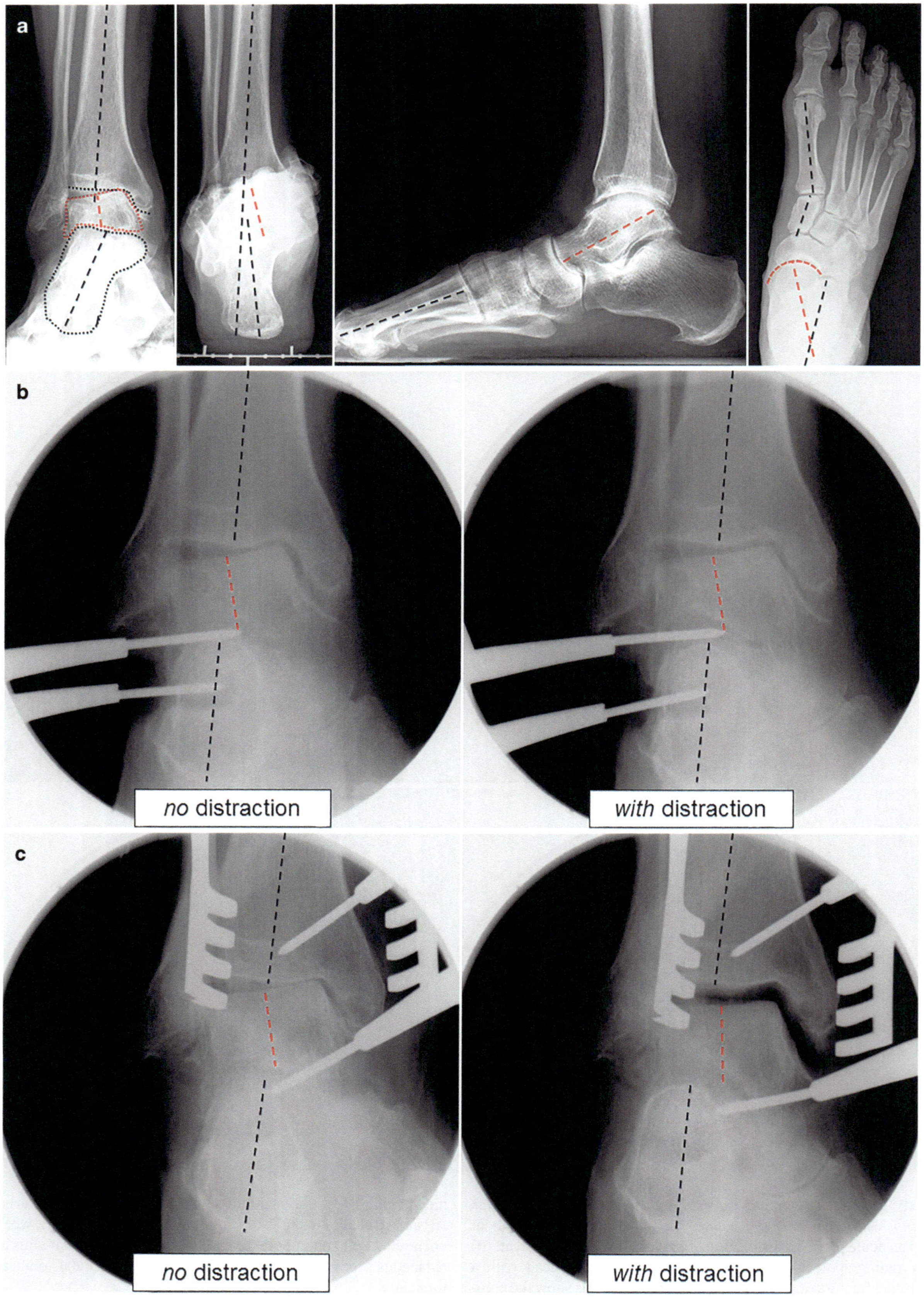

Fig. 7.30 *Surgical technique: intraoperative testing of instability*. A 53-year-old female patient with chronic peritalar instability after a severe ankle sprain 12 years earlier. (**a**) In weight-bearing standard radiographs, the talus is seen to be tilted into varus, while the calcaneus experiences a compensatory valgus tilting movement. The incongruency at the subtalar joint is especially seen in the lateral view. Intraoperative fluoroscopy views show, (**b**) when applying distraction between the talus and calcaneus from the lateral side, little correction at subtalar joint is noticed, whereas (**c**) when applying the distraction from medial side, appropriate realignment is achieved. This suggests that the loss of ligament tension on the medial side may have caused this zigzag deformity

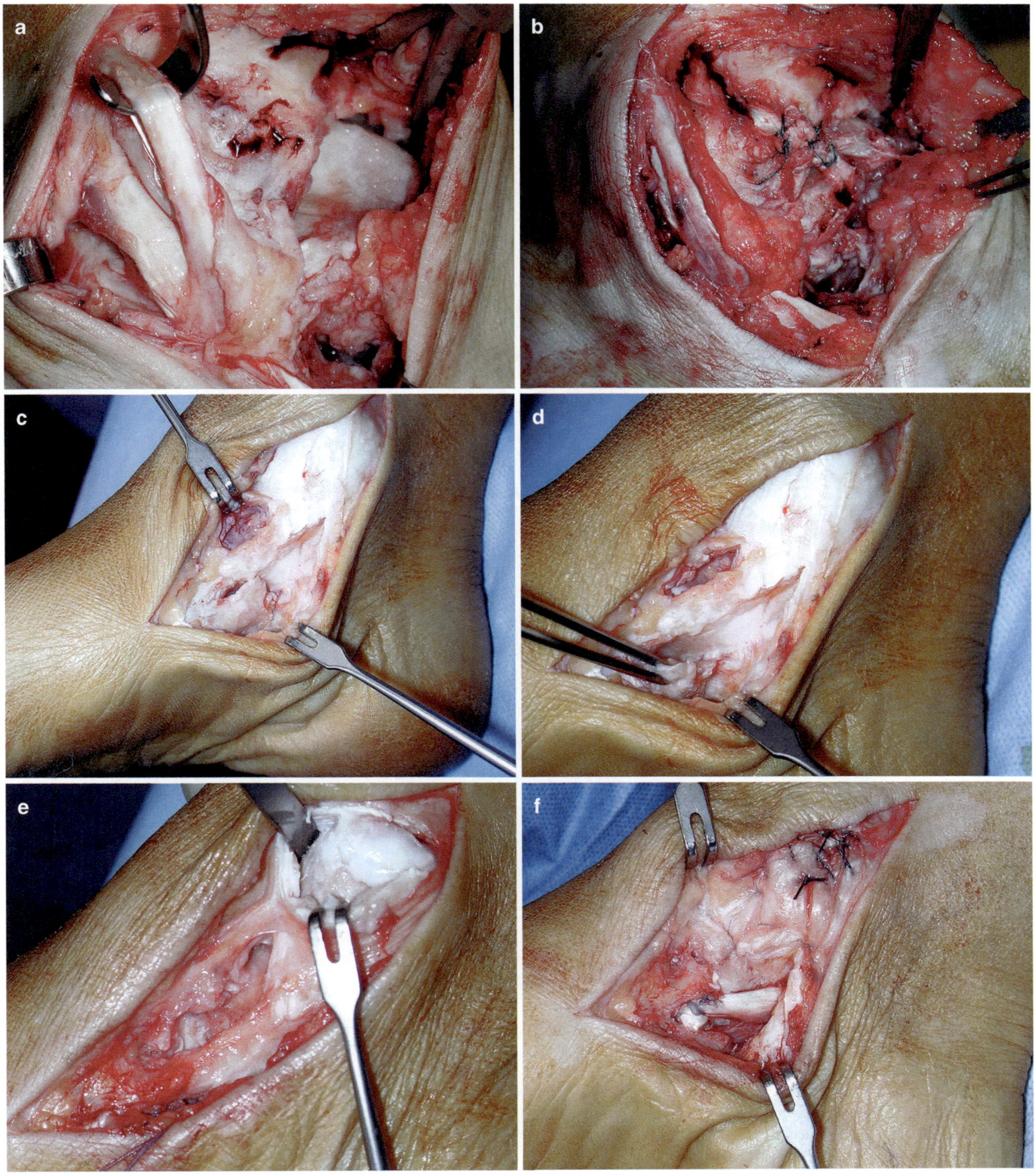

Fig. 7.31 *Surgical technique: surgical treatment of chronic peritalar instability with soft tissue reconstruction.* Intraoperative images of a 54-year-old female patient who sustained a new severe sprain of her right hindfoot besides suffering from chronic peritalar instability. (**a**) On the lateral side, the peroneal tendons are dislocated, associated to a rupture of the lateral ankle ligaments. (**b**) After repositioning the peroneal tendons, the tendon sheath is reconstructed as well as the lateral ankle ligaments. (**c**) On medial side, an old rupture of the PT tendon is found in addition to a rupture of the tibiospring ligament. (**d**) Further exploration shows the distal stump of the PT tendon. (**e**) Further, a complete avulsion of the superficial deltoid ligament is found at its insertion area on the medial malleolus. (**f**) After an FDL transfer and reconstruction of the deltoid ligament (Technique see Fig. 5.57), the ankle is found to be stable during manual testing. Despite a significant improvement and return to previous activities, the peritalar joint remained unstable over time

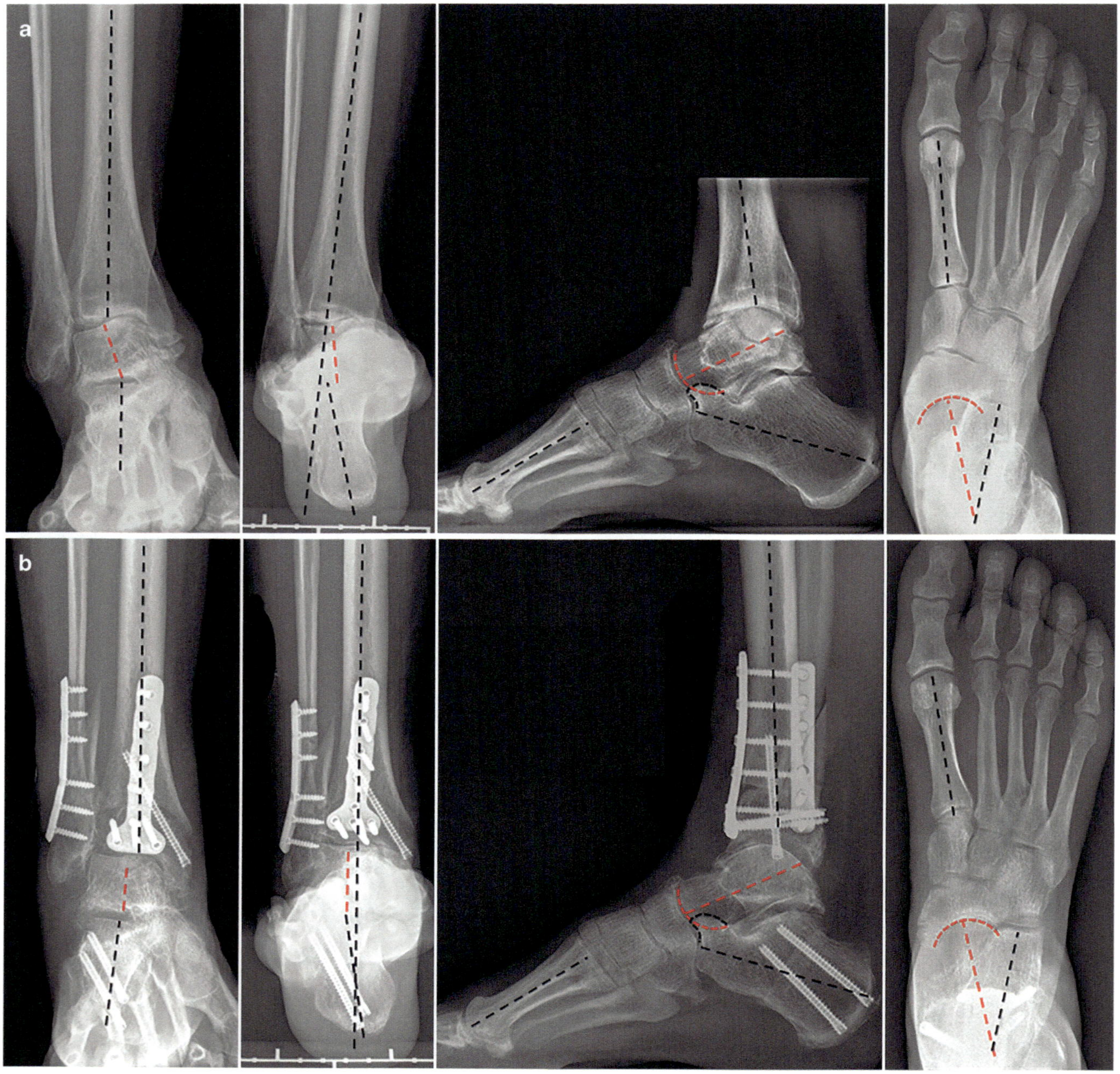

Fig. 7.32 *Surgical technique: surgical treatment of chronic peritalar instability with periarticular osteotomies.* Standard weight-bearing radiographic images of a 59-year-old female patient with increasing pain in her right ankle after recurrent sprains in the past. (**a**) The preoperative radiographs evidenced a varus tilt of the talus with beginning osteoarthritic changes of the medial ankle joint and a compensatory valgus position of the calcaneus due to the peritalar instability. (**b**) Four months after performing bony corrections using a dome shape osteotomy of the distal tibia (Technique see Fig. 2.49) and medial sliding osteotomy of the calcaneus (Technique see Fig. 5.61), the hindfoot was well aligned and the subtalar joint looked repositioned. In this case, combining supra- and inframalleolar correcting osteotomies resulted in well-balanced peritalar joints

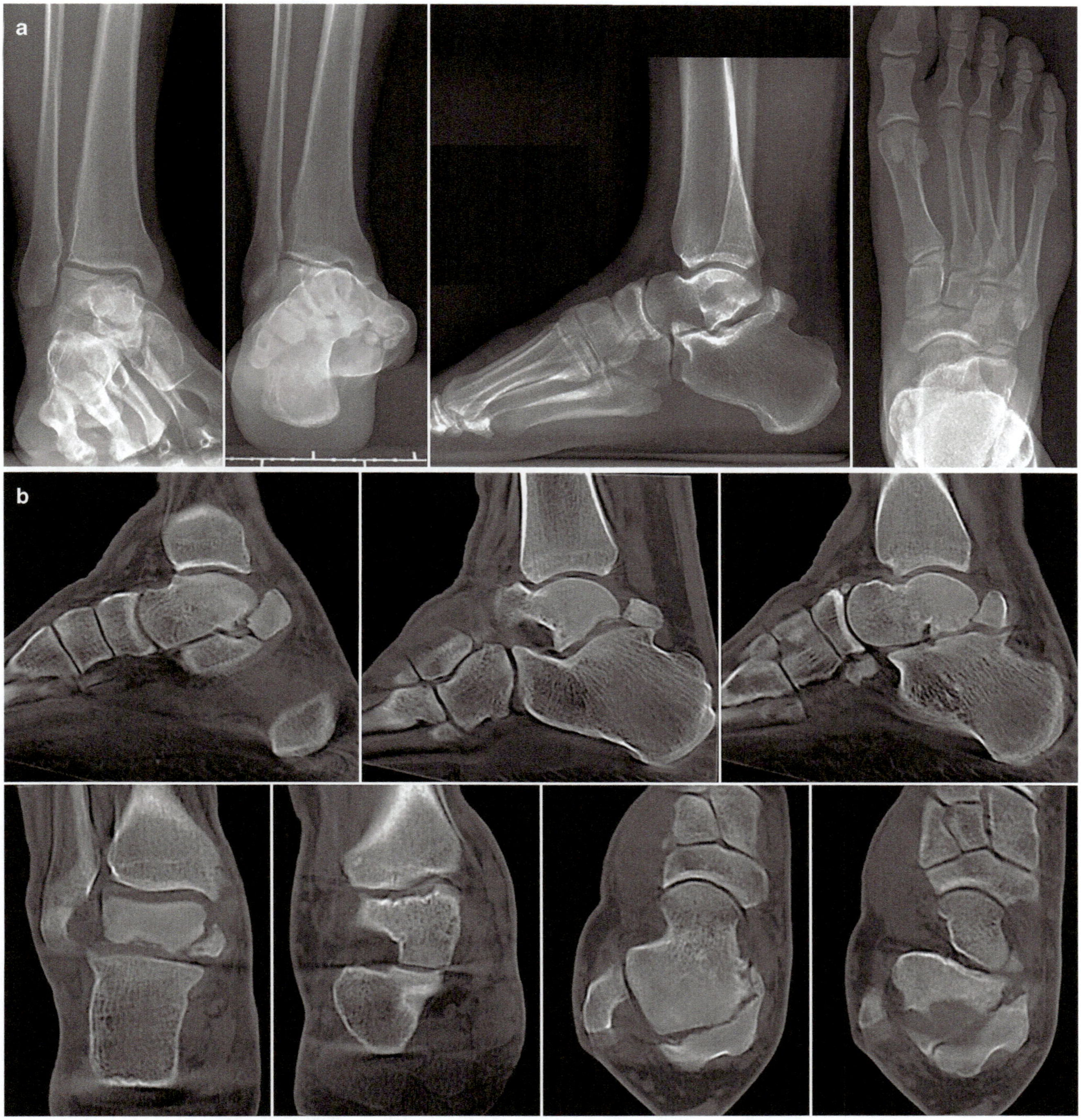

Fig. 7.33 *Surgical technique: surgical treatment of chronic peritalar instability with distraction subtalar arthrodesis through posterolateral approach.* A 28-year-old male patient who sustained a severe hindfoot sprain at the age of 15 years and currently complained about increasing anterior and posterior pain at his right ankle. (**a**) Preoperative radiographs evidenced chronic peritalar instability with anterior displacement and dorsiflexion movement of the talus. In the DP view, the talus is exorotated and in the hindfoot view a distinct varus malalignment of the heel can be seen. (**b**) Weight-bearing CT scans evidenced an old avulsion of the posteromedial talus and a flattening of the articular surfaces of the subtalar joint. (**c**) The subtalar joint is exposed through a posterolateral approach. (**d**) Two K-wires are inserted into talus and calcaneus on each, the medial and lateral side of the incision and used to apply maximal distraction forces to tension the ITCL and thereby reducing the talus on top of the calcaneus. Coronal plane position of the calcaneus is controlled with the two spreaders (Hintermann distractors). (**e**) After having debrided the posterior facets of the subtalar joint, a fresh femoral allograft is inserted. (**f**) Intraoperative fluoroscopy showing the procedure step-by-step, including screw fixation. Notice that full-threaded screws were used to ensure for the achieved position. (**g**) Weight-bearing CT scans after 3 months, showing solid integration of the graft. The patient was permitted to weight-bear his foot as tolerated after 2 weeks, with protection of a boot for 8 weeks

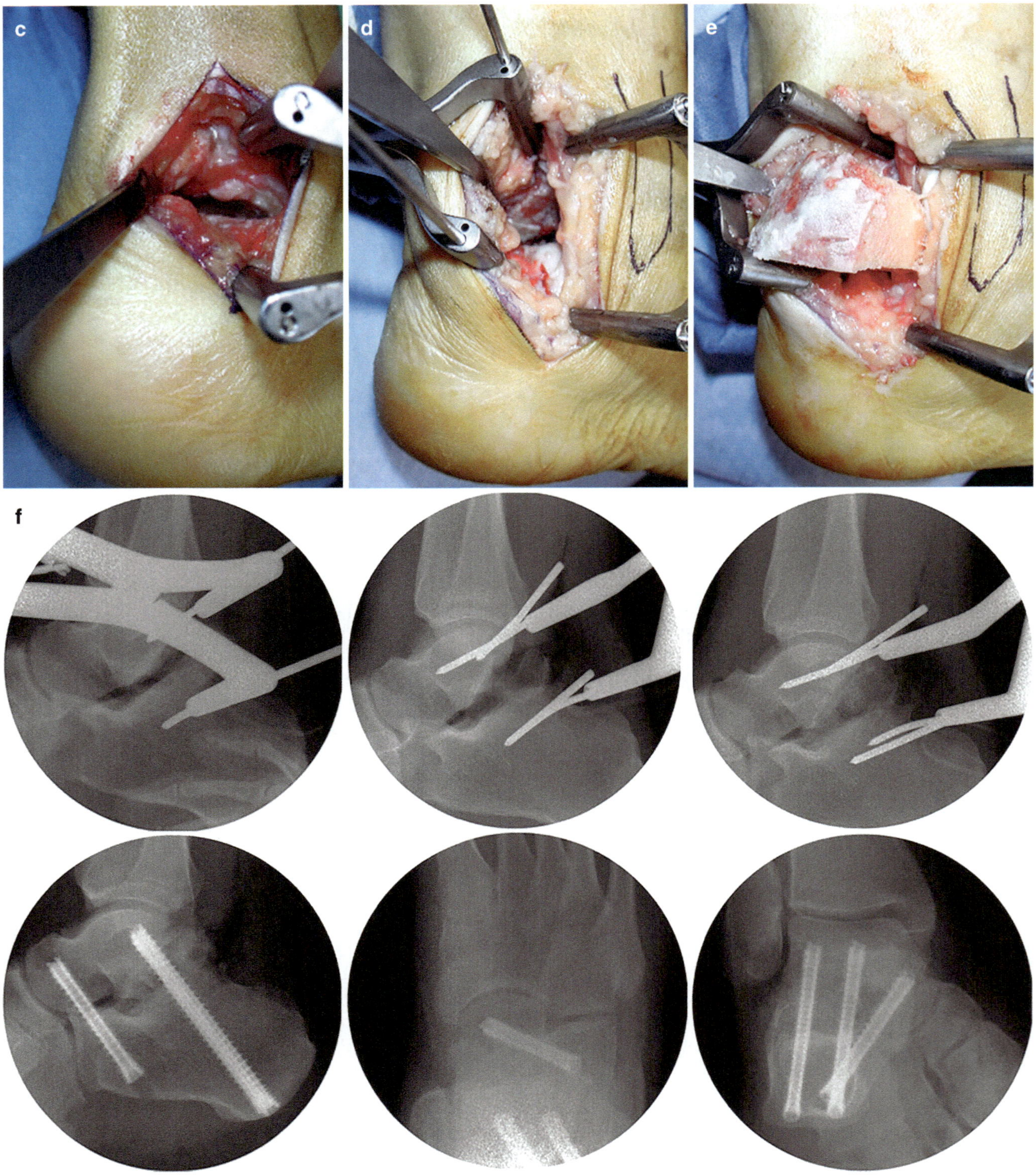

Fig. 7.33 (continued)

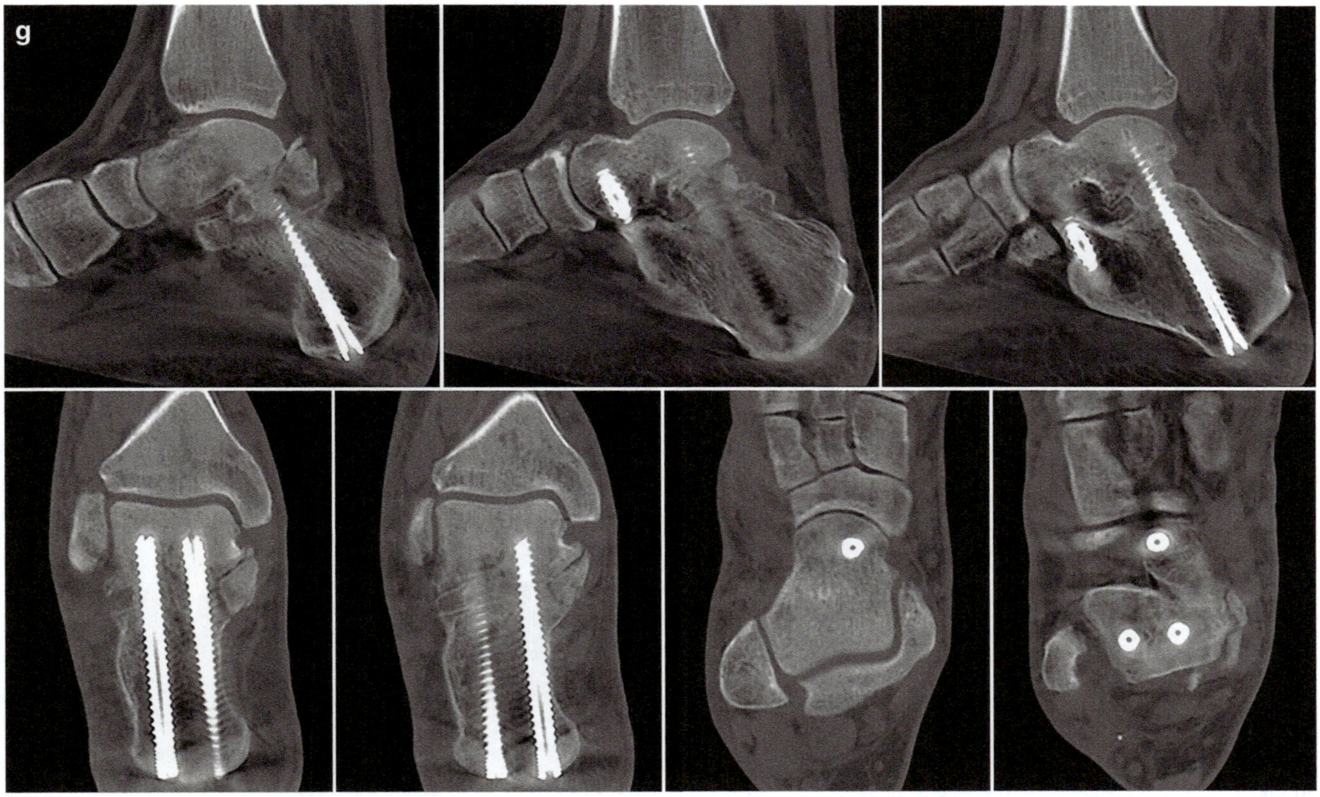

Fig. 7.33 (continued)

7.12 Complications

- Complications mostly include underpowered correction and stabilization that results in recurrent destabilization and deformity.
- Attention must be paid to the stretched tibial nerve in the case of valgus destabilization of the hindfoot that can be injured when attempting to reduce the deformity.

Intraoperative complications include nerve injuries. An important consideration, especially with acute corrections, is the posterior tibial nerve. Varus-to-valgus corrections stretch this nerve, particularly if the center of rotation of angulation is distal to the osteotomy line. Acute tarsal tunnel syndrome can result from acute varus-to-valgus correction. When bony procedures are included in treatment, overcorrection or undercorrection may occur after inappropriate preoperative planning. Delayed or nonunion may result from inappropriate fixation techniques or too aggressive loading of the leg in the early postoperative phase. Loss of correction may occur as a result of implant failure, or inappropriate addressing of concomitant problems such as ligamentous incompetence, muscular dysfunction, and forefoot deformities.

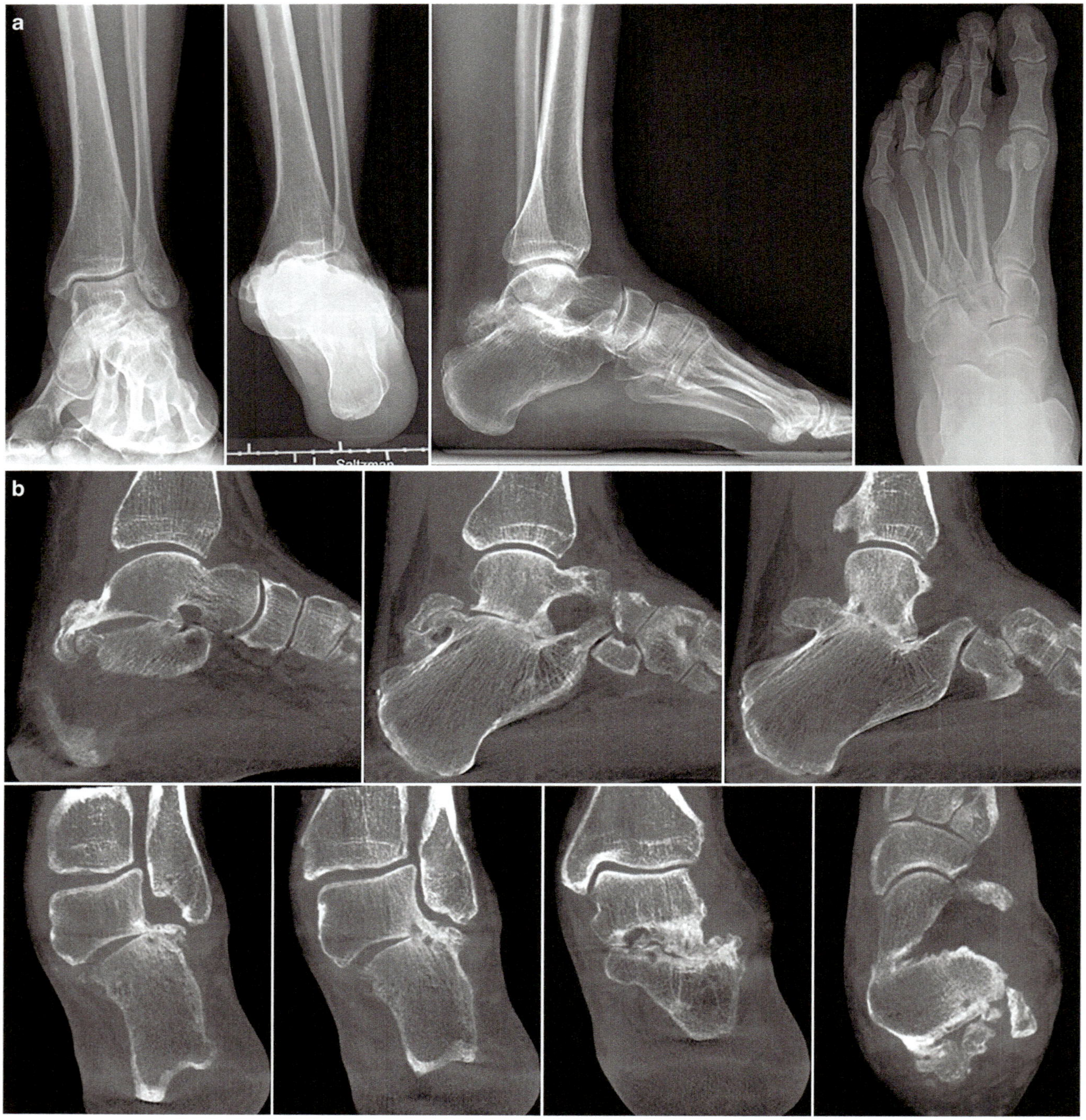

Fig. 7.34 *Surgical technique: surgical treatment of chronic peritalar instability with distraction subtalar arthrodesis through lateral approach.* A 60-year-old male patient with painful end-stage osteoarthrosis of his left subtalar joint subsequent to chronic peritalar instability after having experienced a heavy sprain 15 years earlier. Besides sensing posterior ankle pain, he also indicated anterior impingement of his ankle, therefore arthroscopic surgery was recommended earlier. (**a**) The weight-bearing radiographs showed dorsiflexion position (horizontalization) of the talus and advanced degenerative changes of the posterior subtalar joint. (**b**) Weight-bearing CT scans evidenced in addition a medial translation of the talus on the calcaneus with subsequent subfibular impingement. (**c**) The subtalar joint is approached through a lateral approach and distracted over 2 K-wires. (**d**) An allograft is inserted and (**e**) squeezed between the posterior articular surfaces of the talus and the calcaneus. (**f**) Intraoperative fluoroscopy showing the procedure step-by-step including screw fixation. (**g**) Standard weight-bearing radiographs after 6 months showing solid integration of the graft and regular position of the talus in all three planes. The patient no longer complained about experiencing anterior ankle impingement

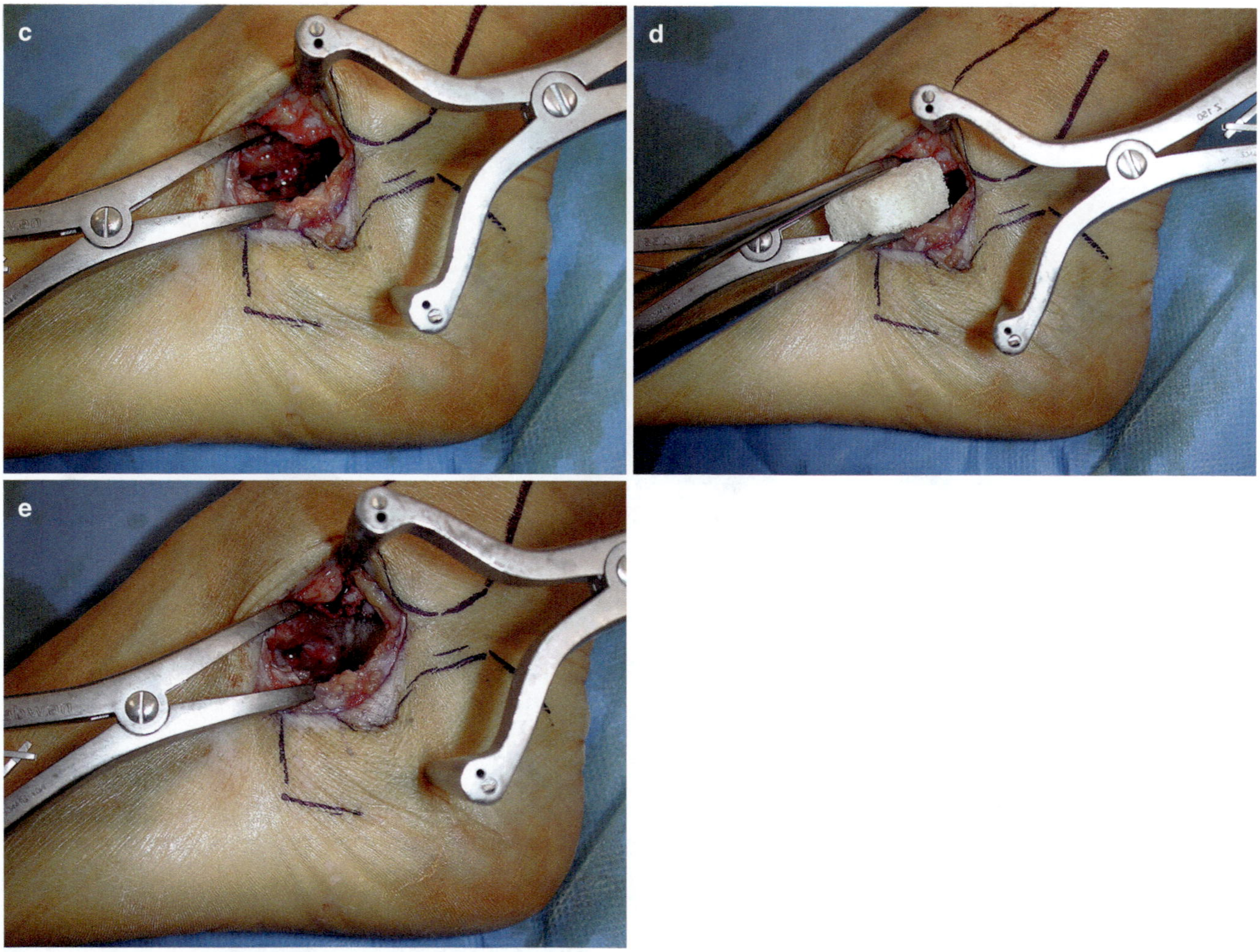

Fig. 7.34 (continued)

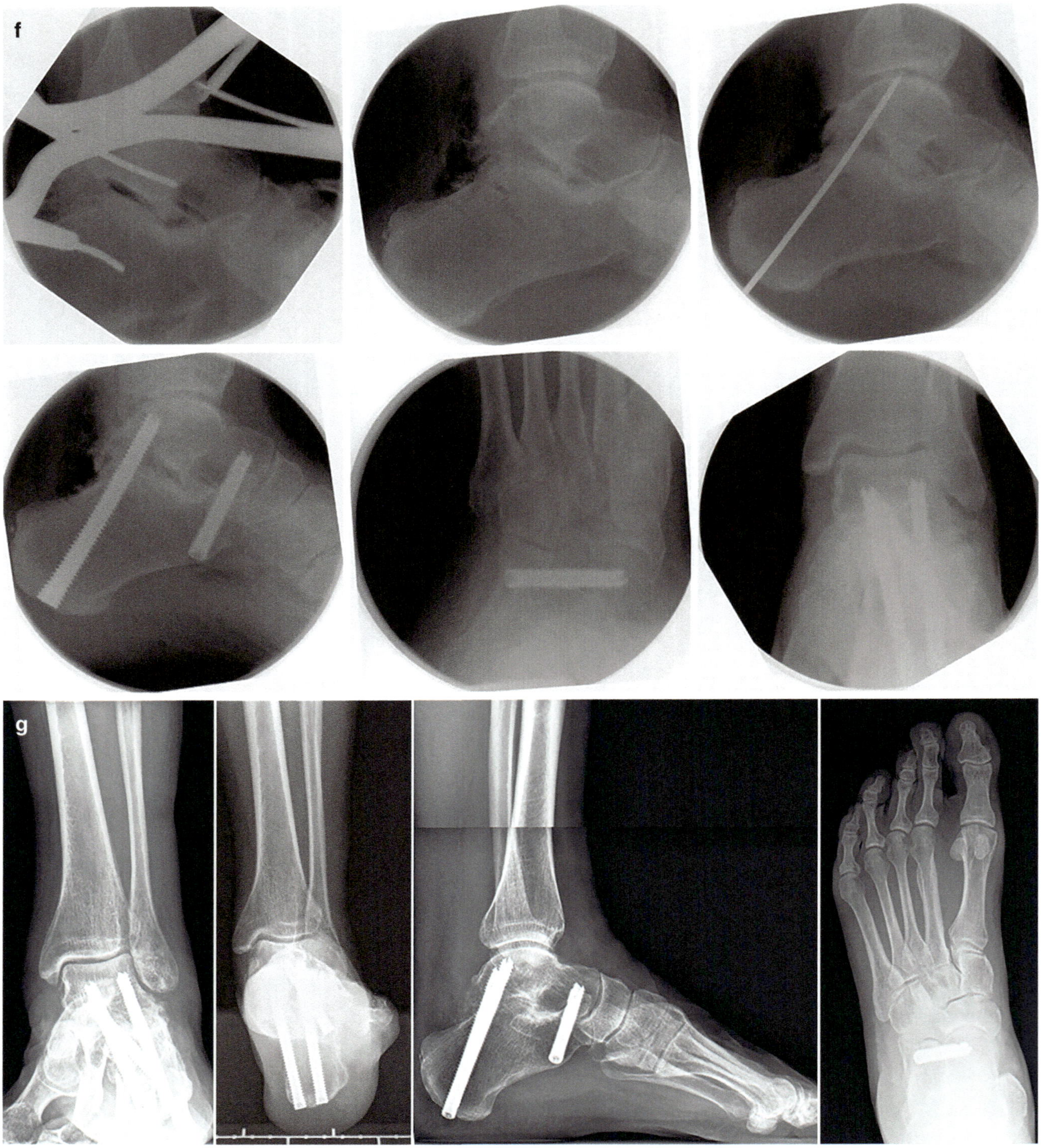

Fig. 7.34 (continued)

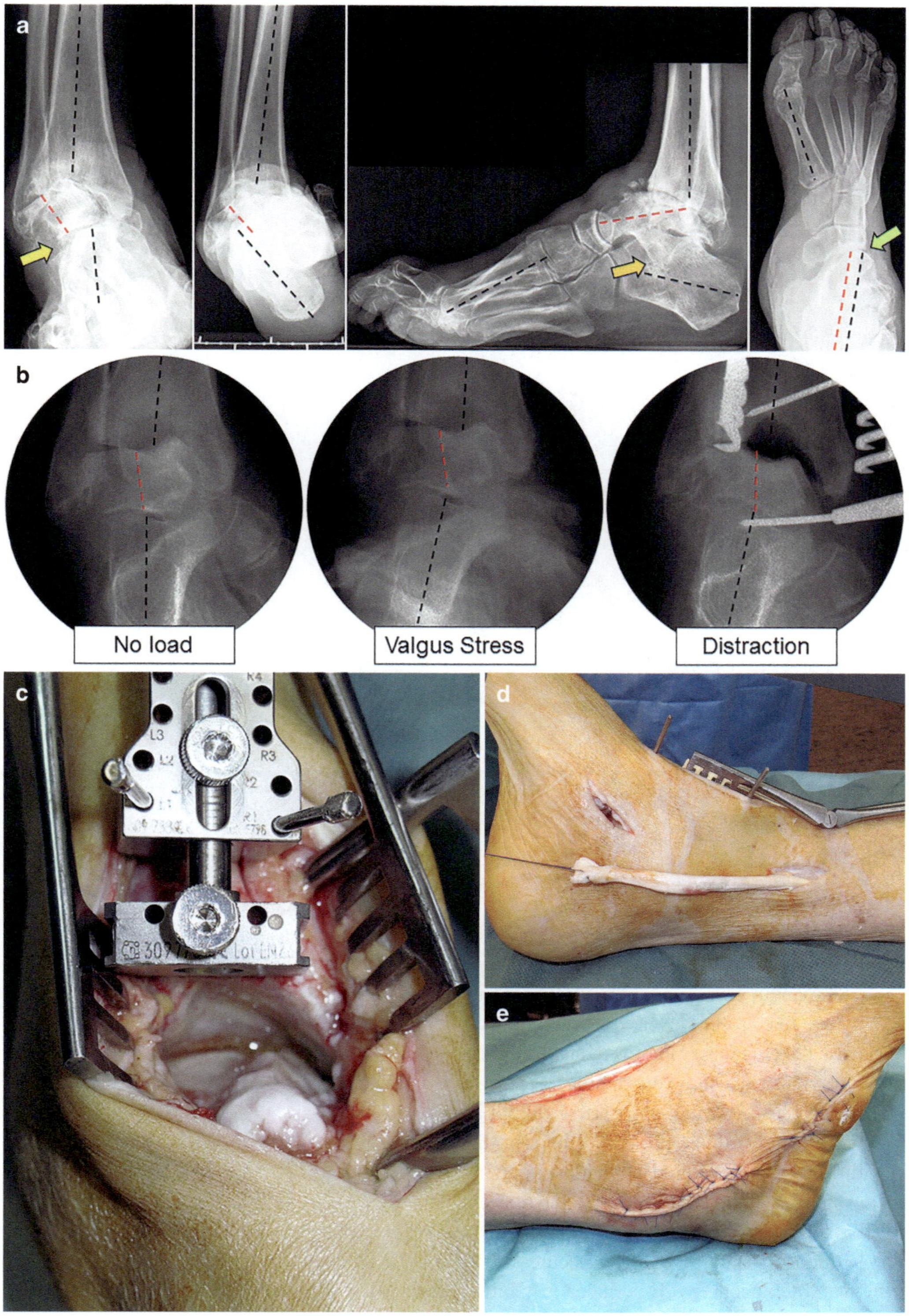

Fig. 7.35 *Surgical technique: surgical treatment of chronic tibiotalar and peritalar instability with secondary ankle osteoarthritis with total ankle replacement and soft tissue reconstruction.* A 61-year-old male patient with chronic lateral ankle instability after having experienced a severe ankle sprain 18 years earlier and recurrent sprains thereafter. (**a**) Weight-bearing radiographs showing the varus deformity with varus tilt and anterolateral extrusion of the talus and peritalar instability (yellow arrow) with significant exorotation of the talus (green arrow). There is also a sinus tarsi impingement (orange arrow). (**b**) Under fluoroscopy, the compensatory valgus tilt is seen at the subtalar joint due to peritalar instability increases with applied valgus stress, whereas it is corrected by applying distraction on the medial side. (**c**) Intraoperative situs of the ankle with applied medial distraction while adjusting the tibial resection bloc. (**d**) The PT tendon is dissected at its distal insertion and brought proximally through a second incision. (**e**) After having brought the PT tendon behind the tibia into the peroneal tendon sheath, it is attached to the peroneus longus tendon. The peroneus longus tendon, in turn, is transferred to the peroneus brevis tendon and fixed to the base of the fifth metatarsal through an additional incision (Technique see Fig. 2.42). (**f**) At the end of surgery, the ankle prosthesis is well aligned, and the ankle joint complex is stable. (**g**) Standard weight-bearing radiographs showing the result after 1 year with a well-balanced ankle. Notice the correction of the subtalar position (yellow and orange arrows) and restoration of the talar position in the horizontal plane (green arrow)

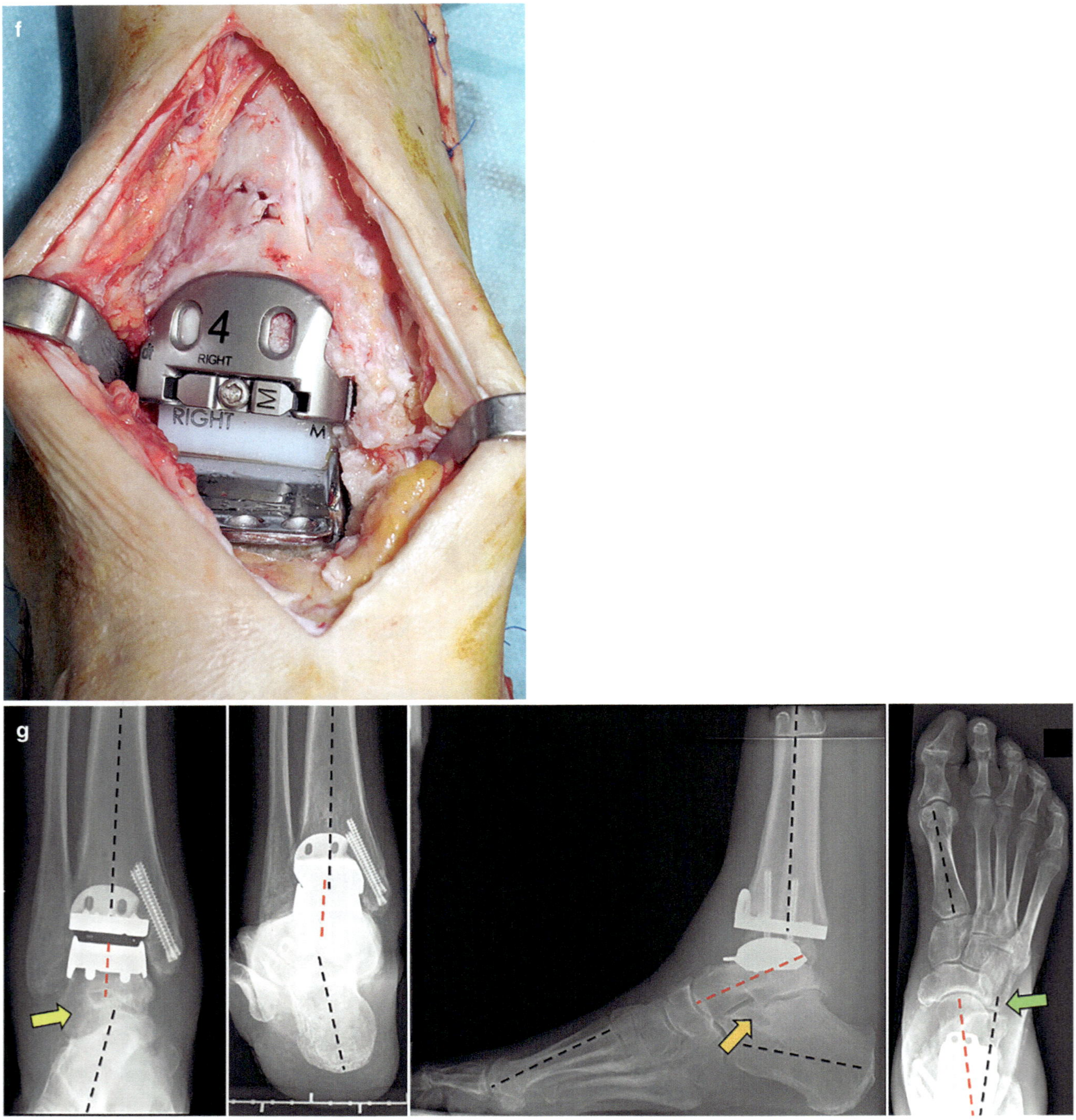

Fig. 7.35 (continued)

7.13 Conclusions and Future Evolution

- Loss of peritalar stability allows the talus to rotate and translate on the calcaneal and navicular bone surfaces, thereby resulting in a three-dimensional positional change and various talar malpositions.
- As articular surfaces may be worn out, isolated ligament reconstruction on the medial and lateral side of the ankle joint may not be able to restore the proper position of the talus within the ankle mortise.
- Osseous balancing by osteotomies and/or arthrodesis may be necessary to properly restore the talar position within the ankle mortise.
- Total ankle replacement with the goal to restore intrinsic stability of the talus in the tibiotalar (ankle) joint may be an interesting approach in the treatment of advanced stages of talar tilt and subsequent asymmetric ankle osteoarthritis, as it also allows to tension the ligaments and thereby to realign the ankle joint complex.

Obviously, loss of peritalar stability allows the talus to rotate and translate on calcaneal and navicular bone surfaces, thereby resulting in a three-dimensional positional change and various talar malpositions. This may be explained by differences in articular geometry, instability pattern of ligaments, and applied forces to the hindfoot complex. Therefore, careful radiographic assessment of the talar position in all three planes is mandatory for success in treatment of peritalar instability. Though being a promising technology for imaging the subtalar joint, weight-bearing CT scans have yet to become a clinical standard. As articular surfaces may be worn out, isolated ligament reconstruction on the medial and lateral side of the ankle joint may not be able to restore proper position of the talus within the ankle mortise. To which extent reconstruction of the ITCL is able to stabilize the subtalar joint at mid- to long term, is not clear yet. Osseous balancing with osteotomies above or below the ankle or subtalar fusion may thus be the main step for successful restoration of the talar position within the ankle mortise. The insertion of an ankle prosthesis may be another method to restore talar position and talar stability by tensioning the attenuated capsular and ligamentous structures, and by providing intrinsic stability at the tibiotalar joint. The key of success is to use all treatment modalities necessary to restore appropriate alignment of the hindfoot complex.

References

1. Sarrafian SK. Anatomy of foot and ankle. 2nd ed. Philadelphia: Lippincott Williams and Wilkins; 1993.
2. Schmidt HM. Shape and fixation of the human sinus tarsi and canalis tarsi ligaments. Acta Anat (Basel). 1978;102(2):184–94.
3. Barg A, Tochigi Y, Amendola A, Phisitkul P, Hintermann B, Saltzman CL. Subtalar instability: diagnosis and treatment. Foot Ankle Int. 2012;33(2):151–60.
4. Cahill DR. The anatomy and function of the contents of the human tarsal sinus and canal. Anat Rec. 1965;153(1):1–17.
5. Harper MC. The lateral ligamentous support of the subtalar joint. Foot Ankle. 1991;11(6):354–8.
6. Stagni R, Leardini A, O'Connor JJ, Giannini S. Role of passive structures in the mobility and stability of the human subtalar joint: a literature review. Foot Ankle Int. 2003;24(5):402–9.
7. Stephens MM, Sammarco GJ. The stabilizing role of the lateral ligament complex around the ankle and subtalar joints. Foot Ankle. 1992;13(3):130–6.
8. Smith JW. The ligamentous structures in the canalis and sinus tarsi. J Anat. 1958;92(4):616–20.
9. Viladot A, Lorenzo JC, Salazar J, Rodriguez A. The subtalar joint: embryology and morphology. Foot Ankle. 1984;5(2):54–66.
10. Karlsson J, Lansinger O. Lateral instability of the ankle joint. Clin Orthop Relat Res. 1992;(276):253–61.
11. Kjaersgaard-Andersen P, Wethelund JO, Helmig P, Soballe K. The stabilizing effect of the ligamentous structures in the sinus and canalis tarsi on movements in the hindfoot. An experimental study. Am J Sports Med. 1988;16(5):512–6.
12. Cass JR, Settles H. Ankle instability: in vitro kinematics in response to axial load. Foot Ankle Int. 1994;15(3):134–40.
13. Burks RT, Morgan J. Anatomy of the lateral ankle ligaments. Am J Sports Med. 1994;22(1):72–7.
14. Goto A, Moritomo H, Itohara T, Watanabe T, Sugamoto K. Three-dimensional in vivo kinematics of the subtalar joint during dorsi-plantarflexion and inversion-eversion. Foot Ankle Int. 2009;30(5):432–8.
15. Sheehan FT, Seisler AR, Siegel KL. In vivo talocrural and subtalar kinematics: a non-invasive 3D dynamic MRI study. Foot Ankle Int. 2007;28(3):323–35.
16. Yamaguchi S, Sasho T, Kato H, Kuroyanagi Y, Banks SA. Ankle and subtalar kinematics during dorsiflexion-plantarflexion activities. Foot Ankle Int. 2009;30(4):361–6.
17. Maceira E, Monteagudo M. Subtalar anatomy and mechanics. Foot Ankle Clin. 2015;20(2):195–221.
18. Hicks JH. The mechanics of the foot. I. The joints. J Anat. 1953;87(4):345–57.
19. Lundberg A, Svensson OK, Bylund C, Goldie I, Selvik G. Kinematics of the ankle/foot complex—part 2: pronation and supination. Foot Ankle. 1989;9(5):248–53.
20. Lundberg A, Svensson OK. The axes of rotation of the talocalcaneal and talonavicular joints. Foot. 1993;3(2):65–70.
21. Gellman H, Lenihan M, Halikis N, Botte MJ, Giordani M, Perry J. Selective tarsal arthrodesis: an in vitro analysis of the effect on foot motion. Foot Ankle. 1987;8(3):127–33.
22. Stormont DM, Morrey BF, An KN, Cass JR. Stability of the loaded ankle. Relation between articular restraint and primary and secondary static restraints. Am J Sports Med. 1985;13(5):295–300.
23. Hintermann B, Knupp M, Barg A. Peritalar instability. Foot Ankle Int. 2012;33(5):450–4.
24. Casillas MM. Operative treatment of peroneus brevis and peroneus longus tendon tears. Oper Tech Sports Med. 2001;9(1):14–9.

25. Hintermann B. Biomechanische Aspekte der Muskel-Sehnen-Funktion [Biomechanical aspects of muscle-tendon functions]. Orthopade. 1995;24(3):187–92.
26. Piazza SJ, Adamson RL, Sanders JO, Sharkey NA. Changes in muscle moment arms following split tendon transfer of tibialis anterior and tibialis posterior. Gait Posture. 2001;14(3):271–8.
27. Karlsson J, Eriksson BI, Renstrom PA. Subtalar ankle instability. A review. Sports Med. 1997;24(5):337–46.
28. Kato T. The diagnosis and treatment of instability of the subtalar joint. J Bone Joint Surg Br. 1995;77(3):400–6.
29. Keefe DT, Haddad SL. Subtalar instability. Etiology, diagnosis, and management. Foot Ankle Clin. 2002;7(3):577–609.
30. Zwipp H, Rammelt S, Grass R. Ligamentous injuries about the ankle and subtalar joints. Clin Podiatr Med Surg. 2002;19(2):195–229, v.
31. Saltzman CL, el-Khoury GY. The hindfoot alignment view. Foot Ankle Int. 1995;16(9):572–6.
32. Heilman AE, Braly WG, Bishop JO, Noble PC, Tullos HS. An anatomic study of subtalar instability. Foot Ankle. 1990;10(4):224–8.
33. Yamamoto H, Yagishita K, Ogiuchi T, Sakai H, Shinomiya K, Muneta T. Subtalar instability following lateral ligament injuries of the ankle. Injury. 1998;29(4):265–8.
34. Meyer JM, Garcia J, Hoffmeyer P, Fritschy D. The subtalar sprain. A roentgenographic study. Clin Orthop Relat Res. 1988;226:169–73.
35. Sugimoto K, Takakura Y, Samoto N, Nakayama S, Tanaka Y. Subtalar arthrography in recurrent instability of the ankle. Clin Orthop Relat Res. 2002;394:169–76.
36. Tochigi Y, Yoshinaga K, Wada Y, Moriya H. Acute inversion injury of the ankle: magnetic resonance imaging and clinical outcomes. Foot Ankle Int. 1998;19(11):730–4.
37. Michels F, Clockaerts S, Van Der Bauwhede J, Stockmans F, Matricali G. Does subtalar instability really exist? A systematic review. Foot Ankle Surg. 2020;26(2):119–27.
38. Niki H, Hirano T, Akiyama Y, Beppu M. Accessory talar facet impingement in pathologic conditions of the peritalar region in adults. Foot Ankle Int. 2014;35(10):1006–14.
39. Pisani G, Pisani PC, Parino E. Sinus tarsi syndrome and subtalar joint instability. Clin Podiatr Med Surg. 2005;22(1):63–77, vii.
40. Barg A, Bailey T, Richter M, de Cesar Netto C, Lintz F, Burssens A, et al. Weightbearing computed tomography of the foot and ankle: emerging technology topical review. Foot Ankle Int. 2018;39(3):376–86.
41. Krahenbuhl N, Siegler L, Deforth M, Zwicky L, Hintermann B, Knupp M. Subtalar joint alignment in ankle osteoarthritis. Foot Ankle Surg. 2019;25(2):7.
42. Apostle KL, Coleman NW, Sangeorzan BJ. Subtalar joint axis in patients with symptomatic peritalar subluxation compared to normal controls. Foot Ankle Int. 2014;35(11):1153–8.
43. Cody EA, Williamson ER, Burket JC, Deland JT, Ellis SJ. Correlation of talar anatomy and subtalar joint alignment on weightbearing computed tomography with radiographic flatfoot parameters. Foot Ankle Int. 2016;37(8):874–81.
44. Colin F, Horn Lang T, Zwicky L, Hintermann B, Knupp M. Subtalar joint configuration on weightbearing CT scan. Foot Ankle Int. 2014;35(10):1057–62.
45. Krahenbuhl N, Tschuck M, Bolliger L, Hintermann B, Knupp M. Orientation of the subtalar joint: measurement and reliability using weightbearing CT scans. Foot Ankle Int. 2016;37(1):109–14.
46. Krahenbuhl N, Zwicky L, Bolliger L, Schadelin S, Hintermann B, Knupp M. Mid- to long-term results of supramalleolar osteotomy. Foot Ankle Int. 2017;38(2):124–32.
47. Kunas GC, Probasco W, Haleem AM, Burket JC, Williamson ERC, Ellis SJ. Evaluation of peritalar subluxation in adult acquired flatfoot deformity using computed tomography and weightbearing multiplanar imaging. Foot Ankle Surg. 2018;24(6):495–500.
48. Probasco W, Haleem AM, Yu J, Sangeorzan BJ, Deland JT, Ellis SJ. Assessment of coronal plane subtalar joint alignment in peritalar subluxation via weight-bearing multiplanar imaging. Foot Ankle Int. 2015;36(3):302–9.
49. de Cesar Netto C, Schon LC, Thawait GK, da Fonseca LF, Chinanuvathana A, Zbijewski WB, et al. Flexible adult acquired flatfoot deformity: comparison between weight-bearing and non-weight-bearing measurements using cone-beam computed tomography. J Bone Joint Surg Am. 2017;99(18):e98.
50. Zhang Y, Xu J, Wang X, Huang J, Zhang C, Chen L, et al. An in vivo study of hindfoot 3D kinetics in stage II posterior tibial tendon dysfunction (PTTD) flatfoot based on weight-bearing CT scan. Bone Joint Res. 2013;2(12):255–63.
51. Ananthakrisnan D, Ching R, Tencer A, Hansen ST Jr, Sangeorzan BJ. Subluxation of the talocalcaneal joint in adults who have symptomatic flatfoot. J Bone Joint Surg Am. 1999;81(8):1147–54.
52. de Cesar Netto C, Godoy-Santos AL, Saito GH, Lintz F, Siegler S, O'Malley MJ, et al. Subluxation of the middle facet of the subtalar joint as a marker of peritalar subluxation in adult acquired flatfoot deformity: a case-control study. J Bone Joint Surg Am. 2019;101(20):1838–44.
53. Ellis SJ, Deyer T, Williams BR, Yu JC, Lehto S, Maderazo A, et al. Assessment of lateral hindfoot pain in acquired flatfoot deformity using weightbearing multiplanar imaging. Foot Ankle Int. 2010;31(5):361–71.
54. Ferri M, Scharfenberger AV, Goplen G, Daniels TR, Pearce D. Weightbearing CT scan of severe flexible pes planus deformities. Foot Ankle Int. 2008;29(2):199–204.
55. Malicky ES, Crary JL, Houghton MJ, Agel J, Hansen ST Jr, Sangeorzan BJ. Talocalcaneal and subfibular impingement in symptomatic flatfoot in adults. J Bone Joint Surg Am. 2002;84-A(11):2005–9.
56. Frey C, Gasser S, Feder K. Arthroscopy of the subtalar joint. Foot Ankle Int. 1994;15(8):424–8.
57. Williams MM, Ferkel RD. Subtalar arthroscopy: indications, technique, and results. Arthroscopy. 1998;14(4):373–81.
58. Frey C, Feder KS, DiGiovanni C. Arthroscopic evaluation of the subtalar joint: does sinus tarsi syndrome exist? Foot Ankle Int. 1999;20(3):185–91.
59. Chen YX, Yu GR, Mei J, Zhou JQ, Wang W. Assessment of subtalar joint neutral position: a cadaveric study. Chin Med J (Engl). 2008;121(8):735–9.
60. Nosewicz TL, Knupp M, Bolliger L, Henninger HB, Barg A, Hintermann B. Radiological morphology of peritalar instability in varus and valgus tilted ankles. Foot Ankle Int. 2014;35(5):453–62.
61. Kim DH, Berkowitz MJ, Pressman DN. Avulsion fractures of the medial tubercle of the posterior process of the talus. Foot Ankle Int. 2003;24(2):172–5.
62. Langer P, Nickisch F, Spenciner D, Fleming B, DiGiovanni CW. In vitro evaluation of the effect lateral process talar excision on ankle and subtalar joint stability. Foot Ankle Int. 2007;28(1):78–83.
63. Shank JR, Benirschke SK, Swords MP. Treatment of peripheral talus fractures. Foot Ankle Clin. 2017;22(1):181–92.
64. Liu C, Jiao C, Hu Y, Guo QW, Wand C, Ao Y. Interosseous talocalcaneal ligament reconstruction with hamstring autograft under subtalar arthroscopy: case report. Foot Ankle Int. 2011;32(11):1089–94.
65. Hintermann B, Knupp M, Barg A. Supramalleolar osteotomies for the treatment of ankle arthritis. J Am Acad Orthop Surg. 2016;24(7):424–32.
66. Knupp M. The use of osteotomies in the treatment of asymmetric ankle joint arthritis. Foot Ankle Int. 2017;38(2):220–9.
67. Knupp M, Stufkens SA, Bolliger L, Barg A, Hintermann B. Classification and treatment of supramalleolar deformities. Foot Ankle Int. 2011;32(11):1023–31.

68. Krähenbühl N, Akkaya M, Deforth M, Zwicky L, Barg A, Hintermann B. Extraarticular supramalleolar osteotomy in asymmetric varus ankle osteoarthritis. Foot Ankle Int. 2019;40(8):936–47.
69. Krähenbühl N, Susdorf R, Barg A, Hintermann B. Supramalleolar osteotomy in post-traumatic valgus ankle osteoarthritis. Int Orthop. 2020;44(3):535–43.
70. Pagenstert GI, Hintermann B, Barg A, Leumann A, Valderrabano V. Realignment surgery as alternative treatment of varus and valgus ankle osteoarthritis. Clin Orthop Relat Res. 2007;462(462):156–68.
71. Scheidegger P, Horn Lang T, Schweizer C, Zwicky L, Hintermann B. A flexion osteotomy for correction of a distal tibial recurvatum deformity. Bone Joint J. 2019;101-B(6):682–90.
72. Zhao HM, Wen XD, Zhang Y, Liang JQ, Liu PL, Li Y, et al. Supramalleolar osteotomy with medial distraction arthroplasty for ankle osteoarthritis with talar tilt. J Orthop Surg Res. 2019;14(1):120.
73. Hintermann B, Ruiz R, Barg A. Novel double osteotomy technique of distal tibia for correction of asymmetric varus osteoarthritic ankle. Foot Ankle Int. 2017;38(9):970–81.
74. Hintermann B, Valderrabano V. Lateral column lengthening by calcaneal osteotomy. Tech Foot Ankle Surg. 2003;2(2):84–90.
75. Knupp M, Horisberger M, Hintermann B. A new Z-shaped calcaneal osteotomy for 3-plane correction of severe varus deformity of the hindfoot. Tech Foot Ankle Surg. 2008;7(2):90–5.
76. Stufkens SA, Knupp M, Hintermann B. Medial displacement calcaneal osteotomy. Tech Foot Ankle Surg. 2009;8(2):85–90.
77. Usuelli FG, Manzi L. Inframalleolar varus deformity: role of calcaneal osteotomies. Foot Ankle Clin. 2019;24(2):219–37.
78. Hintermann B, Barg A, Knupp M. Corrective supramalleolar osteotomy for malunited pronation-external rotation fractures of the ankle. J Bone Joint Surg Br. 2011;93(10):1367–72.
79. Takakura Y, Takaoka T, Tanaka Y, Yajima H, Tamai S. Results of opening-wedge osteotomy for the treatment of a post-traumatic varus deformity of the ankle. J Bone Joint Surg Am. 1998;80(2):213–8.

GPSR Compliance

The European Union's (EU) General Product Safety Regulation (GPSR) is a set of rules that requires consumer products to be safe and our obligations to ensure this.

If you have any concerns about our products, you can contact us on ProductSafety@springernature.com

In case Publisher is established outside the EU, the EU authorized representative is:

Springer Nature Customer Service Center GmbH
Europaplatz 3
69115 Heidelberg, Germany

Batch number: 10731524

Printed by Printforce, the Netherlands